MEDICAL RADIOLOGY
Diagnostic Imaging

Editors:
A. L. Baert, Leuven
K. Sartor, Heidelberg

Springer-Verlag Berlin Heidelberg GmbH

F. Joffre · Ph. Otal · M. Soulie (Eds.)

Radiological Imaging of the Ureter

With Contributions by

M. Bennaceur · L. Bouchard · V. Chabbert · K. Chaumoire · R. Chemali · P. Chemla
M. Claudon · Ph. Devred · G. Escourrou · A. Gozlan · N. Grenier · M. Irsutti
B. Janne D'Othee · F. Joffre · F. Lefevre · B. Malavaud · C. Mazerolles · M. I. Millan
S. Moussouni · Ph. Otal · J. L. Pariente · M. Panuel · P. Plante · P. Rischman · H. Rousseau
J.-P. Sarramon · Ph. Seguin · T. Smayra · M. Soulie · H. Trillaud · G. Victor

Foreword by

A. L. Baert

With 388 Figures in 848 Separate Illustrations, 43 in Color and 13 Tables

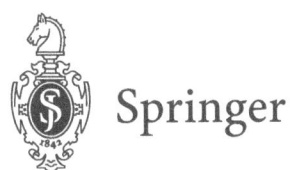 Springer

Francis Joffre, MD
Professor, Chef de Service
Service de Radiologie, Hôpital de Rangueil
1, avenue Jean-Poulhès
31403 Toulouse Cédex 4, France

Philippe Otal, MD
Service de Radiologie, Hôpital de Rangueil
1, avenue Jean-Poulhès
31403 Toulouse Cédex 4, France

Michel Soulie, MD
Service d'Urologie, Hôpital de Rangueil
1, avenue Jean-Poulhès
31403 Toulouse Cédex 4, France

Medical Radiology · Diagnostic Imaging and Radiation Oncology
Series Editors: A. L. Baert · L. W. Brady · H.-P. Heilmann · M. Molls · K. Sartor

Continuation of
Handbuch der medizinischen Radiologie
Encyclopedia of Medical Radiology

ISBN 978-3-540-65521-3

Library of Congress Cataloging-in-Publication Data

Radiological imaging of the ureter / F. Joffre, Ph. Otal, M. Soulie (eds.) ; with
contributions by M. Bennaceur ... [et al.].
    p. ; cm. -- (Medical radiology)
    Includes bibliographical references and index.
    ISBN 978-3-540-65521-3   ISBN 978-3-642-55831-3 (eBook)
    DOI 10.1007/978-3-642-55831-3
    1. Ureters--Radiography. I. Joffre, F. (Francis), 1941- II. Otal, Ph. (Philippe), 1963- III.
Soulie, M. (Michel), 1957- IV. Series.
    [DNLM: 1. Ureteral Diseases--radiography. 2. Diagnostic Imaging--methods. 3.
Ureter--radiography. WJ 400 R129 2003]
    RC922 .R336 2003
    616.6'1--dc21
                         2002036599

http//www. springer.de
© Springer-Verlag Berlin Heidelberg 2003
Originally published by Springer-Verlag Berlin Heidelberg in 2003

Foreword

The rationale to devote a whole volume exclusively to the ureter is the key role this organ plays in the physiology and physiopathology of the kidney and the vulnerability of this thin organ to pathological changes that may occur in the retroperitoneal space.

During the past two decades emphasis in radiological imaging of the ureter has completely shifted from indirect visualisation following classical excretory urography and direct visualisation with retrograde and antegrade pyelography to the new imaging modalities: US, CT and MRI. This book not only describes the classical and modern methods of ureteral imaging but also covers extensively and in great detail all intrinsic diseases of the ureter as well as extrinsic causes of ureteral pathology.

I would like to extend my sincere congratulations to Professor F. Joffre, Dr. P. Otal, and Dr. M. Soulie for preparing this comprehensive overview as well as to the group of outstanding experts in the field who all contributed to this excellent book. I am confident that this outstanding volume will meet with great interest from radiologists, urologists, surgeons, nephrologists and oncologists. I sincerely wish that it will encounter the same success with readers as the previous volumes published in this series.

Leuven   ALBERT L. BAERT

Preface

Ureteral imaging began in 1897, not long after the discovery of X-rays, when TUFFIER developed a ureteral catheter with a rigid metallic stylet, allowing indirect demonstration of the ureter on abdominal films with this catheter inside the ureter (WERSHUB 1970). Thereafter, various attempts at direct ureteral opacification were carried out using bismuth, silver salts, sodium iodide, colloidal silver, thorium, and also air or carbon dioxide. Gradually, these contrast agents were abandoned because of their many drawbacks (DAVIDSON 1985).

The second step in ureteral imaging was taken by OSBORNE and ROWNTREE, dermatologists at the Mayo Clinic who, in 1923, carried out vesical opacification after oral or intravenous administration of 10% sodium iodide, then used mainly in syphilis treatment. However, this technique did not allow any ureteral opacification (OSBORNE et al. 1923).

Intravenous excretory urography (EU) was introduced in 1929 by VON LICHTENBERG and SWICK, who used salts derived from sodium iodide as the contrast medium (VON LICHTENBERG and SWICK 1929). For several decades, EU and techniques of direct ureteral opacification (antegrade and retrograde) were the only methods used to study ureteral pathology. At the beginning of ureteral imaging, retrograde pyelography was the most frequently used technique. However, EU progressively became the gold standard for ureteral imaging, owing to its technical advances and the sustained improvement of contrast media. In return, this significantly reduced the indications for direct imaging in the evaluation of ureteral pathology.

During the past several years, ureteral imaging has changed greatly. EU indications are being restricted for many reasons, chief among them being the exponential growth of ultrasonography. Moreover, the arrival of recent techniques of helical computed tomography (CT) and magnetic resonance imaging (MRI), which allow urographic-like imaging, also greatly contributed to the need for a modified diagnostic algorithm in the evaluation of ureteral pathology.

This fast evolution, as well as these modifications in diagnostic strategy, are the primary factors which led us to produce this work devoted to the imaging of the ureter. It appears indeed useful to take an in-depth look at these new diagnostic techniques and to compare them with "traditional" techniques, which still have their place in certain clinical situations. Moreover, this new, modern ureteral imaging still depends greatly on the extremely rich symptomatology accumulated by the "old" techniques (EU and direct ureteropyelography) during years and years of clinical use.

The second reason for writing this book is the key role played by the ureter in many fields. As the ureter is the organ allowing the transfer of urine from the kidney to the bladder, any pathology involving the ureter can also have an effect on the kidney. Indeed, the majority of obstructive uropathies involving the upper urinary tract have a ureteral origin. The ureter is also a central organ of the retroperitoneal and pelvic cavities: Thus, any pathology involving one of these anatomic regions almost always quickly affects the ureter, and this ureteral involvement may also be the first clinical manifestation. Being the path of migration between the kidney and the bladder, the ureter frequently encloses stones and other rarer pathologies. Given the rich periureteral vascular network, it is also a "vascular bridge" between the pelvic cavity, the retroperitoneum, and the kidney, which may then be part of many pathologic processes, such as metastatic periureteral nodal involvement. These anatomic facts explain the varied and multiple pathologic processes which may involve the ureter and the periureteral space. There are many different ways to explore these pathologies and they must be adapted to particular clinical setting. The writing of this book was driven by the need to form a synthesis between "old" and "new" ureteral imaging. Some will find it too modern, others too traditional. We tried to create a balanced work, which is essential to the integration of technical progress in new imaging techniques in a global ureteral diagnostic strategy without neglecting "old" imaging techniques, which are still indispensable to the understanding of modern imaging.

We received great help and support in the making of this book. Two people initiated this work and must be thanked first. Jean-Michel SUC, nephrology professor and one of the pioneers in nephrology in France, directed one of us (F.J.) towards the field of urinary radiology early in his career. Thanks also go to André DARDENNE, with whom we first conceived this project, but who was not able to conclude the initial work with us. Most of the images were collected during the uroradiology staff meetings that were initiated by Professor SUC during the 1970s and have been held every Wednesday since then. These staff meetings dealt mainly with patient files provided by J. M. SUC, Y. FREGEVU, D. DURAND, J. P. SARRAMON, P. PLANTE, P. RISCHMANN and many others. We are grateful to all the people who have participated in these meetings. We also thank all the authors of this book, mainly PATRICIA CHEMLA, who worked hard on the second reading, MARIA-INES MILLAN, TAREK SMAYRA, BERTRAND JANNE D'OTHEE, and LOUIS BOUCHARD, who took part in the translation process, and ALEXANDRE GOZLAN, who carried out the illustration work. We thank as well all the urologists, nephrologists, and radiologists who entrusted their files or their patients to us. Finally, we want to pay homage to the uroradiological world community, to those who guided us in uroradiology, A. PINET, J. R. MICHEL, and J. TAVERNIER, and also to the great English-speaking authors who partly inspired this work: H. M. POLLACK, H. BERGMAN, L. B. TALNER, and R. C. PFISTER. Finally, SYLVIE DREHER and PATRICIA FRANC handled, with their usual competence and devotion, the huge amount of secretarial work that such a book entails. A. HERNANDEZ and J. M. POUYFOURCAT worked hard to illustrate this book.

Our wish is that this work will interest young people in training as well as active specialists in whatever field: urologists, nephrologists, surgeons, oncologists, and, of course radiologists, in order to help them in the comprehension of ureteral imaging.

Toulouse

FRANCIS JOFFRE
PHILIPPE OTAL
MICHEL SOULIE

References

Davidson A (1985) Urographic contrast material: historical development and chemical characteristics. In: Davidson A (ed) Radiology of the kidney. Saunders, Philadelphia, pp 681–689

Osborne ED, Sutherland CG, Scholl AJ, Rowntree LG (1923) Roentgenography of urinary tract during excretion of sodium iodide. JAMA 80:368

von Lichtenberg A, Swick M (1929) Klinische Prufung des Uroselectans. Klin Wochenschr 8:2089

Wershub LP (1970) Urology from antiquity to the twentieth century. Warren H. Green, St. Louis

Contents

1 Techniques of Ureteral Imaging

Ph. Otal, M. Claudon, F. Joffre, M. Soulie, L. Bouchard, M. I. Millan, M. Bennaceur, and G. Victor

CONTENTS

Ph. Otal, MD
Service de Radiologie, Hôpital de Rangueil, 1, avenue Jean-Poulhès, 31403 Toulouse Cédex, France
M. Claudon, MD
Professor, Service de Radiologie, CHU Nancy Brabois, rue du Morvan, 54511 Vandoeuvre Les Nancy, France
F. Joffre, MD
Professor, Chef de Service, Service de Radiologie, Hôpital de Rangueil, 1, avenue Jean-Poulhès, 31403 Toulouse Cédex 4, France
M. Soulie, MD; M. Bennaceur, MD
Service d'Urologie, CHU Rangueil, 1, avenue Jean-Poulhès, 31403 Toulouse Cédex, France
L. Bouchard, MD
6239 Dumas, Montreal, Québec, H4E 2Z8, Canada
M. I. Millan, MD
Calle A Resid Tamarindo, Apt 92 La Alameda, Caracas 1080, Venezuela
G. Victor, MD
Service de Médecine Nucléaire, CHU Rangueil, 1, avenue Jean-Poulhès, 31403 Toulouse Cédex, France

The screening, diagnosis and evaluation of diseases of the ureter depend almost entirely on radiological examinations. Only the definite diagnosis is obtained, in some cases by biopsy, endoscopic techniques and sometimes after surgical excision and pathological examination of the lesion.

Until the seventies, the main radiological descriptions generally concentrated on the manifestations revealed by ureteral opacification during excretory urography (EU) or direct (antegrade or retrograde) pyelography.

The role of new imaging techniques such as ultrasonography, computed tomography (CT), magnetic resonance imaging (MRI) is expanding and replacing opacification techniques in many situations. Permanent improvement of new imaging techniques is at the origin of extensive debate and many questions are posed in the English and French literature about the best-suited imaging strategy for each patient (Amis 1999; Bigot 1995; Choyke 1992; Moreau 1995).

1.1
Opacification Techniques

Opacification of the ureter with contrast media was proposed shortly after the invention of X-rays. The purpose of opacification of the ureteral lumen is to visualize abnormalities or changes secondary to diseases of the ureteral wall and/or periureteral tissue. Two means of ureter opacification are used: (a) physiological urinary excretion after intravenous injection of contrast media and (b) direct injection of the contrast media into the urinary tract: retrograde ureteropyelography (RUP) or antegrade ureteropyelography (AP).

1.1.1
Excretory Urography

Excretory urography (EU) is the usual method used to visualize the ureter. Improvements in radiological techniques and in contrast media have made the EU a good method for ureteral exploration (HATTERY et al. 1988). For optimal visualization of the ureter, a special technical care is needed.

1.1.1.1
Choice of Contrast Media

A high dose of contrast media (CM) is often necessary because patients usually have an obstructive syndrome. This high dose of contrast can be administrated in one injection if the obstructive syndrome is already known or in two injections if the obstruction is diagnosed during the exam. The dose used can be as high as 200 ml of contrast media, depending on the weight of the patient, generally at a rate of 1–2 ml/kg.

The choice of which contrast media have to be used has led to many discussions (THOMSEN and BUSH 1998). The classic three-iodine ionic high osmolality contrast media (HOCM) have the advantage of a satisfactory opacification of the urinary tract. However, this opacification is associated with a osmotic diuresis induced from the high dose used: it can be excessive, conceals the peristaltic column effect and feigns an overly beautiful image secondary to a moderated obstruction (PFISTER and NEWHOUSE 1978). HOCM also have the disadvantage of a higher risk of minor complications than the lower osmolality contrast media (LOCM). The LOCM have some drawbacks: (a) they provide high opacification of the urinary tract, which could be very dense and conceal small parietal lesions. (b) The reduction of the osmotic diuresis could be responsible for a insufficient filling and a delayed opacification of the ureter. The association of the two types of contrast agents could be beneficial, combining the benefits of both, in particular in cases of obstructive syndrome. In both cases, it seems to be useful to use a high iodine concentration (350–370 mg of iodine per 100 ml).

1.1.1.2
The EU Technique

The EU technique (HATTERY et al. 1988) has two main objectives: searching for a ureteral lesion with optimal opacification and evaluating the effects upstream from the lesion. The plain abdominal film (kidney, ureter, bladder, KUB) is indispensable for the ureter exploration. Some ureteral or periureteral abnormalities can be seen on plain abdominal film: mass effect, fatty radiolucency, abnormal localization of abdominal air, and calci-

fications and stones. Some abnormal images such as calcifications may be concealed after the opacification of the urinary tract. The plain abdominal film must be of good quality and carefully examined: low kilovoltage for higher contrast and lower diffuse radiation (70–80 kV depending on the habitus of the patient), local compression to push away the superposition of the interfering gas, and oblique and lateral incidences to specify the topography of an abnormal opacity.

Three-minute film is indispensable for assessing a functional abnormality. The optimal urinary opacification is usually obtained 10–15 min after injection of the contrast agent (Fig. 1.1). Urinary opacification is improved with the ureteral compression that allows a better filling of the superior portion of the ureter and, after the suspension of the compression, total ureteral opacification (HUGHES and HINE 1991) (Fig. 1.2). Compression is accomplished with a device attached to the table or to the patient, consisting in a belt placed around the abdomen, which maintains a balloon or foam pads upon the abdominal anterior wall at the height of the pelvic brim. The area is compressed after viewing the 5-min films and excluding all obstruction. The area must be compressed routinely after excluding the following categories of patients: those with a painful or tender abdomen, suspicion of aortic aneurysm, renal colic, recent abdominal surgery, or abdominal mass. Its usefulness remains unquestionable when a precise analysis of the ureteral lumen is needed (MAWHINNEY and GREGSON 1987).

Other technical variants are needed in some circumstances. Oblique or profile views are necessary when a ureter displacement is suspected or to suppress superimposition (Fig. 1.3). Delayed films are obtained in case of slow opacification of the ureter. Positioning films are used to facilitate the progression of the contrast media when the urinary tract is dilated. Sedimentation of the contrast media in the lowest zones and the absence of peristalsis slow the opacification. The films in the prone and vertical positions are very useful as well as postvoiding films to study the ending ureter (Fig. 1.4, 1.5). Tomographic views of the ureter and videotape recording of the ureteral peristalsis are rarely used. Localized compression of the ureter with a pad is used to improve visualization of some hidden segments (Fig. 1.6).

Whatever the digital technology, digital X-ray images currently provide the same level of image quality and diagnostic accuracy than classic images (FAJARDO and HILLMAN 1988).

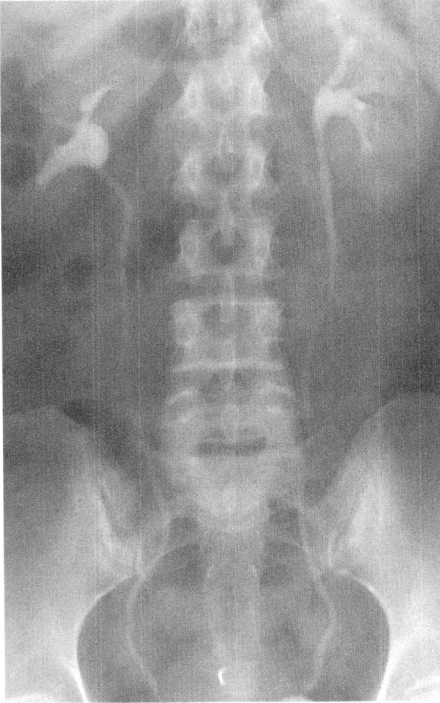
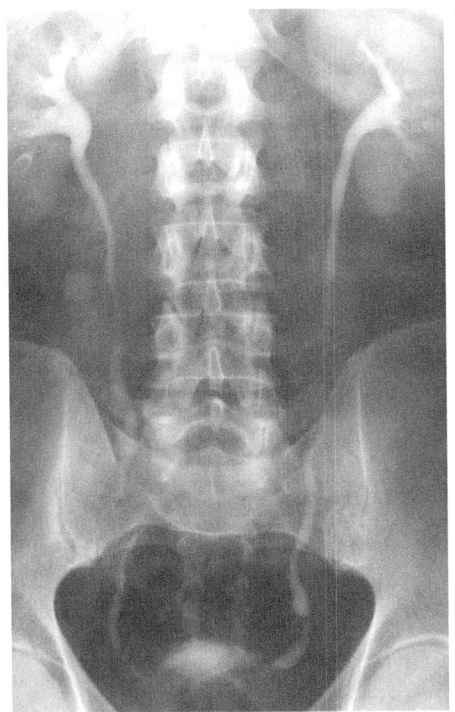

Fig. 1.1a, b. Examples of spontaneous ureteral opacifica-tion during excretory urography (EU)

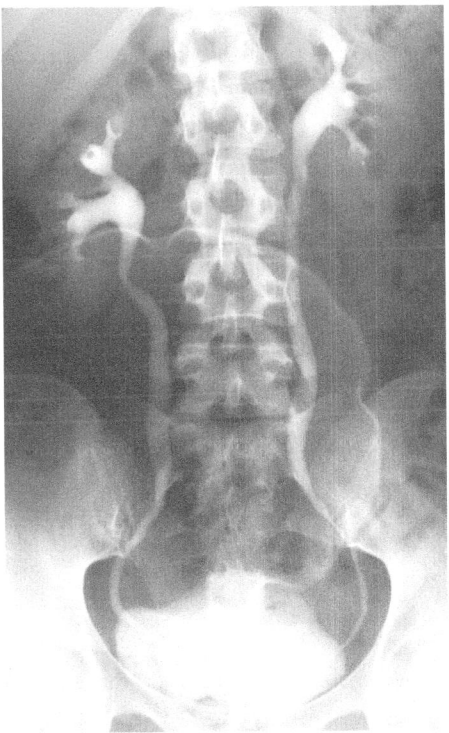

Fig. 1.2. This film was taken immediately after release of the ureteral compression and provides excellent visualization of all the ureteral lumen

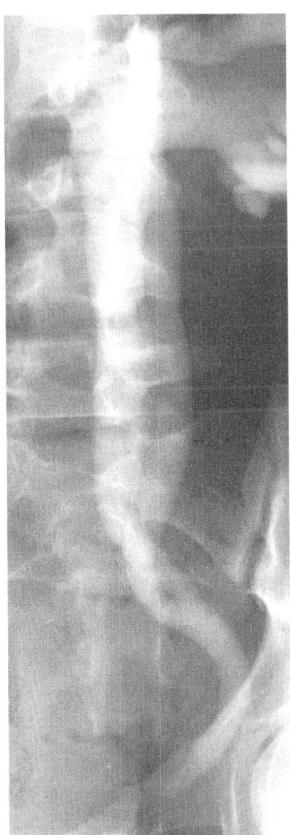
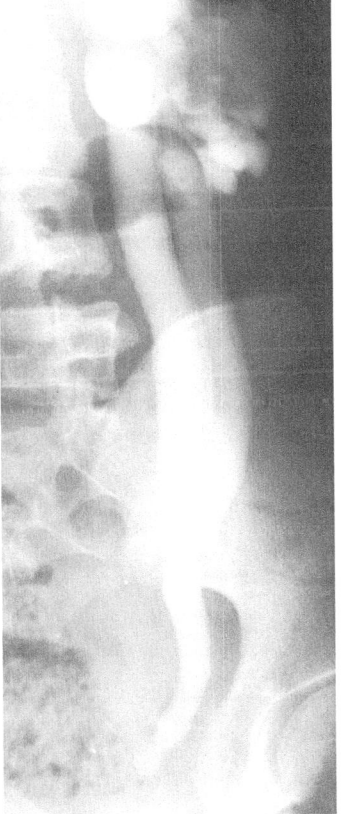

Fig. 1.3a, b. Anterior and posterior oblique views during EU to demonstrate the exact route of both bifid ureters with acute lithiastic obstruction

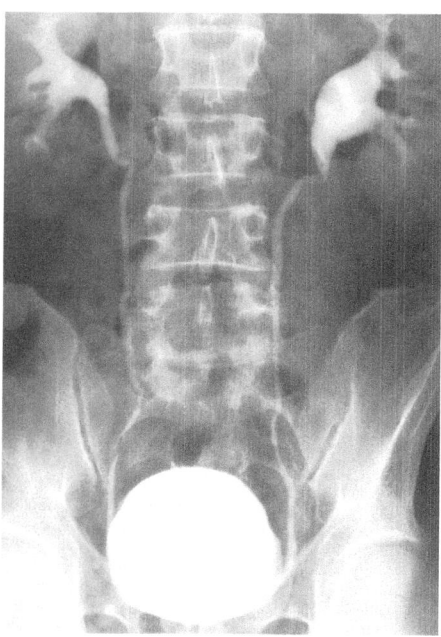

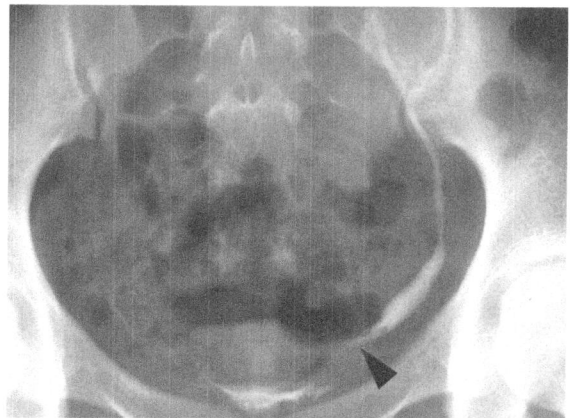

Fig. 1.5. This postvoiding urographic film demonstrates a small radiolucent stone (*arrowhead*) with slight upstream dilatation of the left terminal ureter

Fig. 1.4. EU in prone position showing complete opacification of ureters

The urographic technique of the intermittent obstruction requires a special protocol (Fig. 1.7):
– Higher doses of contrast media
– Hyperdiuresis test with a quick perfusion of a isotonic saline solution or injection of 0.5 mg/kg of furosemide intravenously (DAVIES et al. 1978).

1.1.1.3
Urographic X-ray Pictures Associated with CT

Few authors propose limited CT after a complete EU (PERLMAN et al. 1996). Inversely, taking urographic films of the urinary tract after CT seems to be advisable in many situations, particularly when there is no dilatation, which prevents acceptable 3D reconstruction.

The same technical rules must be followed to obtain excellent opacifications of the ureter (sufficient amount of CM, compression of ureter, positioning films).

1.1.2
Techniques of Direct Opacification

The direct opacification techniques of the upper urinary tract are an important part of radiology history: it was in 1906 that VOELCKER and VON LICHT-ENBERG had the idea of the retrograde opacification of the urinary tract (VOELCKER and VON LICHTEN-

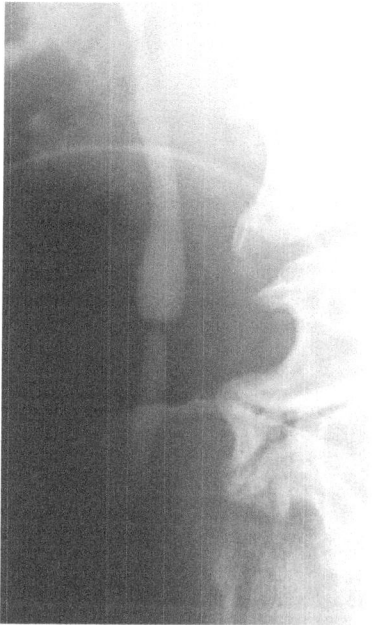

Fig. 1.6. Localized balloon compression of the right ureter during EU making it possible to push away gaseous superimposition to improve visualization of a localized ureteral stenosis

BERG 1906). Ureteral opacification was described by CHEVASSU (1929). He used a bulb-tipped probe for the retrograde opacification of the ureter (Retrograde ureteropyelography, or RUP). In 1955, GOODWIN proposed the puncture of the renal pelvis for its direct anterograde opacification (Anterograde pyelography, or AP) (GOODWIN et al. 1955).

Direct opacification is useful in conditions in which EU does not provide sufficient opacification of the ureter. Currently, 3D reconstructions of urinary

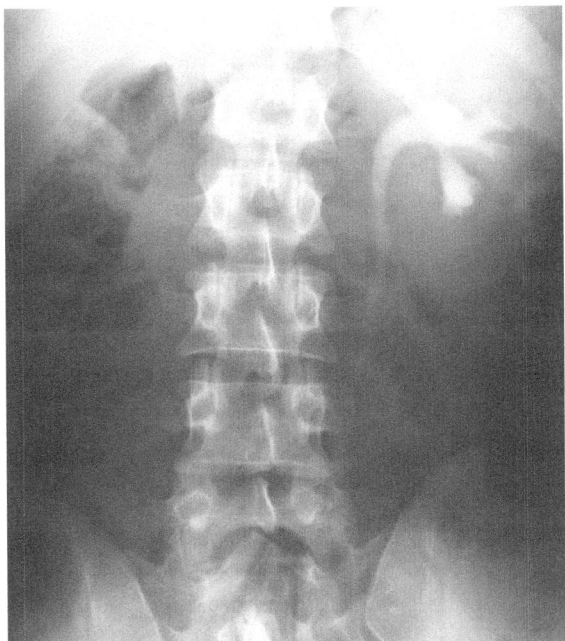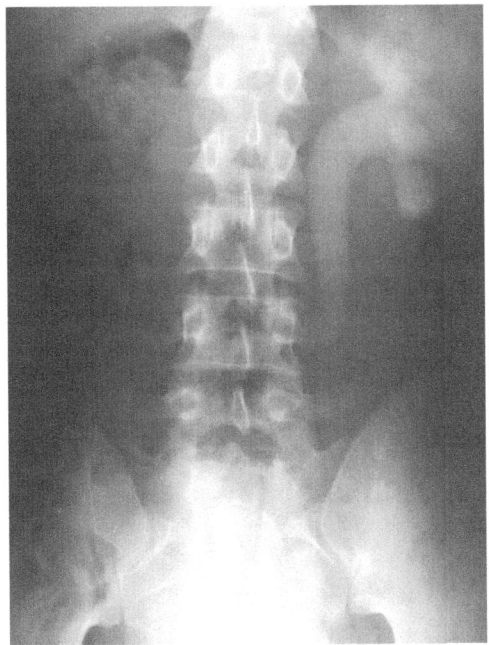

Fig. 1.7a, b. EU with a hyperdiuresis test in a patient with suspected retroperitoneal fibrosis. **a** Discrete stasis on the left side on delayed film. **b** Urographic films after quick perfusion of saline: pyeloureteral dilatation with probable lumbar ureteral obstruction

tract after CT or MRI must reduce indications of these techniques as a diagnostic tool. The main usefulness of direct opacification techniques is to clarify the type of the obstacle. They also have the advantage of allowing other endoureteral interventions such as endoscopy, external or internal drainage of the urinary tract with intubation of the ureter, or pressure measurements and biopsy.

1.1.2.1
Retrograde Ureteropyelography
(IMRAY and LIEBERMAN 1990)

Retrograde ureteropyelography is a radioendoscopic technique requiring special equipment (a uroradiological room with facilities for radiological and endoscopic procedures) as well as hygiene and radioprotection conditions. The image quality is a very important matter and digital imaging from the X-ray intensifier is very useful. The exam is always preceded by a plain abdominal film and performed by cystoscopic catheterization of the ureteral orifice with a Chevassu bulb-tipped probe, which reduces contrast leakage, followed by injection of 5–8 cc of contrast under fluoroscopically guidance. Sometimes more contrast must be injected if the urinary tract is dilated. Low-concentration HOCM with (250 mg of iodine per 100 ml) diluted to 30% is used so that

small filling defect images are not concealed. LOCM do not provide additional advantages. Injection of air as CM to find a radiotransparent calculus is no longer used. The injection of CM must be stopped when a totally and satisfactory opacification of the urinary tract is obtained. If the patient is experiencing pain, or if a lymphatic or pyelotubular reflux is visualized, the injection must be stopped. The films are obtained with a total filling of the ureter in anteroposterior and oblique positions and also at the level of the obstacle with magnification (Figs. 1.8, 1.9). A later film, 5 min after the withdrawal of the catheter, is obtained to be sure of the drainage of the urinary tract.

The procedure could be done under local anesthesia of the urethra, in particular in women. A general anesthesia could be necessary in men and if a therapeutic approach is planned.

The RUP must be interpreted in relation to the retrograde injection of the contrast agent that reduces peristalsis. The films obtained after the withdrawal of the catheter give some physiological information. Using this technique depends on the success of the catheterization of the ureteral meatus. The meatus is inaccessible in case of invasion of the bladder trigone by a tumor, deformation of the bladder by prostatic hypertrophy or meatus stenosis after surgery or radiotherapy. RUP is obviously impossible in case of ureterointestinal anastomosis.

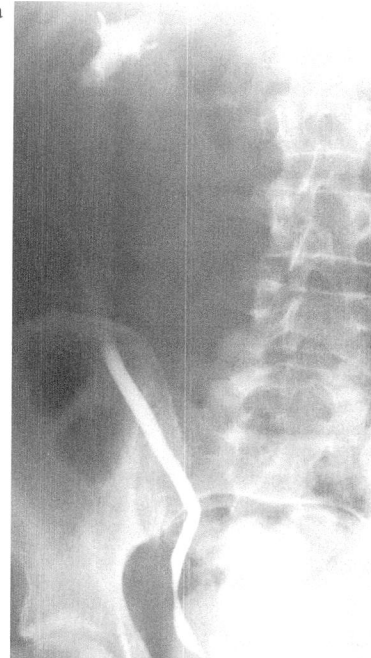
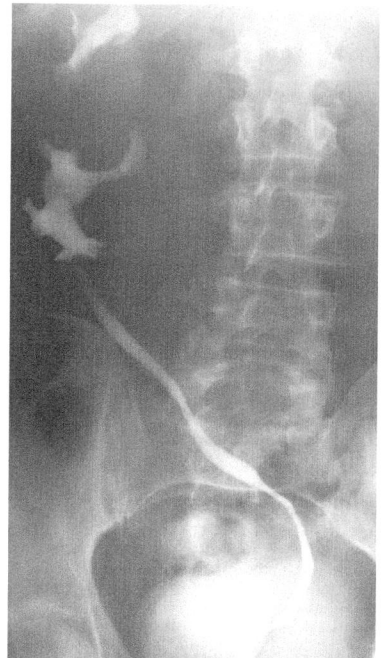

Fig. 1.8a, b. Bilateral retrograde uretero-pyelography (RUP) on a patient with crossed renal ectopia. The bulb-tipped catheter is placed at the meatus level

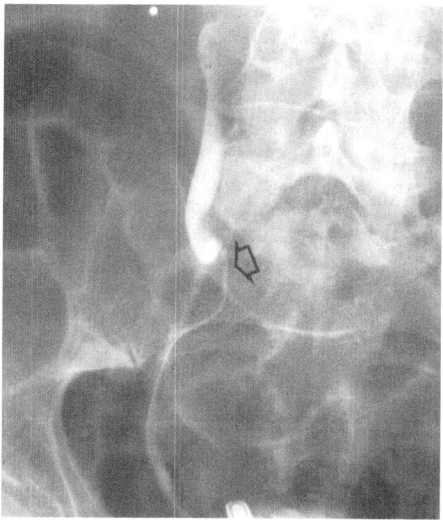

Fig. 1.9. Right retrograde pyelography for obstruction related to calcified iliac artery (*arrow*). The catheter is pushed away up to the stenotic area

With a careful technique, the risk of complications after RUP is limited (2/1000) and consists of: extravasation, ureteral wounds, and sepsis (Goldstein and Conger 1965). RUP must be avoided in cases of urinary infection, except in the preoperative situation or if a drainage is placed. An antibiotic prophylaxis is needed in these situations.

Retrograde opacification of ureterointestinal anastomosis requires a special technique: after a dig-

ital exam of the stoma, a ballooned Foley-type probe is placed at the stoma to block the distal part of the loop of the ileum reservoir. Retrograde injection in the loop under fluoroscopic guidance (loopography) is enough to visualize the urinary tract and to check the patency of the anastomoses, when these anastomoses were made without antireflux anastomosis (Staley 1960) (Fig. 1.10).

1.1.2.2
Anterograde Pyelography

Anterograde pyelography is performed by injecting a contrast media using a nephrostomy catheter or by direct puncture of the pelvis, complementing or substituting RUP. AP also allows the urodynamic study of the urinary tract. Today, it is for the most part the first-step procedure in all percutaneous interventions (Newhouse 1979). The technique depends on whether it is used as a diagnostic or therapeutic approach and also on whether the renal pelvis is dilated. The exam is performed with local anesthesia in the prone position. The puncture could be guided with two modalities, as follows.

Fluoroscopic Guidance. The puncture is done vertically in a posterior approach after the localization of the kidney, 1 cm inside the middle of the bipolar line (Aboulker et al. 1966) (Fig. 1.11). The needle is advanced until a reflux of urine is obtained.

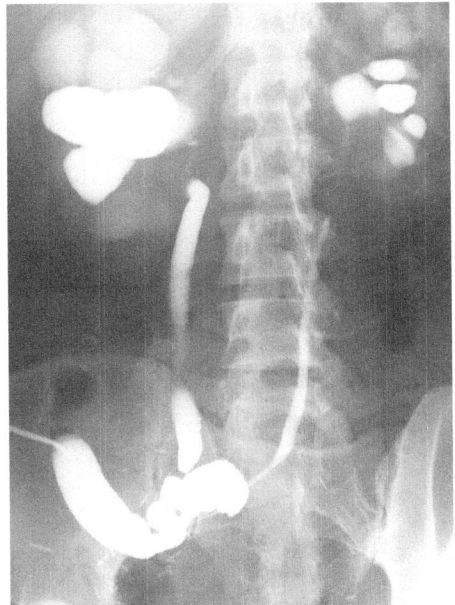
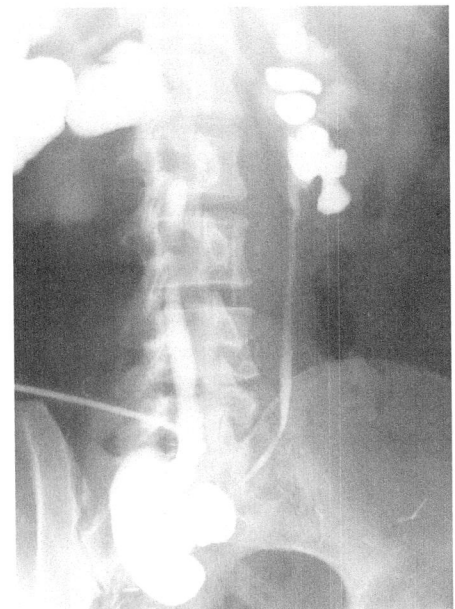

Fig. 1.10a, b. Loopography: retrograde opacification of both ureters by reflux from the ileal reservoir

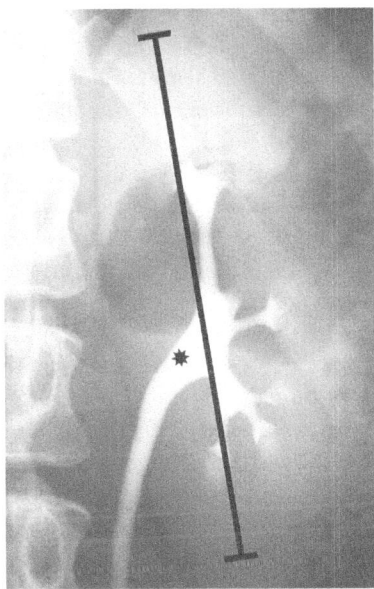

Fig. 1.11. Radiological landmarks for percutaneous puncture. The selected zone of puncture is indicated by the *asterisk*

This technique is used when the renal pelvis is not dilated and allows the opacification of the urinary tract. Intravenous injection of the contrast media can also be used for defining anatomy and position of the kidneys and to directly guide the puncture to a posteroinferior calyx.

More recently, CT technical improvements allow real-time fluoroscopy. CT fluoroscopy provides a precise guidance and an optimal selection of the ade-

quate calyx for antegrade pyelography and further therapeutic intervention on the upper urinary tract via an antegrade route (LEMAÎTRE et al. 2000).

Ultrasonographic Guidance. This is the easiest method when the pelvis is dilated. Ultrasonographic guidance makes it possible to determine the axis of the puncture to the targeted calyx and follows the progression of the needle, avoiding colon, liver and spleen, and confirms its correct position. The puncture, posterior or posterolateral, must be done with a fine CHIBA-type needle. A good position is confirmed with urine aspiration.

Three things must be done when the needle is in a correct position: a bacteriological study of a sample of the urine, pressure measurement (less than 10 cm H_2O) and verification of the needle position after injection of a small quantity of CM. Opacification of the urinary tract is made by the injection of the iodine-diluted CM under fluoroscopic guidance. The quantity of the contrast media that must be administrated depends on the volume of the urinary tract (Fig. 1.12). If the urinary tract is pressurized, it must be drained before opacification. Opacification makes it possible to completely visualize the ureter or just up to the obstacle if it is too tight. The films are made in different incidences. The urinary tract must be emptied before the withdrawal of the needle.

AP is particularly useful for the opacification of the ureter in the transplanted kidney, where the retrograde approach is very difficult and sometimes impossible. The kidney is generally localized and punctured under ultrasonographic guidance.

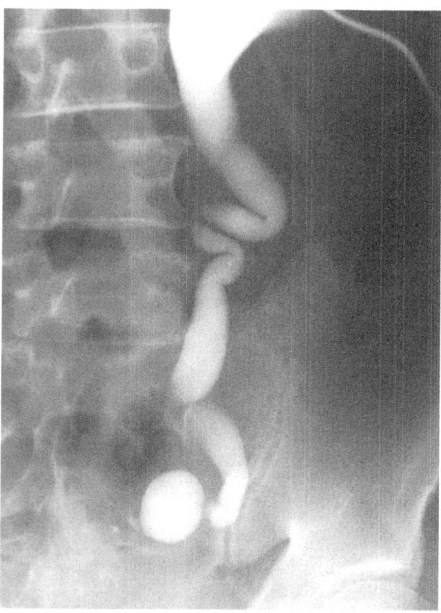

Fig. 1.12. Anterograde pyelography (AP) in a patient with right ureterohydronephrosis (prone position) and obstructive ureterocele. Opacification needs consequent quantity of contrast medium (CM)

The rate of AP failure is very low (less than 0.5%) and generally associated with a small or spastic pelvicaliceal system. Opacification is more physiological than with RUP. Complications are exceptional and rarely serious. Septic shock can occur in case of careless opacification without drainage of an infected pelvicaliceal system under high pressure. A secondary leak of urine before repeated difficult punctures is a cause of failure. A retroperitoneal hematoma is very rare.

Whitaker proposed a concomitant urodynamic test (Whitaker 1973). This technique consists in simultaneous infusion of a solution at a predetermined rate and pressure measurement in the renal pelvis. This technique can be useful in cases of complex surgical procedures or for determining the cause of a dilated ureter of unknown etiology (Newhouse 1979). The indications for this technique are exceptional because of it's complexity.

1.2
New Imaging Techniques

1.2.1
Ultrasound

If the kidneys are easily and reliably evaluated by US, ultrasonography of the ureter is more often limited to the proximal portion of the lumbar ureter and the terminal portion through the bladder. Sonographic examination almost exclusively concerns hydronephrotic kidneys, mostly searching for ureteral stones. To improve analysis of the ureter in these conditions, special US techniques are used.

The proximal portion of ureter can be visualized (in case of dilatation) through the lower pole of the kidney using a posterolateral approach with the patients in supine or oblique position, preferably with a well-distended bladder. Scanning is performed longitudinally and transversally, generally with 3.5 MHz transducer. It is important to use real-time scanning to search for the landmarks of the psoas to explore the retroperitoneum (Fig. 1.13). Great vessels have to be checked with an anterior approach.

The lower lumbar ureter can be explored when it crosses the common iliac vessels, particularly in thin patients. The patient has to lay in a contralateral oblique position and the transducer has to be positioned longitudinally in the iliac fossa. Color Doppler is very helpful in this setting to identify the ureter and differentiate it from the iliac vessels (Grenier et al. 2000; McNeily et al. 1991). Visualization of the lower pelvic ureter requires bladder distension. Suprapubic scanning is performed longitudinally and transversely. A postvoiding scan of the bladder can be useful in some circumstances. Water intake before examination is very useful in creating a diuretic situation with frequent ureteral jets (Onishi et al. 1986). Endorectal and endovaginal approaches have been proposed to improve sensitivity of distal ureter examination (Laing et al. 1994; Lerner 1986). A transperineal route could improve US reliability in detecting abnormalities of this ureteral section (Hertzberg et al. 1994).

Color Doppler ultrasound is useful for measuring the intrarenal resistivity index, which may reflect significant obstruction (Platt et al. 1989). Evaluation consists of spectral samplings at the level of the arcuate arteries of both kidneys. Doppler parameters must include narrow sample gate, low wall filter, and low pulse repetition frequency to optimize the wave forms. At least three measurements are obtained at the upper and lower poles and the middle portion of the kidney (Deyoe et al. 1995). The resistive index (RI) can be calculated as following: (peak systolic frequency – lowest diastolic frequency) peak systolic frequency.

In some circumstances (suspicion of renal colic) another diagnostic tool is the demonstration of ureteral jets on color Doppler ultrasonography (Burge et al. 1991). It is important to know the limitations of demonstrating ureteral jets, which depends on diuresis

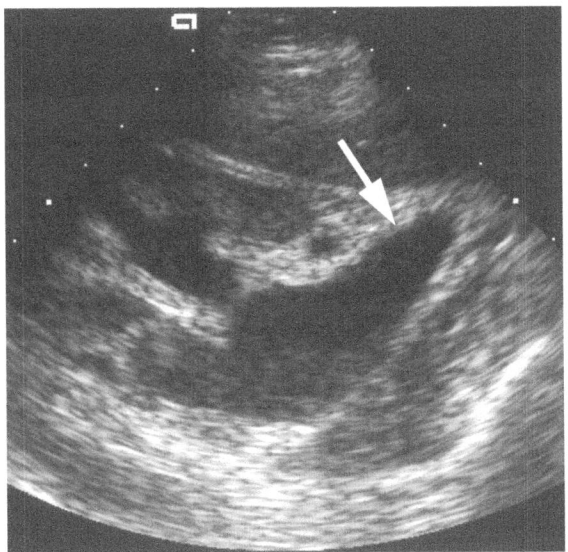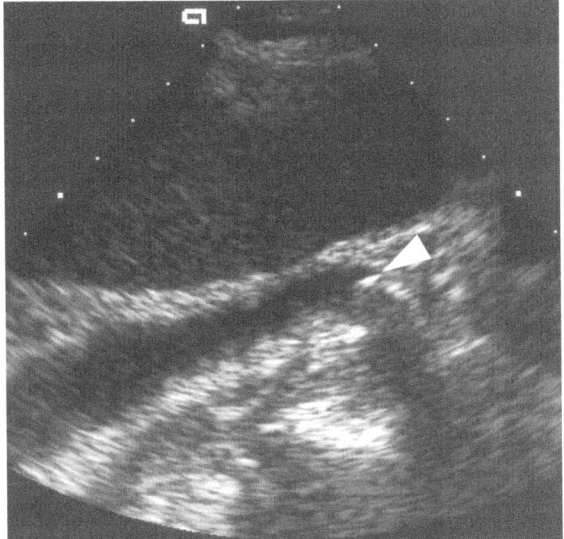

a   b

Fig. 1.13a, b. Ultrasonographic views of ureteral dilatation. **a** Coronal view showing the proximal dilated ureter in front of the psoas muscle (*arrow*). Note the hyperechoic aspect of urine in this patient with pyonephrosis. **b** Coronal view of the dilated lumbar ureter with a stone in the distal part (*arrowhead*)

and urine density differences between the ureter and bladder. The technique requires an incompletely emptied bladder and is very time consuming (5–20 min). Demonstration of twinkling artifacts using color Doppler has been described as a good echographic tool to identify some ureteral stones (CHELFOUH et al. 1998).

1.2.2
Endoluminal Ultrasonography

Endoluminal ultrasonography was recently proposed to evaluate different kinds of disease with ureteral obstruction of unclear etiology (GRASSO et al. 1999). This technique provides a precise demonstration of the ureteral wall and periureteral anatomy. It is performed at the same time as RUP and/or ureteroscopy, but the probe can be also inserted along the anterograde route. A 12.5- or 20-MHz frequency 6.2-F catheter-based transducer gives cross-sectional images by rotating at 30 rpm.

The catheter is placed in the ureter over a hydrophilic guidewire through the cystoscope, monitored using fluoroscopy. Depending on the frequency used, a 3-cm-deep cross-sectional image showing the ureteral wall and periureteral tissue is provided. A computer program reconstructs images into 3D representations (BAGLEY and LIU 1998).

Endoluminal ultrasonography depicts the ureter and surrounding structures with a precision quality not available using other imaging techniques. How-

ever, indications of this technique could be limited by the cost of the probe and evaluation of its true usefulness requires further studies and large clinical trials.

1.2.3
Computed Tomography

1.2.3.1
Contrast Medium Administration

Most of the computed tomography (CT) explorations of the ureter rely on the intravenous administration of contrast medium (CM). The main exception concerns the detection or evaluation of ureteral stone, which has gained wide acceptance among radiologists and referring clinicians in the last few years because of its excellent performance and because there is no need for CM injection (SMITH et al. 1995).

The iodine load is approximately 400 mg iodine per kg of body weight (LEMAÎTRE et al. 2000). When a multiphasic analysis of the renal parenchyma is not indicated on the basis of other radiological or clinical data, an ionic HOCM could be chosen because it results in increased diuresis and subsequently better filling of the excretory system. As helical acquisition is delayed after the injection, a possible intolerance to CM will not interfere with the quality of the breath-hold. Inversely, if the renal parenchyma has to be explored at the cortical and nephrographic phases, nonionic CM is often preferred due to better tolerance. In this case, the CM is administered using a power injector and three or four acquisitions are usually obtained: native, cortical phase, nephrographic phase and excretory time. As the widespread use of helical CT raises the problem of patient irradiation, it could be tempting to prefer a simplified exploration protocol allowing simultaneous visualization of the vascular and excretory systems: immediately after the acquisition of the native slices (if really useful), manual half-dose injection is given for excretory system opacification. Then, 3–5 min later, the remaining dose is injected, followed, after a delay of 30–40 s, by the helical acquisition. The most appropriate method to image the urinary tract is still controversial: further studies are needed to compare the different methods providing post-CT urographic views. Better distension of the collecting system may be obtained by prone exploration and, overall, abdominal compression. McNicholas et al. consider that the opacification of all portions of the collecting system after abdominal compression is at least as good as that seen with EU (McNicholas et al. 1998). These authors also stated that imaging the patient in the prone position resulted in ureteral filling comparable to that of imaging with compression, except for the distal ureter, where compression was superior. Compression CT urography produces equal or improved opacification of the ureter when compared with EU but the accuracy for detecting urothelial lesions needs further evaluation (Heneghan et al. 2001).

A particular technical consideration concerns cases of important urinary tract dilatation, which may lead to sedimentation of the CM in the declive calices and pelvis and to an incomplete opacification of the ureter. In this case, the patient should be placed in prone position, for example, to allow the excreted CM to reach the lower portion of the ureter. This decision should be taken as early as possible during the examination (as soon as detected on native scans or even before if this condition is suspected from previous sonography) in order to reduce the number of acquisitions and, consequently, the patient's irradiation dose.

Some authors advocate the exploration of the urinary tract in the prone position when evaluating stones located in the region of the ureterovesical junction with unenhanced helical CT, because a prone scan can be used to distinguish stones impacted at the ureterovesical junction from stones that have already passed into the bladder (Levine et al. 1999). Selecting a well-adapted window level is important. The window level used for abdominal CT can conceal some endoureteral filling defects. Varying the window setting during interpretation and using high level widths (more than 1000 HU) are mandatory.

1.2.3.2
Technical Parameters (Lemaître et al. 2000)

Exploration of the ureter has benefited tremendously from the developments of helical CT. Even if one of the most recent applications of CT to the ureter – the detection of ureteral stone, as introduced by Smith in 1995 (Smith et al. 1995) – was initially performed with sequential CT, a helical acquisition offers multiple advantages: exploration of the entire abdominal cavity within a single breath-hold, elimination of respiratory misregistration, and a high overlapping reconstruction rate, which warrants high-quality 3D representations.

Examinations are usually performed with a slice thickness of 5 mm, a good compromise between spatial and temporal resolution. The pitch ranges from 1 to 2 (generally 1.5) in order to obtain an acquisition time (from the upper pole of the kidney to the pelvic floor) of 30–40 s. Breath-hold ability is generally not a limiting factor since patients are allowed to breath gently from the iliac crests. The most important parameter of reconstruction is the increment: overlapping slices are mandatory if 3D reconstructions are planned, especially if pitch is higher than 1.5.

The multidetector CT allows optimization of both spatial and temporal resolutions since the same volume is acquired in a shorter time and with thinner slices (Chow and Graham Sommer 2001). It is nowadays possible to examine the whole urinary tract in a single breath-hold with 1- or 1.25-mm slices. A recent experience underlines the usefulness of multislice CT urography performed with abdominal compression (Caoili et al. 2002). The real impact of this technological improvement on patient management requires further evaluation. Moreover, evaluation of radiation of the patient must be a special concern and all technical means to reduce radiation doses must be used.

1.2.3.3
3D Reconstructions (Fig. 1.14)

The emergence of volumetric imaging tools such as helical CT has resulted in the development of 3D rendering techniques. Some of the multidimensional algorithms were available at the time of sequential CT and were applied to immobile structures such as bone. Nevertheless, the emergence of helical CT has made it possible to use them in imaging the retroperitoneum, in particular kidneys and ureters, since acquisition of the entire volume in a single breath-hold is mandatory to avoid respiratory

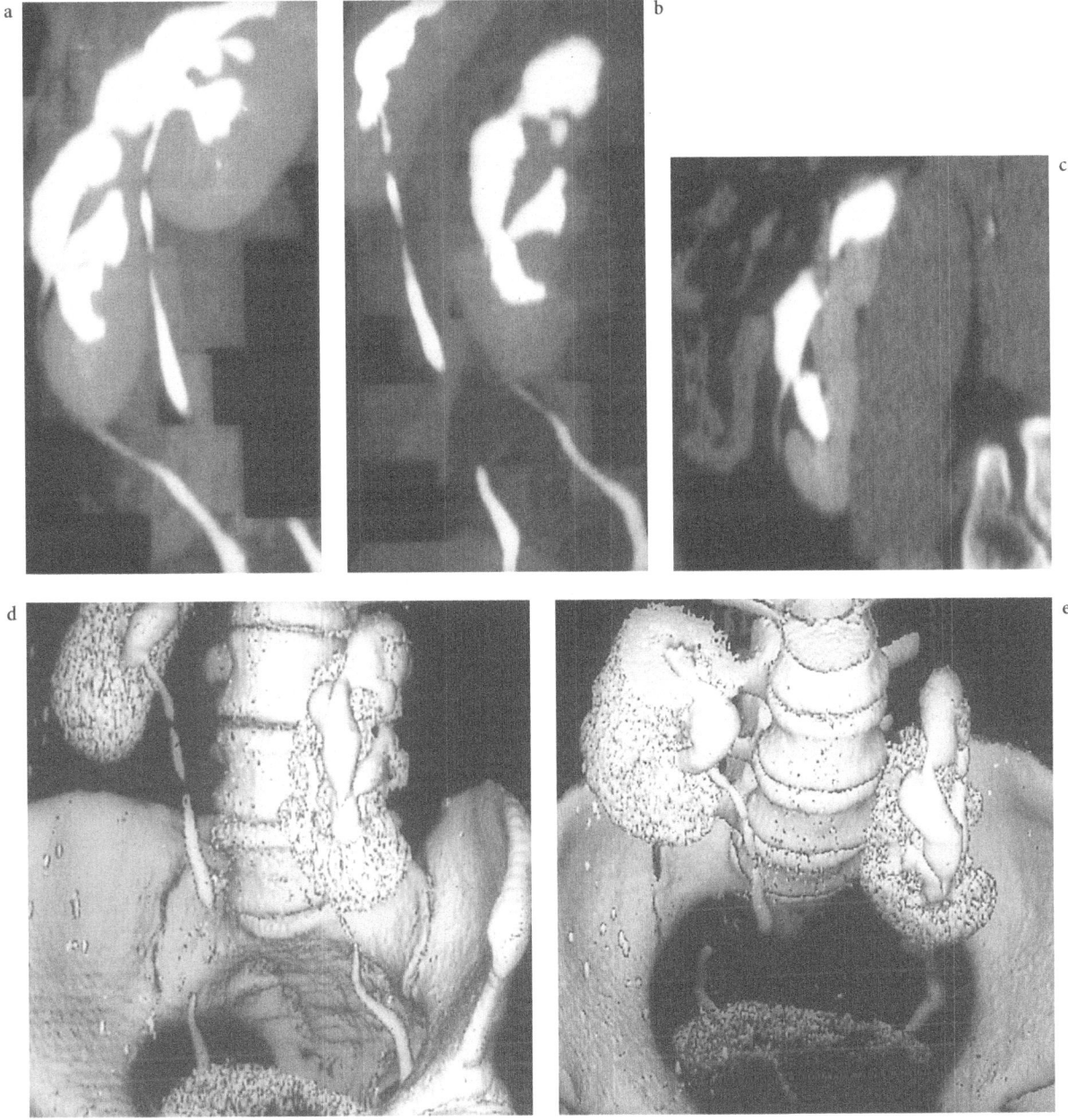

Fig. 1.14a–e. a, b Maximum intensity projection (MIP) reconstructions of both ureters in a patient with bilateral lumbar ectopia and renal malrotation. c Multiplanar reformation (MPR) reconstruction. d, e Shaded surface display (SSD) reconstructions

misregistration. Despite wide availability on most workstations, the application of 3D algorithms to the urinary tract have been the topic of few publications, most of them concerning the anatomy of the lower urinary tract after surgery (FRANCK et al. 1998). The parameters of reconstruction may be adapted to 3D representation by increasing in-plane and longitudinal resolutions (reducing the field-of-view size and increasing the overlapping reconstruction ratio, respectively). When 5-mm-thick slices have

been obtained, the volume should be reconstructed at least every 3 mm in order to reduce the step artifact. The number of slices to be manipulated may become substantial, but recent workstations are more efficient in handling large amounts of data.

The different types of multidimensional reconstructions differ in the rendered effect and the process complexity. In particular, preprocessing of native data such as spatial segmentation may be an important time-consuming factor. Nevertheless, whatever representation mode is chosen, the preliminary analysis of native slices is essential: in the vast majority of cases, multidimensional representation does not add information to native slices. The main interest of 3D reconstructions is to provide clinicians a coronal representation of the whole urinary tract with which they have became familiar after years of prescribing EU.

Shaded surface display (SSD) offers a real 3D representation, even in cases of complex anatomy. The gray scale encodes surface reflection from an imaginary source of illumination. The selection of the voxels participating in the reconstructed image is based on the choice of a density threshold: the pixels integrated into the image are those with densities over the selected threshold. A value in the range of 140–160 Hounsfield units (HU) allows the selection of opacified urine and the elimination of soft tissues. The bony structures are also included in the 3D display; nevertheless, the interactive rotation of the 3D volume makes it possible to limit undesirable superimposition. Otherwise, prerendering editing may be applied in order to remove overlying anatomy that obscures the structures of interest. The anatomic segmentation is based on a region-of-interest drawing or connectivity-based algorithms, depending on the different workstation prototypes. In fact, the main drawback of SSD consists in the influence of the threshold selection on the final image: as observed in CT angiography, the selection of a threshold higher than the density of pixels representing opacified urine results in pseudostenoses or even pseudointerruption of the opaque column. Inversely, an excessively low level may result in the selection of extraurinary pixels, yielding, for example, increased noise. Another limiting factor of SSD is the loss of density information: the gray scale is not allocated to Hounsfield units as on native scans, but to the 3D rendering mode using a shadowing technique. In this condition, opacified urine and ureteral stone may remain undifferentiated with this particular type of 3D display while careful analysis of native scans with interactive windowing is more prone to a correct diagnosis.

Maximum intensity projection (MIP) is probably a more useful tool than SSD, particularly because the gray scale reflects CT attenuation and does not simulate light reflections as does SSD. Consequently, a ureteral stone will be distinguished from the urine as far as its density differs from that of urine and it is not completely surrounded by contrast medium. The MIP image is produced by casting rays through the data volume and displaying the maximum pixel value along each path. As the MIP algorithm projects

the volume on a plane, the resulting image, even if containing information about the whole volume, is two-dimensional. Therefore, the projection incidences have to be multiplied through a rotational axis. The main limiting factor of this mode of display is the initial essential phase of the prerendering editing mode aiming at the removal of all structures other than the urinary tract, which may turn out to be time-consuming if automated tools are not available on the workstation.

When available, the multiplanar volume rendering (MPVR) algorithm may be useful, since it allows an MIP reconstruction of a selected volume with no need for preliminary editing of data. It simply applies the MIP to a volume limited in thickness. The volume is adapted in such a way that it contains as much ureter as possible and avoids inclusion of undesirable structures. Thus, ureters are generally displayed separately, segment by segment.

A volumetric data set with near-isotropic voxels is adapted to the application of virtual endoscopy. This technique is based on threshold image segmentation and surface-rendering algorithms. While the method has been widely applied to colon, tracheobronchial tree and vessels, few data are available on the urinary tract. It is unlikely to detect lesions that are not visible on native scans, but can provide a better image of the lesion (MERRAN 1999).

The volume rendering technique (VRT) is currently the most sophisticated 3D rendering technique and requires high-performance hardware. This technique does not result in information loss since all voxels participate to the calculation. Consequently, no preliminary editing of the data is required. Each voxel is assigned a color and an opacity based on the CT attenuation, making it possible to evaluate the full range of tissue densities and their 3D spatial relationships (RUBIN et al. 1996).

Finally, the most useful tool among the available multidimensional algorithms is probably curved multiplanar reformation (MPR). It can be obtained either without opacification in case of ureteral dilatation or after CM opacification. Simple MPR reconstruction can be used to improve the diagnosis of ureteral stone (Fig. 1.15). It consists in the coronal oblique representation displaying the entire length of the ureter, obtained from the combination of segments of the ureter seen in adjacent CT images, thus depicting the whole ureter and its anatomic relationships on a single image. The delineation of the course of the curved reformation may be obtained from the lateral SSD representation. In the vast majority of cases, both ureters cannot be displayed simultaneously, as they

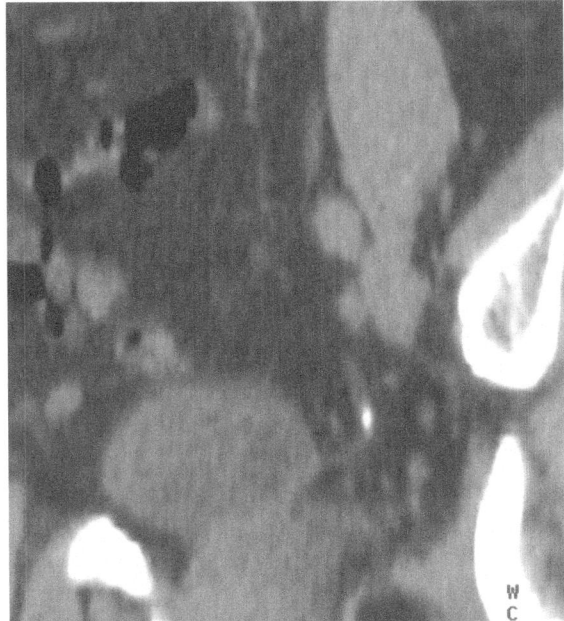

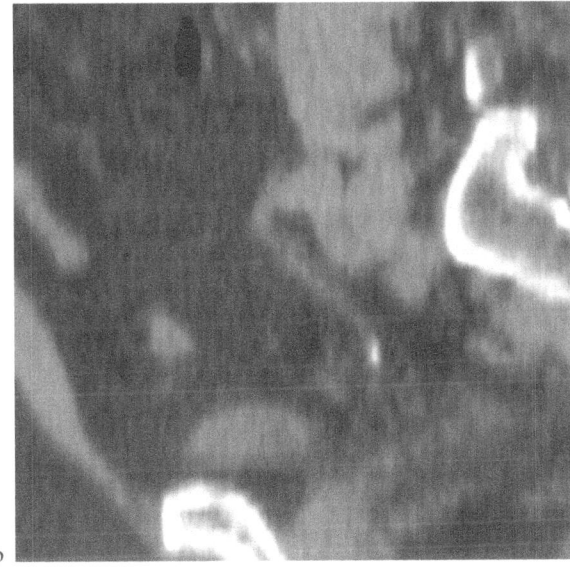

Fig. 1.15a, b. MPR reconstructions of a patient with left renal colic and ureteral stone. Oblique (**a**) and profile (**b**) views spontaneously showing the left ureter and the stone

responding MIP image. Further studies are needed to determine if fine ureteral wall details of EU, not seen on reformatted CT urograms, have a clinical value. If not, EU could be replaced by nonenhanced helical CT to evaluate stones and by CT urography to evaluate for hematuria and other genitourinary disorders (LEVINE et al. 1999; AMIS 1999).

1.2.4
Magnetic Resonance Imaging and MR Urography

In the past 20 years, MRI emerged as a promising, noninvasive imaging method in urology, and more recently, MR urography has been used as an effective imaging method for evaluating abnormalities of the urinary tract. Since the first description of MR urography made by Henning in 1986, its diagnostic capability has been improving with increasingly sophisticated imaging sequences and very short acquisition times (HENNIG et al. 1986; AERTS et al. 1996).

Because of the long T2 of fluid in the collecting system, the first clinical studies were conducted using heavily T2-weighted sequences for visualization of the urine-filled urinary tract (ROY et al. 1994). Excretory MR is a more recent imaging method, similar to that of EU. Based on T1-weighted sequences taken after IV administration of gadolinium chelate, excretory MR provides both morphological and quantitative information about the urinary tract (NOLTE-ERNSTING et al. 1998; ROHRSCHNEIDER et al. 2000a,b). The addition of fast 3D MR angiography provides even more valuable information on renal vasculature in patients in whom abnormal vascular anatomy or vascular diseases affect the urinary tract (LEFEVRE et al. 1998).

Most studies have been performed on a unit with a 1.5-Tesla magnet, but good-quality images have also been obtained at 0.5 Tesla, although longer acquisition times or higher numbers of excitations are required (CATALANO et al. 1999).

1.2.4.1
T2-Weighted Sequences

With heavily T2-weighted sequences, the urine is used as the intrinsic contrast agent, and so IV gadolinium chelate is not needed.

The first studies were conducted using a RARE (rapid acquisition with relaxation enhancement) sequence (ROY et al. 1994; SIGMUND et al. 1991; VINEE et al. 1993). Later, ROTHPEARL used a FSE

do not run in the same plane; consequently two reformations must be obtained. Gray-scale is affected to the display of Hounsfield units; thus the information on density is exactly the same as that contained in the native slice. Notably, the soft-tissue information (for example, the ureter wall) is preserved. The main difficulty remains in the accurate delineation of the center of the lumen while drawing the curve of reconstruction: an apparent stricture of the ureter should be interpreted carefully and compared with the cor-

(fast spin echo) technique, which still required a long acquisition time (ROTHPEARL et al. 1995). More recently, the introduction of stronger and faster gradients permitted ultrafast acquisitions based on HASTE (half-Fourier acquisition single-shot turbo spin-echo), SSFSE or SSTSE (Single shot fast spin echo or turbo spin echo) sequences using a shorter echo-spacing time, while phased array receive coils improved the signal-to-noise ratio (BALCI et al. 1998; O'MALLEY et al. 1997; REUTHER et al. 1997; ROY et al. 1998). Acquisition times range from 0.5 to 8 s, depending on the unit and sequences used (REGAN et al. 1996).

Using T2-weighted sequences, sufficient distension of a nondilated renal collecting system and ureter is an important condition for complete evaluation. Oral hydration prior to the examination is not indicated, because this increases the superimposition of fluid filled bowel loops. IV infusion of saline allows for better distension of nondilated ureters. The injection of a dose of furosemide of 5–20 mg (NOLTE-ERNSTING et al. 1998; HATTERY and KING 1995) a few minutes before the beginning of the examination is very effective, with maximal efficacy 10 min after injection. Compression devices, similar to those used in EU, are rarely used. Voiding before the examination is recommended, except when the study is focused on the bladder itself.

With SSFSE sequences, the use of long effective TEs (approximately 800 ms) produced high contrast, heavily T2-weighted images, resulting in a bright signal from only stationary fluid, and demonstrated urine within dilated or nondilated ureters (Figs. 1.16, 1.17). Calyces, renal pelvis, and ureter were spontaneously completely or partially seen in only 50% and 35% of patients, respectively, while, after injection of furosemide, the structures were well seen in all patients (LEFEVRE et al. 1998).

The HASTE technique, or short effective TEs (approximately 100 ms) on SSFSE sequences, results in less heavily T2-weighted images for analysis of the contents of dilated cavities (such as stones), as well the surrounding soft tissues, including the wall of the ureter and crossing vessels. This can be very helpful in determining the nature of an extrinsic urinary obstruction (LEFEVRE et al. 1998). T2-weighted images also demonstrate a perirenal or periureteral fluid well, which has been described as helpful in the diagnosis of acute urinary obstruction (REGAN et al. 1997). A limitation of the heavily T2-weighted images is related to the superimposition of bowel contents, biliary ducts or CSF on the urinary tract (ROY et al. 1998; GAETA et al. 1999). Multiple oblique views then made it possible to differentiate structures in most cases. Ingestion of ferrite particles has also been suggested in order to suppress signal from bowel loops (HIROHASHI et al. 1997; LECESNE et al. 1998). Moderate blurring artifact can occur, related to long echo train. Another limitation is the occurrence of flow-related filling defect artifacts inside the ureteral lumen in about 50% of cases with these kinds of sequences (GIRISH et al. 2001) (Fig. 1.18).

Recently, in old or critically ill patients, NOLTE-ERNSTING has proposed T1-weighted gradient

a
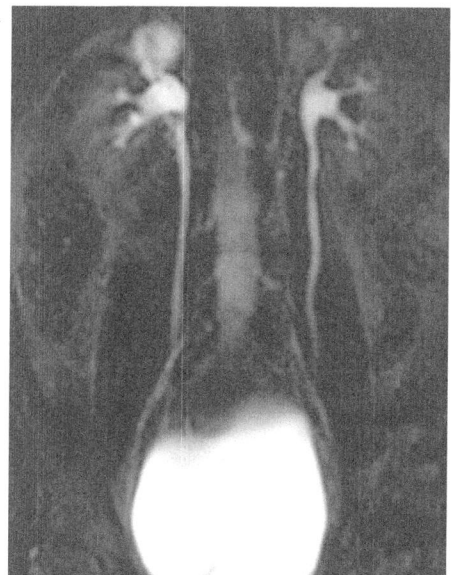
b
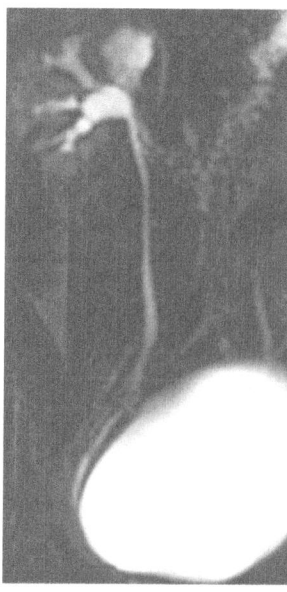

Fig. 1.16a, b. Single-shot strongly T2-weighted images of coronal and oblique views in a normal patient after 20 mg furosemide IV administration. Slice thickness is 30 mm and acquisition time is 900 ms per image. **a** Both upper urinary tracts are well seen, but superimposition of the duodenal bulb makes the evaluation of the upper pole of the right kidney difficult on the coronal view. **b** Oblique view differentiates the renal cavities and the duodenum, and shows the lower ureter behind the filled bladder

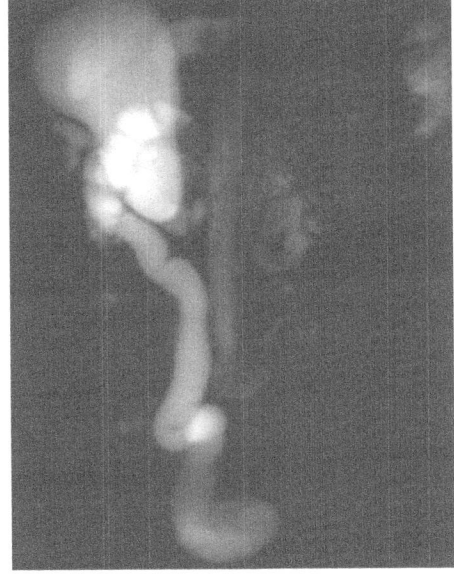
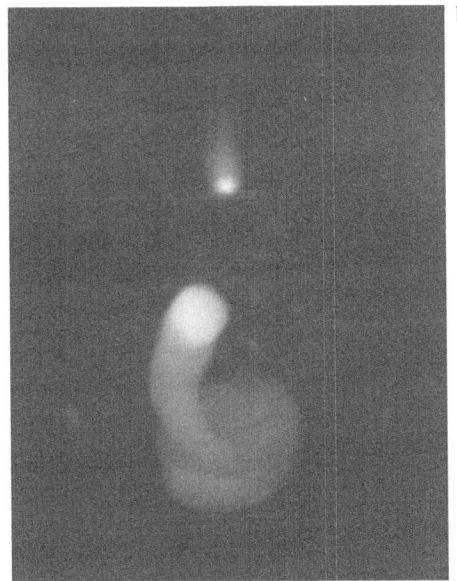

Fig. 1.17a, b. UroMR with single-shot fast spin echo or turbo spin echo (SSTSE) sequences in a patient with right ureterohy-dronephrosis related to ectopic ureter

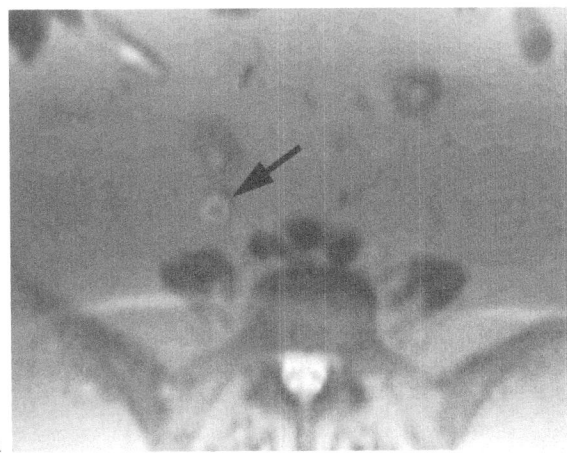
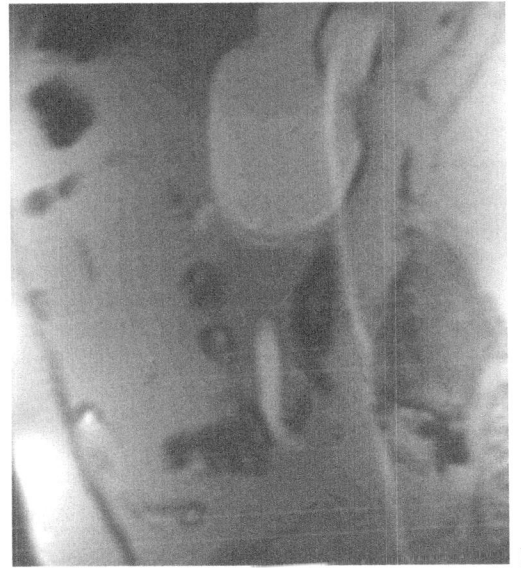

Fig. 1.18a, b. UroMR with HASTE sequences. a Axial view with intra-luminal filling defect artifact in the right ureter (*arrow*) b Absence of the artifact on the sagittal oblique view

echo sequences and echoplanar imaging (EPI) for diuretic-enhanced gadolinium excretory MR urography (NOLTE-ERNSTING et al. 2001b). EPI sequences decrease peristaltic artifacts but morphological studies were less accurate. EPI sequences could be proposed in patients unable to suspend breathing.

1.2.4.2
Excretory MR

Excretory MR urography is based on glomerular filtration of gadolinium chelate. IV administration of a low dose of gadolinium chelate (0.1 mmol/kg)

is sufficient for evaluation of the urinary tract and is characterized by very low nephrotoxicity and also good dialyzability (NOLTE-ERNSTING et al. 1998; ROHRSCHNEIDER et al. 2000a,b).

In excretory MR urography, there is a general gadolinium-related problem, which results from paramagnetic contrast agents leading to a shortening of both the T1 and T2 relaxation times of fluids and tissues. The most effective way to solve this problem is to inject furosemide shortly before the injection of the contrast agent (NOLTE-ERNSTING et al. 1998).

A fast T1-weighted gradient-recalled echo sequence with very short repetition and echo times, demonstrates contrast material-enhanced urine, so that normal and abnormal renal cavities such as the renal pelvis and the ureters can be evaluated at different times and from various views, similarly to EU. Acquisition time is 12 s for the multislice 2D turbo gradient echo sequence, but is significantly reduced by using the single-slice technique.

The repetition of the sequence after the IV administration of gadolinium chelate up to 40–60 min, in an oblique coronal plan adjusted on the long axis of kidneys, provides both morphological and at least gross functional information about the urinary tract. Time-intensity curves obtained from parenchymal ROI are similar to those obtained during renal scintigraphy and may permit assessment of urinary excretion (ROHRSCHNEIDER et al. 2000a,b). An additional dose of furosemide can be administrated intravenously 20 min after IV injection of gadolinium chelate, as is usually done with renal scintigraphy (ROHRSCHNEIDER et al. 2000a,b). Comparative analysis may reveal asymmetry in the kinetics of enhancement of the kidneys. However, precise quantification is limited since there is no simple linear relationship between measured signal intensity and renal perfusion (BORTHNE et al. 1999).

The practicality of gadolinium-enhanced T1-weighted MR urography depends on renal excretory function. Good urographic effect is regularly obtained up to a serum creatinine concentration of 2 mg/dl (NOLTE-ERNSTING et al. 1998).

Due to longer acquisition times compared with T2-weighted sequences, image quality can be degraded by patient motion, especially in children (BORTHNE et al. 2000). Finally, the most recent studies show the superiority of the gadolinium-enhanced MR urography over static fluid imaging in evaluation of acute flank pain (SUDAH et al. 2001).

1.2.4.3
MR Angiography

Another option is to inject gadolinium chelate as a bolus, using a power injector and automatic detection of contrast within the abdominal aorta. A 3D gradient-recalled echo (GRE) sequence then makes it possible to acquire multiple images in the coronal plane in the arterial phase, during a breath-hold, with a mean acquisition time of approximately 20 s. High-quality images, obtained after reconstruction of data in oblique views, demonstrate aorta, iliac and renal arteries, so that the relationship between the vessels and the urinary tract can be analyzed, and to demonstrate an arterial cause of urinary obstruction such

as a crossing vessel causing UPJ obstruction or artery aneurysm compressing of the ureter (Fig. 1.19).

With such an initial arterial 3D phase study, a complete functional study cannot be conducted. However, later coronal or multiple-view GRE acquisitions can still be obtained for morphological evaluation of renal parenchyma enhancement.

1.2.4.4
Scanning and Postprocessing Techniques

Coil placement needs to be adjusted so that the field of view (FOV) covers the entire urinary tract from the top of the kidneys to the base of the bladder. Smaller FOV may be useful for complementary, focused examination. Asking patients to keep upper limbs above the head during the examination eliminates phase wrap artifacts.

The use of breath gating, or respiratory compensation, should reduce artifacts from breathing, which can significantly degrade images. However, single-breath-hold acquisition seems better than respiratory triggering, as long as the patient is able to suspend breathing during the acquisition time (NOLTE-ERNSTING et al. 1998). The use of prospective or retrospective navigator gating may also improve image quality (BORTHNE et al. 2000).

For T1-weighted sequences or short TE effective T2-weighted sequences, the adjunct of fat saturation, using STIR technique (ROHRSCHNEIDER et al. 2000a) or presaturation bands, can be useful in order to eliminate signal from fatty tissues surrounding ureters. However, this increases the acquisition time and decreases the signal-to-noise ratio.

Two acquisition protocols may be used to cover the entire volume of the urinary tract. The first protocol uses multiple one-slice, interleaved acquisitions obtained in various scanning planes, rotating in a stepwise manner from the coronal to the lateral view. The slice thickness usually ranges from 30 to 60 mm, and makes it possible to evaluate the entire ureter in different views. The main limitation of this thick-slice technique is a potential lack of spatial resolution due to partial volume effect.

The second approach is to obtain multiple, 2D, thin slices and to subsequently acquire MIP reconstruction images of the entire urinary tract. The in-slice spatial resolution is optimal, but details such as small filling defects can also be removed on MIP images, although they are clearly visible on the individual source slices (ROY et al. 1994). This technique is also more sensitive to artifacts from breathing (NOLTE-ERNSTING et al. 2001b).

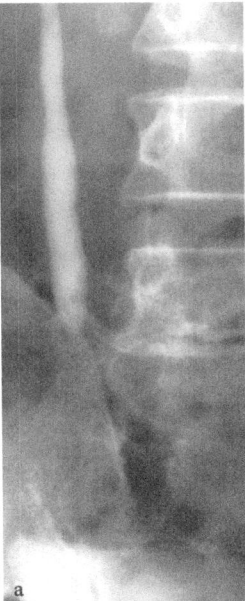 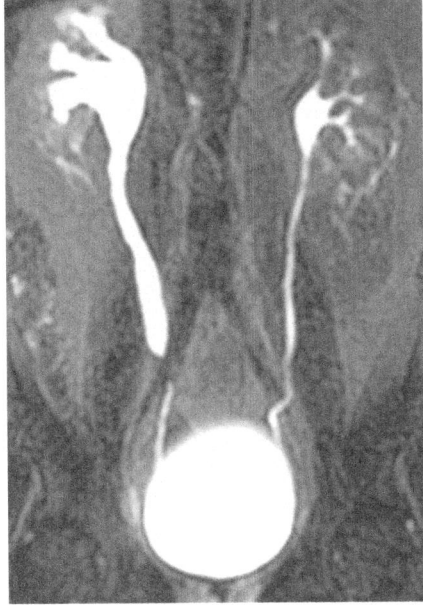 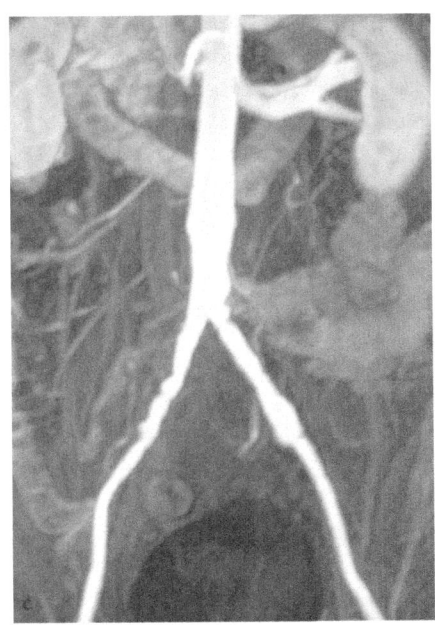

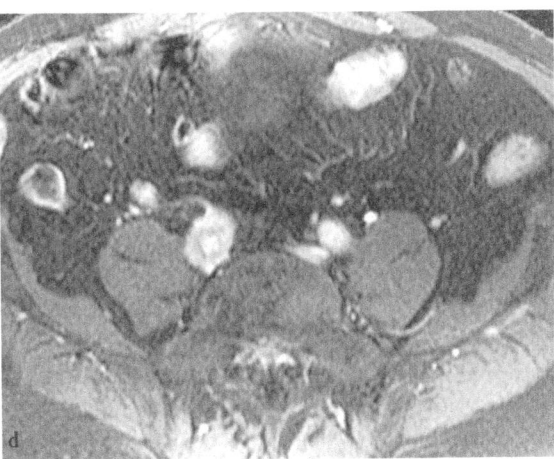

Fig. 1.19a–d. Compression of the ureter by an inflammatory aneurysm of the right iliac artery. a EU demonstrates a right ureterohydronephrosis and shows the level of the obstruction. b T2-weighted images shows the dilatation of the right renal calyces, renal pelvis and upper ureter, and suggests that the obstruction is located at the level of the right iliac artery. Normal lower ureter is clearly seen. c 3D MR angiography reveals diffuse atheromatosis of the aorta and both iliac arteries. d Delayed transverse T1-weighted images show inflammatory changes around the right iliac artery extending to the ureter. Compression of the ureter by a small inflammatory iliac aneurysm was confirmed by surgery

Unenhanced MR urography can be associated with virtual endoscopy of the upper urinary tract. Feasibility was demonstrated in all cases with dilatation but only in 43% of cases without dilatation (NERI et al. 2000). Lumen abnormalities (masses and stenosis) can be visualized but further studies are required to demonstrate improvement of diagnostic accuracy.

MR urography is now a viable alternative to EU and contrast-enhanced CT in selected patients such as those allergic to iodinated contrast agents, pregnant women, or patients for whom radiation exposure is of great concern (LI et al. 1997). Recent technical improvements show that this technique is able to offer a highly accurate morphological and comprehensive functional diagnostic evaluation of the urinary tract in most conditions. It has the potential to become the preferred imaging modality for the

diagnosis of suspected ureteral disease, significantly decreasing the need for EU and retrograde pyelography (NOLTE-ERNSTING et al. 2001a).

1.2.5
Nuclear Medicine

Renal scintigraphy allows for both evaluation of urodynamics and measurement of tubular cell viability and global renal function.

1.2.5.1
Urodynamics

Urodynamics is evaluated by diuresis renography. This noninvasive test tracks a high endogenous rate of urine flow obtained after stimulation by administration of furosemide (TAYLOR 1999; FINE 1999). The protocol has been standardized by the recommendations of the International Consensus Committee on diuresis renography (O'REILLY et al. 1996; PRIGENT et al. 1999). Mag3 labeled with technetium is the preferred tracer because of its most efficient extraction. Hydration consists of 10 ml/kg body weight over 1 h prior to the study. The patient should void immediately prior to the examination. The most usual choice for furosemide administration is 20 min after the radiotracer injection (F+20) but administration of diuretic 15 min before the radiotracer is an alternative procedure (F–15). The consensus quantitative criterion of differentiation between obstructive and nonobstructive pyelocaliectasis is the half-time ($T_{1/2}$) of renal pelvic provocative emptying. Kidneys able to excrete more than half of the radioisotope in less than 10 min are considered unobstructed and those requiring more than 20 min are considered obstructed.

Depending on the technique, a $T_{1/2}$ between 10 and 20 min is considered inconclusive. This result can occur due to a distended bladder or to the failure of a poorly functioning kidney to respond to furosemide. A poor response to diuresis may also be seen in severe pelvic dilatation. The rate of equivocal or false-positive results is approximately 10%–15%. This percentage of inconclusive studies is only 7% using the (F–15) method. Presently diuretic renography is used as the gold standard for the diagnosis of obstruction (SHOKEIR et al. 1996; BARTHEZ et al. 1999).

Impaired renal function is a well-known cause of an unreadable diuretic renogram. In this case the third phase of the renogram curve does not accurately reflect radiopharmaceutical excretion from the kidney but depends upon continuing tracer uptake. A recent approach allows for calculation of the Renal Output Efficiency (ROE) independently of the variations in the uptake rate (CHAIWATANARAT et al. 1993; SPICER et al. 1999; SAUNDERS et al. 1997). ROE is the integrated output as a percentage of the integrated input which is the integral of the blood clearance curve fitted as a part of the rising second phase of the background corrected kidney curve. The furosemide protocol is a (F–10) test. ROE has been shown to be an accurate parameter in the assessment of outflow obstruction in native kidneys in both the adult and pediatric populations and in renal transplants patients. It improves diagnostic accuracy when investigating obstruction in patients with impaired renal function.

1.2.5.2
Functional Evaluation

Renal scintigraphy can play an important role in the evaluation of the global renal function and obstruction before and after surgical procedures or in diagnosing unilateral acute tubular necrosis as a complication of acute ureteral obstruction (MOHSIN and KIM 1996; TIEL-VAN BUUL et al. 1998).

Fast frame renography is also a noninvasive technique for imaging ureteric peristalsis and renal drainage. Peristalsis is determined from the condensed image of each ureter in which sloping lines of activity represent individual boluses of urine moving down the ureter. The mean normal frequency of peristalsis is 1.3 boluses/min (BROUGH et al. 1998).

Besides urodynamics, another type of information is brought by renal cortical scintigraphy using technetium-labeled dimercaptosuccinic acid (DMSA). It is performed to assess the renal sequelae of urinary tract infection. It is the most reliable technique in the diagnosis of chronic renal cortical scarring. In cases of obstructive pyelocaliectasis, the measurement of tubular cell viability by DMSA allows for a choice between nephrectomy, conservative surgery and nonsurgical treatments (CHOI et al. 1999).

References

Aboulker P, Steg A, Zorzos SI (1966) La ponction du bassinet et la pyélo-urétérographie descendante. J Urol Nephrol 72: 485–491

Aerts P, Van Hoe L, Bosmans H et al (1996) Breath-hold MR urography using the HASTE technique. AJR Am J Roentgenol 166:543–545

Amis ES Jr (1999) Epitaph for the urogram. Radiology 213: 639–640

Bagley DH, Liu JB (1998) Three-dimensional endoluminal ultrasonography of the ureter. J Endo Urol 12:411–416

Balci NC, Mueller-Lisse UG, Holzknecht N et al (1998) MR urography: comparison between HASTE and RARE in healthy volunteers. Eur Radiol 8:925–932

Barthez PY, Smeak DD, Wisner ER et al (1999) Effect of partial ureteral obstruction on results of renal scintigraphy in dogs. Am J Vet Res 60:1383–1389

Bigot JM (1995) Que reste-t-il de l'urographie en 1995? J Radiol 76:987–989

Borthne A, Nordshus T, Reiseter T et al (1999) MR urography: the future gold standard in paediatric urogenital imaging? Pediatr Radiol 29:694–701

Borthne A, Pierre-Jerome C, Nordshus T et al (2000) MR urography in children: current status and future development. Eur Radiol 10:503–511

Brough RJ, Lancashire MJR, Prince JR et al (1998) The effect of diclofenac (Voltarol) and pethidine on ureteric peristalsis and the isotope renogram. Eur J Nucl Med 25:1520–1523

Burge HJ, Middleton WD, McClennan BL et al (1991) Ureteral jets in healthy subjects and in patients with unilateral ureteral calculi: comparison with color Doppler ultrasound. Radiology 180:437–442

Caoili EM, Cohan RH, Korobkin M (2002) Urinary tract abnormalities: initial experience with multi-detector row CT urography. Radiology 222:353–360

Catalano C, Pavone P, Laghi A et al (1999) MR pyelography and conventional MR imaging in urinary tract obstruction. Acta Radiol 40:198–202

Chaiwatanarat T, Padhy AK, Bomanji JB et al (1993) Validation of renal output efficiency as an objective quantitative parameter in the evaluation of upper urinary tract obstruction. J Nucl Med 34:845–848

Chevassu M (1929) L'urétero-pyélographie rétrograde. XXIX Congrés Français d'urologie. DOIN, Paris, pp 539–552

Chelfouh N, Grenier N, Migueret D et al (1998) Characterization of urinary calculi: in vitro study of «twinkling artifact» revealed by color-flow sonography. AJR 171:1055–1060

Choi H, Oh SJ, So Y et al (1999) No further development of renal scarring after antireflux surgery in children with primary vesicoureteral reflux: review of the results of 99m technetium dimercapto-succinic acid renal scan. J Urol 162:1189–1192

Chow LC, Graham Sommer F (2001) Multidetector CT urography with abdominal compression and three-dimensional reconstruction. AJR 177:849–855

Choyke PL (1992) The urogram: are rumors of its death premature? Radiology 184:33–36

Davies P, Woods KA, Evans CM et al (1978) The value of provocative and acute urography in patients with intermittent loin pain. Br J Urol 50:227–232

Deyoe LA, Cronan JJ, Bareslaw BH et al (1995) New technique of ultrasound and color Doppler in the prospective evaluation of acute renal obstruction. Do they replace the intravenous urogram? Abdom Imaging 20:58–63

Fajardo LL, Hillman BJ (1988) Image quality, diagnostic certainty and accuracy: comparison of conventional and digital urograms. Urol Radiol 10:72–74

Fine EJ (1999) Interventions in renal scintirenography. Sem Nucl Med 29:128–145

Frank R, Stenzl A, Frede TH et al (1998) Three-dimensional computed tomography of the reconstructed lower urinary tract: technique and findings. Eur Radiol 8:657–663

Gaeta M, Blandino A, Scribano E et al (1999) Diagnostic pitfalls of breath-hold MR urography in obstructive uropathy. J Comput Assist Tomogr 23:891–897

Girish G, Chooi WK, Morcos SK (2001) Filling defect artifacts in magnetic resonance urography (abstract). Radiology 221:634

Goldstein AG, Conger KB (1965) Perforation of the ureter during retrograde pyelography. J Urol 94:658–664

Goodwin WE, Casey WC, Woolf W (1955) Percutaneous Trocar (needle) nephrostomy in hydronephrosis. J Am Med Assoc 157:891–894

Grasso M, Li S, Liu JB (1999) Examining the obstructed ureter with intraluminal sonography. J Urol 162:1286–1290

Grenier N, Pariente JL, Trillaud H et al (2000) Dilatation of the collecting system during pregnancy: physiologic VS obstructive dilatation. Eur Radiol 10:271–279

Hattery RR, King BF (1995) Technique and application of MR urography (editorial; comment). Radiology 194:25–27

Hattery RR, Williamson MD Jr, Hartman GW et al (1988) Intravenous urographic technique. Radiology 167:593–599

Heneghan JP, Kim DH, Leder RA et al (2001) Compression CT urography: a comparison with IVU in the opacification of the collecting system and ureters. J Comput Assist Tomogr 25:343–347

Hennig J, Nauerth A, Friedburg H (1986) RARE imaging: a fast imaging method for clinical MR. Magn Reson Med 3: 823–833

Hertzberg BS, Kliewer MA, Paulson EK et al (1994) Distal ureteral calculi, detection with transperineal sonography. AJR 163:1151–1153

Hirohashi S, Hirohashi R, Uchida H et al (1997) MR cholangio-pancreatography and MR urography: improved enhancement with a negative oral contrast agent. Radiology 203: 281–285

Hughes TH, Hine AL (1991) The most advantageous timing of external ureteric compression during intravenous urography. Br J Radiol 64:314–317

Imray TJ, Lieberman RP (1990) Retrograde pyelography. In: Pollack HM (ed) Clinical urography: an atlas and textbook of uroradiological imaging, vol 1. Saunders, Philadelphia, pp 244–255

Laing FC, Benson CB, Di Salvo DN et al (1994) Distal ureteral calculi detection with vaginal US. Radiology 192:545–548

Lecesne R, Drouillard J, Cisse R et al (1998) Contribution de l'abdoscan dans la cholangiopancréatographie et l'urographie par IRM. J Radiol 79:573–575

Lefevre F, Debelle L, Gaucher H et al (1998) Coronal Mr Uro-angio-nephrography (MR-UAN) in upper urinary tract diseases. Scientific Exhibit: 84th Scientific Assembly and Annual Meeting of Radiological Society of North America, Chicago, 209:590

Lemaître L, Ala Edine C, Dubrulle F et al (2000a) Retroperitoneum and ureters. In: Terrier F, Grossholtz M, Becker CD (eds) Spiral CT of the abdomen. Springer, Berlin Heidelberg New York, pp 277–316

Lemaître L, Mestdagh P, Marecaux-Delomez J et al (2000b) Percutaneous nephrostomy: placement under laser guidance and real time CT fluoroscopy. Eur Radiol 10:892–895

Lerner RM (1986) Distal ureteral calculi: diagnosis by transrectal sonography. AJR 147:1189–1191

Levine J, Neitlich J, Smith RC (1999) The value of prone scanning to distinguish ureterovesical junction stones from ureteral stones that have passed into the bladder: leave no stone unturned. AJR Am J Roentgenol 172:977–981

Li W, Chavez D, Edelman RR et al (1997) Magnetic resonance urography by breath-hold contrast-enhanced three dimensional FISP. J Magn Reson Imaging 7:309–311

Mawhinney RR, Gresson RHS (1987) Is ureteric compression still necessary? Clin Radiol 38:179–180

McNeily AE, Goldenberg SL, Allen GJ (1991) Sonographic visualisation of ureter in pregnancy. J Urol 146:298–301

McNicholas MMJ, Raptopoulos VD, Schwartz RK et al (1998) Excretory phase CT urography for opacification of the urinary collecting system. AJR Am J Roentgenol 170:1261–1267

Merran S (1999) Virtual endoscopy of the urinary tract (abstract). Radiology 213:475

Mohsin J, Kim CK (1996) Renal scintigraphy in a patient with retroperitoneal fibrosis. Clin Nucl Med 21:390–391

Moreau JF (1995) Defense et illustration de l'urographie. J Radiol 76:989–990

Neri E, Boraschi P, Caramella D et al (2000) MR virtual endoscopy of the upper urinary tract. AJR 175:1697–1702

Newhouse JH (1979) Interventional percutaneous pyeloureteral techniques I. Antegrade pyelography and ureteral perfusion. Radiol Clin North Am 17:341–352

Nolte-Ernsting CC, Bucker A, Adam GB et al (1998) Gadolinium-enhanced excretory MR urography after low-dose diuretic injection: comparison with conventional excretory urography. Radiology 209:147–157

Nolte-Ernsting CC, Adam GB, Gunther RW et al (2001a) MR urography: examination techniques and clinical applications. Eur Radiol 11:355–372

Nolte-Ernsting CC, Tacke J, Adam GB et al (2001b) Diuretic-enhanced gadolinium excretory MR urography: comparison of conventional gradient echo sequence and echoplanar imaging. Eur Radiol 11:18–27

O'Malley ME, Soto JA, Yucel EK et al (1997) MR urography: evaluation of a three-dimensional fast spin-echo technique in patients with hydronephrosis. AJR Am J Roentgenol 168: 387–392

Onishi K, Watanabe H, Ohe H et al (1986) Ultrasound findings in urolithiasis in the lower ureter. Ultrasound Med Biol 12: 577–579

O'Reilly P, Aurell M, Britton K et al (1996) Consensus on diuresis renography for investigating the dilated upper urinary tract. Radionuclides in Nephrourology Group. J Nucl Med 37:1872–1876

Perlman ES, Rosenfield AT, Wexler S et al (1996) CT urography in the evaluation of urinary tract disease. J Comput Assist Tomogr 20:620–626

Pfister RC, Newhouse JH (1978) Radiology of ureter. Urology 1:15–39

Platt JF, Rubin JM, Ellis JH (1989) Duplex Doppler US of the kidney: differentiation of obstructive with nonobstructive dilatation. Radiology 171:515–517

Prigent A, Cosgriff P, Gates GF et al (1999) Consensus report on quality control of quantitative measurements of renal function obtained from the renogram: International Consensus Committee from the Scientific Committee of Radionuclides in Nephrourology. Sem Nucl Med 29:146–159

Regan F, Bohlman ME, Khazan R et al (1996) MR urography using HASTE imaging in the assessment of ureteric obstruction. AJR Am J Roentgenol 167:1115–1120

Regan F, Petronis J, Bohlman M et al (1997) Perirenal MR high signal – a new and sensitive indicator of acute ureteric obstruction. Clin Radiol 52:445–450

Reuther G, Kiefer B, Wandl E (1997) Visualization of urinary tract dilatation: value of single-shot MR urography. Eur Radiol 7:1276–1281

Rohrschneider WK, Becker K, Hoffend J et al (2000a) Combined static-dynamic MR urography for the simultaneous evaluation of morphology and function in urinary tract obstruction. II. Findings in experimentally induced ureteric stenosis (in process citation). Pediatr Radiol 30: 523–532

Rohrschneider WK, Hoffend J, Becker K et al (2000b) Combined static-dynamic MR urography for the simultaneous evaluation of morphology and function in urinary tract obstruction. I. Evaluation of the normal status in an animal model (in process citation). Pediatr Radiol 30:511–522

Rothpearl A, Frager D, Subramanian A et al (1995) MR urography: technique and application (see comments). Radiology 194:125–130

Roy C, Saussine C, Jahn C et al (1994) Evaluation of RARE-MR urography in the assessment of ureterohydronephrosis. J Comput Assist Tomogr 18:601–608

Roy C, Saussine C, Guth S et al (1998) MR urography in the evaluation of urinary tract obstruction. Abdom Imaging 23:27–34

Rubin GD, Beaulieu CF, Argiro V et al (1996) Perspective volume rendering of CT and MR images: applications for endoscopic imaging. Radiology 199:321–330

Saunders C, Choong K, Larcos G et al (1997) Assessment of pediatric hydronephrosis using output efficiency. J Nucl Med 38:1483–1486

Shokeir AA, Provoost AP, El-Azab M et al (1996) Renal Doppler ultrasound in children with obstructive uropathy: effect of intravenous normal saline fluid load and furosemide. J Urol 156:1455–1458

Sigmund G, Stoever B, Zimmerhackl LB et al (1991) RARE-MR-urography in the diagnosis of upper urinary tract abnormalities in children. Pediatr Radiol 21:416–420

Smith RC, Rosenfield AT, Choe KA et al (1995) Acute flank pain: comparison of unenhanced-enhanced helical CT and intravenous urography. Radiology 194:789–794

Spicer ST, Chi K-K, Nankivell BJ et al (1999) Mercaptoacetyltriglycine diuretic renography and output efficiency measurement in renal transplant patients. Eur J Nucl Med 26:152–154

Staley C (1960) Retrograde ileopyelography. Surg Gynecol Obstet 111:243–244

Sudah M, Vanninen R, Partanen K et al (2001) MR urography in evaluation of acute flank pain: T2-weighted sequences and gadolinium-enhanced three dimensional FLASH compared with urography. AJR 176:105–112

Taylor A (1999) Radionuclide Renography: a personal approach. Sem Nucl Med 29:102–127

Tiel-Van Buul M, Aronson D, Groothoff J et al (1998) The role of renal scintigraphy in the diagnosis and follow-up of unilateral ATN after complete bilateral distal ureteral obstruction as a complication of acute appendicitis. Clin Nucl Med 23:141–145

Thomsen HS, Bush WH Jr (1998) Adverse effects of contrast media: Incidence, prevention and management. Drugs Safety 19:313–324

Vinee P, Stover B, Sigmund G et al (1993) L'urographie «RARE» par IRM: une alternative à l'UIV? Ann Radiol 36:109–113

Voelcker F, Von Lichtenberg A (1906) Pyelographie (Röntgenographie des nieren beckens nach collargolfüllung). Munch Med Wochenschr 53:105

Whitaker RH (1973) Methods of assessing obstruction in dilated ureters. Br J Urol 45:15–22

2 The Normal Ureter

M. Claudon, F. Joffre, G. Escourrou, M. Mazerolles, J. P. Sarramon

CONTENTS

Diseases of the ureter are related to its anatomy, physiology, and structure, and to the relationships established along its pathway through the retroperitoneal and pelvic space. Radiological analysis of ureteral abnormalities is based upon a good knowledge of its anatomy, physiology, histology, and normal radiological aspects and variants.

2.1
Anatomy
(Joffre and Russ 1997; Olsson 1986)

The ureter starts at the uretero-pelvic junction (UPJ) and courses in a caudal direction through the retroperitoneum to reach the posterior wall of the bladder (Fig. 2.1). The length of the adult ureter varies from 28 to 32 cm. Its diameter varies from 4 to 6 mm (outer diameter), and from 2 to 4 mm (inner diameter), depending on the level at which it is measured.

In the absence of peristaltic activity, three normal narrowings are described: The first one is at the uretero-pelvic junction, the second is where the ureter crosses the iliac vessels, and the third corresponds to the intramural portion. The ureter is divided into three parts: the abdominal or lumbar, the iliac, and the pelvic portion.

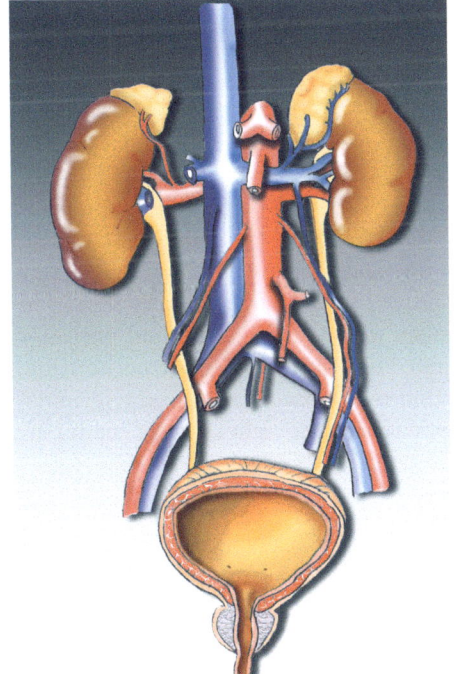

Fig. 2.1. General topographic anatomy and main relationships of the ureters (Netter 1973)

M. Claudon, MD
Service de Radiologie, CHU Nancy Brabois, rue du Morvan, 54511 Vandoeuvre Les Nancy, France
F. Joffre, MD
Service de Radiologie, Hôpital de Rangueil, 1, avenue Jean-Poulhès, 31403 Toulouse Cédex 4, France
G. Escourrou, MD
Service d'Anatomo-pathologie, CHU Rangueil, 1, avenue Jean-Poulhès, 31403 Toulouse Cédex 4, France
M. Mazerolles, MD
Service d'Anatomo-pathologie, CHU Purpan, place Baylac, 31059 Toulouse Cédex, France
J. P. Sarramon, MD
Service d'Urologie, CHU Rangueil, 1, avenue Jean-Poulhès, 31403 Toulouse Cédex, France

2.1.1
The Abdominal Portion (Kabalin 1992)

The abdominal portion is approximately 15 cm in length. It starts at the uretero-pelvic junction and courses vertically to the pelvic rim. The initial part of the abdominal ureter is located at the level of the transverse process of the second lumbar vertebra and lies, surrounded by fat, on the fascia iliaca, which separates the ureter from the body of the psoas muscle. The genitofemoral nerve branch of the lumbar plexus is in direct relation to the ureter at the level of the third lumbar vertebra. The genitofemoral nerve crosses the ureter from below (Weinberg 1967).

On the right, the ureter is behind the second part of the duodenum and the line of attachment of the mesentery. On the left, the ureter is in relation to the left mesocolon. Gonadal vessels (testicular or ovarian) are directly in contact with the ureter. The gonadal artery crosses the ureter from above at the level of the third lumbar vertebra. The gonadal veins have a different course: The left gonadal vein is located outside and courses along the ureter, crossing it from above near the UPJ; the right gonadal vein crosses the ureter from above at the level of the third lumbar vertebra.

Medially, the lumbar ureters are situated outside the aorta on the left and the inferior vena cava on the right.

2.1.2
The Iliac Portion

The iliac portion crosses the brim of the pelvis, usually over the bifurcation of the common iliac vein on the right side and over the common iliac artery on the left side. The iliac portion is a very short and narrow segment, with a slight lateral and posterior concave course. Through the posterior peritoneum, the iliac portion is in close relation to the terminal ileum and appendix on the right side and the mesosigmoid colon on the left.

2.1.3
The Pelvic Ureter

The pelvic portion measures about 14 cm. Immediately after crossing the iliac vessels, the ureter runs backward and laterally in a vertical course along the side wall of the true pelvis, just lateral and anterior to the internal iliac artery until the level of the ischial spine. Then it turns forward and medially towards the bladder in a horizontal course, just medial to the obturator nerve and superior vesical artery. The ureteral ending lies below the tip of the coccyx.

The vertical portion courses between the obturator muscle and the peritoneum. The anatomical relationships differ between male and female subjects for both the vertical and the horizontal portion.

2.1.3.1
The Female Pelvic Ureter

The relations of the female pelvic ureter are complex. In its vertical portion, the ureter is dorsal to the ovary, medial to the ovarian vessels, and lateral to the sacrouterine ligament. The horizontal portion is located inside the broad ligament and runs close to the uterine artery, which goes obliquely forward. After crossing the broad ligament, the ureter lies lateral to the uterine cervix and above the lateral fornix of the vagina. During its course, the ureter is accompanied by the vaginal artery, venous plexus, and lymphatics, and it is crossed below by the round ligament.

2.1.3.2
The Male Pelvic Ureter

In its vertical portion, the male pelvic ureter is located lateral to the rectum and is crossed ventrally by the vas deferens at the level of the ischial spine. In its horizontal portion, the ureter turns medially and enters the posterolateral wall of the bladder, lateral to the seminal vesicles. It is crossed below by the vesicoprostatic arteries.

2.1.4
Intramural Vesical Ureter

The ureter crosses the vesical wall obliquely, so that it creates a complex anatomical system to prevent vesicoureteral reflux (Hutch 1967). The length of the intramural ureter is about 15 mm. It runs through longitudinal and circular muscular layers of the bladder inside the so-called sheath of the ureter, which links the ureteral wall to the bladder wall. After crossing the vesical wall, the ureter becomes an intravesical structure for about 1 cm. This portion lies directly under the mucosa and can be collapsed by increase of the bladder pressure.

2.1.5
Blood Supply, Lymphatics, Nerves
(WILLIAMS and WARWICK 1980)

The rich vascularization of the ureteral wall explains the frequency of metastatic disease around and along the ureter (MARINCEK et al. 1993). Ureteral blood vessels are also used as collateral pathways in case of occlusion of arterial or venous retroperitoneal vessels.

Arterial supply is provided by branches of the renal artery, the gonadal artery, the common iliac artery, and the vesical or uterine arteries. This supply is variable, particularly in its upper part. In the lumbar part arterial supply is provided by a branch of the renal and gonadal arteries and by a direct aortic branch. The pelvic portion is supplied by branches that may arise from the common iliac artery or from the internal iliac artery (vesical, uterine, middle rectal, or vaginal). Ureteral arteries form a continuous longitudinal plexus in the adventitia, supplying the muscularis and mucosa by smaller perpendicular branches (SHAFIK 1972).

Similarly, venous drainage is assumed by subadventitial plexuses, which drain into lumbar, iliac, renal, vesical, and gonadal veins. Venous plexuses are particularly well developed in the lowermost part of the ureter, allowing communications between vesical and internal iliac veins.

Lymphatic drainage is important and in continuity with lymphatics of the bladder and the kidney (HARRISON and CLOUSE 1985). It consists of widely anastomosed vessels located mainly in the adventitia and communicating freely along the entire ureter (MARINCEK et al. 1993).

Nerves are derived mainly from the renal testicular or ovarian and hypogastric plexus.

2.2
Histology

Like other segments of the urinary tract, the ureteral wall is composed of three distinct layers: mucosa, muscularis, and adventitia (WINALSKI 1990) (Fig. 2.2). Thickness and characteristics of the different layers are variable according to the ureteral level. Thus diameter and wall thickness are not uniform (VELARDO 1967).

The mucosa is the inner layer and consists of urothelial transitional epithelium with four to six cell layers, like other parts of the urinary tract. Longitudinal folds appear when the ureter is contracting, giving a stellate pattern to the lumen. This mechanism allows stretching of the wall without risk of rupture. The uro-

thelial epithelium rests on a fibrous "lamina propria" which contains elastic and collagenous fibers.

The muscularis is made of outer and inner longitudinal and circular smooth muscle bundles. Distribution of the bundles is variable according to the portion.

The adventitia is the outer layer of the ureteral wall and is composed of fibroelastic connective tissue with a large number of blood vessels, lymphatics, and nerves (DE SOUSA 1966). The adventitia is in continuity with the renal capsule and the bladder adventitia.

2.3
Physiology

The ureter has a single function, which is to propel urine from the kidney to the bladder. According to Sherwood, three forces are involved in the transport of urine: gravity when the patient is in an upright position, filtration pressure from the nephron, and peristalsis (SHERWOOD 1979). Peristalsis is the most important mechanism. It is initiated by "pacemaker" cells, probably located at the fornix of minor calices. The rate of contraction is dependent on the volume of urine, with the frequency varying from two to six waves per minute. The mechanism of contraction seems to be myogenic and autonomous rather than neurogenic. This fact is attested to by the persistence of peristalsis after transplantation or progressive reestablishment of contraction after ureteral surgical anastomosis (O'REILLY 1985).

The role of gravity is minimal and comes into play only in case of very high flow rate in normal subjects (SHERWOOD 1979).

Measurement of ureteral pressure shows a varia-

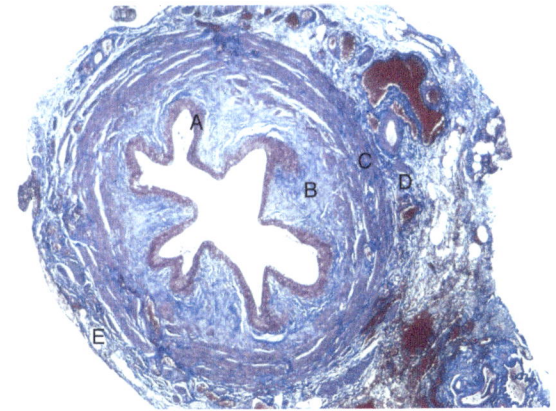

Fig. 2.2. Cross section of a human ureter: *A* mucosa, *B* lamina propria, *C* muscularis, *D* adventitia, *E* periureteral vessel

tion between periods of rest and contraction. The mean values vary from 0 to 15 mmHg. Many factors may influence the pressure level: urine flow, position of the patient, environment, bladder repletion, anesthesia, psychologic state (SHOPFNER 1976).

2.4
Normal Radiological Aspects and Variants

The ureter can be imaged by indirect EU (excretory urography) or direct opacification (antegrade or retrograde pyelography) and by cross-sectional imaging techniques (mainly CT).

2.4.1
EU and Direct Opacification (FRIEDENBERG 1990)

In the usual incidence of EU or direct opacification (anteroposterior view in supine position), ureters appear as opacified conduits approximately 25–30 cm long located bilaterally and symmetrically outside the spine.

The diameter varies from 0 to 7 mm, depending on the level and timing of contraction. Peristaltic activity changes the size and shape of the ureter. Because of contraction, the entire length is not usually visualized on a single radiographic exposure during EU (Fig. 2.3). Peristaltic waves begin at the pelvis and move downward to the bladder. They may simulate stricture on a single X-ray view but, unlike stricture, the morphology changes from film to film. Between waves the ureter seems slightly dilated, mainly in its abdominal portion, and may be spindle-shaped.

Many physiological factors described elsewhere may produce high-flow diuresis, decrease peristalsis, and simulate dilatation, e.g., high-dose contrast media (mainly HOCM), pregnancy, full bladder, and hyperdiuresis states (SHOPFNER 1976).

Besides the variations of caliber, the normal ureter shows three areas of narrowing: the uretero-pelvic junction, the crossing of the iliac vessels, and the vesico-ureteral junction (RIGGS et al. 1970; ROSENFIELD et al. 1977).

The abdominal portion starts at the UPJ, which generally projects at the extremity of the transverse process of the second lumbar vertebra. Its course is straight or slightly concave inside. It lies over the

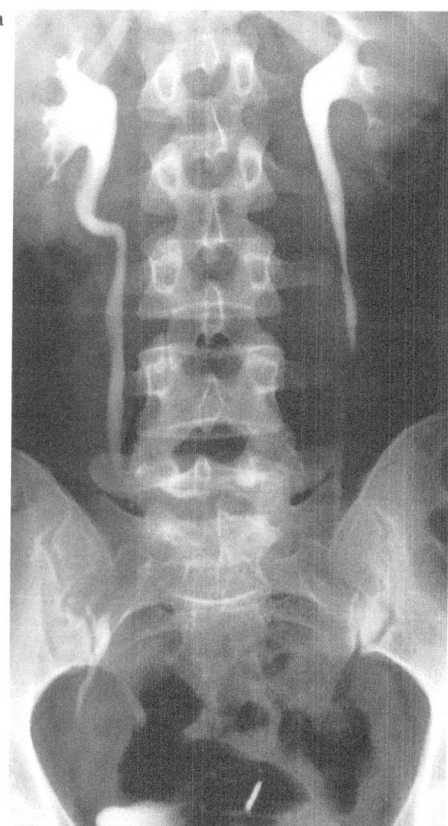
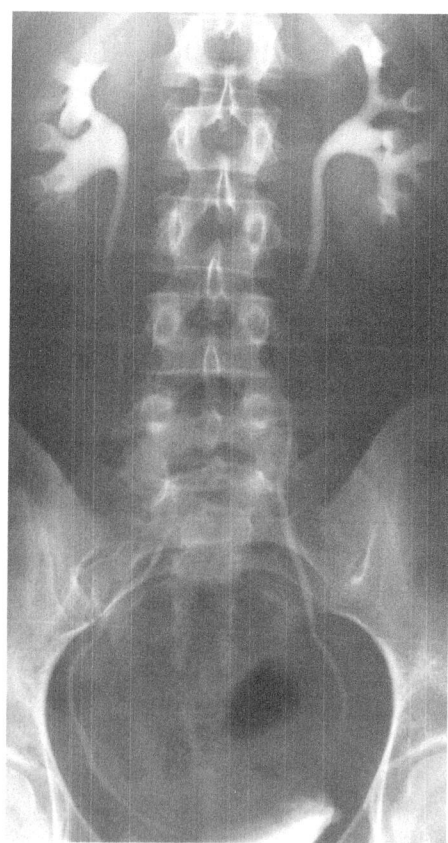

Fig. 2.3a, b. Normal aspects of the ureter on EU: discontinuous and asymmetrical opacification of both ureters

anterior surface of the psoas muscle. On a lateral view, the ureter projects behind the anterior margin of the lumbar vertebral body at the L1-2 level and becomes superimposed to the anterior margin at the L4-5 level.

The iliac portion is situated at a variable level depending on the characteristics of the iliac vessels (ectasias, curves) medial to the sacroiliac joint. This portion is usually short, poorly opacified, and slightly concave outside (Fig. 2.4).

The pelvic portion has a curved course with an anterior and medial concavity. It runs lateral until the ischial spine and after that turns medial toward the bladder. The uretero-vesical junction is narrow where the ureter crosses the bladder wall.

The ureteral jet was described on EU as a stream of densely opacified urine into the bladder, which contains dilute unopacified urine (KALMAN et al. 1955) (Fig. 2.5). It can also be seen on real time and color Doppler sonography as a stream of low-level or colored echoes entering the bladder. In adequate conditions, this phenomenon is seen asymmetrically four to five times per minute (DUBBINS et al. 1981) (Fig. 2.6a,b).

Patterns on direct antegrade or retrograde uretero-pyelography are similar, but these techniques are not

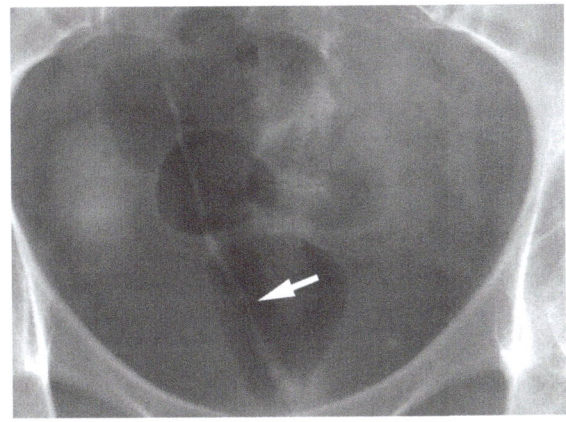

Fig. 2.5. Aspect of right ureteral jet on EU (*arrow*)

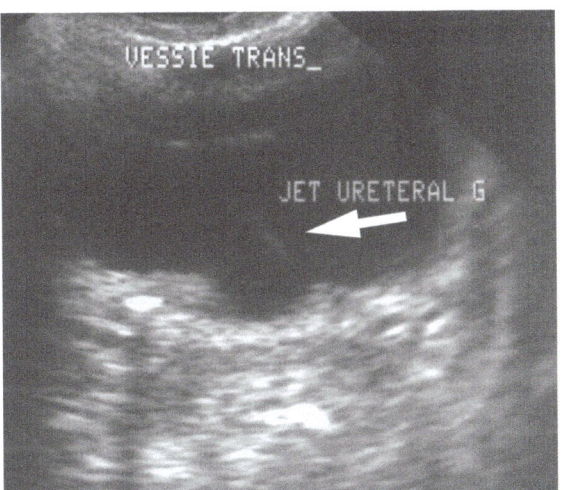

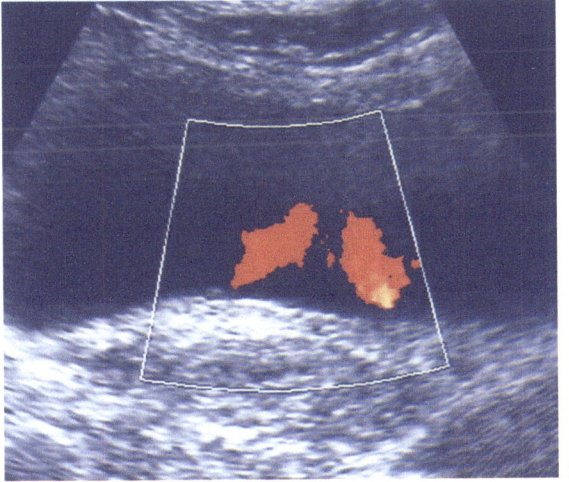

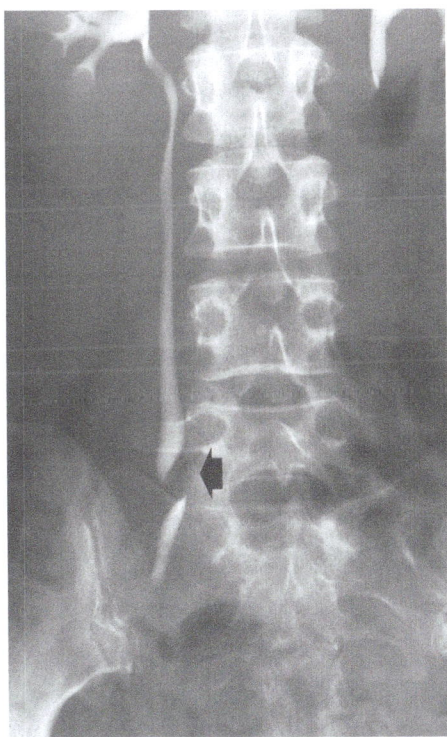

Fig. 2.4. Crossing of the iliac vessels. Urographic opacification shows an extrinsic vascular imprint with sharp margins (*arrow*)

Fig. 2.6a, b. Ultrasonographic aspects of normal ureteral jet. **a** Real-time B-mode echography: low level echoes, entering the bladder lumen from the left meatus (*arrow*). Note Stone on the right side. **b** Color Doppler sonography: bilateral and symmetrical ureteral jets

physiological owing to antegrade or retrograde pressure injection which leads to distortion of the anatomy. Peristaltic activity, physiological strictures, and vascular impressions decrease or disappear (Fig. 2.7).

2.4.2
Computed Tomography and MRI

The unopacified normal ureter is difficult to identify in both the abdominal portion and the pelvic portions (BECHTOLD et al. 1988). In the abdominal portion, it is generally situated in front of the psoas muscle beneath the anterior renal fascia and has a diameter of 2–4 mm without visible internal lumen. It is impossible to differentiate from gonadal veins: surrounded by retroperitoneal fat, they appear as similar rounded opacities with tissular density. The pelvic portion is difficult to detect without injection of contrast medium (Fig. 2.8).

Following i.v. opacification, the lumen becomes visible but visualization may be transient, according to the peristalsis (Fig. 2.9). The wall is often undetectable and has a thickness less than 1 mm. If the orientation of the ureter is oblique in relation to the scanning plane, eccentric false thickening of the wall

can be present (BECHTOLD et al. 1998). Opacification allows better identification of the ureter and surrounding venous structures.

The abdominal portion is contiguous to the gonadal veins, which are located inside at the third lumbar vertebra level and then become more lateral after crossing the ureter anteriorly. 3D reconstruction techniques allow a pseudo-urographic visualization of the ureters and virtual endoureteral endoscopic views (Figs. 2.10-a–c, 2.11a–d, 2.12a,b). Normal aspects on uro-MRI are similar and depend on the sequence used (Fig. 2.13) (see Chap. 1).

2.4.3
Endoluminal Sonography

Endoluminal ultrasonography (Fig. 2.14) provides cross-sectional images of the ureteral wall, and in most cases it is possible to delineate the three layers with different echogenicity (LIU et al 1997). The anechoic lumen surrounds the probe, which is associated with acoustic shadowing. The inner layer is hyperechoic and corresponds to the mucosa. The muscularis propria appears as a fine, punctate, hypoechoic structure. The adventitia is hyperechoic and generally merges with the hyperechoic periureteral fat. Periureteral vessels and lymph modes are discernable as hypoechoic structures until 2–3 cm from the ureteral wall, depending on the frequency of the transducer. The precise anatomical relationship between the ureteral wall and the detrusor can be analyzed at the UVJ level but differentiation of the muscular layers is not always possible (ROSHANI et

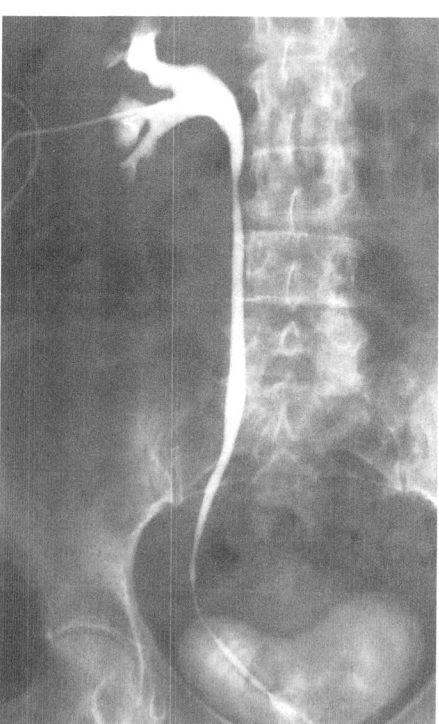

Fig. 2.7. Right antegrade pyelography: normal opacification of the ureter with disappearance of physiological strictures

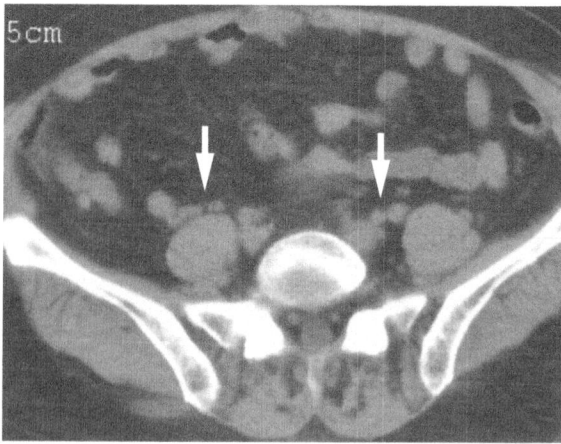

Fig. 2.8. Unenhanced CT slice at the pelvic brim level: Ureters are located in front of the psoas muscle and are impossible to differentiate from vascular structures (*arrows*)

Fig. 2.9a–k. Unenhanced CT shows opacification of ureter at different levels

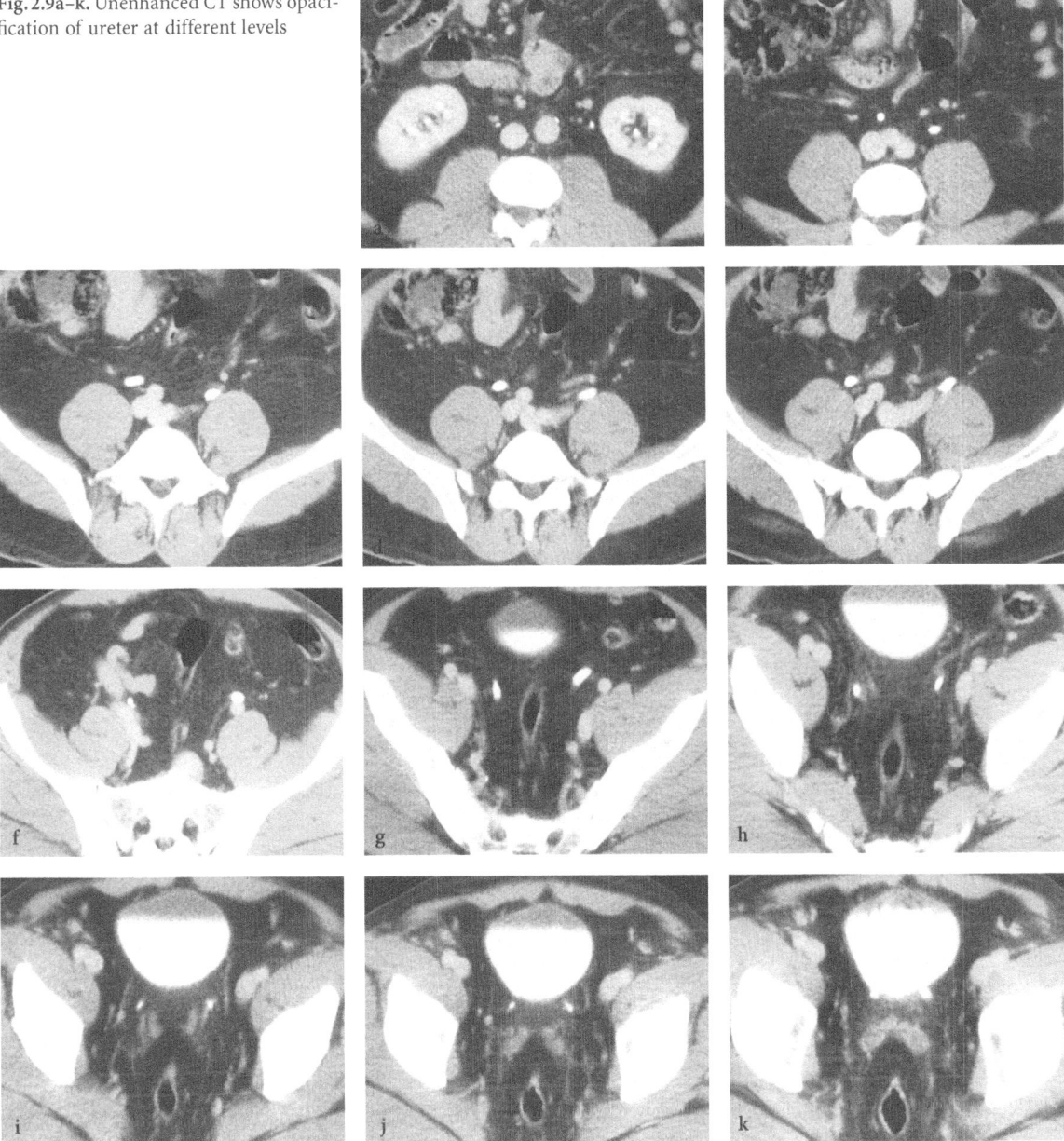

al 1999). Variations in caliber of the lumen along the ureteral course and during peristalsis can be seen. Three-dimensional reconstruction of the images can show longitudinal appearance of the different ureteral segments (BAGLEY and LIU 1998).

2.4.4
Variants

Variations of Caliber of the Abdominal Portion. Ureteral dilatation proximal to the common iliac vessels is quite common and is easily recognized as a variant of normal patterns. At this level, the ureter is slightly displaced medially, and in some cases, mainly in women, a transient dilation above can occur. A clinically significant obstruction may be easily eliminated if there are changes from films to films and no delay in evacuation in erect or prone views.

Vascular Impressions. Arteries as well as veins may produce extrinsic defects on the ureter. Intraluminal or intramural defects are usually eliminated by the use of oblique views and/or abdominal ureteral

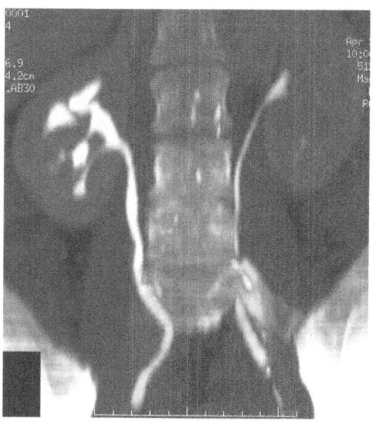

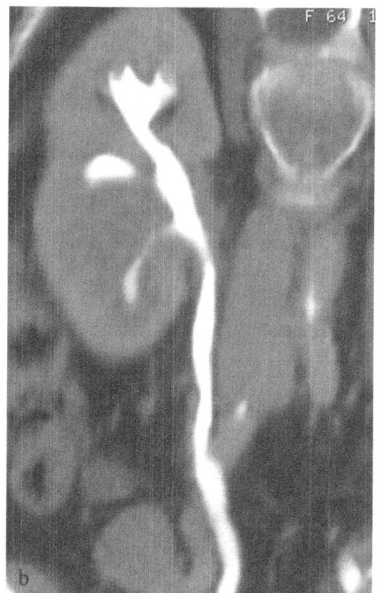

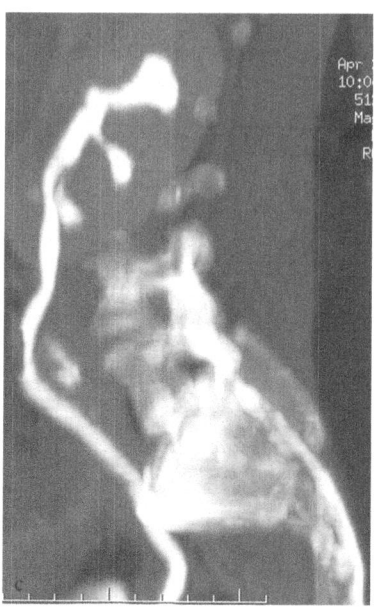

Fig. 2.10a–c. Normal aspects of the ureter on uro-CT (MIP reconstructions). **a** Frontal view. **b, c** Right ureter: frontal and lateral view

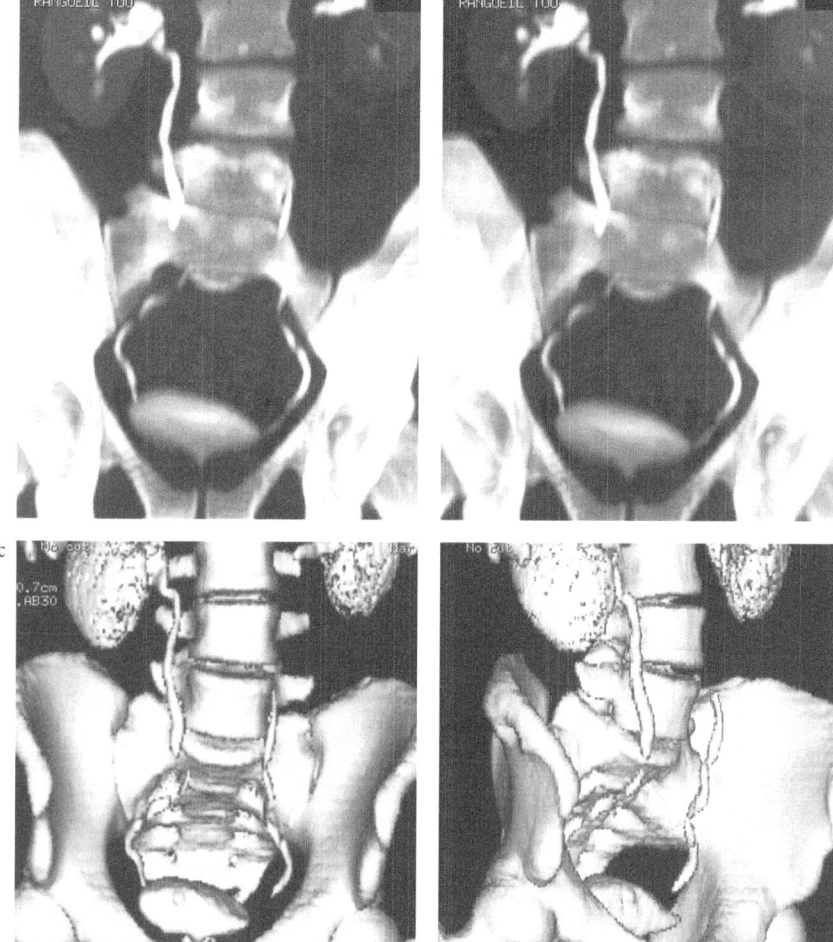

Fig. 2.11a–d. Normal aspects of the ureter on uro-CT. **a, b** MIP reconstructions; **c, d** SSD reconstructions

a

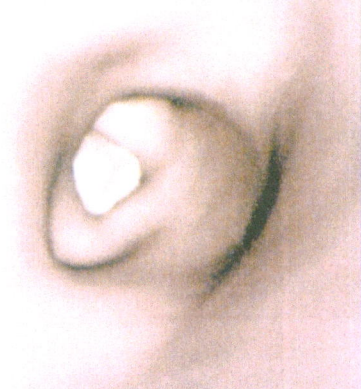

b

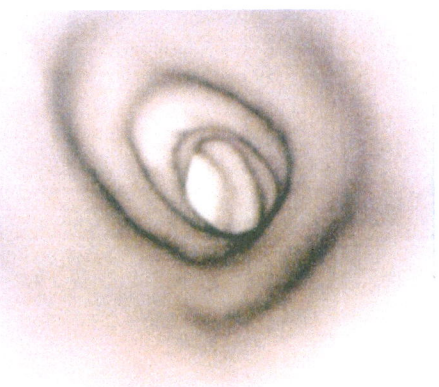

Fig. 2.12a, b. Virtual endoscopy of normal ureter (courtesy of S. Merran, Paris)

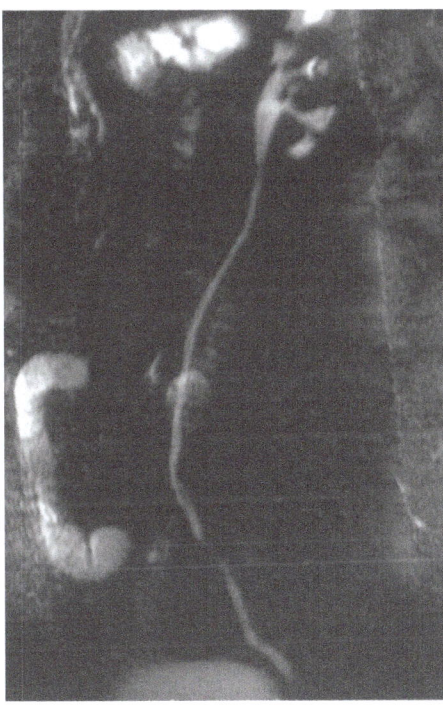

Fig. 2.13. Normal left ureter on uro-MRI (heavily T_2-weighted turbo spin-echo sequence)

compression. Beyond crossing with iliac vessels, the most frequent vascular impression corresponds to the right ovarian vein (Figs. 2.15a–e, 2.16). Normal imprints by anterior branches of the internal iliac artery are rarer (Fig. 2.17a–d). The different patterns of ureteral vascular impressions are described in Chap. 11.

Ureteral Valves. Frequent in young infants, ureteral valves are uncommon in adults (KIRKS et al. 1978). Nonobstructive (Fig. 2.18), they represent folds of

mucosa or kinks in the wall of the ureter and can take a corkscrew configuration when they are multiple.

Displacement of the Ureter. The ureter usually is within 1 cm of the transverse processes. A position more than 15 mm lateral to the margin of the transverse process or medial to the pedicle must raise suspicion of a pathological displacement (DROUILLARD et al. 1977).

Medial deviation of the abdominal portion is the most frequent normal variant (Fig. 2.19) (SALDINO and PALUBINSKAS 1972). Its incidence varies between 15% and 20% and is related largely to race (ADAM et al. 1985). A prospective study has found a frequency of 54% in patients of African origin. The reason for this racial difference is not clear. In all races, the displacement is more frequent in younger patients, in males, and on the right side.

Except in case of postoperative changes, normal external deviation of the abdominal portion generally is secondary to psoas muscle hypertrophy (Figs. 2.20, 2.21a,b). On a lateral view, the ureters are displaced anteriorly (DROUILLARD et al. 1977). Psoas muscle hypertrophy can also result in a medial course of the abdominal portion, mainly on the right side (BREE et al. 1976).

Variation of Length and Route. Some abnormalities can lead to changes of length and route of the whole ureter. In case of renal ptosis, and particularly on the right side, the ureter has a sinuous route, and curves and kinks can occur in both the abdominal and the pelvic portion (Fig. 2.22).

Urinary malformations such as ectopia and horseshoe kidney are often associated with changes of the route the ureter follows. Its length can be shortened in case of lumbar or pelvic ectopia (Fig. 2.23).

On a single CT slice, a ureteral sinuosity can appear as a duplicated ureter (Fig. 2.24a,b). Isolated

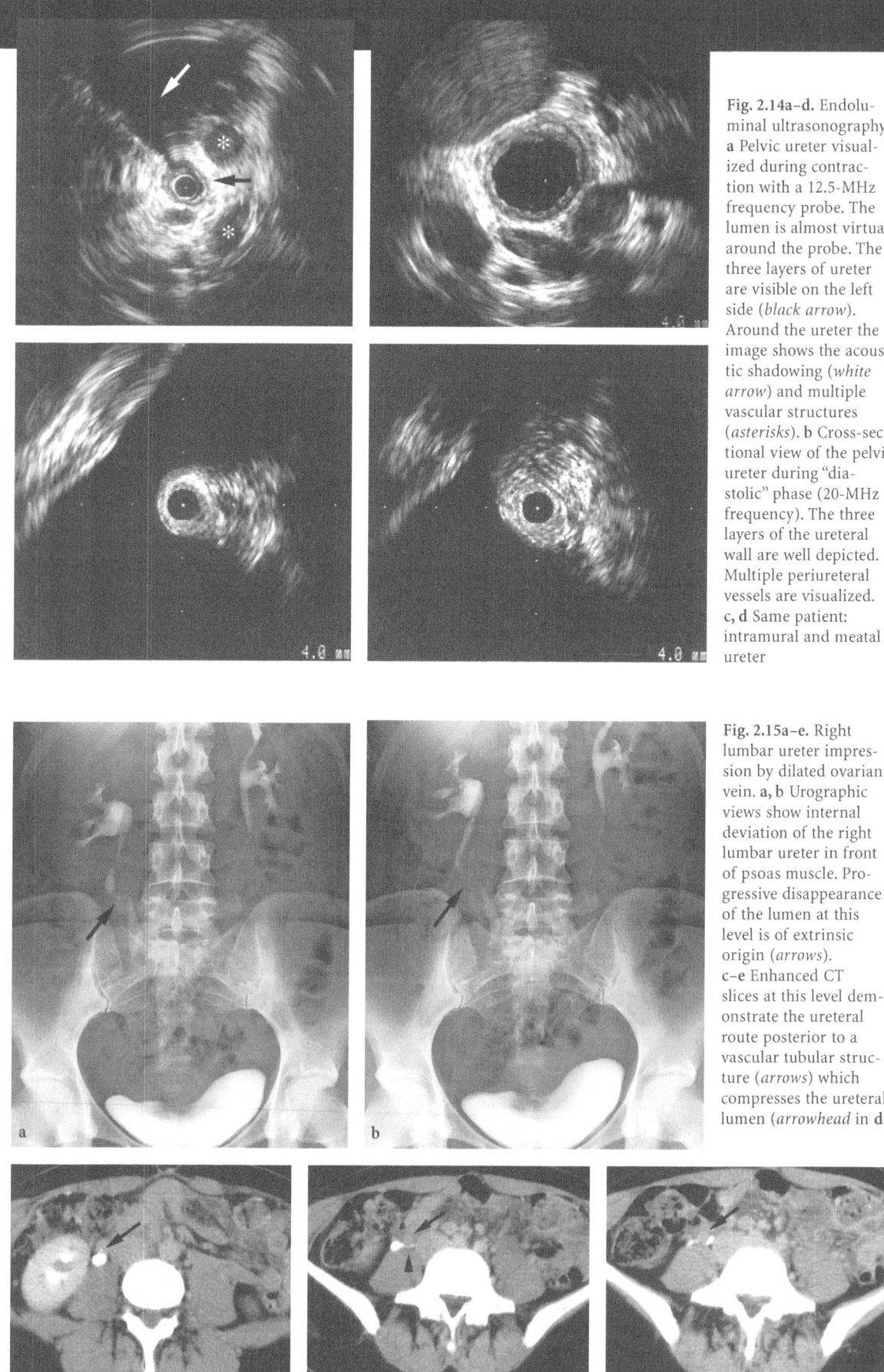

Fig. 2.14a–d. Endoluminal ultrasonography. **a** Pelvic ureter visualized during contraction with a 12.5-MHz frequency probe. The lumen is almost virtual around the probe. The three layers of ureter are visible on the left side (*black arrow*). Around the ureter the image shows the acoustic shadowing (*white arrow*) and multiple vascular structures (*asterisks*). **b** Cross-sectional view of the pelvic ureter during "diastolic" phase (20-MHz frequency). The three layers of the ureteral wall are well depicted. Multiple periureteral vessels are visualized. **c, d** Same patient: intramural and meatal ureter

Fig. 2.15a–e. Right lumbar ureter impression by dilated ovarian vein. **a, b** Urographic views show internal deviation of the right lumbar ureter in front of psoas muscle. Progressive disappearance of the lumen at this level is of extrinsic origin (*arrows*). **c–e** Enhanced CT slices at this level demonstrate the ureteral route posterior to a vascular tubular structure (*arrows*) which compresses the ureteral lumen (*arrowhead* in **d**)

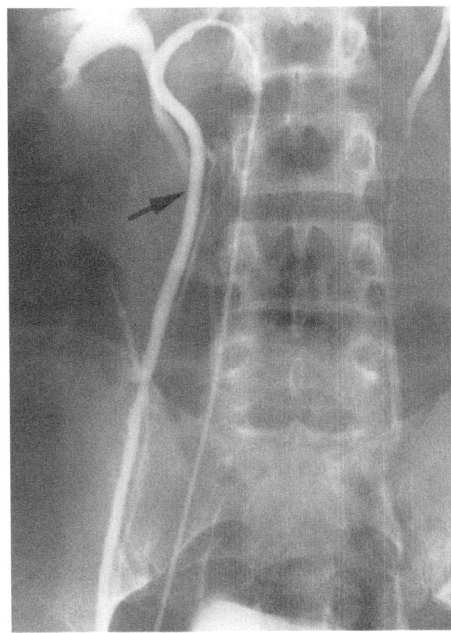

Fig. 2.16. Right ovarian selective phlebography showing the crossing with lumbar ureter (*arrow*)

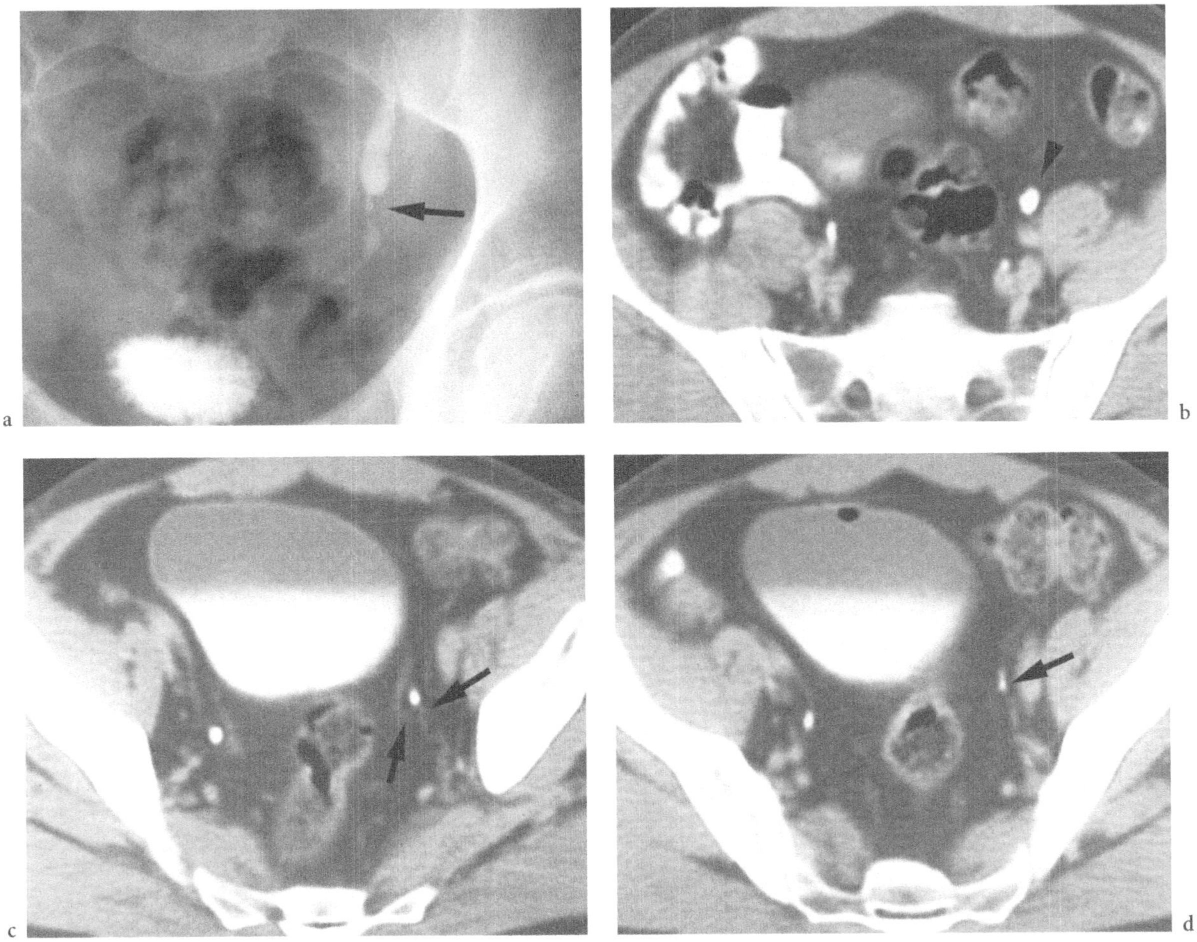

a

b

c

d

Fig. 2.17a–d. Crossing with internal iliac artery branch. **a** EU shows a discrete dilatation of the left pelvic ureter with external compression (*arrow*). **b–d** CT slices demonstrate the dilated left ureter (*arrowhead*), the crossing with anterior branches of ureteral iliac arteries (*arrows*), and the nondilated downstream ureter (*arrow*)

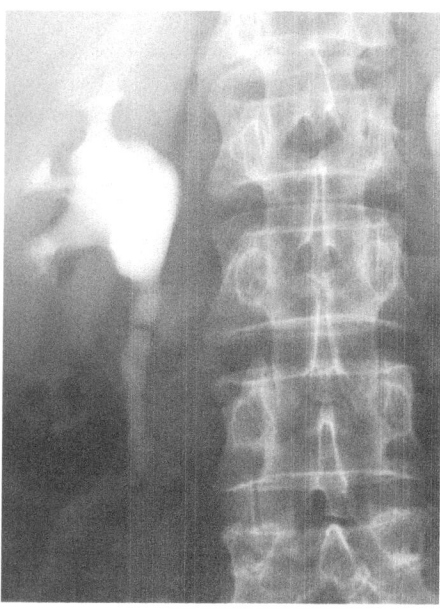

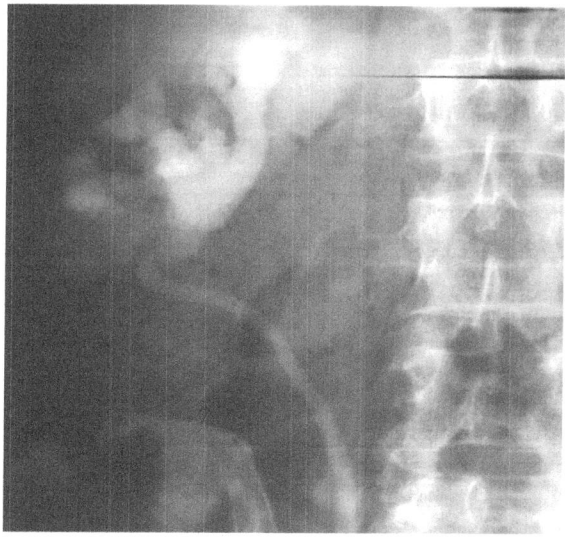

Fig. 2.20. External deviation of the initial right lumbar ureter related to previous surgical pyelolithotomy

Fig. 2.18. Nonobstructive and asymptomatic valve of the right lumbar ureter

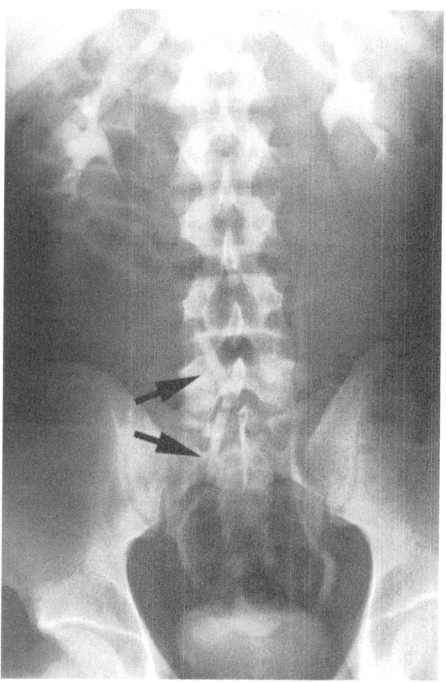

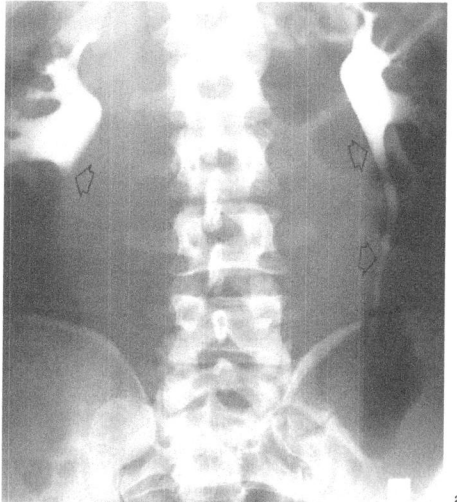

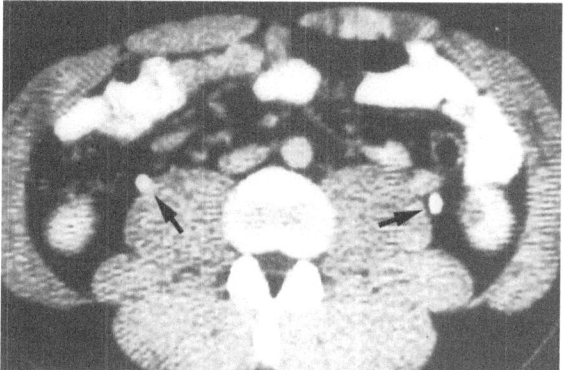

Fig. 2.19. Medial deviation of the right ureter without evident causes and consequences

Fig. 2.21. a EU shows external deviation of both lumbar ureters (*arrowheads*). **b** CT demonstrates the lateral position of both ureters secondary to psoas muscle hypertrophy (*arrows*)

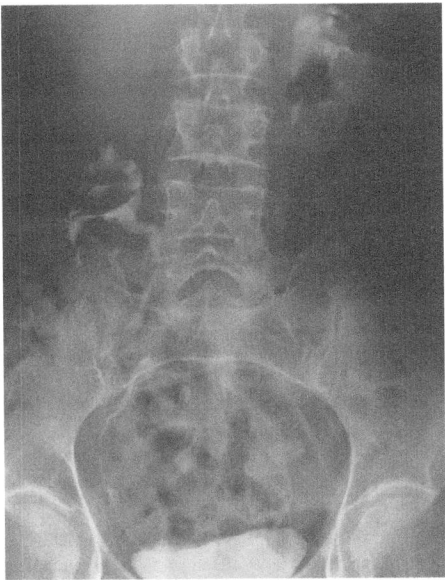 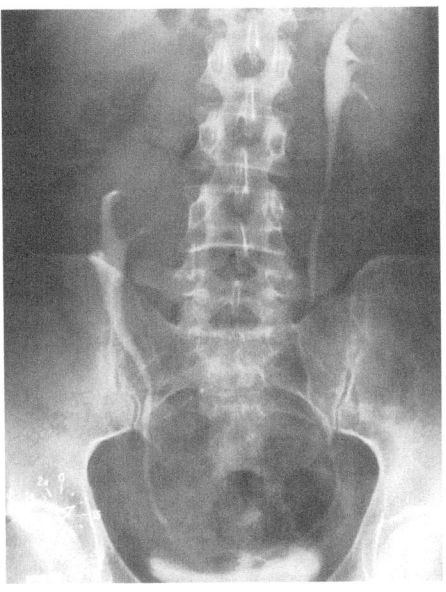

Fig. 2.22. Right renal ptosis with sinuous route of the right ureter

Fig. 2.23. Ureteral variant related to urinary malformation: urographic view of a patient with right lumbar ectopia. The ureter is short and presents a normal route

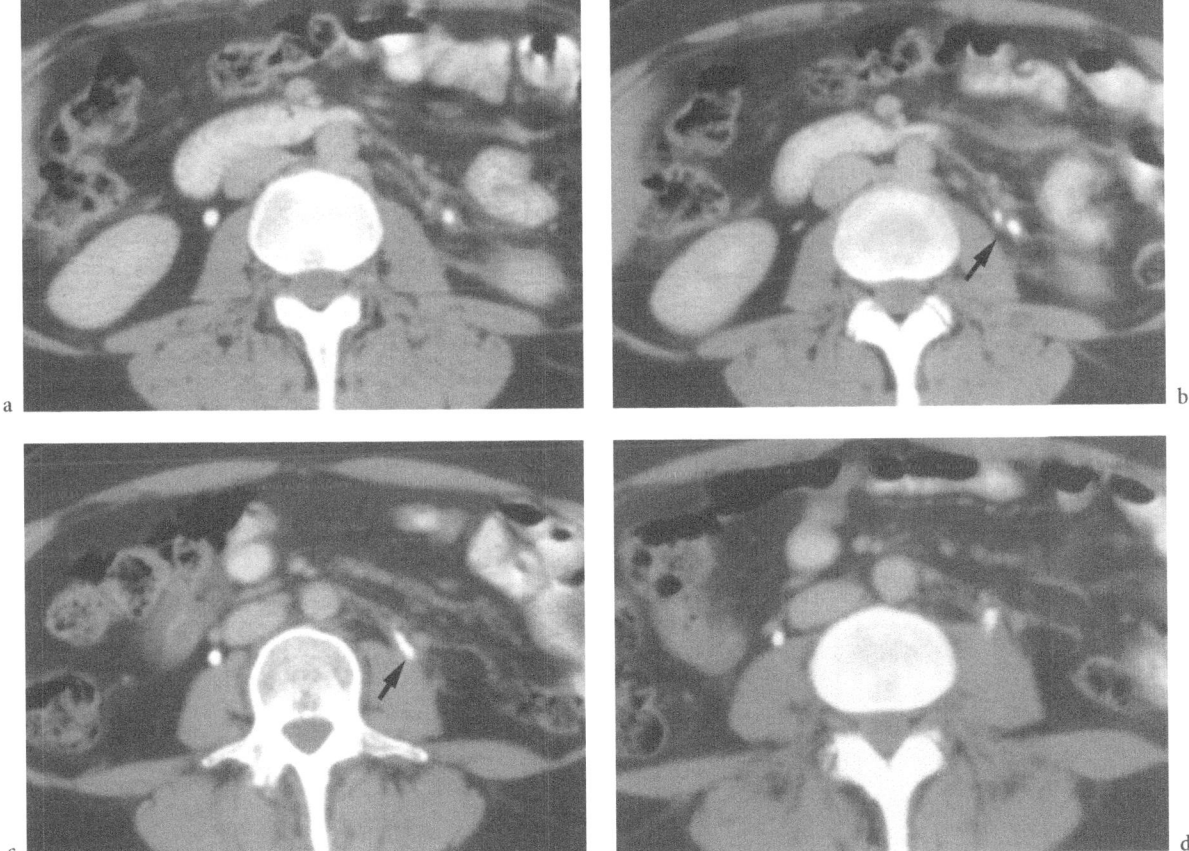

Fig. 2.24a–d. CT aspect of ureteral sinuosity. Note in **b** a false aspect of duplicated ureter (*arrow*) and in **c** the ureteral route parallel to the axial plane (*arrow*)

duplication of the upper urinary tract must be identified prior to interventional endoscopy or a surgical procedure on the upper urinary tract (Fig. 2.25).
Visualization of both opacified ureteral lumen from
the pelvis up to the junctional zone or the bladder is
needed (Fig. 2.26a–c).

Localized increased density can be seen when
the sinuosity is visualized end-on during its course
in an axis tangent to the X-ray beam. This pattern
can simulate calculus disease (Fig. 2.27). Without any
clear explanation, both normal pelvic ureters may be
straight, with an absence of concavity or convexity. In
all these situations, an absence of obstruction makes
it possible to rule out true ureteral disease.

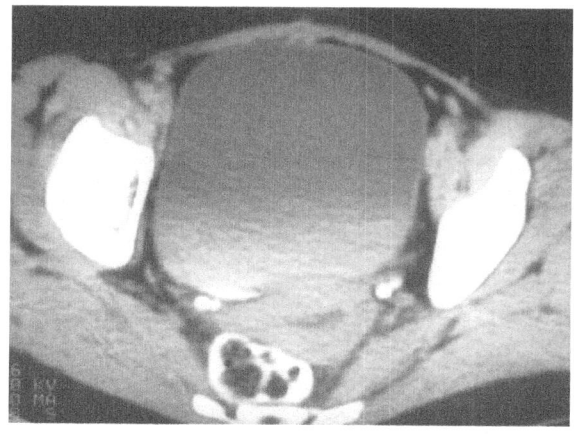

Fig. 2.25. CT aspect of bilateral duplication of ureter

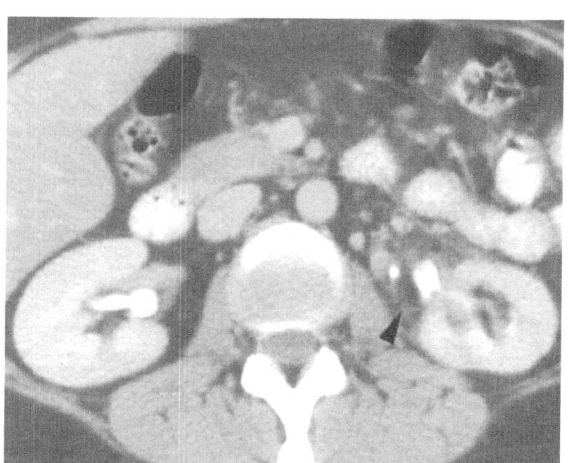

a

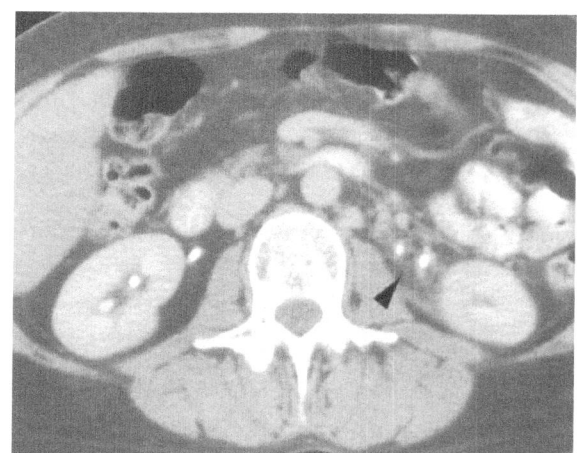

b

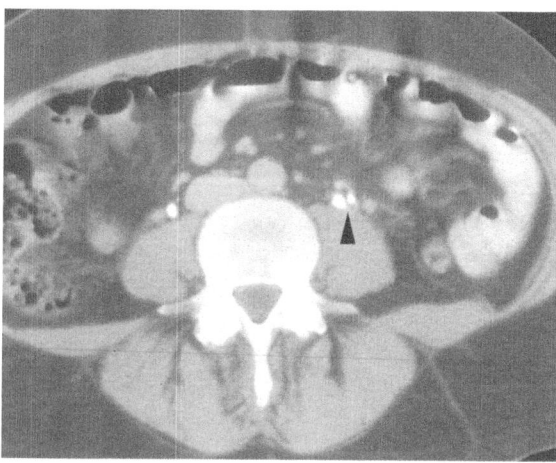

c

Fig. 2.26a–c. Left ureteral duplication on CT slices at different
levels (*arrowheads*)

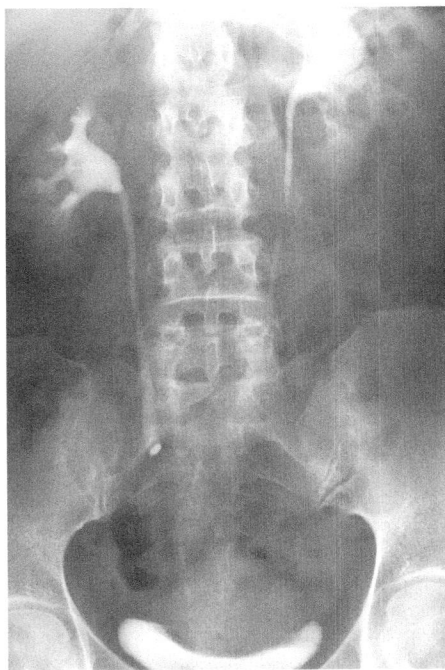

Fig. 2.27. Right ureteral hyperdensity related to a sinuosity immediately before crossing with iliac vessels

References

Adam EJ, Desai SC, Layton G (1985) Racial variations in normal ureteric course. Clin Radiol 36:373–375

Bagley H, Liu JB (1998) Three-dimensional endoluminal ultrasonography of the ureter. J Endourol 12:411–416

Bechtold RB, Chen MYM, Zagoria RJ (1998) CT of the ureteral wall. AJR Am J Roentgenol 170:1283–1289

Bree RL, Green B, Keiller DL, et al (1976) Medial deviation of the ureter secondary to psoas muscle hypertrophy. Radiology 118:691–695

De Sousa LA (1966) Micro-angiographic aspects of the ureter. J Urol 95:179–183

Drouillard J, Bruneton JN, Resca JR, et al (1977) La déviation urétérale lombaire et l'hypertrophie des psoas. Ann Radiol (Paris) 20:557–562

Dubbins PA, Kurtz AB, Darby J, et al (1981) Ureteric jet effect: the echographic appearance of urine entering the bladder. Radiology 140:513–515

Friedenberg RM (1990) Excretory urography in the adult. In: Pollack HM (ed) Clinical urography: an atlas and textbook of uroradiological imaging, vol 1. Saunders, Philadelphia, pp 101–103

Harrison DA, Clouse M (1985) Normal anatomy. In: Crouse ME, Wallace S (eds) Lymphatic imaging: lymphography, computed tomography and scintigraphy, 2nd edn. Williams & Wilkins, Baltimore, pp –26-33

Hutch JA (1967) Vesico-ureteral reflux. In: Bergman H (ed) The ureter. Harper and Row, New York, pp 465–507

Joffre F, Russ PD (1997) Anatomy and conventional imaging of the kidneys and upper urinary tract. In: Weill FS, Manco-Johnson M (eds) Imaging of abdominal and pelvic anatomy. Churchill Livingstone, New York, pp 248–278

Kabalin JN (1992) Anatomy of the retroperitoneum and kidney. In: Walsh PC, Retic AB, Stamey TA, Vaughan ED (eds) Campbell's urology, 6th edn. Saunders, Philadelphia, pp 3–39

Kalman EH, Albers DD, Dunn JH (1955) Ureteral jet phenomenon: stream of opaque medium simulating anomalous configuration of the ureter. Radiology 65:933–935

Kirks DR, Currarino G, Weinberg AG (1978) Transverse folds in the proximal ureter. A normal variant in infants. AJR Am J Roentgenol 130:463–464

Liu JB, Bagley DH, Conlin MJ, et al (1997) Endoluminal sonographic evaluation of ureteral and renal pelvic neoplasms. J Ultrasound Med 16:515–512

Marincek B, Scheidegger JR, Studer UE, et al (1993) Metastatic disease of the ureter: patterns of tumoral spread and radiologic findings. Abdom Imaging 18:88–94

Netter FH (1973) Kidney, ureters and urinary bladder. In: The CIBA collection of medical illustrations, vol 6. CIBA, Summit, NJ

Olsson CA (1986) Anatomy of the upper urinary tract. In: Walsh PC, Gittes RF, Perremuter AD, Stamey TA (eds) Campbell's urology, 5th edn. Saunders, Philadelphia

O'Reilly PH (1985) Introduction and general considerations. In: O'Reilly PH (ed) Obstructive uropathy. Springer-Verlag, Berlin Heidelberg New York, pp 3–12

Riggs W jr, Hagood JH, Andrews AE (1970) Anatomic changes in the normal urinary tract between supine and prone urograms. Radiology 94:107–113

Rosenfield AT, Littner MR, Ulreich S, et al (1977) Respiratory effects of excretory urography. A preliminary report. Invest Radiol 12:295

Roshani H, Dabhoiwala NF, Verbeek FJ, et al (1999) Anatomy of the uretero-vesical junction and distal ureter studied by endoluminal ultrasonography in vitro. J Urol 161: 1614–1619

Saldino RM, Palubinskas AJ (1972) Medial placement of the ureter. A normal variant which may simulate retroperitoneal fibrosis. J Urol 101:582–583

Shafik A (1972) A study of the arterial patterns of normal ureter. J Urol 107:720–722

Sherwood J (1979) The dilated upper urinary tract. Radiol Clin North Am 17:333–340

Shopfner CE (1976) Nonobstructive hydronephrosis and hydroureter. AJR Am J Roentgenol 98:172–180

Velardo JT (1967) Histology of the ureter. In: Bergman H (ed) The ureter. Harper and Row, New York, pp 22–35

Weinberg SR (1967) Applied anatomy of the ureter. In: Bergman H (ed) The ureter. Harper and Row, New York, pp 36–47

Williams PL, Warwick R (1980) Gray's anatomy, 36th edn. Saunders, Philadelphia

Winalski CS, Lipman JC, Tumeh SS (1990) Ureteral neoplasms. Radiographics 10:271–283

3 Ureteral Malformations

M. Panuel, Ph. Otal, Ph. Devred, K. Chaumoire, F. Joffre, N. Grenier, V. Chabbert

CONTENTS

M. Panuel, MD; K. Chaumoire, MD
Service d'Imagerie Médicale Hôpital Nord Chemin des Bourrelys, 13915 Marseille Cedex 20, France
Ph. Otal, MD; F. Joffre, MD; V. Chabbert, MD
Service de Radiologie, Hôpital de Rangueil, 1 avenue Jean Poulhes, 31403 Toulouse Cedex 4, France
Ph. Devred, MD
Service de Radiologie, Hôpital Enfant de la Timone, 264 rue Saint Oierre, 13385 Marseille Cedex 05, France
N. Grenier, MD
Service de Radiologie, B.G.H. Pellegrin Tripode, Place Amélie Raba Léon, 33076 Bordeaux Cedex, France

Ureteral malformations are common malformations of differing degrees of severity. They are much more often found in young children or antenatally than in adults. Knowledge of normal and abnormal development of the ureter allows an understanding of the imaging findings. In this chapter, congenital anomalies of the uretero-pyelic junction will not be considered as true ureteral malformations.

3.1 Development of the Ureter

3.1.1 Normal Ureteral Development

During the fourth week of embryonic life, the ureteral bud arises as a diverticulum of the mesonephric, or wolffian, duct from the urogenital sinus (Fig. 3.1). Several days later, the caudal part of the urogenital sinus narrows and elongates to form the proximal part of the urethra and the neck of the bladder (Fig. 3.2). The ureteral bud grows laterally and invades the metanephric blastema, the primordial renal tissue. The ureteral bud and the metanephric blastema represent the metanephros, which will become the mature kidney and the collecting system. The meeting of these two tissues causes changes in both. The metanephric blastema forms glomeruli, proximal tubules, and distal tubules. The ureteral bud divides and branches, forming the renal pelvis, infundibula, calices, and collecting tubules which will provide a conduit for urine drainage in the mature kidney.

The development of the bladder leads the meso-nephric duct and the ureter to be incorporated into the base of the bladder and the proximal urethra (Fig. 3.2). The mesonephric duct and the ureter rotate so that the ureter meets the bladder cephalad to the point at which the mesonephric duct meets the urethra (Fig. 3.3). In males, the mesonephric duct becomes the epididymis, the vas deferens, the seminal vesicle, and the ejaculatory duct and drains into the posterior urethra through the verumonta-num (Fig. 3.4). In females, the mesonephric duct regresses and the ureter alone remains, draining into the bladder (Fig. 3.5). The paramesonephric, or müllerian, duct develops parallel and lateral to the mesonephric duct and crosses it ventrally to reach the contralateral müllerian duct and become the uterus (Fig. 3.6) (Moore 1988; Tanagho 1976).

The ureteral bud presents a membrane called the Chwalla membrane at its junction with the meso-nephric duct. Normally, this membrane ruptures after the ureteral bud becomes incorporated into the urogenital sinus and separates from the mesonephric duct, allowing the free passage of urine.

Urine formation begins early in the second tri-mester. As the fetal urine drains into the bladder, patency of the ureter is maintained. Smooth muscles developing in the ureteral wall will generate and propagate peristaltic contractions to conduct urine from the kidney to the bladder.

3.1.2
Abnormal Ureteral Development

Disturbances in any of these concurrent and complex developmental steps may produce several abnormalities involving the ureter and/or the kidney. Moreover, due to the close relationships of the precursors, genital and urinary tract malformations may frequently coexist.

3.1.2.1
Renal Agenesis

Absence of a kidney is due to failure of the ureteral bud to form, failure to grow and thus to encounter the metanephric blastema, or absence of the metaneph-ric blastema. In the first condition, the ureteral orifice of the bladder and the ipsilateral hemitrigone are also absent. In the latter two conditions, a blind ureter may be encountered. In some males, the mesonephric duct may fail to form. In this case, neither a kidney nor a vas deferens and epididymis will form; the testis may descend to its normal position in the scrotum or may

be absent or hypoplastic. In some females, develop-ment of the mesonephric (wolffian) duct and of the paramesonephric (müllerian) duct may be altered. In these girls, renal agenesis may be associated with uterine anomalies (agenesis, hypoplasia, unicornuate or bicornuate) and/or aplasia of the vagina.

3.1.2.2
Renal Dysplasia and Hypoplasia

These conditions result from a quantitative and/or qualitative deficiency in the ureteral bud and the metanephric blastema. The kidney may be ectopic, small, poor, or nonfunctioning; it may also present a multicystic pattern.

3.1.2.3
Ectopic Ureter

Ureteral ectopia is related to a cephalic location of the ureteral bud on the wolffian duct. The higher the ureteral bud, the lower it will be incorporated into the urogenital sinus. This condition may result in renal dysplasia, as described above. The ureter will come to lie medial and distal to its normal position in the mature bladder, at the bladder neck, or in the urethra. Ectopic ureter may drain also into all the derivatives of the wolffian duct. In males, the ureteral ectopic ending may be located in the ejaculatory duct, the seminal vesicle, or the vas deferens (Fig. 3.7). In females, the ectopic ureter may drain into the vestibule or the distal vagina. It may also be located in a remnant of wolffian duct, Gartner's duct, which is in the vaginal wall, the cervix, and the broad ligament (Fig. 3.8).

3.1.2.4
Ureterocele

If rupture of the Chwalla membrane is delayed, drain-age of urine from the fetal kidney will be obstructed. Because the Chwalla membrane lies on the interior of the musculature of the developing bladder, the distal ureter will be enlarged. Such an enlargement of the ureter within the bladder is called a ureterocele. Ureterocele may also be encountered with ectopia of the ureter.

3.1.2.5
Vesicoureteral Reflux

The ureteral bud may arise from the mesonephric duct nearer to the urogenital sinus than it should. As the rotational incorporation of the mesonephric

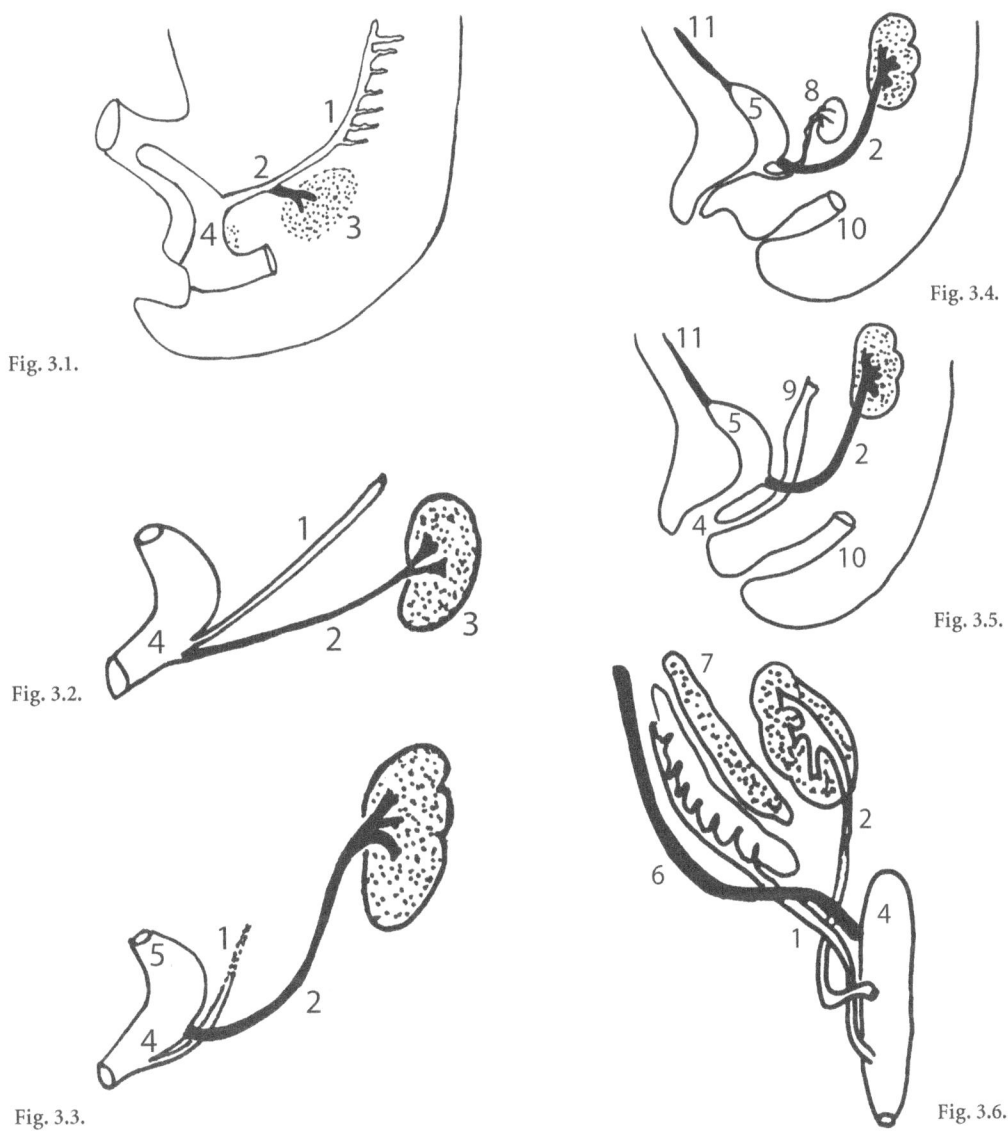

Figs. 3.1–3.6. Normal development of the ureter (adapted from MOORE 1988). 1 Fifth week of embryonic life (lateral view). 2 Sixth week of embryonic life (lateral view). 3 Later, longitudinal rotation of the ending of the mesonephric duct and of the ureteral bud (lateral view). 4 Twelfth week of embryonic life in male (lateral view). 5 Twelfth week of embryonic life in female (lateral view). 6 Frontal view in female before development of the uterus. 1 mesonephric duct (wolffian duct); 2 ureteral bud, 3 metanephric blastema; 4 urogenital sinus; 5 urinary bladder; 6 paramesonephric duct (müllerian duct); 7 ovary; 8 testis; 9 uterus; 10 rectum; 11 urachus

duct and ureter into the developing bladder progresses, the ureteral orifice will finally lie lateral and cephalad to the normal position in the developed bladder (Fig. 3.9). In such cases, the tunnel through which the ureter travels to the bladder will be abnormally short. Vesicoureteral reflux (VUR) may result because the tunnel is too short to make a competent distal ureteral valve. In addition, abnormal development of the ureteral bud may induce renal dysplasia. This may explain why many

kidneys with high-grade reflux function poorly. On the other hand, a more caudal ectopic ending of the ureter, particularly into the bladder neck, may also lead to reflux.

In cases where the ectopia is subtle, particularly in a cephalad position, elongation of the submucosal segment is a characteristic of growth and development in infants and young children. This explains why the frequency of VUR is inversely related to age.

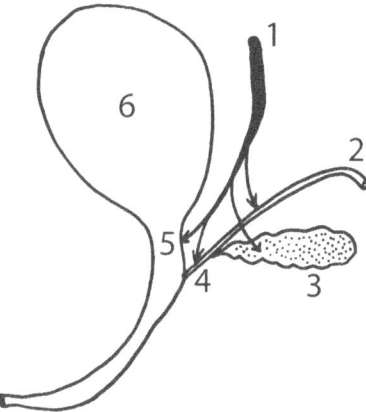

Fig. 3.7. Ectopic ureter in male: *1* ureter; *2* vas deferens; *3* seminal vesicle; *4* ejaculatory duct; *5* posterior urethra; *6* bladder

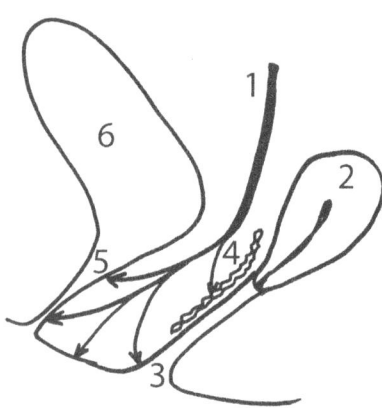

Fig. 3.8. Ectopic ureter in female: *1* ureter; *2* uterus; *3* vagina; *4* Gartner's duct; *5* urethra; *6* bladder

3.1.2.6
Megaureter

The musculature of the distal ureter is both circular and longitudinal. Where the musculature is deficient or abnormal (particularly the longitudinal fibers), that portion of the ureter will not conduct peristaltic waves (TANAGHO 1973). Although the lumen of the ureter is of normal caliber, the lack of peristalsis effectively obstructs the flow of urine. The backup of urine proximal to this aperistaltic segment will cause dilation of the upper ureter and renal pelvis. This condition is referred to as primary megaureter.

3.1.2.7
Duplication

When two independent ureteral buds arise from the mesonephric duct, complete duplication occurs. The ureter draining the upper pole of the kidney has an ectopic distal insertion at a point caudal and medial to that of the ureter draining the lower pole. The latter inserts into the bladder either at a normal site in the trigone or more cranially and laterally, with susceptibility to VUR. These relationships of the two ureters are expressed in the Weigert-Meyer law (Fig. 3.10). The ureter draining the upper pole may be obstructed or may present a ureterocele (ectopic ureterocele).

Partial duplication of the ureter is related to a division of the ureteral bud which occurs too early. There is a single ending of the ureter, usually in an orthotopic or a cephalad position. In some cases, one of the duplicated ureters ends upward blindly. Triplication of the ureter may also occur, but it is a very rare anomaly.

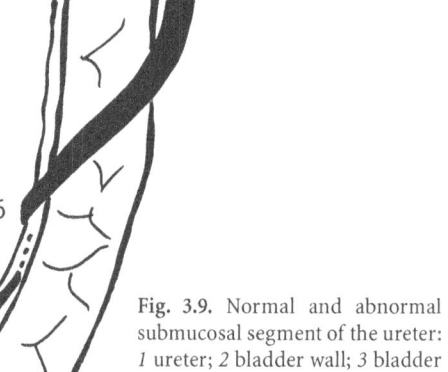

Fig. 3.9. Normal and abnormal submucosal segment of the ureter: *1* ureter; *2* bladder wall; *3* bladder mucosa; *4* normal situation; *5, 6* abnormal positions with short submucosal segment

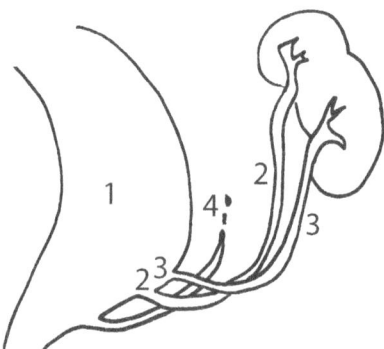

Fig. 3.10. Embryologic development of complete duplication of the ureter (Weigert-Meyer law): *1* urogenital sinus; *2* ureter draining the upper pole; *3* ureter draining the lower pole; *4* mesonephric duct

3.2
Clinical Findings in Neonates, Infants and Children

Ureteral malformations may be asymptomatic or may be found in various conditions. The most frequent conditions are urinary tract dilation diagnosed antenatally by ultrasonography and urinary tract infection.

Clinical symptoms of urinary tract infection, such as vomiting, failure to thrive, or recurrent fever, are nonspecific, particularly in young children. A urinary tract infection exists when there are more than 100,000 bacteria per milliliter of properly collected urine, when the organism is single, and when there is leukocyturia.

In girls, urinary incontinence may be encountered when the ureter drains below the external sphincter; when the child is toilet-trained, this symptom is pathognomonic of an ectopic ureter. On the other hand, incontinence is never related to an ectopic ureter in boys, because there are no wolffian duct remnants below the external sphincter. Epididymo-orchitis is a very rare condition in young boys; when it occurs, it may be related to an ectopic ureter. A pelvic mass may also be related to an abnormal ureter (ureterocele, Gartner's cyst, or hydrometrocolpos).

Ureteral malformations may be encountered during the evaluation of associated anomalies such as VAC-TERL association (vertebral anomalies, anal atresia, congenital heart disease, tracheo-esophageal fistula or esophageal atresia, reno-urinary anomalies, and limb defects), or MURCS association (müllerian duct, unilateral renal agenesis, and anomalies of the cervicothoracic somites) or anorectal and cloacal malformations (RITTLER et al. 1996; BRAUN-QUENTIN et al. 1996).

3.3
Imaging Findings

3.3.1
Imaging Methods

3.3.1.1
Ultrasonography

Ultrasonography is an important tool for assessing an ureteral abnormality, antenatally and in children; it offers a good evaluation of the renal parenchyma, the collecting system, the bladder, and the genital tract. Concerning the detection of transient dilatation such as in VUR, its sensitivity is poor (BLANE et al. 1993; DAVEY et al. 1997; EVANS et al. 1999). However, thickening of the wall of the renal collecting system by more than 0.8 mm should be considered pathological, despite the lack of specificity; thickening may be related to urinary tract infection, intermittent dilatation (e.g., VUR) or dilatation in the recent past, such as primary megaureter or pyelectasis (ROBBEN et al. 1999). Moreover, careful and meticulous ultrasound examination in neonates to search for signs such as caliceal or ureteral dilatation, pelvic or ureteral wall thickening, absence of the corticomedullary differentiation and signs of renal dysplasia (small kidney, thinned or hyperechoic cortex, and cortical cysts) enables prediction of VUR in 87% of cases (AVNI et al. 1997). These data are not valid for older children (DIPIETRO et al. 1997). Attempts have been made to improve the sensitivity of ultrasonography using an echo-enhancing agent instilled into the bladder (cystosonography), but this method is not yet widely used (DARGE et al. 1999; MENTZEL et al. 1999).

3.3.1.2
Voiding Cystourethrography

Voiding cystourethrography (VCUG) is commonly used in the evaluation of the lower urinary tract and particularly for the screening of VUR. The retrograde route through the urethra into the bladder is usually chosen, but in some instances, such as in male neonates with suspected posterior urethral valves or in some patients with neurogenic bladder, the suprapubic puncture is preferable. Cyclic filling of the bladder increases detection of VUR (PALTIEL et al. 1992; GELFAND et al. 1999). Irradiation is a classical drawback of VCUG, although the real hazard is hard to evaluate; new equipment allows for significant reduction of the radiation exposure (CLEVELAND et al. 1992; KLEINMAN et al. 1994; BOURLIÈRE-NAJEAN et al. 1994; GONZALEZ et al. 1995). In our opinion, this examination is still required in the first evaluation of situations in which ureteral abnormalities are suspected.

3.3.1.3
Excretory Urography

Excretory urography (EU) or intravenous pyelography is easily performed in children; the cost is low, and it is reliable for the estimation of ureteral morphology if renal function is good. However, it is being used less and less frequently.

3.3.1.4
Nuclear Imaging

Nuclear imaging has a significant place in the armamentarium for imaging pediatric urinary tract disease. For the evaluation and follow-up of a dilated collecting system, ^{99m}Tc-mercaptotriacetylglycine (MAG3) scans quantify the physiological significance of a radiologically detected abnormality. ^{99m}Tc-dimercaptosuccinic acid (DMSA) may show renal functional abnormalities due to pyelonephritis or dysplasia associated with VUR or obstructive uropathy (BONNIN et al. 1998). For some authors, direct radionuclide cystography is useful for follow-up of VUR (WILLI and TREVES 1983). Moreover, nuclear imaging carries low radiation hazards (TAYLOR et al. 1994).

3.3.1.5
Magnetic Resonance Imaging

Magnetic resonance imaging is a new tool in the diagnosis of urinary tract abnormalities. Used here are fast MR imaging techniques enhancing the signal intensity of static fluid, such as T_2-weighted fast spin-echo, RARE (rapid acquisition with relaxation enhancement), and HASTE (half-Fourier acquisition single-shot turbo spin-echo) sequences. These provide very good anatomical details of dilated structures (BORTHNE et al. 1999; KLEIN et al. 1998; TANG et al. 1996; SIGMUND et al. 1991). Moreover, gadolinium and furosemide administration offers an

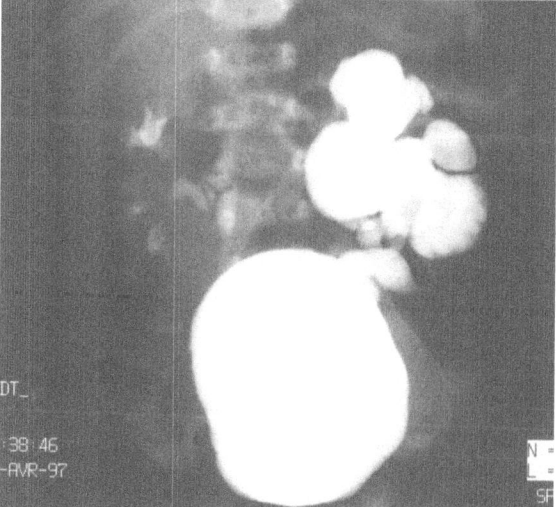

Fig. 3.11. Bilateral vesicoureteral reflux in a neonate with antenatal diagnosis of dilatation of the left ureter and postnatal confirmation. VCUG (fluoroscopic view): right grade II reflux, left grade IV reflux (normal urethra)

evaluation of the renal function (NOLTE-ERNSTING et al. 1998). However, MR imaging cannot distinguish between VUR and nonrefluxing megaureter, and, in young patients, sedation is mandatory to avoid movement.

3.3.1.6
Other Imaging Methods

Other imaging methods may be helpful in some instances. Percutaneous pyelography and nephrostomy may be used to drain an infected dilated collecting system. Vaginography may be used to evaluate associated genital anomalies.

3.3.2
Pathological Findings in Neonates, Infants and Children

3.3.2.1
Vesicoureteral Reflux

Vesicoureteral reflux is a very common abnormality involving the ureter in children. The most common form is related to a maldeveloped or ectopic ureterovesical junction (see above). Other causes are abnormality of the bladder wall, such as in the prune-belly syndrome, bladder outlet obstruction, such as in posterior urethral valves, voiding dysfunction, or neurogenic bladder; the reflux may also be iatrogenic. The pathogenesis of VUR has also been suggested to differ between the sexes. Transient anatomical obstruction during fetal life has been proposed as the cause of gross VUR in males (AVNI and SCHULMAN 1996). In older girls, reflux is more often related to voiding dysfunction (SILLEN 1999).

VUR is usually found in two situations: workup of uropathy detected in utero and workup of urinary tract infection. In neonates, evaluation of dilatation found in utero may reveal a VUR in 25% to 40% of cases (ZERIN et al. 1993; DEVAUSSUZENET et al. 1997; PAL et al. 1998) (Fig. 3.11).

VUR is the main abnormality found in children with urinary tract infection. Reflux may be found in 60% of cases (RING and ZOBEL 1988); in our experience this value is 35%, and, as a rule, it is seen most often in younger patients (Fig. 3.12). However, infection does not cause reflux (GROSS and LEBOWITZ 1981), but effects of reflux on renal parenchyma may be worsened by infection. Indeed, renal damage is more often found in patients with VUR and urinary tract infection than in children with antenatal diagnosis but without infection (SHERIDAN and JENKES GOUGH 1991; ASSAEL et al. 1998). Moreover, a significant number of end-stage renal diseases in children are related to a VUR (ARANT 1991; VALLEE et al. 1999). The role of a pre-existing dysplasia is very likely (Fig. 3.13).

An international grading system of VUR in children based on VCUG findings is widely used (LEBOWITZ et al. 1985). It offers an efficient comparison of the severity in the same child and from child to child. Reflux is graded on a scale of I–V, as follows.

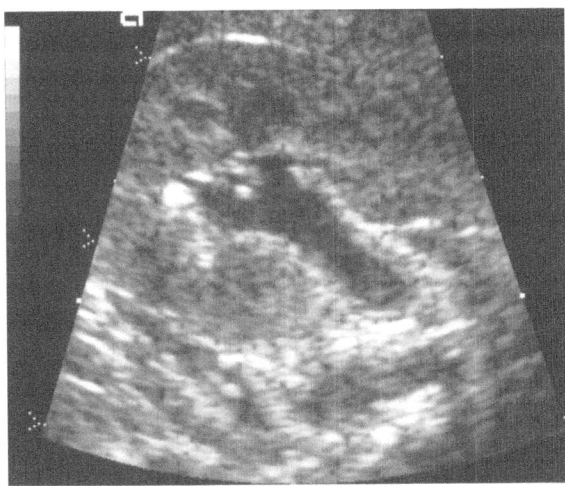

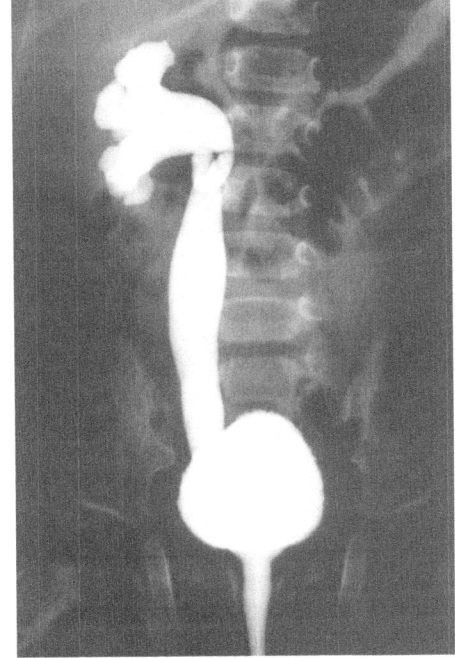

Fig. 3.12a, b. Vesicoureteral reflux in a 4-month-old girl with urinary tract infection. a Ultrasonography of the right kidney: moderate dilatation of the pelvis, thickening of the pelvic wall, hyperechogenicity of the sinus. b VCUG: grade IV vesicoureteral reflux

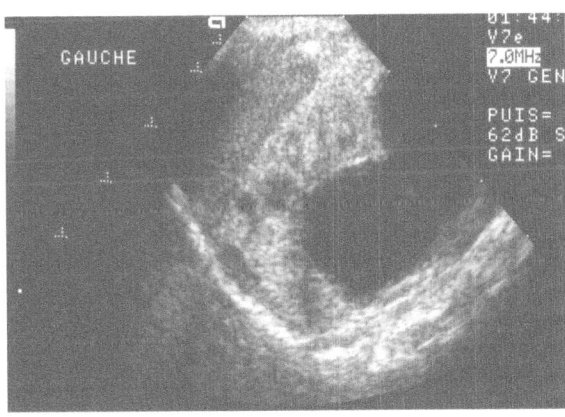

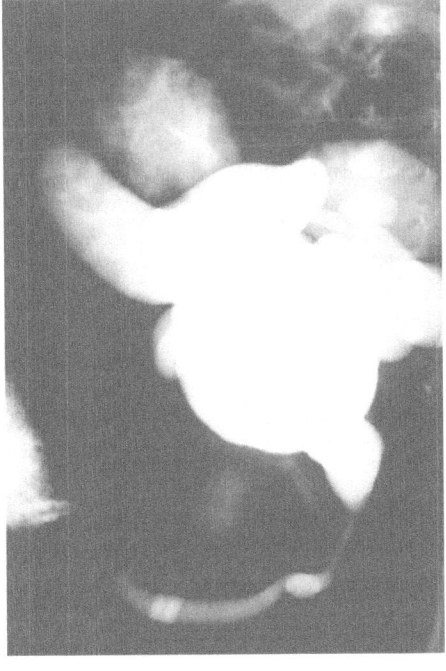

Fig. 3.13a, b. Prune-belly syndrome in a 2-day-old boy with antenatal diagnosis of urinary tract dilatation. At birth, the syndrome was diagnosed on the basis of the wrinkled appearance of the abdominal wall. a Ultrasonography of the left lumbar fossa: dilatation of the left pelvis, hyperechogenicity of the renal parenchyma with small cysts (renal dysplasia); same findings on the right side (not shown). b VCUG: large-capacity bladder, huge bilateral reflux, dilatation of the posterior urethra without obstruction

Grade	Description
I	Ureter only
II	Ureter, pelvis and calices; no dilatation; normal fornices
III	Ureter, pelvis and calices; mild dilatation; normal fornices
IV	Ureter, pelvis and calices; moderate dilatation; tortuosity of the ureter; unsharp fornices; normal papilla
V	Gross distension; effaced papilla

Two cystographic findings should be looked for: Intrarenal reflux, which is the reflux of urine into renal tubules, occurs more often from compound calices and commonly at the poles of the kidney (Fig. 3.14). This may explain why renal scars tend to be polar. One may meticulously depict the presence of a paraureteral diverticulum of the bladder known as a Hutch diverticulum (Fig. 3.15). This occurs as a result of a congenital deficiency of the posterolateral wall of the bladder; in some cases, the diverticulum may incorporate the ureteral ending.

Controversies exist over the screening of VUR, the main questions being "How?" and "When?".

- *How?* VCUG is a specific and quite sensitive method for depicting VUR. In our opinion, it remains the tool of choice for the first evaluation. For follow-up, radionuclide cystography or cysto-

sonography would be useful. Reflux is a dynamic phenomenon, and whatever the modality chosen to detect it, one should keep this fact in mind.

- *When?* Children with urinary tract infection, particularly the very young, undoubtedly require VCUG. Children with other uropathies such as renal agenesis, ureteropelvic junction obstruction, multicystic dysplastic kidney, or fused kidneys should also undergo VCUG because of a high risk of associated reflux (Avni et al. 1998). On the other hand, should VCUG be performed on neonates with an antenatal diagnosis of mild dilatation of the collecting system and with normal ultrasound studies during the first month of life or with mild dilatation? The question remains unanswered. Asymptomatic siblings of children with documented reflux, particularly those under the age of 4 years, need a screening for reflux; ultrasonography of the urinary tract and radionuclide cystography seem to be adequate (Connolly et al. 1997; Schulman and Snyder 1993) (Fig. 3.15).

Another controversy is related to the treatment of VUR (surgical versus long-term antibiotic therapy); no significant difference in outcome was found between the two methods in terms of growth and weight gain in children, or in terms of development of renal lesions (Smellie et al. 1992; Wingen et al. 1999). Here again, imaging follow-up must

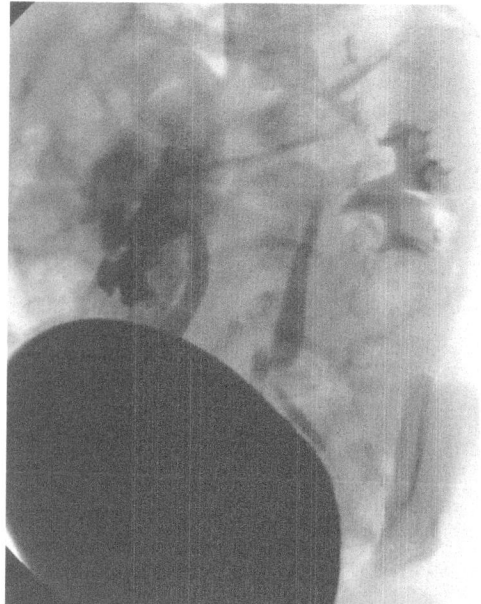
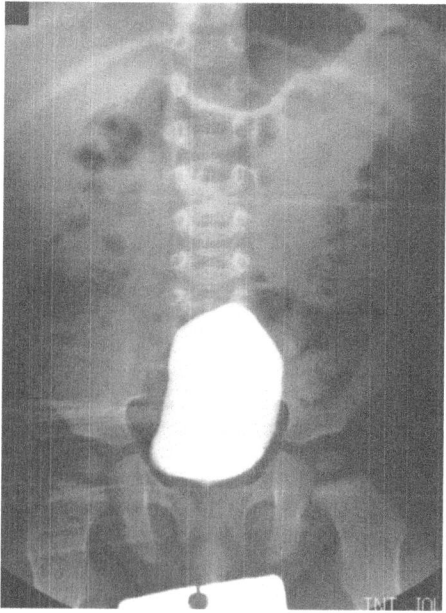

Fig. 3.14a, b. Intrarenal reflux of the right kidney in a 2-month-old boy with urinary tract infection. **a** VCUG: bilateral reflux (right grade IV, left grade III), opacification of renal tubules of the right kidney. **b** VCUG 6 months later following antibiotic therapy: normal findings

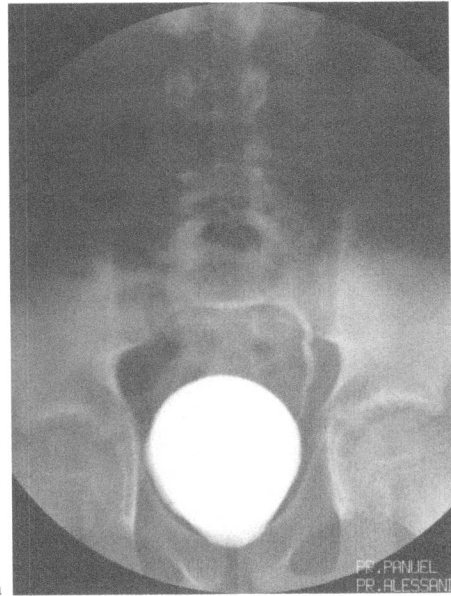

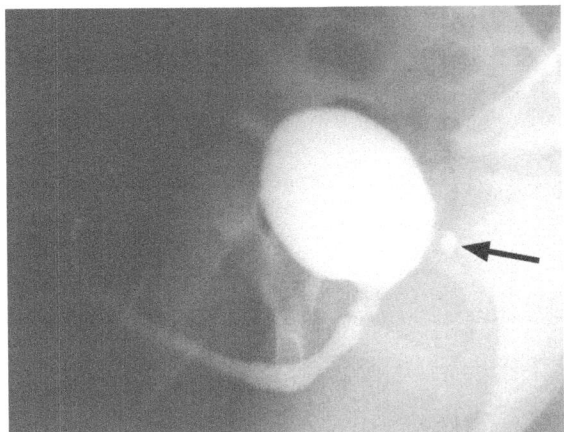

a

b

Fig. 3.15a, b. Transient vesicoureteral reflux and Hutch diverticulum in an asymptomatic 12-year-old boy whose brother had VUR with urinary tract infection. Sonography (not shown) revealed a small left kidney. VCUG (fluoroscopic views). **a** Filling phase: grade I reflux in the left ureter; **b** voiding phase: Hutch diverticulum (*arrow*), reflux no longer visible (transient reflux)

use less invasive methods, such as ultrasonography and/or nuclear imaging; however, in some instances, repeated VCUG may be necessary (Fig. 3.14).

3.3.2.2
Megaureter

The term megaureter refers to ureteral dilatation. The megaureter may be secondary or primary. Several conditions may induce a megaureter, such as reflux or obstruction. Obstruction may be related to a developmental anomaly such as an ectopic ending or a ureterocele, to a bladder outlet obstruction (e.g., posterior urethral valves) or a neurogenic bladder, or to urolithiasis, or it may be iatrogenic.

Primary megaureter is related to a distal adynamic segment (see above); it may be also refluxing. The dilatation may involve mainly the lower segment of the ureter or, more rarely, the whole ureter and the pelvocaliceal system (MEYER and LEBOWITZ 1992). The renal parenchyma is often normal, but in more severe cases renal dysplasia may be found. The anomaly may be bilateral and involves boys more often than girls. Spontaneous improvement has been described.

Diagnosis of primary megaureter is usually made by ultrasonography. The sonographic findings are more or less severe dilatation of the ureter and increased peristalsis of the lower segment with a to-and-fro motion (SIEGEL 1995) (Fig. 3.16). EU, MAG3 scintigraphy, or MRI may also demonstrate this anomaly (Fig. 3.17). On EU, the dilated distal ureter ends with a threadlike pattern (Fig. 3.18).

3.3.2.3
Ureteral Duplication

Ureteral duplication is a common anomaly occurring in 0.7% of the population. Duplication is twice as common in girls as in boys; bilateralism is present in 40% of patients; both kidneys are affected equally. Duplications range from partial to complete forms (see above).

3.3.2.3.1
Partial Duplication

Partial duplication ranges from a bifid renal pelvis to a ureteral junction within the intramural ureter (V-type). Bifurcation that takes place above the bladder has been referred to a Y-type ureter. Uretero-ureteral reflux may occur, known as the yo-yo phenomenon. The clinical significance of this is not clearly established. On sonography, the duplicated kidney is larger than normal, with two separate sinuses. However, diagnosis of partial duplication is usually made on EU. In some instances, when the junction is very low, it may be difficult to clearly define it. In very rare cases, one branch of the partially duplicated ureter ends blindly.

3.3.2.3.2
Complete Duplication

Complete duplication is frequently symptomatic (antenatal diagnosis, urinary tract infection, incon-

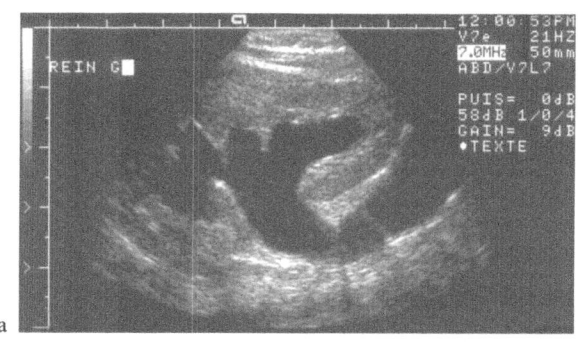

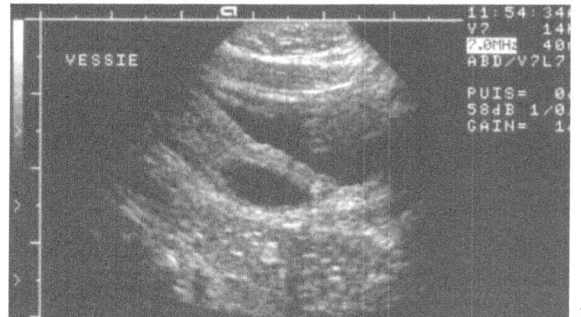

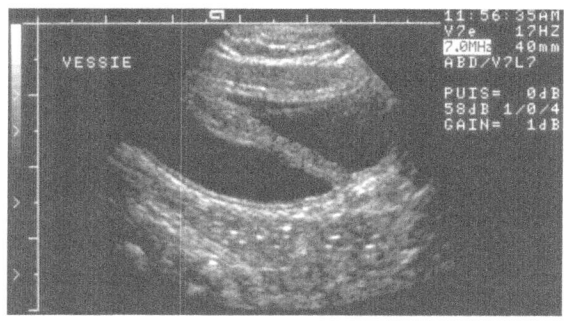

Fig. 3.16a–c. Primary megaureter in a 2-month-old boy with antenatal diagnosis of urinary tract dilatation. **a** Ultrasono-graphic longitudinal view of the lumbar fossa: dilatation of the calices, pelvis, and proximal ureter. **b, c** Ultrasonographic longitudinal views of the pelvis: peristalsis of the dilated distal ureter

01mn46   03mn32   05mn18   07mn05

08mn51   10mn37   12mn23   14mn10

15mn56   17mn42   19mn28   21mn15

Fig. 3.17. Bilateral primary megaureter in a 3-month-old boy with antenatal diagnosis of urinary tract dilatation. ^{99m}Tc-MAG3 scans after furosemide administration: dilatation of the ureters with delayed uptake of the bladder

23mn01   24mn47   26mn33   28mn20

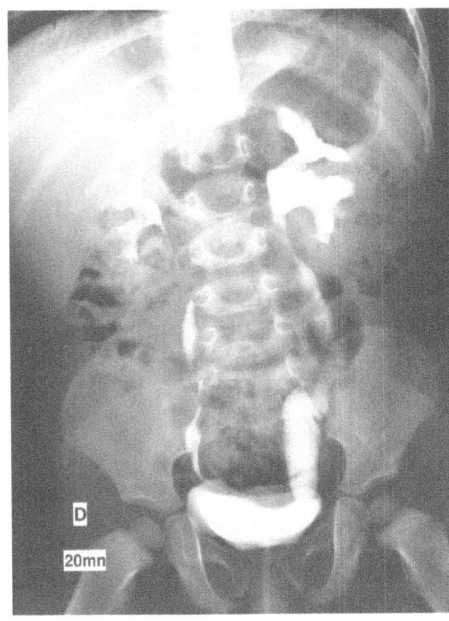

Fig. 3.18. Primary megaureter in a 3-year-old girl with urinary tract infection.EU: dilatation of the left ureter, predominantly in its distal segment; no reflux at VCUG (not shown)

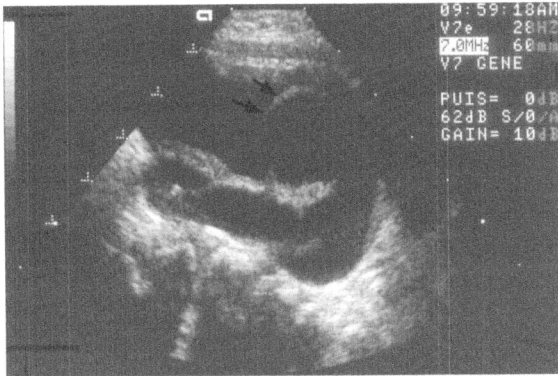

Fig. 3.19. Intravesical ectopic ureterocele in a male neonate with antenatal diagnosis of urinary tract dilatation. Ultrasonographic longitudinal view of the pelvis: intravesical cyst-like formation with an echogenic wall (*arrows*), dilated distal ureter

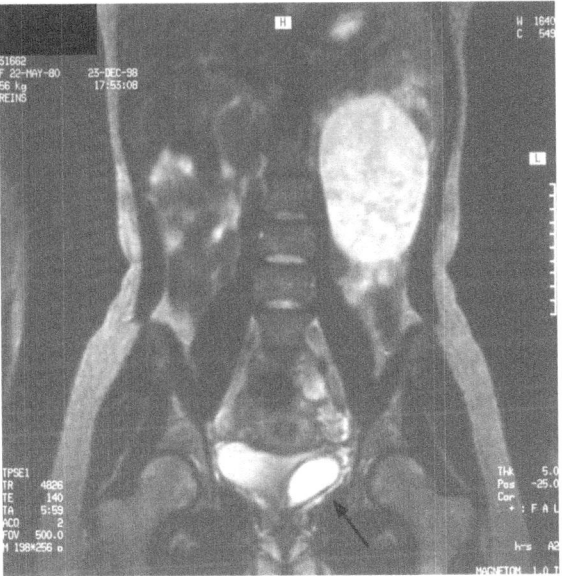

Fig. 3.20. Complete duplication with ectopic ureterocele in a 16-year-old girl with left flank pain. MR T_2-weighted fast spin-echo coronal image: clearly defined ureterocele (*arrow*), huge dilation of the ureter of the upper pole in its lumbar segment

tinence) and much more frequent in girls. As we saw above, the lower pole is predisposed to VUR because of the location of the ending of its ureter. The upper pole is predisposed to more complex situations: ectopic ending into the distal bladder or the posterior urethra leading or not to an ectopic ureterocele; ectopic ending with more or less obstruction in the genital tract in males, in the distal urethra, the distal vagina, or the wolffian remnants in girls; and renal dysplasia.

The imaging features differ according to the anatomical conditions. Diagnosis can be made by ultrasonography, but a complete workup requires other imaging methods.

The upper pole may present a normal finding, or a dilatation with thinning of the parenchyma and sometimes small cysts, or it may be hypoplastic without dilatation of the collecting system. The ureter draining the upper pole may be dilated and tortuous. An ectopic ureterocele appears on ultrasonography or on MRI as a cyst-like formation within the bladder and, on VCUG, as a filling defect of the bladder (Figs. 3.19, 3.20). If the ending of the ureter is ectopic but without ureterocele, retrovesical dilatation of the ureter may be seen (Fig. 3.19). During the voiding phase of VCUG, ectopic ureterocele may prolapse into the urethra or even backward simulating a large Hutch diverticulum (BELLAH et al. 1995; CURRARINO et al. 1993). In some instances, the parenchyma of the upper pole is so dysplastic that it cannot be recognized by imaging methods; this condition is known as ureterocele disproportion (DACHER et al. 1997) (Fig. 3.21). The functional value of the upper pole is better assessed by nuclear imaging than by EU. Moreover, the therapeutic approach depends on the quality of the upper pole (MONFORT et al. 1992; MOSCOVICI et al. 1999).

The lower pole may be normal or dilated secondary to reflux (Figs. 3.21, 3.22). In severe cases, the ectopic ureterocele may even obstruct the ureter on

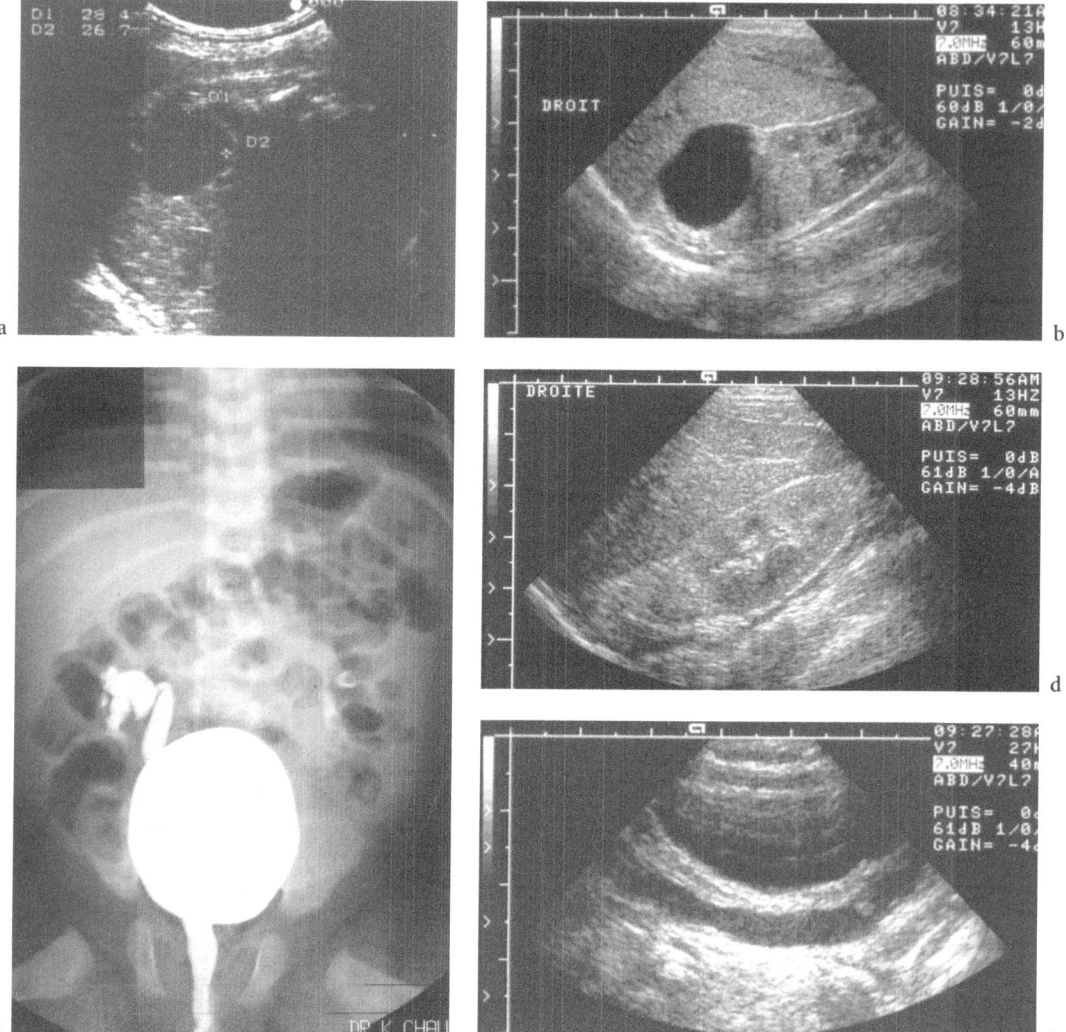

Fig. 3.21a–e. Complete bilateral duplication with the ureterocele disproportion phenomenon on the right side in a young girl. **a** Antenatal ultrasonographic view at 34 weeks of fetal life: cystic formation in the right lumbar fossa (28.4+26.7 mm). **b** Ultrasonography of the right lumbar fossa at 5 weeks of age: decrease in size of the cystic formation (20.6+18.3 mm), dilatation of a right ureter (not shown). **c** VCUG at 6 weeks of age: bilateral vesicoureteral reflux in lower poles of complete duplication. **d** Ultrasonography of the right lumbar fossa at 8 months of age: no dilatation ("pseudo-adrenal" finding). **e** Ultrasonography of the pelvis at 8 months of age: dilatation of the ectopic ureter of the right lower pole without ureterocele

the contralateral side (SIEGEL 1995) or may induce bladder dysfunction (ABRAHAMSSON et al. 1998). In rare cases, ureteropelvic junction obstruction may affect the upper or the lower pole.

3.3.2.4
Simple Ureterocele

Simple ureterocele is much more frequent in adults than in children. This suggests that in many instances this condition is acquired. In this anomaly, the ureter is single and ends in a normal position (orthotopic ureterocele). In children, simple ureterocele is com-

monly associated with dilatation of the ureter. Diagnosis is easily made by ultrasonography: Ureterocele appears as an intravesical anechoic and thin-walled mass near the lateral margin of the trigone. EU is also diagnostic, with the well-known "cobra-head" pattern of the terminal ureter (Fig. 3.23).

3.3.2.5
Ectopic Ureter

Ectopic ureter is much more common in girls than in boys. Nonduplicated ectopic ureter is very rare compared with duplicated ectopic ureter. The

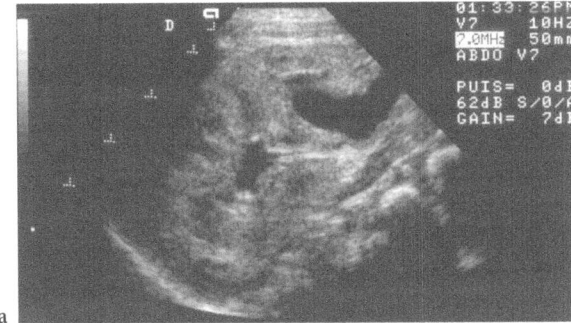

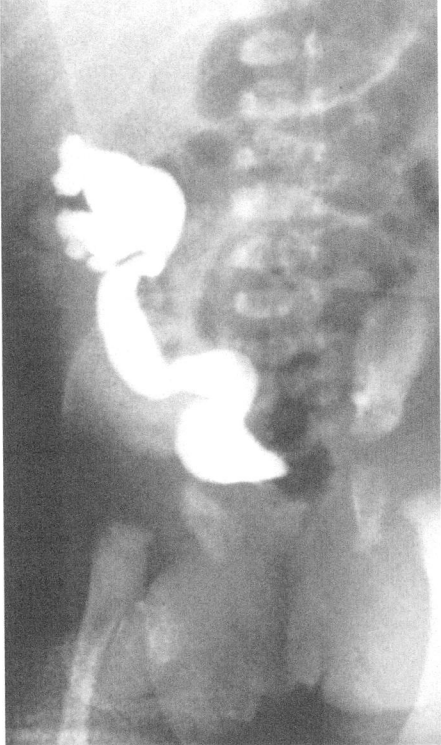

Fig. 3.22a, b. Complete duplication with reflux in the lower pole in a male neonate with antenatal diagnosis of right urinary tract dilatation. a Ultrasonographic view of the right kidney: moderate dilatation of the lower pole with thinning of the parenchyma; visualization of the upper pelvis with normal parenchyma. b VCUG, post-voiding fluoroscopic film: grade IV reflux in the lower pole; note lateral displacement of the collecting system

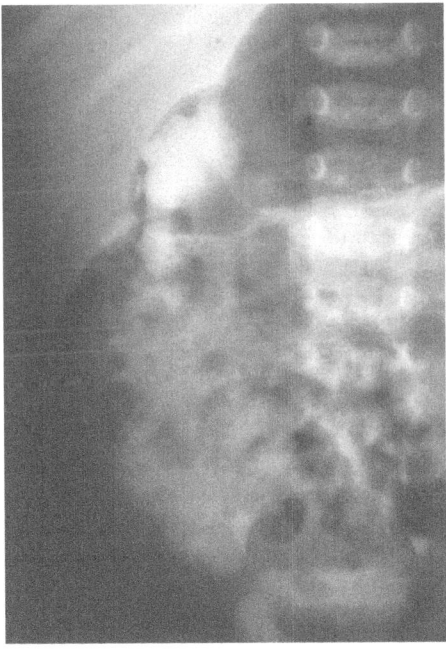

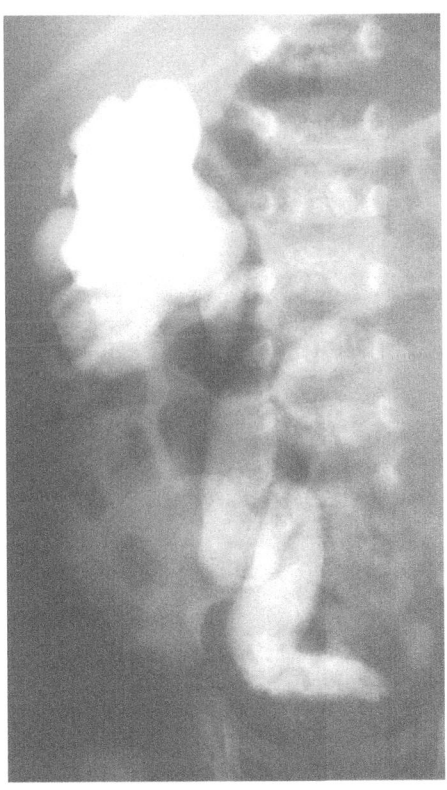

Fig. 3.23a, b. Simple ureterocele in a 2-month-old boy with antenatal diagnosis of urinary tract dilatation. a Eight-minute film EU: dilatation of the right ureter with filling defect of the bladder. b Delayed film: "cobra-head" pattern of the distal ureter

renal parenchyma drained by the ectopic ureter is often dysplastic and, in some cases, may be not found (Fig. 3.24). An ectopic ureter draining into a Gartner's cyst may be confused with an ectopic ureterocele (SUMFEST et al. 1995) (Fig. 3.25). In girls with continuous urine loss, the role of EU has been stressed (CARRICO and LEBOWITZ 1998).

3.3.2.6
Other Rare Conditions

Ureteral triplication is a rare anomaly; one, two, or three ureters may enter the bladder. Triplication is usually unilateral, but duplication of the contralateral system may occur (Fig. 3.26). This condition may be associated with other renal anomalies such as fused kidneys (GOLOMB and EHRLICH 1989).

Persisting mesonephric duct is a very rare anomaly occurring in boys; in this condition, the vas deferens joins the ipsilateral ureter. Diagnosis may be made on the basis of VUR with opacification of a tortuous structure looping down toward the inguinal canal (MERROT and ALESSANDRINI 1996) (Fig. 3.27).

Retrocaval ureter, although congenital, usually manifests in adult life. Sonography may demonstrate mild or moderate dilatation of the right proximal ureter; EU or other imaging methods confirm the diagnosis, showing the abnormal course of the ureter at the level of the third or fourth lumbar vertebral bodies (DEVRED et al. 1995).

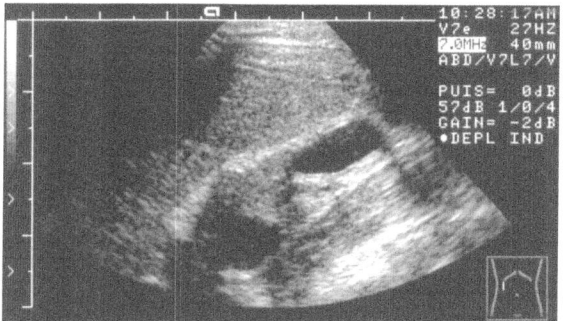
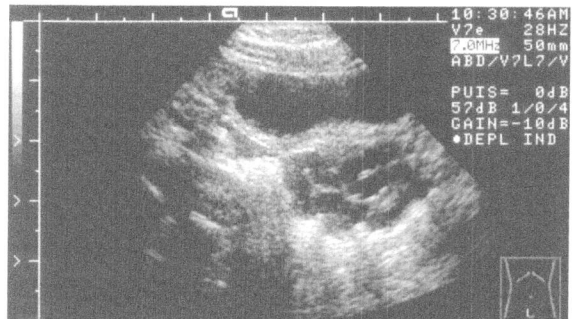

Fig. 3.24a, b. Ectopic ureter draining into the seminal vesicle in a 6-month-old boy referred for suspected epididymo-orchitis. **a** Ultrasonographic longitudinal view of the right lumbar fossa: dysplastic kidney with dilated ureter. **b** Ultrasonographic longitudinal view of the pelvis: retrovesical serpiginous formation. Diagnosis was confirmed at surgery

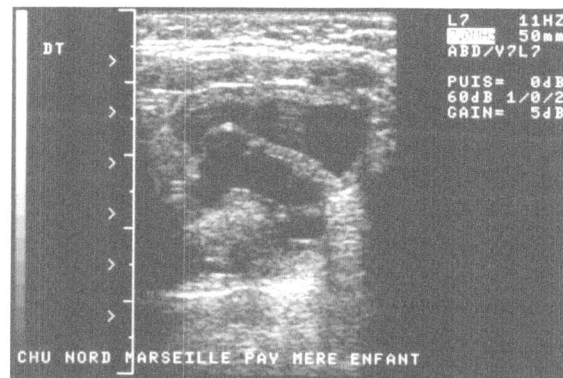
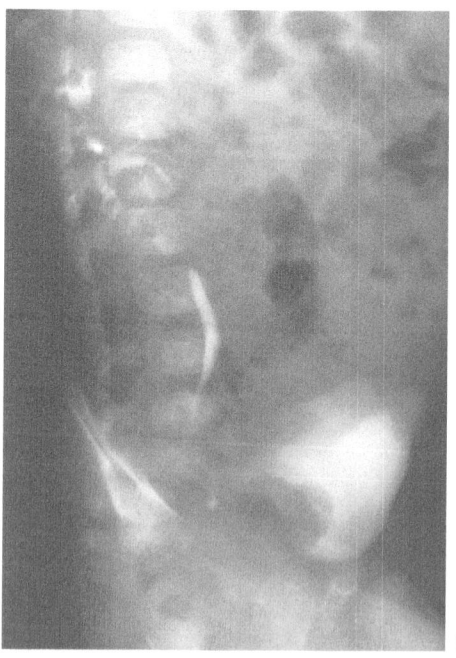

Fig. 3.25a, b. Ectopic ureter draining into a Gartner's cyst in a 3-month-old girl with urinary tract infection and antenatal diagnosis of right ectopic and dysplastic kidney. **a** Ultrasonographic transverse view of the pelvis: retrovesical tortuous anechoic formation corresponding to the Gartner's cyst. **b** EU: no excretory urogram on the right side, filling defect of the bladder ("pseudo-ureterocele"). Diagnosis was confirmed at surgery

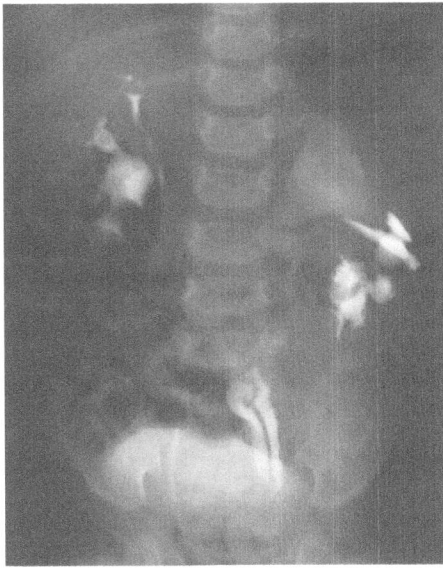

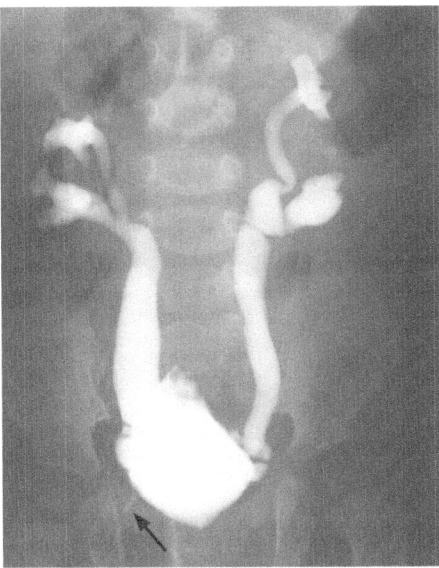

Fig. 3.26. Triplication of the left ureter in a 4-month-old girl with urinary tract infection. EU: dilatation of the left upper collecting system due to ectopic ending; partial duplication of the right kidney. (Courtesy P. Alessandrini, Marseille)

Fig. 3.27. Persisting mesonephric duct in an 8-month-old boy with VACTERL association. VCUG: bilateral reflux in incomplete duplicated system with likely renal dysplasia, opacification of the right vas deferens (*arrow*). Diagnosis was confirmed at surgery for bilateral inguinal hernia. (Courtesy P. Alessandrini and T. Merrot, Marseille)

3.4
Specific Patterns in Adult

Ureteral malformations are typically discovered in infancy and childhood, though many of them remain clinically silent for a long time and may be first identified in adulthood.

As in pediatric cases, the diagnosis can be made incidentally by EU but more commonly by ultrasonography or computed tomography. Nonspecific presentations in symptomatic patients include UTI and loin pain. Some abnormalities are found mainly in adults and will be more developed. They concern mostly the ureter and its distal part.

3.4.1
Anomalies of the Ureter (CHATEIL et al. 1991)

Bifid ureters are commonly encountered in adults and are mostly asymptomatic (Fig. 3.28). The morphology of the ureteral bifurcation is similar to that in pediatric cases with V- and Y-type. A yo-yo phenomenon with uretero-ureteral reflux can exist, owing to distal stenosis or to the different pressure state of the upper and lower moiety (FRIEDLAND et al. 1990). Inverted Y duplication of the ureter is extremely rare (Fig. 3.29). It is characterized by the

proximal fusion of two distal ureteral limbs which occur at a variable level (MOSLI et al. 1986).

As with children, double ureters are more commonly found in adult females, but they are more often asymptomatic. Their exact frequency is unknown.

Blind-ending bifid ureters (FRIEDLAND et al. 1990) are frequently asymptomatic. They are often detected as an incidental finding on EU (Fig. 3.30). They are not an uncommon ureteral anomaly, as is generally believed (HAWAS et al. 1987). They can arise from all ureteral parts with similar frequency. The diagnosis is easy on EU, the anomalies being opacified by uretero-ureteral reflux. It shows a tubular, pseudo diverticular structure of variable length caudally oriented parallel to the ureter. It is often dilated at its extremity and makes an acute angle with the ureter. However, opacification is sometimes intermittent, so the diagnosis can be overlooked. A CT scan can demonstrate a pattern of localized double ureter but the diagnosis also can easily go unrecognized.

A true ureteral diverticulum is very rare and is usually solitary. It has a saccular shape, perpendicular to the ureteral lumen, and a variable size. It has to be differentiated from ureteral pseudo-diverticulosis, which is probably acquired (see Chap. 9).

Congenital ureteral valves and strictures (Fig. 3.31) are very rare in adults because they are most often symptomatic in infants. They have to be differentiated

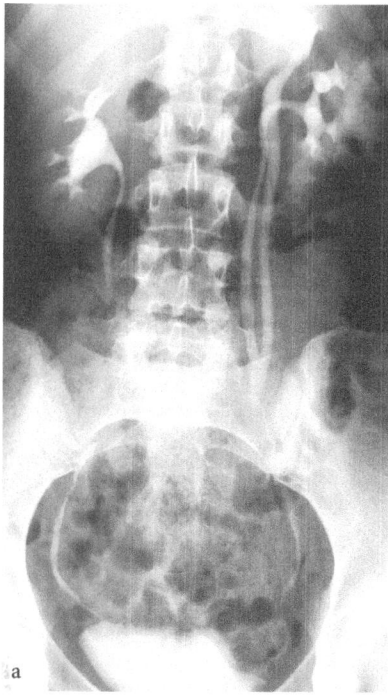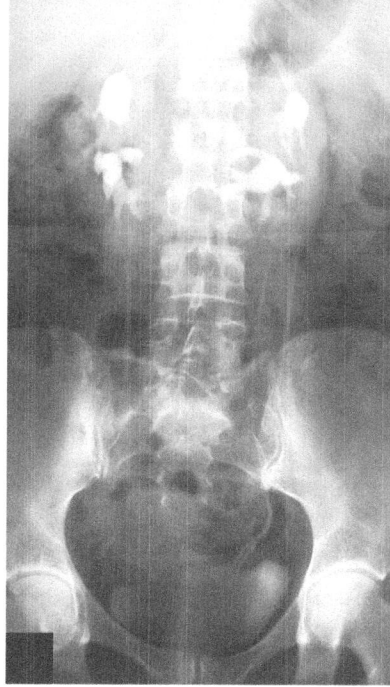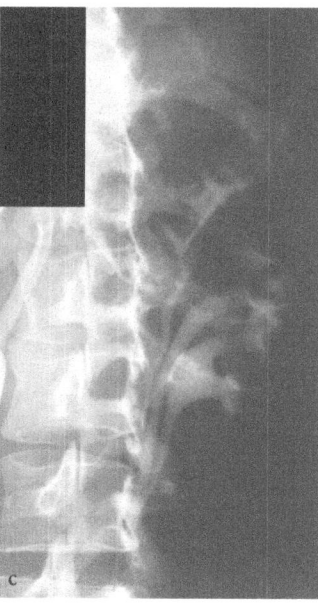

Fig. 3.28a–c. Asymptomatic anomalies of number in adults. **a** Bifid ureters on the left side. **b** Complete duplication on the left side of a patient with horseshoe kidneys. **c** Partial triplication of the left ureter

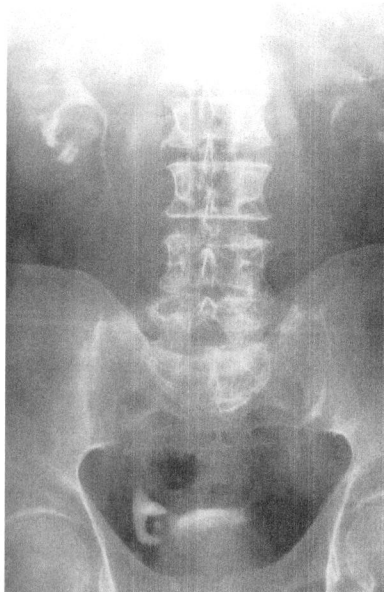

Fig. 3.29. Inverted Y duplication. Incidental finding during EU for left abdominal pain

from normal mucosal folds, which are generally not obstructive. A tortuous and kinked ureter can simulate a valve but it is generally dilated below and above the stenotic image. Ureteral ring has been described in adults, with a slight female preponderance. It is most often located in the upper third of the ureter and is nonobstructive. It is believed to result from the contraction of hypertrophied circular muscular layers (Dure-Smith et al. 1999).

3.4.2
Abnormalities of the Ureteral End

3.4.2.1
Vesicoureteral Reflux

VUR is found less frequently in adults than in infants. It can be related to a congenital abnormality (malformation of the ureteral orifice, ectopic uretero-vesical junction) or more often is secondary to acquired conditions. Bladder carcinoma, iatrogenic injury, or postsurgical changes of the ureteral orifice generally lead to unilateral VUR. Benign or neoplastic prostatic hypertrophy, hypertrophic cystitis, bladder neck obstruction, neurogenic bladder, traumatic or inflammatory urethral strictures, and all other causes

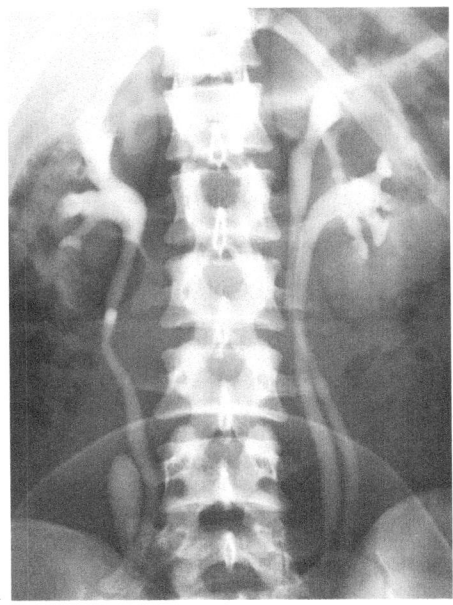
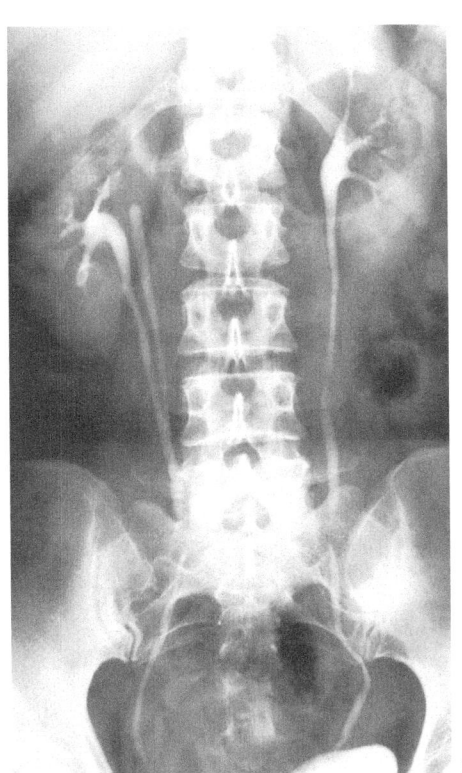

Fig. 3.30a, b. Blind-ending bifid ureters in adults. a Short pseudodiverticular and sacciform structure parallel to the right lumbar ureter. b Long, tubular, caudally oriented structure parallel to the right lumbar ureter. Bifid ureter on the left

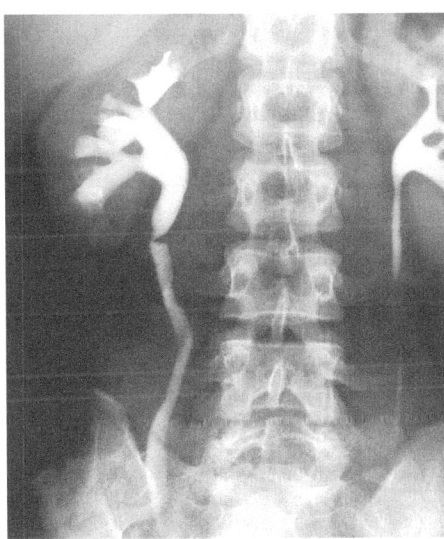

Fig. 3.31. Ureteral valve. Transverse and linear filling defect of the proximal ureter with moderate dilatation of the upper urinary tract in a young woman with history of recurrent acute pyelonephritis

of bladder outlet obstruction can lead to bilateral VUR. Clinical and pathological consequences for the urinary tract are similar to those in the pediatric population.

Radiological diagnosis is based on VCUG, and the need for surgical correction is still the subject of controversy.

3.4.2.2
Primary Megaureter

Primary megaureter is a rare congenital anomaly related to the presence of a short adynamic segment of the distal ureter. The exact cause of this functional obstruction remains unknown. The ureter becomes dilated proximal to this segment, with involvement of the whole or, more frequently, the distal part of the ureter (HAMILTON and FITZPATRICK 1987). Almost half of the cases are first discovered in adulthood (PFISTER and HENDREN 1978).

Diagnosis is usually made incidentally by EU, which shows fusiform dilatation of the pelvic segment of the ureter proximal to the adynamic segment (TALNER 1990). The junction between the dilated and the adynamic segments is tapered (Fig. 3.32). The distal aperistaltic portion is about 1.5–2 cm in length. If the dilatation involves the whole ureter, the

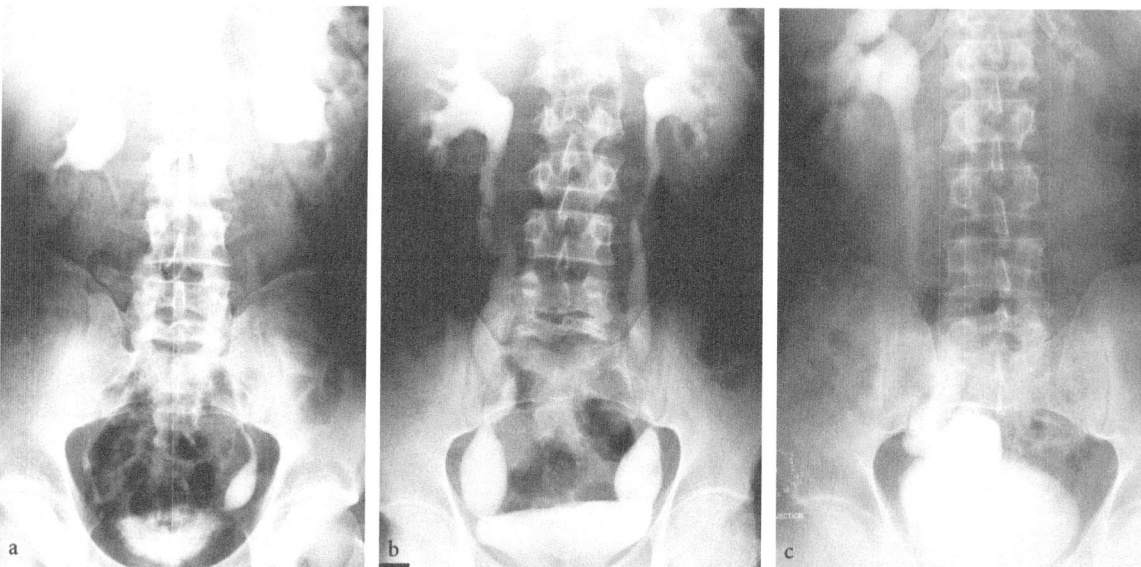

Fig. 3.32a–c. Primary megaureters in adults. **a** Moderate and asymptomatic dilatation of the lower centimeters of the left ureter without dilatation of the proximal ureter. **b** Bilateral fusiform dilatation of the distal part of both ureters; moderate obstruction of the upper urinary tract. **c** Fusiform dilatation of the right terminal ureter with ipsilateral obstruction

distal ureter is the most dilated. Hyperperistalsis may be noted (PFISTER and HENDREN 1978). Rarely, primary megaureter causes severe obstruction with loss of renal function (Fig. 3.33). VCUG should always be performed because the condition can be associated with VUR. Calculi may be found as a consequence of obstruction.

No treatment is mandatory in asymptomatic cases. Complications such as repeated infections or symptomatic lithiasis may require surgical treatment with ureteroneocystostomy.

3.4.2.3
Ectopic Ureter and Ureterocele
(GLASSBERG et al. 1984)

Ectopic implantation of the ureter is defined as an implantation to a site on the proximal lip of the bladder neck or beyond (TALNER 1990). Ureterocele corresponds to a dilatation of the distal end of the ureter.

Nonduplicated ectopic ureter and/or ureterocele are very rare compared with the duplicated type, which represents more than 80% of cases. The incidence in females is approximately twice that in males. Ectopic ureter and/or ureterocele may be complicated by reflux or obstruction, as observed in the pediatric population (AMITAI et al. 1992).

The main symptoms in adults are pain, symptoms related to sexual activity in males (pain during ejaculation, epidydimitis). Recurring UTI is more frequent in females. Incontinence never occurs in males and is rare in adult females.

The goals of imaging are to demonstrate the importance of obstruction and/or destruction of parenchyma of the upper moiety, the site of implantation of the ectopic ureter and, if present, the type of ectopic ureterocele (intravesical or extravesical). Because of the possibility of other causes of obstruction in the adult duplicated urinary tract, a careful examination of the retroperitoneum has to be performed.

Most often, the upper segment functions poorly, indicating parenchymal destruction and/or dysplastic changes. EU shows indirect signs: drooping-lily appearance of the lower pole, spherical filling defect in the bladder (BLAIR et al. 1987) (Fig. 3.34).

Ultrasonography can show the upper pole as a multilocular pseudocystic mass. Careful examination of the pelvis, possibly by the transrectal or transvaginal route, can demonstrate the dilated ureter and its ectopic orifice (ENGIN et al. 2000). A CT scan can also demonstrate the hypoplastic or hydronephrotic upper pole (Fig. 3.35). The dilated ureter can also be followed to the pelvis but it may be difficult to assess the exact position of the ectopic orifice and the presence or not of ureterocele. Multiplanar reconstruction may give better information about the distal ureter. MR urography with fast, heavily T_2-weighted or contrast-enhanced sequences allows accurate imaging with multiplanar visualization of the urinary tract form the upper pole to the pelvis (Figs. 3.36, 3.37). Thus, it may become extremely useful

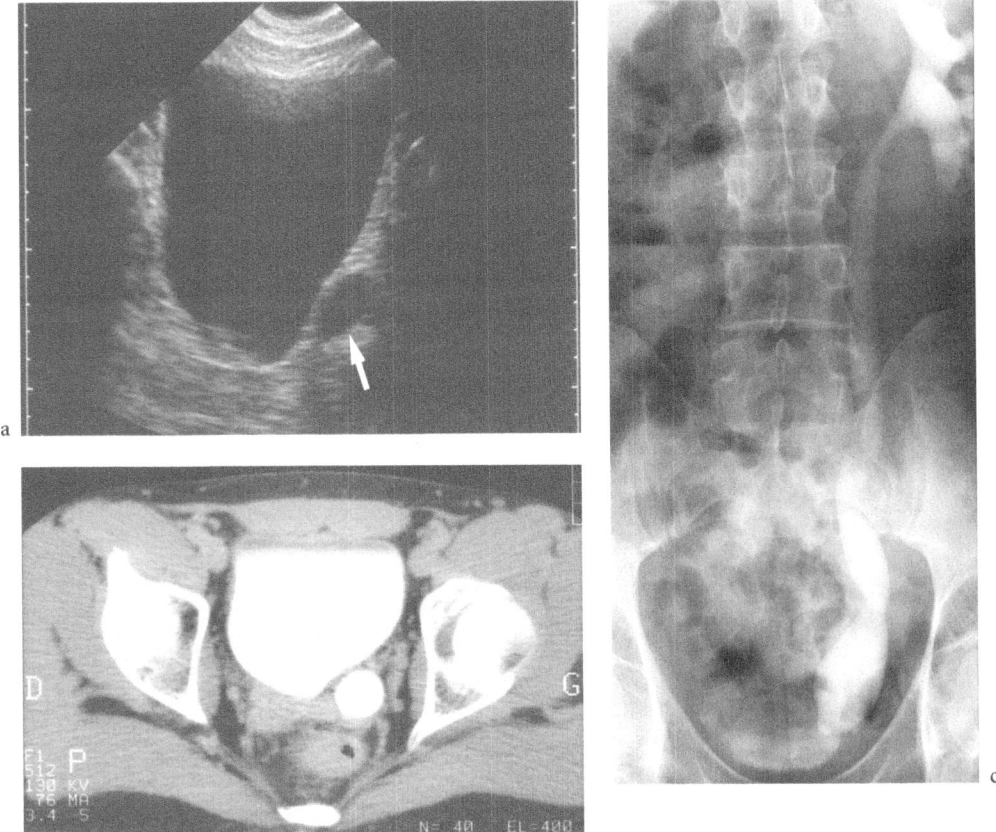

Fig. 3.33. Primary megaureter in an adult. **a** Bladder ultrasonography in a 25-year-old male patient with urinary tract infection. Presence of rounded echo-free structure lateral to the bladder corresponding to the dilated left ureter (*arrow*). **b** CT after intravenous opacification of the dilated left ureter lateral to the bladder. **c** Post-voiding view during EU, showing important dilatation of left upper urinary tract

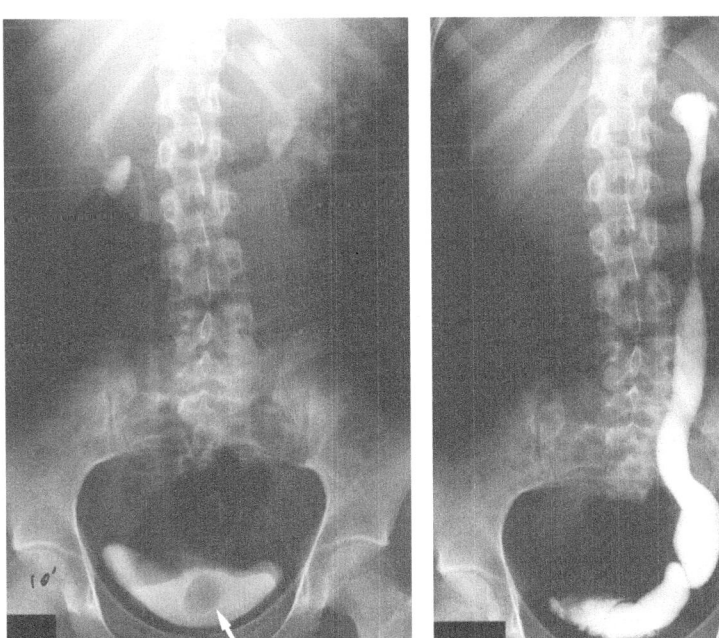

Fig. 3.34a, b. Intravesical ureterocele with duplication in an adult. **a** EU in a 30-year-old male patient demonstrates a large radiolucent filling defect within the urinary bladder. **b** Retrograde cystoureterography shows a reflux into the left ureter with opacification of the upper calix. The left ureter is dilated, and a "cobra-head" pattern is demonstrated at its end

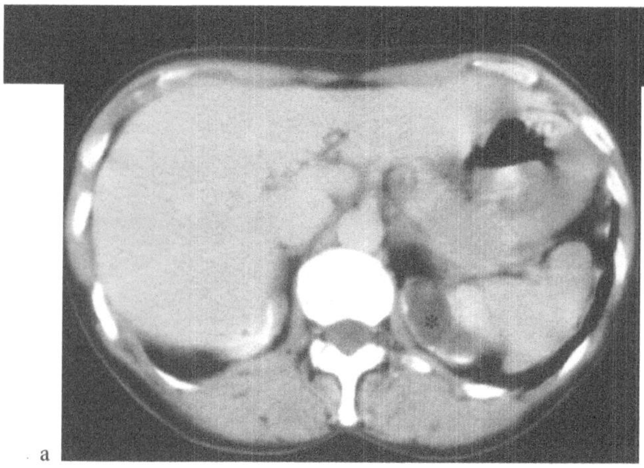

Fig. 3.35a–d. Ectopic ureter in an adult. **a–c** CT at different levels of the upper urinary tract in a 26-year-old woman with back pain. **a** Dilatation of the upper pole with parenchymal atrophy of the left kidney (*asterisk*). **c** Dilatation of the whole left ureter until the bladder (*asterisk*). **d** Voiding cystouretrography shows reflux in the left ureter due to ectopic opening into the urethra

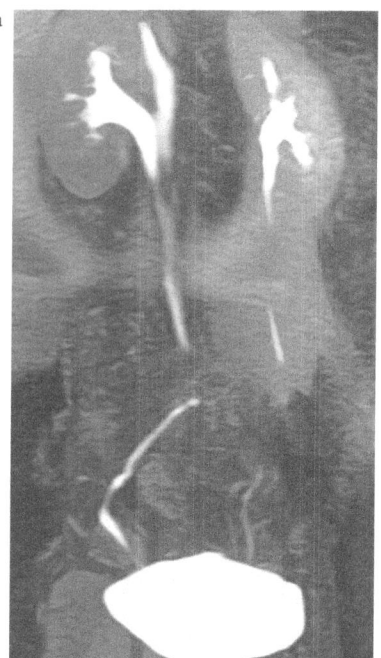
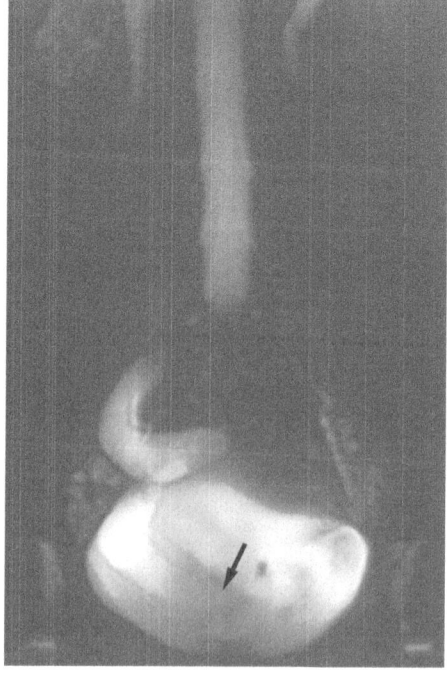

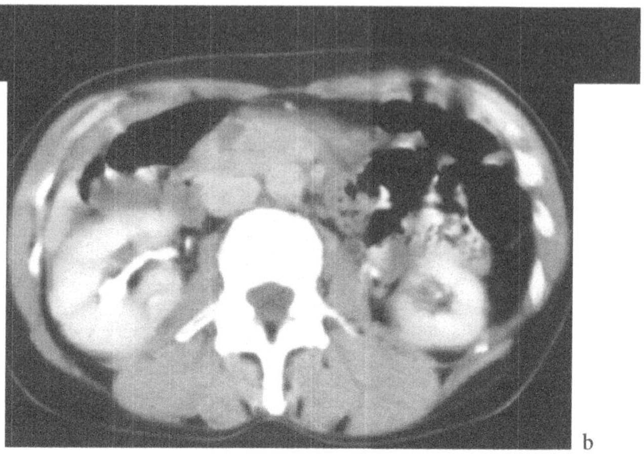

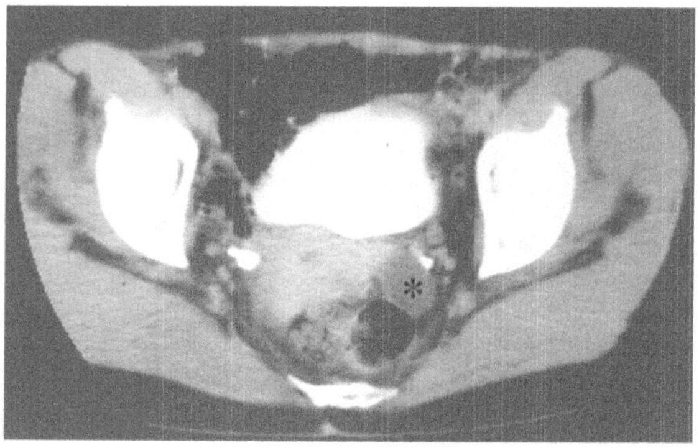

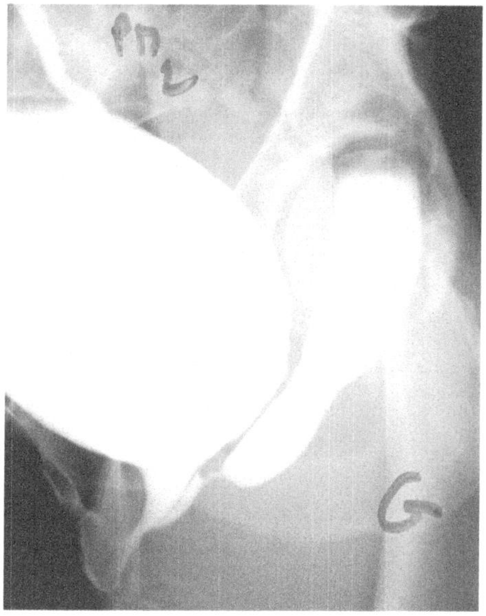

Fig. 3.36a, b. Ectopic ureter in an adult. **a** MR urography (MIP projection of a gadolinium enhanced T_1-weighted coronal sequence) in a young woman with incontinence demonstrates right duplication with dilatation of the upper calix. **b** Coronal acquisition with single-shot RARE sequence. Dilatation of the pelvic right ureter with ectopic orifice in vaginal topography (*arrow*)

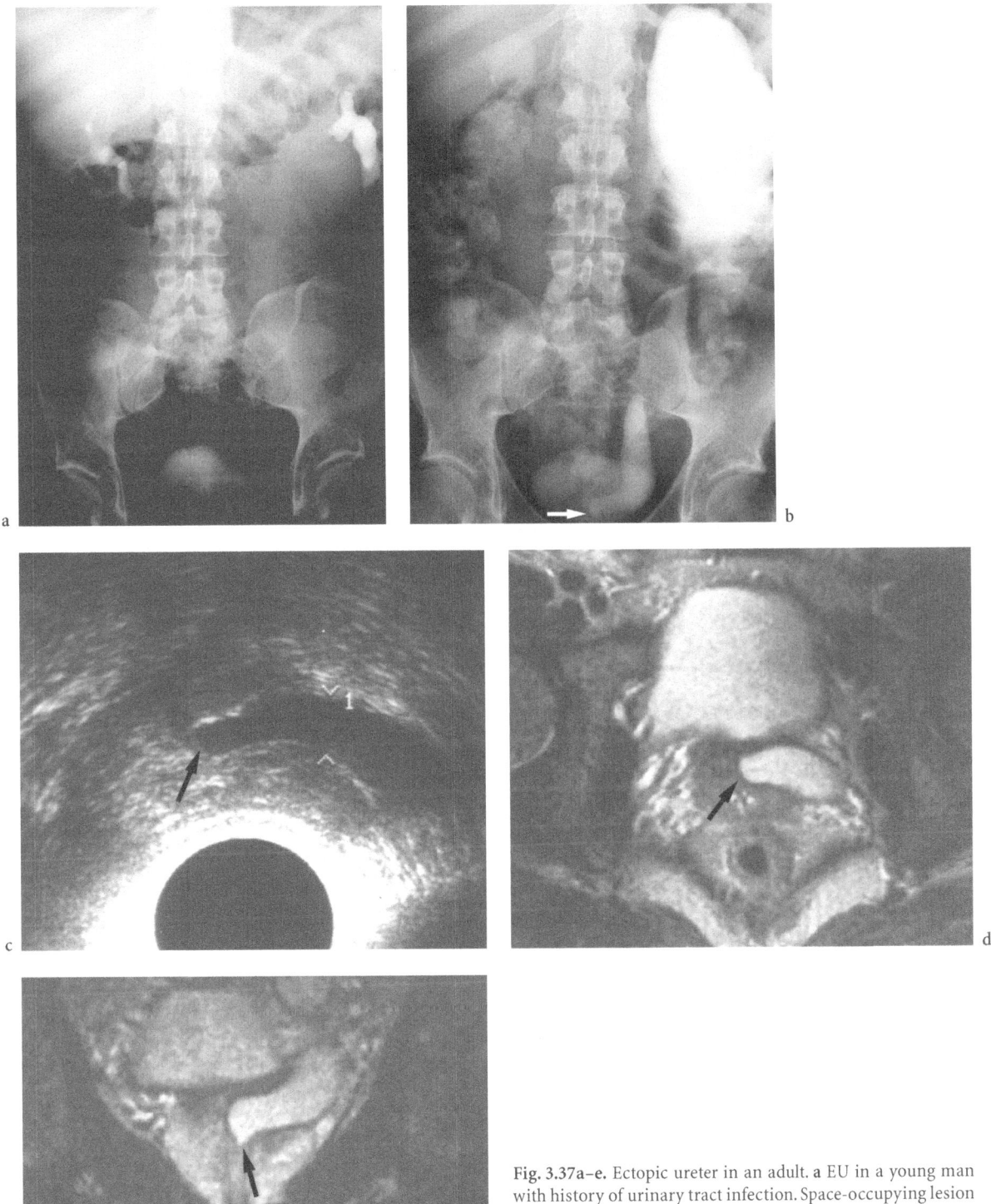

Fig. 3.37a–e. Ectopic ureter in an adult. **a** EU in a young man with history of urinary tract infection. Space-occupying lesion with displacement of the left upper urinary tract and left ureter. Absence of opacification of the upper calices. **b** Late film of EU shows opacification of a huge upper moiety of upper urinary tract and the left ureter with a medial implantation (*arrow*). **c** Transrectal ultrasonography; transprostate urethral implantation of a dilated left ureter (*arrow*). **d, e** Transverse and coronal views of MRI (SE T_2-weighted sequences). Visualization of the dilated left ureter with ectopic opening in the prostatic urethra (*arrows*)

after ultrasonography (ENGIN et al. 2000). VCUG is always necessary to rule out a VUR.

Treatment depends on the functional status of the related kidney: removal of the upper moiety and ureter or ureteroneocystostomy or transurethral incision of the ureterocele (ALBERS et al. 1995).

3.4.2.4
Intravesical Ureterocele

Intravesical ureterocele is much more frequent in adults than in children. Its exact etiology, congenital or acquired, is not clearly determined.

Insertion is usually orthotopic and most intravesical ureteroceles are incidental findings. It is rarely symptomatic. When large, it may obstruct the bladder neck or be responsible for urinary tract obstruction. The risk of infection and stones is increased (Fig. 3.38). Because renal function is more often normal, ureterocele is opacified during EU with the classical cobra-head pattern due to a thin, lucent line inside the bladder surrounding the dilated ureteral lumen. A local or diffuse thickness of the halo suggests the so-called pseudo-ureterocele due to contiguous diseases (bladder carcinoma, ureteral calculus, edema, hypertrophic cystitis) (MITTY and SCHAPIRA 1977). The wall of the ureterocele may be demonstrated by ultrasonography as a rounded echogenic line inside the bladder lumen (cyst-like formation near the lateral margin of the trigone) (Fig. 3.39). CT may also show a "cobra-head" inside the opacified bladder (Figs. 3.40, 3.41).

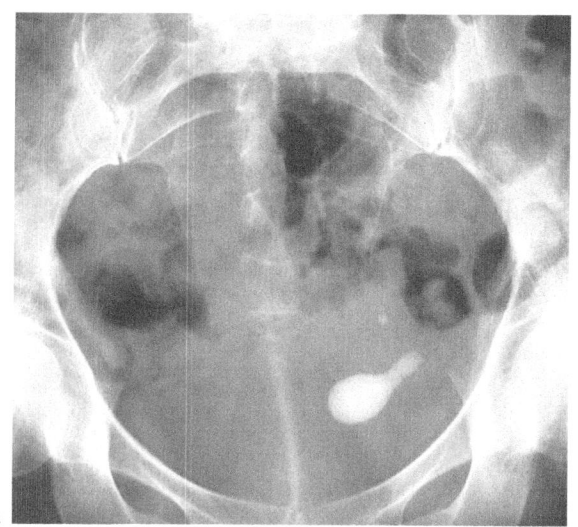

a

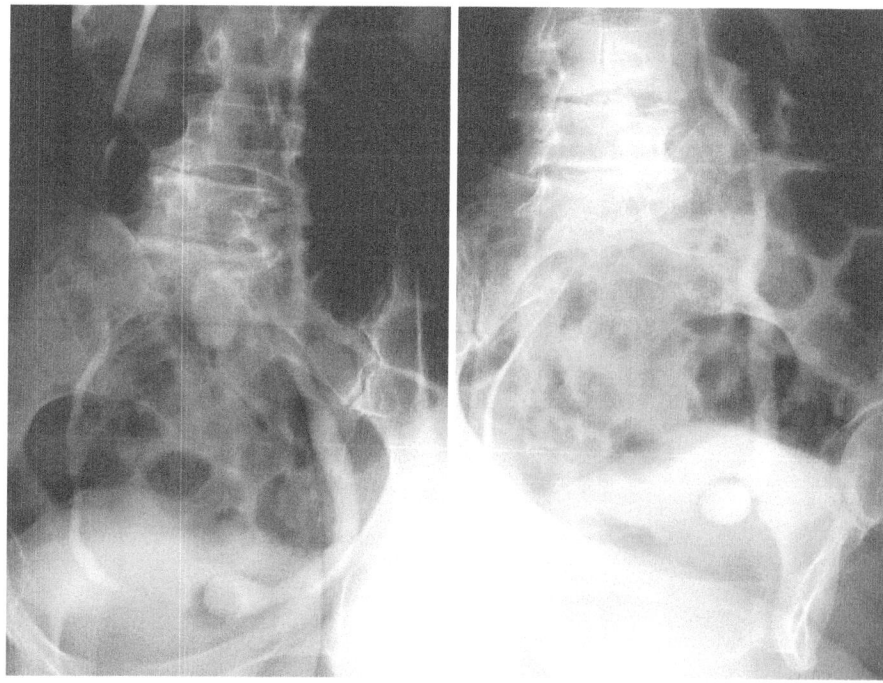

b

Fig. 3.38a, b. Intravesical ureterocele plus lithiasis. **a** KUB shows an oval-shaped pelvic calcification in projection with the left part of the bladder area. **b** EU shows a dilatation of the left ureter with a typical aspect of ureterocele on frontal and oblique views, with casting of the stone

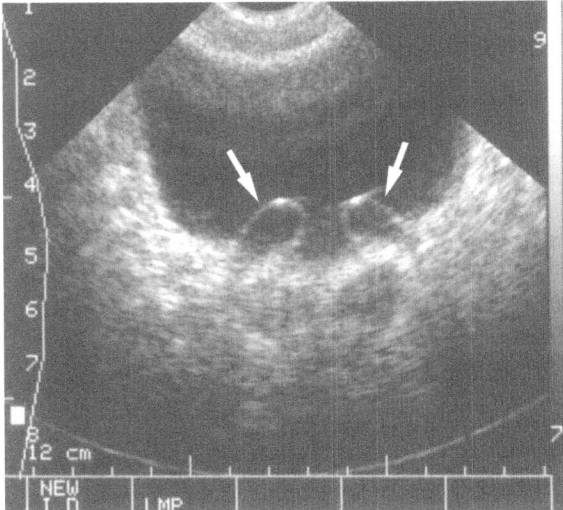
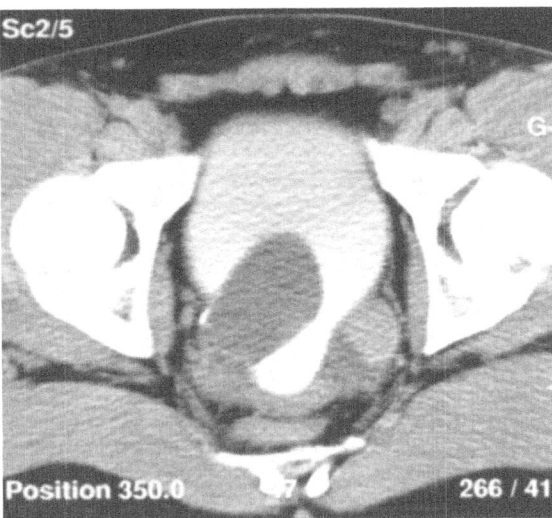

Fig. 3.39. Intravesical ureterocele in adult. Transverse ultrasonogram shows bilateral intravesical ureterocele (*arrows*)

Fig. 3.40. Intravesical ureterocele in an adult. CT after intravenous injection of contrast medium: rounded right lacunar intravesical image corresponding to a intravesical ureterocele with ipsilateral mute kidney

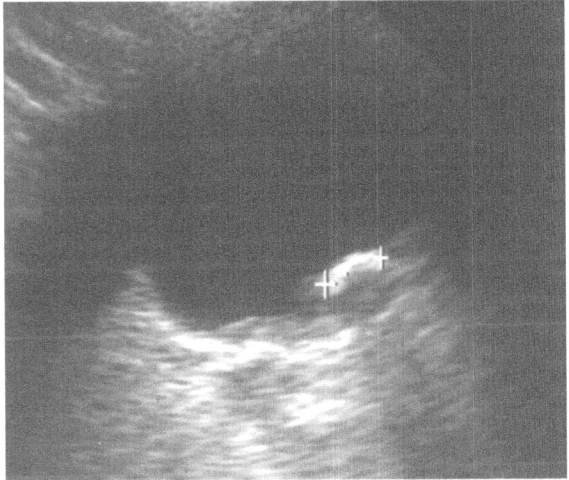
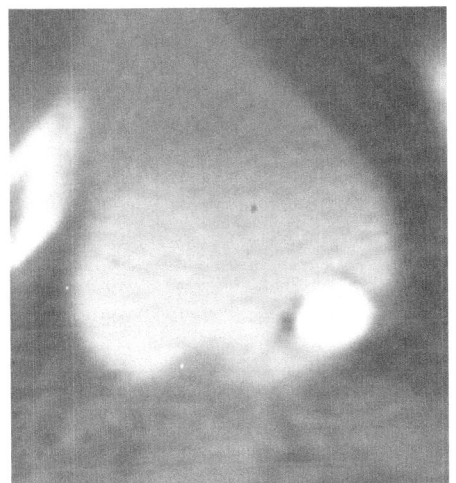

a

b

Fig. 3.41a, b. Intravesical ureterocele plus lithiasis. a Ultrasonography shows a typical pattern of a stone in the ureterocele. b Computed tomography after intravenous injection of CM

References

Abrahamsson K, Hansson E, Sillen U, et al (1998) Bladder dysfunction: an integral part of the ectopic ureterocele complex. J Urol 160:1468–1470

Albers P, Foster RS, Bihrle R, et al (1995) Ectopic ureters and ureteroceles in adults. Urology 45:870–874

Amitai M, Hertz M, Jonas P, et al (1992) Ectopic ureterocele in adults with a comparison of the anomaly in children. Urol Radiol 13:181–186

Arant BS jr (1991) Vesicoureteric reflux and renal injury. Am J Kidney Dis 17:491–511

Assael BM, Guez S, Marra G, et al (1998) Congenital reflux nephropathy: a follow-up of 108 cases diagnosed perinatally. Br J Urol 82:252–257

Avni EF, Schulman CC (1996) The origin of vesico-ureteric reflux in male newborns: further evidence in favour of a transient fetal urethral obstruction. Br J Urol 78:454–459

Avni EF, Ayadi K, Rypens F, et al (1997) Can careful ultrasound examination of the urinary tract exclude vesicoureteric reflux in the neonate? Br J Radiol 70:977–982

Avni FE, Hall M, Schulman CC (1998) Congenital uronephropathies: is routine voiding cystourethrography always warranted? Clin Radiol 53:247–250

Bellah RD, Long FR, Canning DA (1995) Ureterocele eversion with vesicoureteral reflux in duplex kidneys: findings at voiding cystourethrography. AJR 165:409–413

Blair D, Rigsby C, Rosenfield AT (1987) The nubbin sign on computed tomography and sonography. Urol Radiol 9: 149–151

Blane CE, Dipietro MA, Zerin JM, et al (1993) Renal sonography is not a reliable screening examination for vesicoureteral reflux. J Urol 150:752–755

Bonnin F, Le Stanc E, Lottmann H, et al (1998) Urology and nuclear medicine in children. Experience from a series of 1200 renal scintigraphies. Ann Urol (Paris) 32:186–190

Borthne A, Nordshus T, Reiseter T, et al (1999) MR urography: the future gold standard in paediatric urogenital imaging? Pediatr Radiol 29:694–701

Bourlière-Najean B, Panuel M, Faure F, et al (1994) Comparison of radiation dose between conventional and digital cystography in children. Rev Im Med 6:687–689

Braun-Quentin C, Billes C, Bowing B, et al (1996) MURCS association: case report and review. J Med Genet 33:618–620

Carrico C, Lebowitz RL (1998) Incontinence due to an intrasphincteric ectopic ureter: why the delay in diagnosis and what the radiologist can do about it? Pediatr Radiol 28: 942–949

Chateil JF, Diard F, Castell JF (1991) Uropathies et malformations du haut appareil. EMC Radiognost Urogynecol 34570, A10

Cleveland RH, Constantinou C, Blickman JG, et al (1992) Voiding cystourethrography in children: value of digital fluoroscopy in reducing radiation dose. AJR 158:137–142

Connolly LP, Treves ST, Connolly SA. et al (1997) Vesicoureteral reflux in children: incidence and severity in siblings. J Urol 157:2287–2290

Currarino G, Wood B, Majd M (1993) The genitourinary tract and retroperitoneum. In: Silverman FN, Kuhn JP (eds) Caffey's pediatric X-ray diagnosis. Mosby, St. Louis, pp 1145–1318

Dacher JN, Douvrin F, Monroc M, et al (1997) Mid-ureteric cyst: a variant of ureterocele disproportion. Pediatr Radiol 27:559

Darge K, Troeger J, Duetting T, et al (1999) Reflux in young patients: comparison of voiding US of the bladder and retrovesical space with echo enhancement versus voiding cystourethrography for diagnosis. Radiology 210:201–207

Davey MS, Zerin JM, Reilly C, et al (1997) Mild renal pelvic dilatation is not predictive of vesicoureteral reflux in children. Pediatr Radiol 27:908–911

Devaussuzenet V, Dacher JN, Eurin D, et al (1997) Postnatal echography and cystography after prenatal diagnosis of minor dilatation of the kidney pelvis. Prospective study of 89 cases. J Radiol 78:27–31

Devred P, Bourlière-Najean B, Meyrat B, et al (1995) Pathologie malformative. In: Devred P (ed) Imagerie de l'appareil urinaire de l'enfant. Masson, Paris, pp 55–106

Dipietro MA, Blane CE, Zerin JM (1997) Vesicoureteral reflux in older children: concordance of US and voiding cystourethrographic findings. Radiology 205:821–822

Dure-Smith P, Wiley TE III, Suh RD, et al (1999) The ureteric ring Abdom. Imaging 24:426–428

Engin G, Esen T, Rozanes I (2000) MR Urography findings of a duplicated ectopic ureter in an adult man. Eur Radiol 10: 1253–1256

Evans ED, Meyer JS, Harty MP, et al (1999) Assessment of increase in renal pelvic size on post-void sonography as a predictor of vesicoureteral reflux. Pediatr Radiol 29: 291–294

Friedland GW, Devries PA, Ninq-Murlia M (1990) Congenital anomalies of the urinary tract. In: Pollack HM (ed) Clinical urography: an atlas and textbook of uroradiological imaging, vol 1. Saunders, Philadelphia, pp 653–710

Gelfand MJ, Koch BL, Elgazzar AH, et al (1999) Cyclic cystography: diagnostic yield in selected pediatric populations. Radiology 213:118–120

Glassberg KI, Braren V, Duckett JW, et al (1984) Suggested terminology for duplex systems, ectopic ureters and ureteroceles. J Urol 132:1153–1154

Golomb J, Ehrlich RM (1989) Bilateral ureteral triplication with crossed ectopic fused kidneys associated with the VACTERL syndrome. J Urol 14:1398–1399

Gonzalez L, Vano E, Ruiz MJ (1995) Radiation doses to paediatric patients undergoing micturating cystourethrography examinations and potential reduction by radiation protection optimization. Br J Radiol 68:291–295

Gross GW, Lebowitz RL (1981) Infection does not cause reflux. AJR 137:929–932

Hamilton S, Fitzpatrick JM (1987) Primary nonobstructive megaureter in adults. Clin Radiol 38:181–185

Hawas N, Noah M, Pattel PJ (1987) Blind-ending bifid ureter: clinical significance? Analysis of 13 cases with review of the literature. Eur Urol 13:39–43

Klein LT, Frager D, Subramanium A, et al (1998) Use of magnetic resonance urography. Urology 52:602–608

Kleinman PK, Diamond DA, Karellas A, et al (1994) Tailored low-dose fluoroscopic voiding cystourethrography for the reevaluation of vesicoureteral reflux in girls. AJR 162: 1151–1154

Lebowitz RL, Olbing H, Parkkulainen K, et al (1985) International system of radiographic grading of vesicoureteric reflux. International Reflux Study in Children. Pediatr Radiol 15:105–109

Mentzel HJ, Vogt S, Patzer L, et al (1999) Contrast-enhanced sonography of vesicoureterorenal reflux in children: preliminary results. AJR 173:737–740

Meyer JS, Lebowitz RL (1992) Primary megaureter in infants and children: a review. Urol Radiol 14:296–305

Merrot T, Alessandrini P (1996) Bilateral persistence of the common mesonephric duct in children. Prog Urol 6: 582–586

Mitty HA, Schapira HF (1977) Ureterocele and pseudoureterocele: cobra versus cancer. J Urol 177:557–561

Monfort G, Guys JM, Coquet M, et al (1992) Surgical management of duplex ureteroceles. J Pediatr Surg 27:634–638

Moore KL (1988) The developing human: clinically oriented embryology, 4th edn. Saunders, Philadelphia

Moscovici J, Galinier P, Berrogain N, et al (1999) Management of ureteroceles with pyelo-ureteral duplication in children. Report of 64 cases. Ann Urol (Paris) 33:369–376

Mosli HA, Schillinger JF, Futter N (1986) Inverted Y duplication of the ureter. J Urol 135:126–127

Nolte-Ernsting CC, Bucker A, Adam GB, et al (1998) Gadolinium-enhanced excretory MR urography after low-dose diuretic injection: comparison with conventional excretory urography. Radiology 209:147–157

Pal CR, Tuson JR, Lindsell DR, et al (1998) The role of micturating cystourethrography in antenatally detected mild hydronephrosis. Pediatr Radiol 28:152–155

Paltiel HJ, Rupich RC, Kiruluta HG (1992) Enhanced detection of vesicoureteral reflux in infants and children with use of cyclic voiding cystourethrography. Radiology 184:753–755

Pfister RC, Hendren WH (1978) Primary megaureter in children and adults. Clinical and pathological features of 150 ureters. Urology 2:160–176

Ring E, Zobel G (1988) Urinary infection and malformations of urinary tract in infancy. Arch Dis Child 63:818–820

Rittler M, Paz JE, Castilla EE (1996) VACTERL association, epidemiologic definition and delineation. Am J Med Genet 63:529–536

Robben SG, Boesten M, Linmans J, et al (1999) Significance of thickening of the wall of the renal collecting system in children: an ultrasound study. Pediatr Radiol 29:736–740

Schulman SL, Snyder HM (1993) Vesicoureteral reflux and reflux nephropathy in children. Curr Opin Pediatr 5: 191–197

Sheridan M, Jenkes Gough DCS (1991) Reflux nephropathy in the first year of life: the role of infection. Pediatr Surg Int 6:214–216

Siegel MJ (1995) Urinary tract. In: Siegel MJ (ed) Pediatric sonography. Raven, New York, pp 357–435

Sigmund G, Stoever B, Zimmerhackl LB, et al (1991) RARE-MR-urography in the diagnosis of upper urinary tract abnormalities in children. Pediatr Radiol 21:416–420

Sillen U (1999) Vesicoureteral reflux in infants. Pediatr Nephrol 13:355–361

Smellie JM, Tamminen-Mobius T, Olbing H, et al (1992) Five-year study of medical or surgical treatment in children with severe reflux: radiological renal findings. The International Reflux Study in Children. Pediatr Nephrol 6:223–230

Sumfest JM, Burns MW, Mitchell ME (1995) Pseudoureterocele: potential for misdiagnosis of an ectopic ureter as a ureterocele. Br J Urol 75:401–405

Talner LB (1990) Specific causes of obstruction. In: Pollack HM (ed) Clinical urography: an atlas and textbook of uroradiological imaging, vol 2. Saunders, Philadelphia, pp 1629–1751

Tanagho EA (1973) Intrauterine fetal ureteral obstruction. J Urol 109:169–203

Tanagho EA (1976) Embryologic basis for lower ureteral anomalies: a hypothesis. Urology 7:451–464

Tang Y, Yamashita Y, Namimoto T, et al (1996) The value of MR urography that uses HASTE sequences to reveal urinary tract disorders. AJR Am J Roentgenol 167:497–502

Taylor AJR, Clark S, Ball T (1994) Comparison of Tc-99m MAG3 and Tc-99m DTPA scintigraphy in neonates. Clin Nucl Med 19:575–580

Vallee JP, Vallee MP, Greenfield SP, et al (1999) Contemporary incidence of morbidity related to vesicoureteral reflux. Urology 53:812–815

Willi U, Treves S (1983) Radionuclide voiding cystography. Urol Radiol 5:161–173

Wingen AM, Koskimies O, Olbing H, et al (1999) T Growth and weight gain in children with vesicoureteral reflux receiving medical versus surgical treatment: 10-year results of a prospective, randomized study. International Reflux Study in Children (European Branch). Acta Paediatr 88:56–61

Zerin JM, Ritchey ML, Chang AC (1993) Incidental vesicoureteral reflux in neonates with antenatally detected hydronephrosis and other renal abnormalities. Radiology 187: 157–160

4 Ureteral Obstruction

T. Smayra, Ph. Otal, L. Bouchard, B. Janne D'Othee, F. Lefevre,
M. Claudon, M. Irsutti, F. Joffre

CONTENTS

Whitaker has suggested a practical and useful definition of urinary tract obstruction: "A narrowing of the urinary tract, such that the proximal pressure must be raised to transmit the usual flow through it" (Whitaker 1978b). The key factor of obstruction is blockade of urine flow, which leads to increased pressure in the collecting system.

T. Smayra, MD; Ph. Otal, MD; L. Bouchard, MD;
B. Janne D'Othee, MD; M. Irsutti, MD; F. Joffre, MD
Service de Radiologie, Hôpital de Rangueil, 1, avenue Jean Poulhès, 31403 Toulouse Cedex 4, France
F. Lefevre, MD; M. Claudon, MD
Service de Radiologie, CHU Nancy Brabois, rue de Morvan, 54511 Vandoeuvre Les Nancy, France

Ureteral lesions are among the most important causes of urinary obstruction (Table 4.1). Early and confident diagnosis of ureteral obstruction is war-

Table 4.1. Main etiologies of ureteral obstruction

	Type of obstruction	
Congenital	Primary mega-ureter	
	Ureterocele	Intravesical
		Ectopic
	Ureteral valve	
	Circumcaval ureter	
	Ectopic ureter	
Acquired		
Intraluminal	Ureteral calculi	
	Blood clot	
	Sloughed papilla	
	Fungus ball	
Parietal	Ureteral tumors	Urothelial tumors
		Ureteral metastasis
	Inflammatory ureteral diseases	Tuberculosis
		Malakoplakia
		Schistosomiasis
		Systemic diseases (amyloidosis, polyarteritis)
	Strictures	Postoperative
		Post-radiation
		Post-traumatic
Extraluminal	Pelvic and retroperitoneal tumors	Direct invasion, encasement, external compression, periureteral metastasis
	Benign and malignant retroperitoneal fibrosis	
	Pelvic lipomatosis	
	Gynecological	Endometriosis, hydronephrosis of pregnancy, prolapse, pelvis abscesses
	Gastrointestinal	Crohn's disease, appendicitis, diverticulitis, fecal impaction
	Vascular	Perianeurysmal fibrosis, post aorto-iliac surgery
	Ureteral hernia	
	Urethral or vesical	

(see table 4.4)

ranted to prevent damage to the urinary tract. Long-term evolving ureteral obstruction leads to infection, stone formation, renal failure, and progressive renal parenchymal destruction.

The role of the radiologist is essential in the evaluation of a patient with ureteral obstruction. The aim of imaging is, by allowing the earliest and most accurate possible diagnosis, to obtain maximal information on the cause of obstruction and its morphological and physiologic impact in order to propose the best therapeutic choice. Treatment must aim to suppress the cause of obstruction and restore normal urinary tract physiology to prevent loss of renal function. New imaging modalities are causing considerable changes in the evaluation of ureteral obstruction, allowing a shorter, more efficient, and less invasive diagnostic strategy. The need for excretory urography (EU) and direct opacification is reduced, but interventional endoureteral procedures have provided major clinical benefits for the patient in the same time period.

The issue of "wide ureter" will be developed in this chapter (FLOWER 1977). This problem, that involves the adult as well as the infant, is a real challenge for the uroradiologist and has been the subject of numerous publications and discussions (SHOPFNER 1966; SHERWOOD 1979; PFISTER et al. 1986). This issue raises many questions: (a) Is there an obstruction in the low ureter? (b) Is there a congenital reflux or secondary vesicoureteral reflux? (c) Is there a bladder outflow obstruction? (d) Is it an isolated dilation without evident cause? In every case all these questions must be answered to allow adequate therapeutic management and prevent useless surgery.

Urinary tract dilation is a classical phenomenon during pregnancy secondary to physiological phenomena or an possible pathologic obstruction. The discussion about these difficult diagnostics will be presented in Chap. 8.

4.1
Terminology

A lot of confusion is created by the inappropriate use of several terms which can lead to false clinical implications.

4.1.1
Obstruction vs Dilatation

The term "obstruction" means that there is an increased resistance to normal urinary flow evacuation. The uri-nary tract adapts itself by raising the urinary pressure. A "dilatation" corresponds to an increase in urinary tract volume. It may appear without obstruction and/or pressure elevation (nonobstructive dilatation). An obstruction can be accompanied or not by dilatation.

4.1.2
Organic vs Functional Obstruction

Organic obstruction is always secondary to a narrowing of the ureteral lumen. Functional obstruction corresponds to a urinary pressure elevation without ureteral narrowing. The latter is generally secondary to a dyssynergy of ureteral peristalsis (e.g., primary megaureter).

4.1.3
Hydronephrosis vs Ureterohydronephrosis

Hydronephrosis corresponds to renal calices and pelvis dilatation. When renal collecting system dilatation is accompanied by a variable ureteral dilation with or without obstruction, it is called ureterohydronephrosis. As hydronephrosis is not associated with ureteral disorder, it will not be discussed in this book. In the same way, hydroureter or ureterectasis are used to describe an obstructive or nonobstructive ureteral dilatation. The term megaureter is reserved for congenital lesions.

4.2
Pathophysiology

The presence of a ureteral obstruction leads to functional and morphological modifications of the upstream urinary tract (obstructive uropathy) and to structural, functional, and metabolic alterations of the nephron (obstructive nephropathy). These effects are the function of different factors: uni-or bilateral, acute or chronic, complete or partial obstruction (GILLENWATER 1986). Other factors are implicated: the level of obstruction, morphology of the urinary tract above the obstruction (for example, extrasinusal pelvis), association with urinary tract infection, and pre-existing nephropathy (O'REILLY and RICKARDS 1986). The different anomalies secondary to obstruction have been demonstrated in animal models and correlate well with clinical observations (HODSON et al. 1969).

4.2.1
Acute Obstruction

In an acute ureteral obstruction, many phenomena appear (Whitaker 1978a, Djurrhus and Stage 1978):
1. Important fivefold rise of intrapelvic pressure, from 10 mmHg to 50–60 mmHg
2. Temporary hyperperistalsis, followed by diminished activity or disappearance of peristalsis
3. Drop in glomerular filtration rate and renal blood flow, probably in relation with preglomerular vasoconstriction. Alteration of renal blood flow is one of the main factors responsible for serious parenchymatous damage. Following an early and transient increase in the renal blood flow, the arteriolar vasoconstriction occurs 3–5 h after the beginning of obstruction and persists for 24 h even if the pressure in the collecting system has returned to normal level (Klahr 1991).

Fornix tears are frequent and allow the intrapelvic pressure to drop and the glomerular filtration to raise again. Successive periods of hyperpressure alternating with relatively low pressure periods in relation to urine extravasation are seen if the obstruction is not suppressed.

Thus progressive loss of nephrons appears after a long period of obstruction with progressive and generally uniform atrophy of the kidney. Canine kidneys tolerate 7 days of total obstruction without damage (Kerr 1956). Past this threshold, the kidney recovers its function only partially, and after 6 weeks of total obstruction it can be considered nonfunctional. Although some cases of return of significant renal function after long periods of total obstruction (several weeks to several months) have been described, these events are rarely encountered.

4.2.2
Chronic Obstruction

By definition, chronic obstruction is always incomplete. Experimentally, it is difficult to reproduce the phenomena occurring during chronic obstruction and thus they remain relatively misunderstood. The functional response to chronic obstruction is extremely variable: Some chronic obstructions may last for years without important functional impairment, whereas others lead to progressive renal atrophy (Platt 1996).

After a transient rise in pressure, an equilibrium is found between the glomerular filtration rate and uri-

nary tract dilation, and the urinary pressure returns to normal levels.

Dilatation depends on the renal pelvis anatomy (ampullary, extrasinusal) and compliance of the urinary tract wall, as well on the level, severity, and duration of obstruction. Severe chronic obstruction usually leads to renal loss with major cortical atrophy, but uncertainties remain about the possibility of renal damage reversibility.

4.2.3
Intermittent Obstruction

Patients with moderate narrowing of the urinary tract may have normal urine evacuation when the flow is normal. However, during periods of high urinary flow an acute obstruction can appear. The best example is intermittent obstruction at the ureteropelvic junction (UPJ) after excessive beer intake.

Between acute obstructive periods a mild dilation remains, with an acceptable ureteral patency. No renal parenchyma alteration or definitive functional damage occurs in this situation.

The presence of an intermittent obstruction is, however, exceptional in case of ureteral disease, UPJ being excluded from the group of ureteral diseases.

4.3
Acute Obstruction

Ureteral stone is a common disease, affecting up to 10% of the entire population in industrialized countries. Only 10% of patients with urinary lithiasis will present with symptoms, usually pain. Renal colic is a clinical syndrome characteristic enough to allow, in most cases, the prescription of ambulatory medical treatment. Radiological imaging is performed in a relatively low number of cases, particularly when the patient is admitted to the emergency department or when the clinical syndrome is atypical. Its role is to confirm the diagnosis, to determine the number, location, size and, if possible, the chemical composition of the calculus/calculi, to rule out complications, and to detect predisposing factors.

The two main factors conditioning the spontaneous elimination of the stone are its size and location. The probability of spontaneous passage is 22%, 44%, or 71%, respectively, if the stone is located in the upper, middle, or lower third of the ureter (Morse and Resnick 1991). The chance of spontaneous passage is about 80% if the calculus is smaller than 4 mm in diameter and only 21% if it is larger than 6 mm (VENO et al. 1977).

EU is theoretically the best examination to characterize most of these stone parameters. Its relative invasiveness (use of ionizing radiation and need for CM intravenous injection) has led US to be, along with KUB (kidneys, ureters, bladder), a first-line diagnostic technique in the evaluation of renal obstruction, even if it leaves many questions unanswered. More recently, unenhanced CT has became an effective technique for diagnosing renal and ureteral calculus disease and other causes of acute abdominal pain. Finally, MRI can be useful in the diagnostic approach to ureteral colic.

The aim of this chapter is to assess the current advantages, drawbacks, and performance of the different imaging modalities in the diagnosis of acute renal obstruction and to propose a practical diagnostic strategy.

4.3.1
KUB

In the past several years, the role of KUB as a first-line emergency examination for renal colic has been debated (Fig. 4.1a, b). Other imaging techniques are still needed to confirm the diagnosis. Ileus accompa-

nying clinical manifestations, could strongly limit its diagnostic efficacy, and smaller pelvic phleboliths are often misleading. Other structures potentially interfering with the visualization of ureteral stones are the sacrum and stools. Despite the high rate (90%) of calcified stones (HERRING 1962), sensitivity ranges from about 45% to 74% and specificity is evaluated at 77% (LAING et al. 1985; LEVINE et al. 1997). The CT scout radiograph can be used instead of baseline KUB. The percentage of stone detection is similar to that with conventional KUB (CHU et al. 1999). Despite its relatively poor diagnostic value, KUB is still useful in most cases in order to prescribe urine alkalization if the stone is proven radiolucent, to predict spontaneous passage or visibility for further ESWL, and for the surveillance of the patient (ZAGORIA et al. 2001).

4.3.2
Excretory Urography

Introduced in 1923 for this indication, EU remains for many authors the gold-standard exploration technique in renal colic. Unlike other diagnostic modalities, it allows both anatomic and physiologic evaluation. Functional information (delayed excretion of CM in the obstructed kidney, increased and prolonged nephrogram, silent kidney, extravasation of CM) is used to define the severity of obstruction

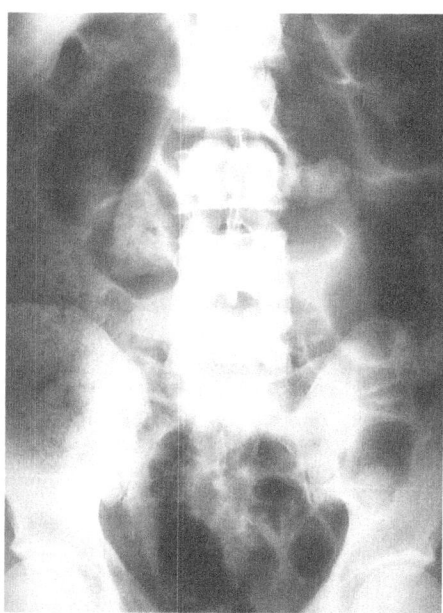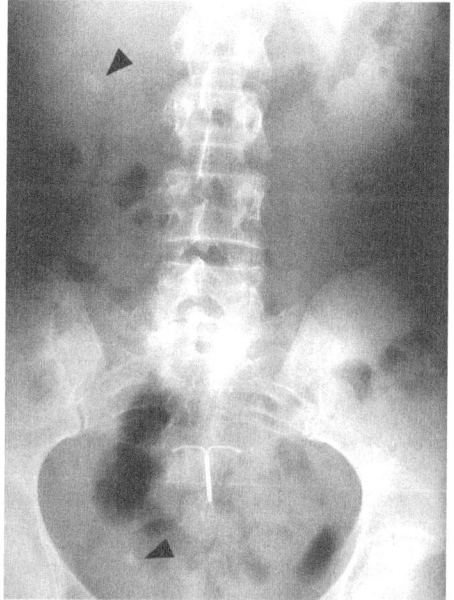

a   b

Fig. 4.1a, b. Two examples of KUB. **a** The large amount of intestinal air prevents accurate identification of stone in this patient with right renal colic. **b** In another patient with right renal colic, KUB allows identification of a right renal stone and a right ureteral stone (arrowheads)

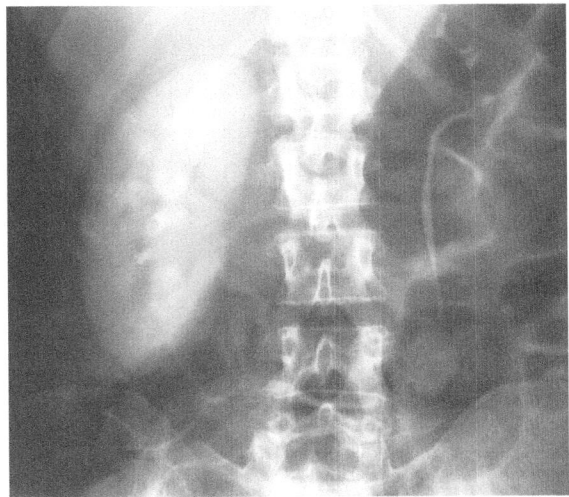

Fig. 4.2. EU for right renal colic (10 min): This image shows hyperdense nephrogram and delayed opacification of dilated calices

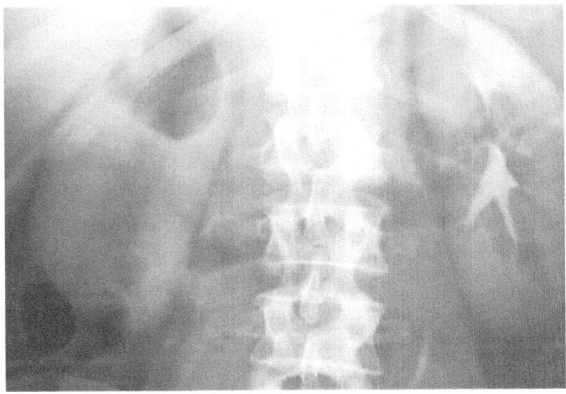

Fig. 4.3. EU for right renal colic (10 min): absence of opacification of the upper urinary tract

and influences the type and timing of treatment (Figs. 4.2, 4.3, 4.4a, b). The upstream ureter is dilated and the intraluminal stone is characterized by a filling defect of variable density. Excretion is sometimes so delayed that films have to be repeated up to 24 h after i.v. injection in order to correctly depict the site and nature of obstruction (Fig. 4.5a, b). Urinary tract dilation may be moderate or even absent but is nevertheless associated with tensed cavities imaged before hydronephrosis (Fig. 4.6). Inversely, dilatation is not specific of obstruction, since not all dilated cavities are tensed. Thus, the absence of delayed excretion makes it possible to eliminate the diagnosis of acute obstruction.

Accuracy of EU is excellent for the diagnosis of obstruction. It is always abnormal during the crisis and the following hours; it is sometimes difficult to differentiate a ureteral stone from spasm secondary to a spontaneous stone passage. Despite the use of LOCM, the i.v. injection causes increased urinary pressure in the excretory cavities and, consequently, exacerbation of the pain. The current decline in the use of EU in the exploration of suspected renal colic is explained somewhat by the risks of contrast-induced nephrotoxicity and fear of a life-threatening anaphylactoid reaction. Besides the need for CM injection and ionizing radiation, other EU drawbacks are its limited use in case of silent kidney and sometimes long duration (up to 24 h), which prevents rapid patient evaluation in emergency settings. Furthermore, as with KUB, the diagnostic quality of EU can be limited by the presence of stools, bowel gas, or bony superpositions. Finally, it does not provide extraurinary information.

a

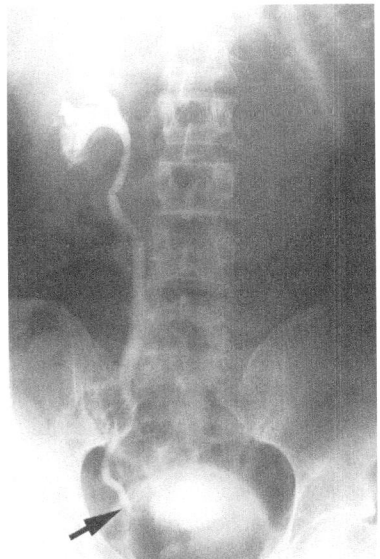

b

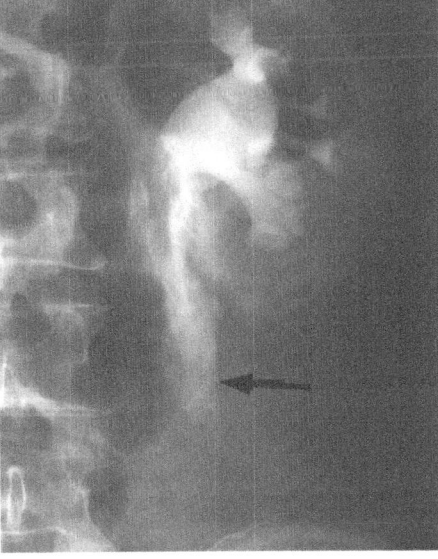

Fig. 4.4a, b. Two examples of extravasation during renal colic. **a** Intrasinusal extravasation probably secondary to fornix rupture with late opacification and mild dilatation of the upper urinary tract. The stone is located in the terminal portion of the ureter (*arrow*). Asymmetrical opacification of the bladder with probable edema of the meatal area (Vespignani's sign, see Chap. 5). **b** Peripelvic and periureteral extravasation secondary to a ureteral stone (*arrow*)

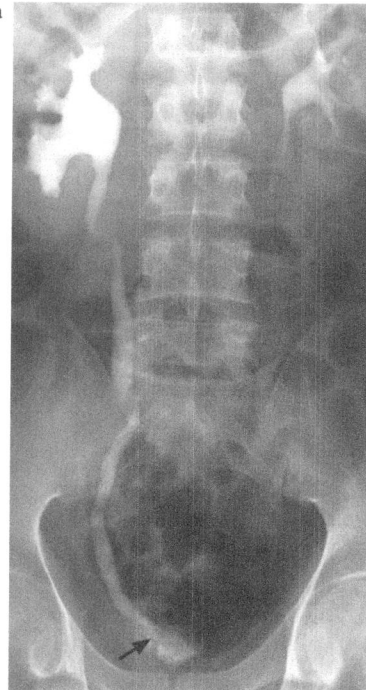

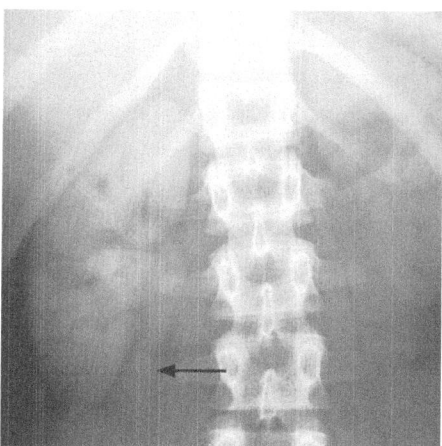

Fig. 4.5a, b. Delayed X-ray films during EU. **a** Post-voiding X-ray film, 30 min after the CM injection showing mild dilatation of the upper urinary tract until the stone (*arrow*). **b** Delayed X-ray film 6 h after CM injection. Persistent nephrogram, poor opacification of dilated pelvicaliceal cavities and proximal ureter until the stone (*arrow*)

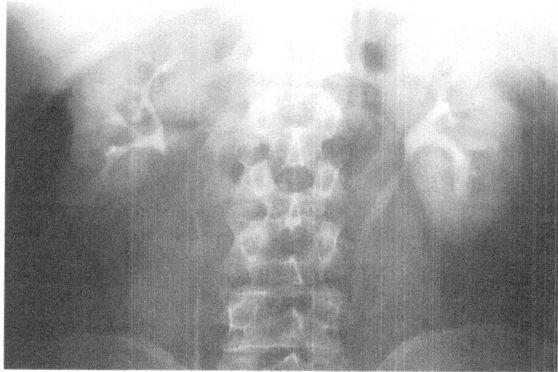

Fig. 4.6. EU in a patient with left renal colic shows dense nephrogram but absence of dilatation of upper urinary tract

4.3.3
Ultrasonography

Examination by US offers many attractive features compared with the relatively more invasive EU: absence of known side effects, no need for CM injection and ionizing radiation. The diagnosis depends essentially on depiction of dilated excretory cavities. Ultrasonography distinguishes three grades of dilatation (Fig. 4.7a–c): 1 = minimal pyelocaliceal dilatation, 2 = moderate, 3 = severe with a decrease of the parenchymal thickness (ELLENBOGEN et al. 1978). In grade

1 the echographic diagnosis can be difficult, and other methods are necessary to provide further information to establish the diagnosis of obstruction (Fig. 4.8). In the other grades, diagnosis of hydronephrosis is not technically difficult and can be made by demonstrating the dilated branching fluid-filled collecting system within the hyperechogenic sinus. However, many situations can lead to a false-positive diagnosis of excretory system dilatation on ultrasound (Table 4.2). Extrasinusal pelvis is a relatively common normal variant that mimics a dilated renal pelvis. Confluent renal sinus (peripelvic) cysts may also be wrongly interpreted as renal pelvis and calyx dilatation, especially when they have a branching appearance (Fig. 4.9a, b). A contrast study is then the only way to distinguish between the two conditions. Mild dilatation of the excretory system may be the result of a full bladder. In this particular case, the urinary tract dilation is bilateral and should resolve after voiding. Prominent renal hilum vascular structures, particularly on the left side, are easily distinguished from excretory cavities by means of color Doppler sonography. False-negative ultrasonography is rare but possible in the early period of acute obstruction and in case of an intrasinusal collecting system. Repeated urine extravasation by fornix rupture may also be responsible for the absence of dilatation, but ultrasonographic detection of abnormal intrasinusal or perirenal presence of hypoechoic urine is an argument in favor of acute obstruction (Fig. 4.10).

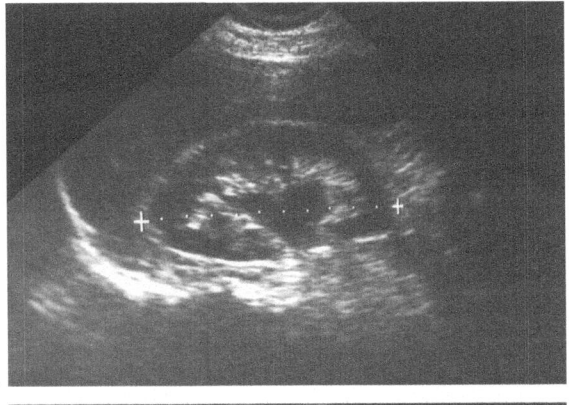

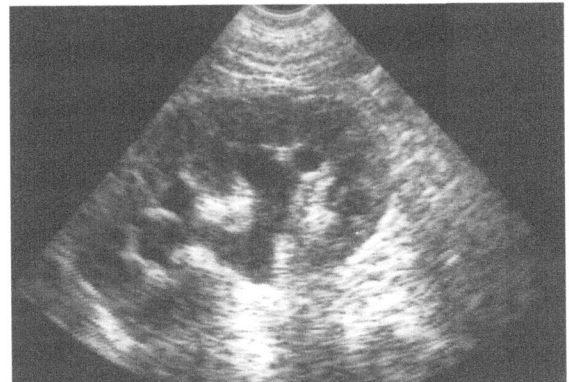

a

b

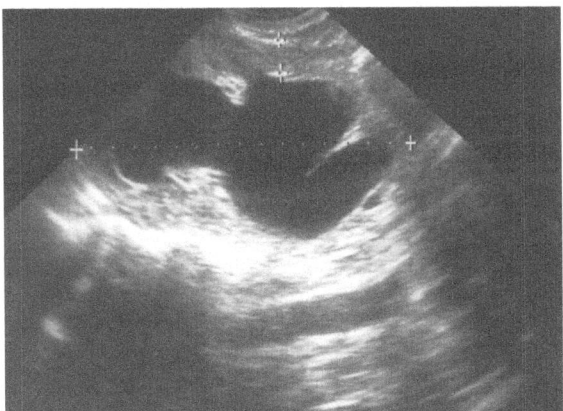

c

Fig. 4.7a–c. Ultrasonographic aspects of dilatation of the excretory cavities: a minimal dilatation; b moderate dilatation; c severe dilatation with decrease of parenchymal thickness

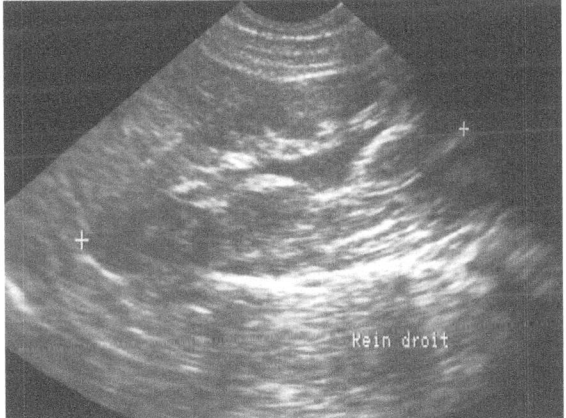

Fig. 4.8. Ultrasonographic aspect of dilatation in acute obstruction. Visualization of the nondilated pyelocaliceal system in a patient with renal colic; this aspect alone is insufficient for the diagnosis

Table 4.2. Causes of error of US diagnosis of acute obstruction

Error	Causes
False positive	Extrasinusal pelvis
	Dilatation of left renal vein
	Peripelvic sinus cysts
	Increased flow of urine
	Full bladder with retained micturition
	Dilatation without obstruction or hypotonia
	Vesicoureteral reflux
	Megacalicectasis
False negative	Early acute obstruction
	Intrasinusal pelvis
	Infiltration of renal pelvis by tumoral or inflammatory tissue
	Repeated fornix ruptures
	Hypovolemia

Stone detection remains the most difficult part of the ultrasound examination, since even for the most experienced sonographer the visualization of the entire ureteral length is generally impossible. The inferior pole of the kidney represents a good acoustic window for examination of the first ureteral centimeters. Color Doppler US is useful to localize the ureter crossing the iliac vessels. Visualization of a dilated ureter crossing the iliac vessels always means that a pathological downstream obstruction is pres-

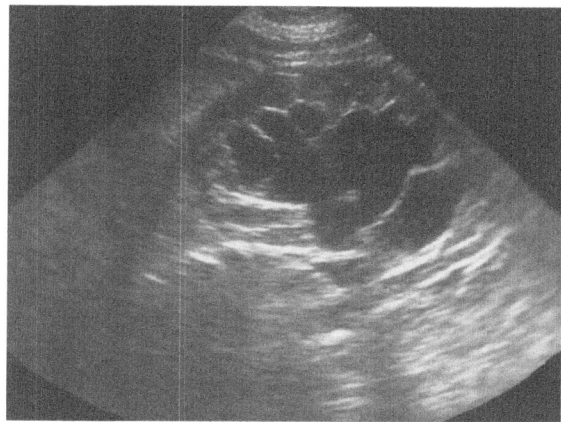
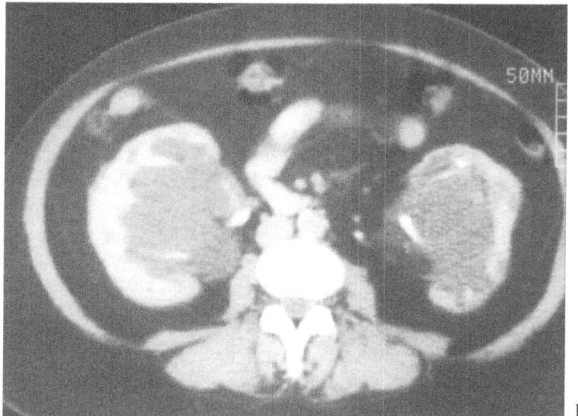

a   b

Fig. 4.9a, b. Peripelvic cysts can simulate dilatation of upper urinary tract on ultrasonography. a Presence of confluent anechoic cavities interpreted as pelvicaliceal dilatation. b CT shows absence of bilateral dilatation of the urinary tract and allows the diagnosis of bilateral peripelvic cysts

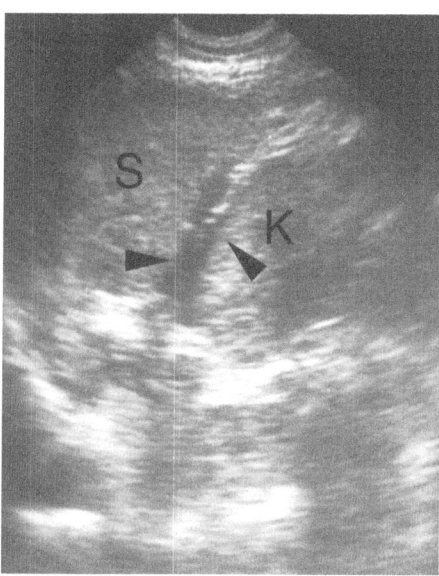

Fig. 4.10. Perirenal extravasation: This ultrasonographic view of the left flank shows a crescent-like anechoic image between the spleen (S) and the left kidney (K) (arrowheads) corresponding to perirenal extravasation of urine. This sign allows the accurate diagnosis of obstruction

ent. Furthermore, a partial bladder filling allows the detection of vesicoureteral junction stones (OHNISHI et al. 1986) (Fig. 4.11). Careful bladder exploration can show edema of the meatus area (echographic Vespignani's sign) which allows a retrospective diagnosis of renal colic after passage of the stone. This sign can persist for 24 h (Fig. 4.12). If the bladder cannot be filled, a transrectal or a transvaginal exploration may be helpful (LERNER and RUBENS 1986;

LAING et al. 1994). Nevertheless, the entire examination of the remaining ureteral portions requires a more tedious and time-consuming technique, such as a prone exploration.

As expected, the performance of US in terms of stone detection is not excellent: Sensitivity ranges from 10% (HADDAD et al. 1992) to 89% (SOYER et al. 1990) When associated with KUB, the sensitivity is estimated between 80% and 100% (AL-HASSAN et al. 1991; DALLA PALMA et al. 1993; HILL et al. 1985). False-negative cases are not only related to missed stones: If the examination is performed shortly after the onset of symptoms, US is not able to detect the tensed cavities before hydronephrosis occurs. Inversely, dilated but nontensed cavities lead to a false-positive diagnosis. Thus, specificity ranges from only 78% to 90%. Compared with unenhanced CT, the association of ultrasonography and KUB has a lower sensitivity (77% vs 92%), negative predictive value (68% vs 87%), and overall accuracy (83% vs 94%) (CATALANO et al. 2002).

The lack of physiologic information using the gray-scale sonogram has prompted several authors to complement the anatomic examination with a functional study based on Doppler. The utility of the intrarenal resistive index (RI) (peak systolic velocity minus diastolic velocity, divided by the peak systolic velocity) measurements relies on the hemodynamic changes induced by the urinary tract obstruction. Experimental animal studies have demonstrated that the first 5 h following an acute obstruction are characterized by an increased flow related to prostaglandin-mediated vasodilatation. If obstruction persists beyond that time, a phase of arteriolar vasoconstriction occurs,

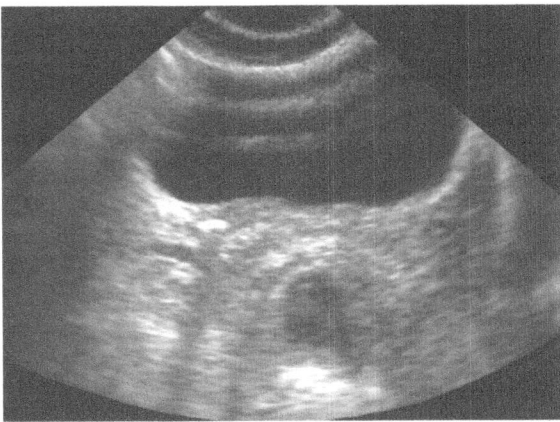

Fig. 4.11. Ultrasonographic visualization of a ureteral stone: presence of a hyperechoic area with a posterior acoustic shadow in the area of the right terminal ureter

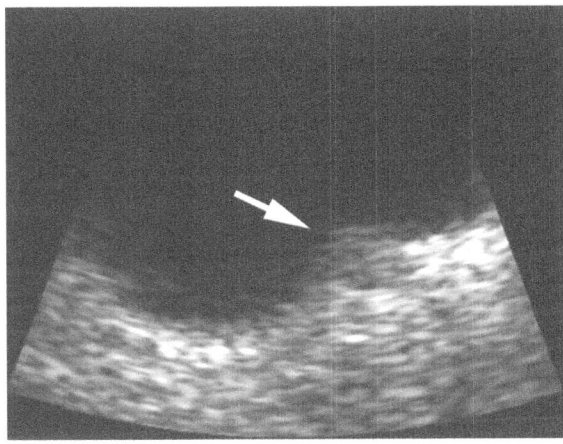

Fig. 4.12. Echographic Vespignani's sign. This transversal ultrasonographic view of the bladder shows edema of the left meatus (*white arrow*) which allows a retrospective diagnosis of renal colic after passage of the stone

resulting in a reduced flow and, consequently, an elevated RI (Fig. 4.13a, b). The maximal RI value is reached between the 6th and 48th hours. Two modes of measurement are proposed in the literature: the absolute RI value (the pathologic threshold generally being fixed at 0.7) and the gradient compared with the opposite kidney (the threshold varying between 0.07 and 0.1) (PLATT et al. 1993). This technique is sometimes technically difficult: Some patients are not able to hold their breath, especially when they are examined during the acute phase of renal colic.

PLATT was the first author to promote this technique and reported a sensitivity of 86% and a specificity of 92% (PLATT et al. 1993). Nevertheless, some criti-

cisms must be expressed from a methodological point of view: RI was measured on films and not directly on screen during the examination, and some patients had Doppler ultrasound after contrast injection for EU, which is known to induce an RI elevation. More recent studies have had disappointing results. In the series reported by TUBLIN, Doppler sensitivity and specificity were estimated at about 44% and 82%, respectively, as compared with 79% and 100% for US. Doppler allowed the detection of a gray-scale US false-negative diagnosis in only one case (TUBLIN et al. 1994).

There are several factors that explain the disappointing results of RI measurements. If the patient is explored during the first 6 h after the acute crisis onset, the response of renal vascularization to obstruction is a vasodilatation, thus decreasing the RI. Similarly, an intermittent obstruction may not induce an elevated RI. In case of forniceal rupture the collecting system urinary pressure decreases, thus limiting the renal blood flow alteration. Furthermore, multiple extrinsic factors may influence RI values: Some painkillers (NSAIDs), for example, are known from animal studies to alter the hemodynamic changes secondary to obstruction. On the other hand, a rise in RI is not specific of obstruction and may be associated with pyelonephritis, pre-existing nephropathy, acute renal vein thrombosis, etc.

Doppler analysis of ureteral jets may be helpful and is not technically difficult (Fig. 4.14). It is performed by a transabdominal axial approach through a moderately filled bladder in a well-hydrated patient. Color Doppler helps to depict the urine jet from the trigone toward the opposite side, searching for asymmetrical jets. In case of obstruction, flow is either absent or weak and continuous, as opposed to the peristalsis-induced periodic urine spurts observed on the opposite side (BURGE et al. 1991). The role of this exploration is to reduce the rate of false-positive obstruction on gray-scale imaging by allowing an additional argument, in case of hydronephrosis, in favor of an obstructing mechanism. Jets are often normal in case of low-grade obstruction or nonobstructing stones. Several authors have suggested that a state of hyperdiuresis could increase the accuracy of this technique. Color Doppler can also be helpful for detecting small pelvic ureteral stones, using the twinkling artifact even if an acoustic shadow is not visible (CHELFOUH et al. 1998) (Fig. 4.15a, b). Recently, Bateman reported the usefulness of color Doppler of the venous flow during acute renal colic. According to his group, measurements of peak venous flow show earlier and more significant changes than arterial flow (BATEMAN and CUGANESAN 2002).

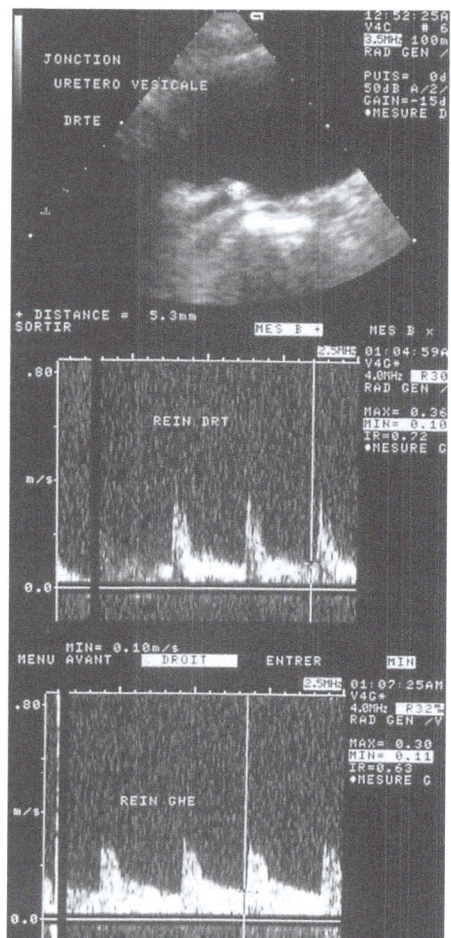

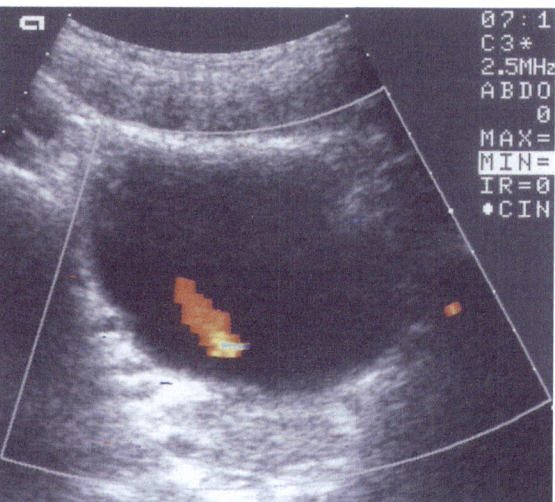

Fig. 4.14. Ureteral jet: Absence of right ureteral jet in a patient with left renal colic

a

b

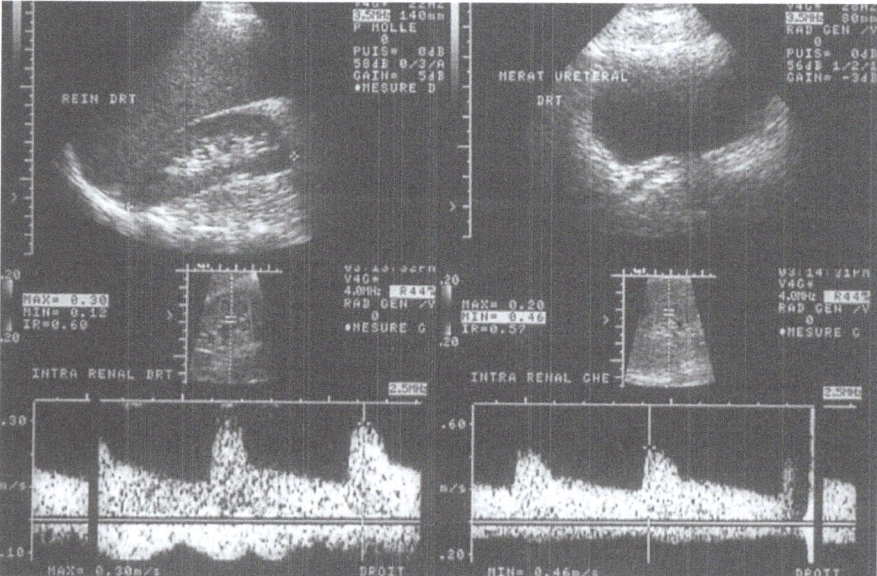

Fig. 4.13a, b. Examples of resistive index measurement in a case of acute obstruction. **a** Right renal colic related to a stone visualized at the terminal ureteral level: RI of the right kidney = 0.72; RI of the left kidney = 0.63. **b** Ultrasonographic study after passage of the stone: RI of the right kidney = 0.60; RI of the right kidney = 0.57

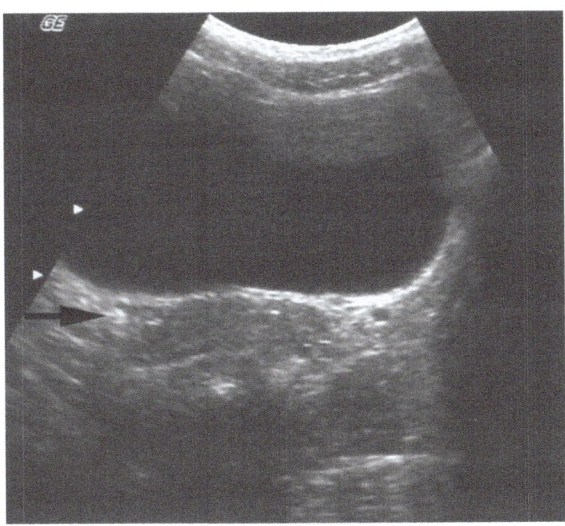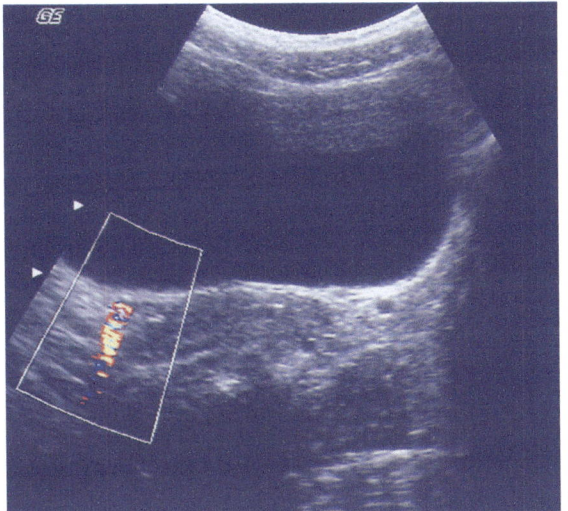

a   b

Fig. 4.15a, b. Ultrasonography of a patient with right renal colic. **a** Hyperechoic zone behind the posterior wall of the bladder without evident acoustic shadowing (*arrow*). **b** Visualization of a twinkling artifact of this area allowing an accurate diagnosis of ureteral lithiasis

In summary, US in suspected acute renal obstruction can depict intrarenal signs of ureteral obstruction but is often limited for specific calculus detection. It requires careful examination of the kidney, but also of the ureterovesical junction and all the ureteral segments visible in between. Despite the use of additional tools such as the transvaginal approach, intrarenal RI measurement, or ureteral jets, Doppler analysis ultrasonographic diagnosis of renal colic may be unreliable. Moreover, ultrasonography of acute obstruction requires an optimal US unit, a cooperative patient, and an experienced radiologist. Thus, at some centers US has not succeeded in replacing the time-honored EU as the initial diagnostic imaging modality in cases of renal colic, except in pregnant women and in patients with contraindications to i.v. injection of contrast medium.

4.3.4
Unenhanced Computed Tomography

Unenhanced CT has emerged as an effective modality for the imaging of renal colic since the pioneering publication by SMITH in 1995 (SMITH et al. 1995). The main advantages of this technique are its great sensitivity in detection of ureteral stone and indirect obstructive signs, with a protocol acquisition requiring no preparation and particularly no CM injection. Currently, CT proves to be superior to EU to diagnose acute lithiasis obstruction and to demonstrate

ureteral stones, providing a differential diagnosis in patients with acute flank pain.

The first patients in the Smith series were explored with incremental CT, but urinary tract CT exploration obviously benefits from helical acquisition technology, notably because it guarantees the absence of respiratory misregistration, whatever the breath-hold quality. The acquisition protocol usually consists of a 5-mm collimation with a 1.5 pitch, without any oral preparation or intravenous injection. If the patient is not able to hold his breath as long as required by the acquisition time, gentle breathing is allowed during lesser pelvis acquisition because it remains relatively immobile during respiration. Multislice CT allows an increased spatial and temporal resolution, since the same volume may be acquired with thinner slices and in a shorter period of time. In selected cases, when the first acquisition does not permit determination of whether a ureteral stone is impacted at the ureterovesical junction or has already migrated into the bladder, a second limited acquisition should be performed in the prone or lateral position (LEVINE et al. 1999). In order to limit pelvis irradiation and duration of examination, some authors suggest performing a single acquisition directly in the prone position. Multiplanar reconstructions play a role only in selected cases, where they may help to precisely determine the intraureteral location of a calcification.

The radiological signs are classified into two groups (Fig. 4.16a, b), i.e., direct (the calculus) and indirect signs of obstruction. All stones, even radiolucent uric acid stones, are hyperdense (MOSTAFAVY

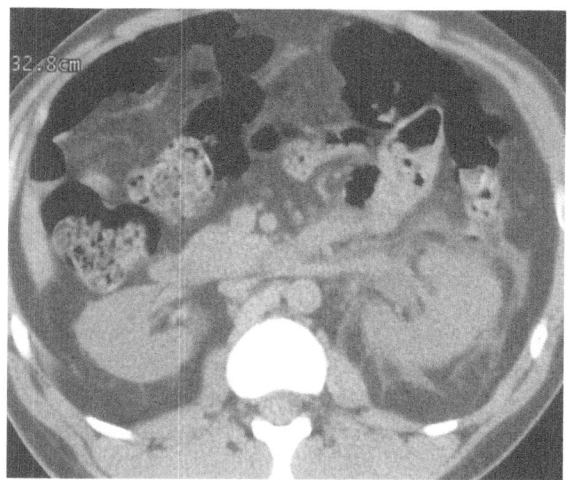
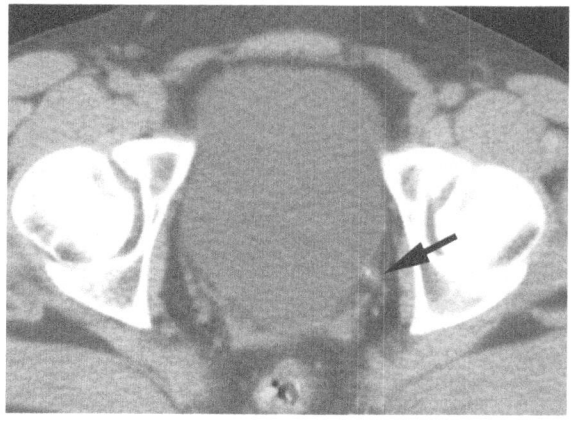

Fig. 4.16a, b. Unenhanced CT in a patient with left renal colic. **a** Slice at the kidney level showing a slightly enlarged left kidney with discrete pelvis dilatation and multiple perirenal and linear soft-tissue densities related to edema and urine extravasation. **b** This slice shows a small stone in the terminal ureter with moderate thickening of the ureteral wall (*arrow*)

et al. 1998), the only exception being stones in HIV patients undergoing "indinavir" therapy (BLAKE et al. 1998). Diagnosis is therefore easy when a dilated ureter is followed downstream to an area of hyperdense, intraluminal structure. CT, owing to its excellent tissue contrast resolution, is highly accurate in distinguishing an intraureteral calculus from a neoplasm, a blood clot, or an extrinsic cause of obstruction. Indirect signs are related to the secondary effects of even mild obstruction on ureter and kidney (Fig. 4.17a–c): moderate hydronephrosis, perirenal fat stranding (probably related to edema and/or urine resorption via local lymphatics), perirenal effusion (manifestation of a fornix rupture), or kidney enlargement, the contralateral side serving as an intrinsic control (KATZ et al. 1994).

It can be difficult to distinguish a ureteral stone from nonureteral calcified structures such as arterial calcifications and phleboliths. Several tools exist to overcome these diagnostic difficulties (see also Chap. 5). First, a careful evaluation of the ureteral course by scrolling through the images on the CT console (rather than reading the films) may help to define the relationship between the suspected stone and ureter. When ureteral dilatation is absent or when patients have little retroperitoneal fat, some authors advocate the use of a multiplanar reformat, with the aim of demonstrating the intraureteral calculus, but even this technique is subject to the same difficulties regarding the low amount of periureteral fat.

The tissue-rim sign is useful in differentiating ureteral calculi from extraurinary calcifications (Fig. 4.18). It represents the thickened wall of the

ureter at the stone level. The sensitivity of this sign for the diagnosis of ureteral stone varies from 50% to 77% (KAWASHIMA et al. 1997; SMITH et al. 1996; HENEGHAN et al. 1997). Inversely, it is highly specific (92%–100%); the rare false-positive diagnoses have been attributed to certain phleboliths with central calcification and a noncalcified wall. It is sometimes difficult to establish whether this sign is present or not, particularly when retroperitoneal fat around the stone is lacking. The presence of a tissue-rim sign seems to be inversely correlated to the stone size. The most likely explanation is that the ureteral wall, even if it is edematous, may be stretched by a large stone.

The "comet" sign usually indicates that a phlebolith is present (BORIDY et al. 1999b). Phleboliths often have a radiolucent center, as known from KUB. With CT, the detection of the radiolucent center can be optimized by a density histogram profile (BELL et al. 1998). Nevertheless, this feature is neither sensitive nor specific and is of limited clinical value. Of higher diagnostic value is the "comet" sign, characterized by a calcification seen in the continuity of a vascular structure running in the transverse plane: This sign has 21% sensitivity and 100% positive predictive value rates for phlebolith diagnosis (TRAUBICI et al. 1999).

As stated above, the less abundant the retroperitoneal fat, the more difficult is the distinction between ureteral stones and phleboliths. The level of confidence in ureteral stone diagnosis is reinforced when indirect signs are present, which is usually the case when the ureteral stone is obstructive. Nevertheless, the indirect signs are not necessarily related to the calcified structure, for example, in the case of a

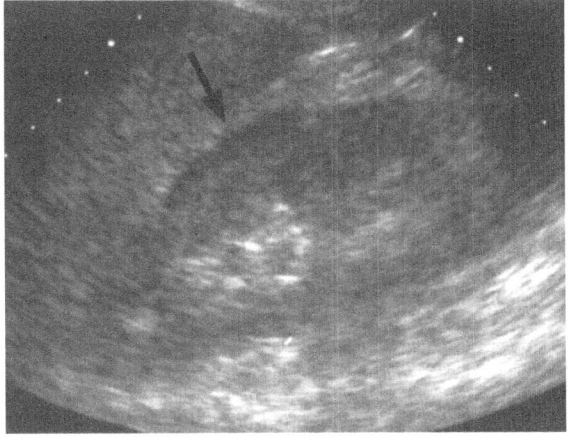
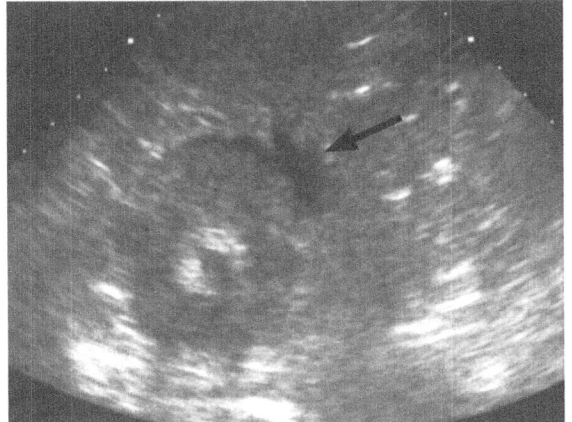
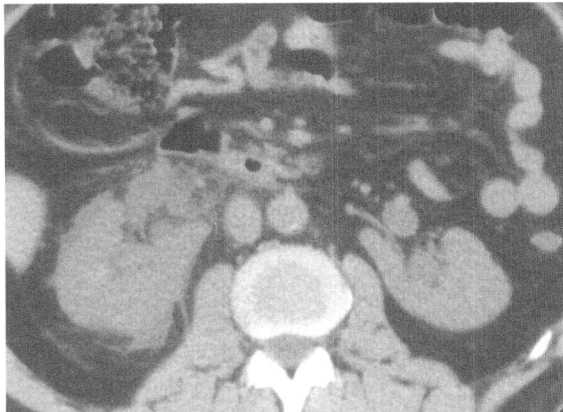

Fig. 4.17a–c. Patient with right renal colic. Axial (a) and transverse (b) ultrasonographic views showing perirenal extravasation (*arrows*). c Unenhanced CT with discrete pelvis dilatation and perirenal standing

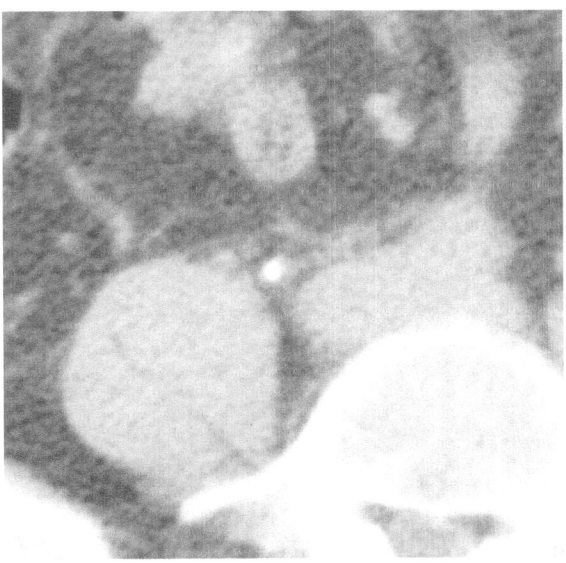

Fig. 4.18. CT example of a rim sign around a right ureteral stone

spontaneous stone passage. This is the reason why Heneghan et al. (Heneghan et al. 1997) do not recommend relying on indirect signs to distinguish a ureteral stone from a phlebolith. Their interpretation algorithm is based on the tissue-rim sign. A calcification is likely to be a stone if the tissue-rim sign is present, whereas the calcification is probably extraurinary if, when the tissue-rim sign is negative, the calcification is less than 4 mm and no indirect sign is present. In fact, the roles of rim and comet-tail signs are discussed by many authors. Rim sign is rarely isolated and the presence or not of this sign and the comet-tail sign is not the main indication of the presence of stones. Interobserver agreement for identification of these signs is low and the presence of secondary signs of acute obstruction (perirenal stranding, renal enlargement, hydronephrosis) are more reliable for the diagnosis (Guest et al. 2001).

If no urinary abnormality is seen, a careful analysis of the abdominal cavity is mandatory, as alternative diagnoses may be considered. As kidney pain fibers are shared with other adjacent organs, a wide range of diseases present clinically with an acute flank pain syndrome. Many of these diseases may be diagnosed with CT, even unenhanced: e.g., appendicitis, sigmoiditis, abdominal aortic aneurysm, pelvic mass torsion, biliary obstruction, and pancreatitis.

Another important limitation of unenhanced CT is its inability to detect renal infarction and renal vein thrombosis, which may sometimes manifest clinically as ureteral colic. In the absence of macroscopic hematuria, a normal CT may be misleadingly comforting. In those selected cases where clinical symptoms are highly suggestive of renal disease and the CT scan is normal or demonstrates only perirenal fat stranding or renal swelling, a second acquisition after intravenous contrast injection should be considered.

In his pioneering study, SMITH postulated that, compared with EU, unenhanced CT was as accurate in the diagnosis of urinary tract obstruction, and even superior in the demonstration of ureteral stone disease (SMITH et al. 1995). Further series have confirmed the excellent performance of CT, with sensitivity and specificity evaluated at about 97%–98% and 95%–98%, respectively (YILMAZ et al. 1998) (SHELEY et al. 1999). CT is now considered the gold standard for the detection of ureteral stone, since it is able to detect calculi as small as 1 mm wide that may be missed by EU when overlying bone or other dense structures are present (SOURTZIS et al. 1999).

CT is more accurate than KUB in measurement of stone size, which has, as already mentioned, a great influence on patient management: When a multiplanar reformat is used, the error rate in stone size measurement is 3.6%, compared with 16% for conventional imaging techniques (OLCOTT et al. 1997). Finally, the CT scout view may constitute a baseline study for patient follow-up and also for treatment planning before lithotripsy or other intervention. In the series of CHU, approximately 50% of ureteral stones were visible on the scout view, and large stones not visible on the scout view were likely composed of uric acid or xanthine (CHU et al. 1999). These authors considered that the need for obtaining a KUB at the time of diagnosis could be limited to cases with medium-size stones (5–9 mm). Investigators from the same institution compared KUB with unenhanced CT in the detection of ureteral calculi and showed that KUB sensitivity was only 45%, based on the report made prior to the CT scan, and rose to only 59% after retrospective reading, even unblinded to CT examination (LEVINE et al. 1997).

Besides its excellent diagnostic performance, CT has several other advantages: It is technically simple, and the patient stays in the radiological department usually less than 15 min compared with the several hours required for EU. Physician presence is not required during the examination since no CM is injected: As long as the raw data of the helical acquisition are not deleted, a retrospective reconstruction using overlapping thin sections (aimed at optimizing multiplanar reformation in the difficult diagnostic cases) can be performed at any desired level after the patient has left the radiological department (Fig. 4.19a, b). The learning curve is rather brief, especially when compared with that for US. The extraobserver variability is low,

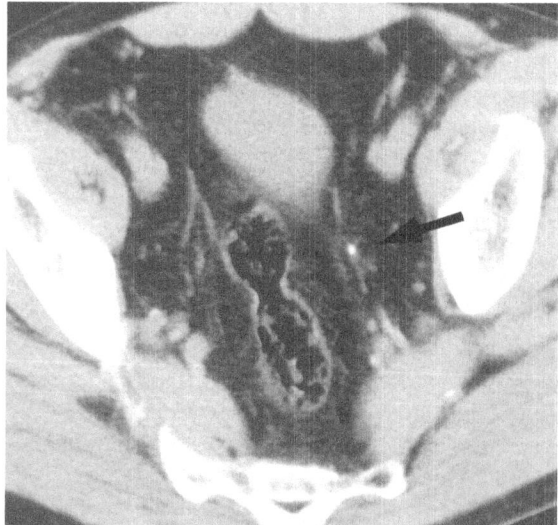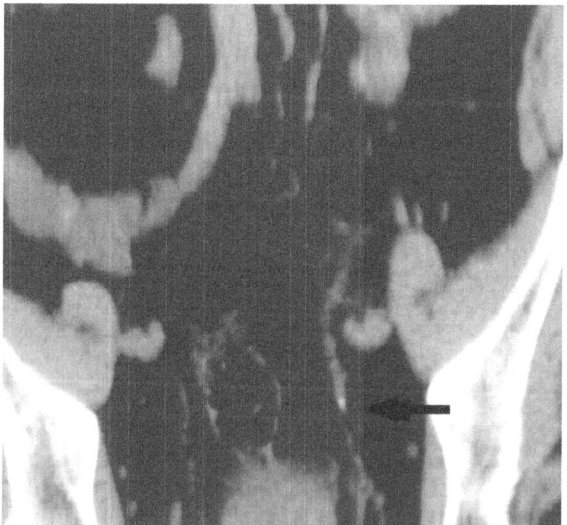

a   b

Fig. 4.19a, b. CT demonstration of a ureteral stone by coronal reconstruction (*arrows*)

even when less experienced readers are tested (FREED et al. 1998). Some of the alternative diagnoses, such as appendicitis and sigmoiditis, would require a significantly longer exploration time with US. Since no oral or i.v. CM is used, unenhanced CT of the urinary tract does not interfere with any further imaging modality. Its overall cost is similar to that of EU (DALLA PALMA et al. 2001). Finally, helical CT provides essential information in case of suspected severe complications of acute urinary obstruction, such as rupture of the urinary tract or infected or uninfected urinoma (Figs. 4.20a, b, 4.21a–c).

One of the main limitations of CT is the absence of functional information provided. Urologists, who base the nature and timing of treatment more or less on the importance of delayed excretion of CM on EU, may criticize the inability of unenhanced CT to determine the degree of obstruction. However, BORIDY et

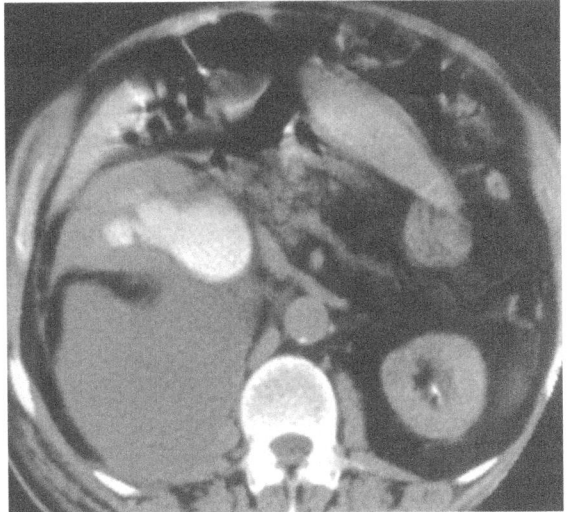

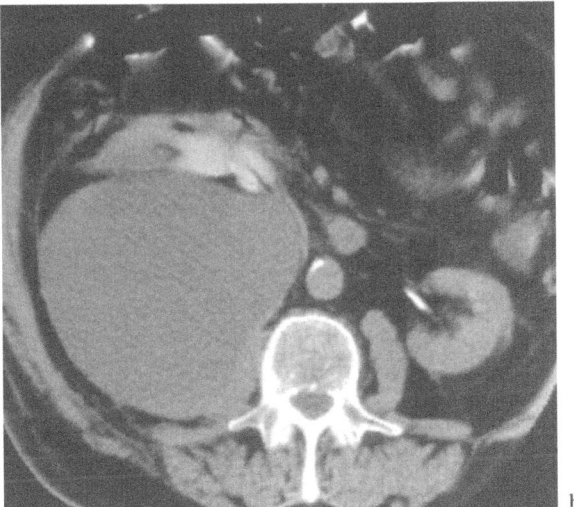

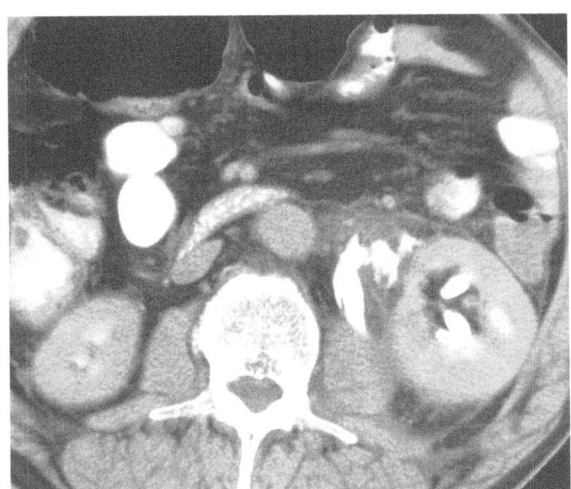

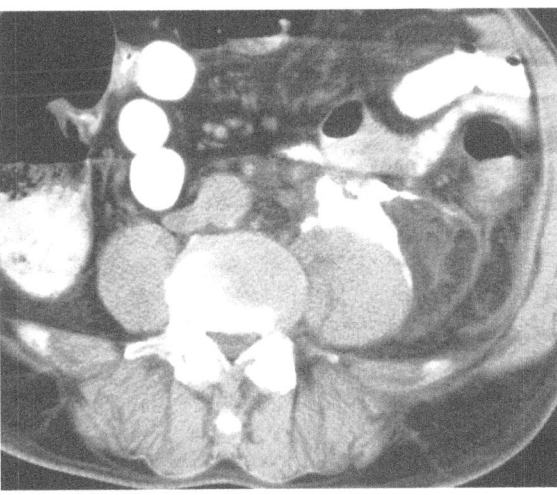

Fig. 4.20a, b. CT demonstration of severe perirenal and retroperitoneal extravasation of urine and contrast medium

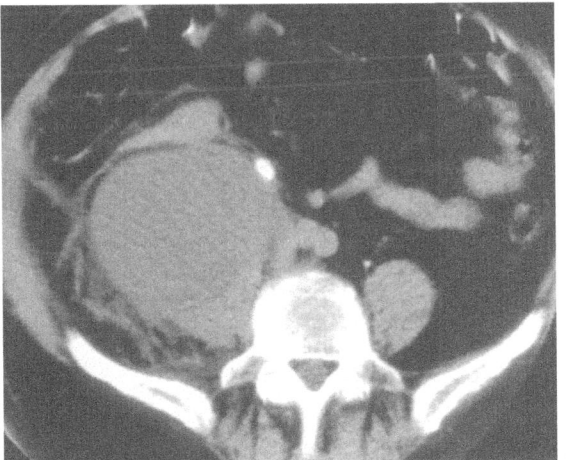

Fig. 4.21a–c. CT demonstration of a retroperitoneal urinoma after right renal colic. Large liquid mass developed in the psoas compartment with important displacement of the right kidney and compression of the ureter

al. have proven that the importance of perirenal edema can be used to predict the degree of ureteral obstruction with an accuracy of 94% (BORIDY et al. 1999a). A previous study from the same institution stated showed that perirenal stranding was more prominent in patients whose stones migrated spontaneously (TAKAHASHI et al. 1998). The authors proposed the hypothesis that abundant perirenal stranding was positively correlated with increased pressure in the collecting system, which is considered to be the most important factor conditioning stone migration.

A final point of discussion is the radiation dose. CT scanning is a widely available and effective diagnostic tool, but it also entails significant patient irradiation; this could become worrying in recurrent lithiasis, which is not uncommon. Thus, radiologists and clinicians should be aware of the dose delivered by a standard examination, particularly in young women. The values reported in the literature vary on several points (units, CT protocol). On average, the mean dose of exposure of CT is two fold superior to EU dose (DALLA PALMA et al. 2001). A protocol using a high pitch (more than 1.5) and reduced slice thickness (3 mm) allows an acceptable compromise between performance and radiation dose (DALLA PALMA et al. 2001).

4.3.5
Magnetic Resonance Imaging

MRI is theoretically applicable for renal colic exploration, given its ability for coronal representation of the urinary tract, particularly if the sequences initially developed for MR cholangiopancreatography are used. These sequences allow a "urographic" effect and are also very sensitive in the depiction of perirenal inflammation or extravasation. Stone appears as a signal void at the tip of the dilated ureter (REGAN et al. 1996).

Perirenal and periureteral hyperintensity, commonly observed in acute urinary obstruction, may represent edema, lymphatic distension, or free fluid from a fornix rupture (REGAN et al. 1997). Diagnosis of ureteral stones can be difficult because it may be hidden by the surrounding urine hyperintensity, particularly with heavily T_2-weighted turbo spin-echo sequences (HASTE). (GAETA et al. 1999). The use of gadolinium-enhanced MR urography (with three-dimensional flash sequence) improves the evaluation of patients with suspected acute renal colic and improves the detection of stones compared with EU, with a sensitivity and a specificity between 95% and 100 % (SUDAH et al. 2001). SUDAH et al. compared the

performance of MR urography with that of unenhanced helical CT (SUDAH et al. 2002). The sensitivity and specificity were comparable for ureteral stone detection and diagnosis of acute obstruction. Advantages of helical CT are short imaging time, better evaluation of the stone size, and easier differential diagnosis with phleboliths. MR urography allows better functional evaluation and an improved visualization of perirenal stranding and extravasation. MR urography may also be of interest for detecting stones in HIV patients. Conversely, as the diagnosis of a stone is being based on the presence of a filling defect, this technique does not allow a differential diagnosis with clots or ureteral tumor.

Even if MRI is of a certain clinical interest in this indication, its use will remain limited by the problems of cost-effectiveness and availability, especially in an emergency setting. The most obvious clinical use concerns the pregnant woman, who may benefit, in selected cases remaining unresolved after US, from this nonirradiating exploration (Fig. 4.22a, b).

4.3.6
Strategy

Three types of diagnostic tool (EU, US, CT) theoretically are in competition in the evaluation of acute flank plain in cases where the referring clinician considers a radiological exploration to be necessary (OTAL et al. 2001). Among them, EU is considered the most invasive, because of the use of ionizing radiation and CM injection. US, combined with KUB, can be considered less invasive but has a higher rate of false-positive (dilated, nontensed cavities) and false-negative (tensed, nondilated cavities) diagnoses. These two approaches are less effective than CT for the diagnosis of ureteral stone. However, CT has limited availability in some centers and entails a radiation dose at least equal or superior to that of EU. Nevertheless, fast CT evaluation facilitates correct triage in the emergency department. Furthermore, CT often eliminates the need for further diagnostic imaging, since it allows many differential (urinary and extraurinary) diagnoses. Since CT has proven to be an effective technique in the evaluation of these differential diagnoses, it is gaining rapid and wide acceptance by referring clinicians as first-line examination of abdominal pain of uncertain origin. The broadening of clinical criteria leading to unenhanced CT was noticed by CHEN, who explained this phenomenon by a somewhat inappropriate patient selection and increased physician awareness of the value of unenhanced helical CT to

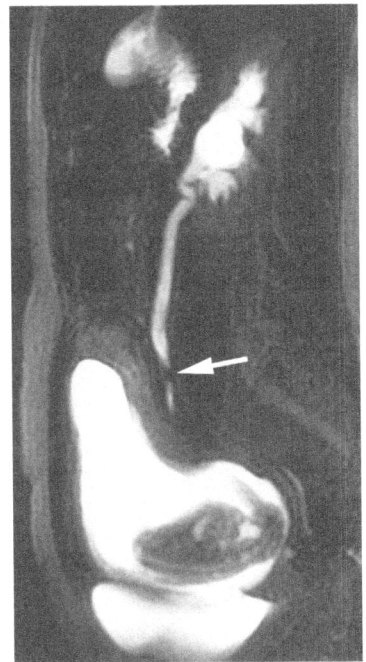
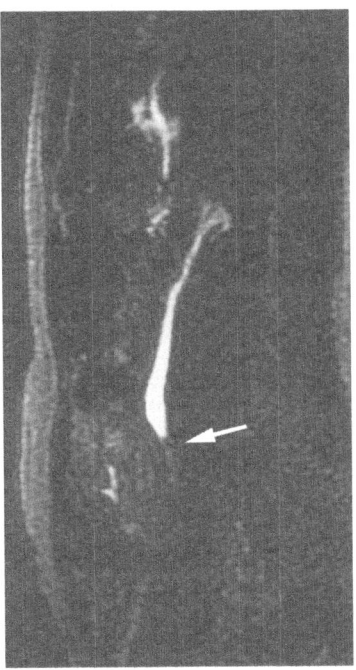

Fig. 4.22a, b. MR urography in a pregnant women with right renal colic. Oblique views with a single-shot fast spin-echo sequence showing moderate dilatation and absence of signal in the stone area (*white arrow*)

establish the source of the patient's symptoms (CHEN et al. 1999). The shift of the indications was reflected by the statistically significant increase in extraurinary lesions and the decreasing rate of ureteral stone detection when two consecutive series of patients were compared. If the increase in prescription of CT for any acute abdominal pain, even if not suggestive of renal colic, is confirmed, it will probably lead to a wider use of contrast media, since an increased number of unenhanced CT scans will reveal unexplained or incomplete findings. Appendicitis and sigmoiditis may generally be diagnosed on unenhanced CT performed for the evaluation of renal colic, inasmuch as intra-abdominal fat tissue is sufficiently abundant. This is not the case with other differential diagnoses: The problem of renal infarction has already been mentioned. Other conditions such as renal infection or carcinoma, pancreatitis, and visceral ischemia are diagnosed more confidently with CM injection.

In conclusion, we propose a decision algorithm which has to be modulated according to the equipment available and expertise at a given institution (Fig. 4.23):

- A simple and noncomplicated renal colic does not require urgent imaging and must be treated medically. US combined with KUB can be postponed and performed on an outpatient basis.
- In case of intense or persisting pain despite medical treatment, oligoanuria, or undetermined diagnosis, an unenhanced CT should be performed if available, leading in most case to urologic treatment.
- The cases remaining unexplained after US will certainly benefit less from EU than from unenhanced CT, which is highly effective in both stone detection and alternative diagnosis. CM injection should be considered in selected cases (suspicion of renal infarction, renal carcinoma, pyelonephritis).

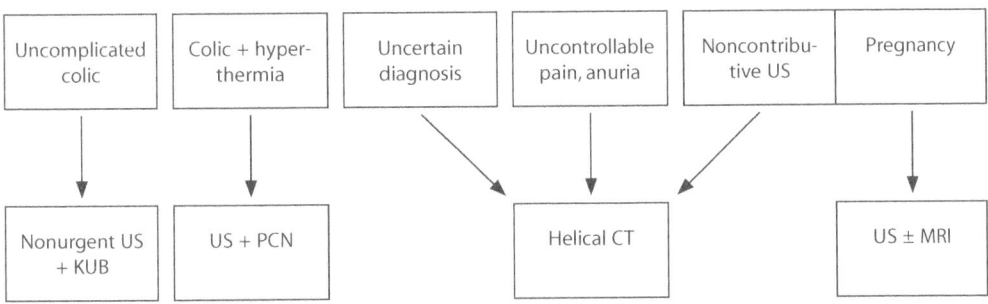

Fig. 4.23. Suggested decisional algorithm of imaging modalities according to the different clinical presentations of renal colic (PCN= percutaneous nephrostomy)

• Evaluation of acute flank pain in pregnant women relies essentially on US. Unresolved cases will benefit from an MRI examination rather than limited EU (GRENIER et al. 2000).

• When the renal colic is associated with fever US is essential, as it is an effective and fast imaging modality in the diagnosis of pyonephrosis, which indicates a prompt urine drainage.

• EU may still be indicated in exceptional unresolved cases. MR urography can replace EU in situations where the latter is contraindicated or undesirable (SUDAH et al. 2000).

It was recently demonstrated that unenhanced CT improves clinicians' diagnostic confidence and thus their deciding between discharge with medical treatment or intervention. It also allows unexpected alternative diagnoses (ABRAMSON et al. 2000).

4.4
Chronic Obstruction

Imaging techniques must depict two types of information:
1. Information about the impact of the obstruction on the upstream urinary tract from an anatomic and functional point of view. This allows evaluation of the possibilities for functional recovery after treatment.
2. Information on the etiology of the obstruction, developed in the next chapters

4.4.1
Excretory Urography

Urographic modifications in chronic obstruction depict the secondary functional disturbances as well as morphological modifications on the urinary tract and renal parenchyma (TALNER 1990a,b; O'REILLY and RICKARDS 1986).

4.4.1.1
Functional Changes

The main functional sign is delayed contrast excretion, which may be quite variable in time (see Fig. 4.24a–c). In case of severe destruction of the renal parenchyma, minimal or no urinary tract opacification occurs even with high-dose nephrotomography techniques. Due to the reduction of ureteral peristalsis, ureteral opacifi-

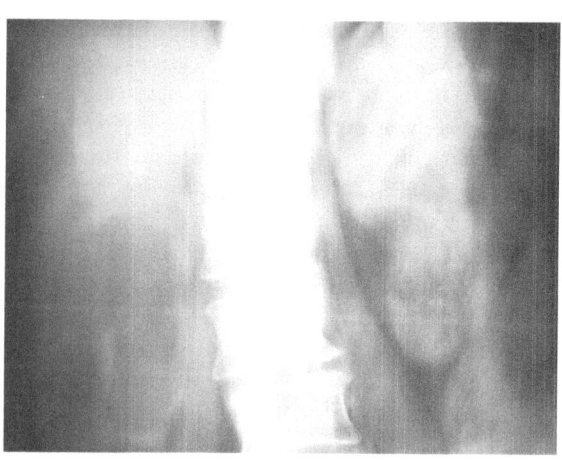

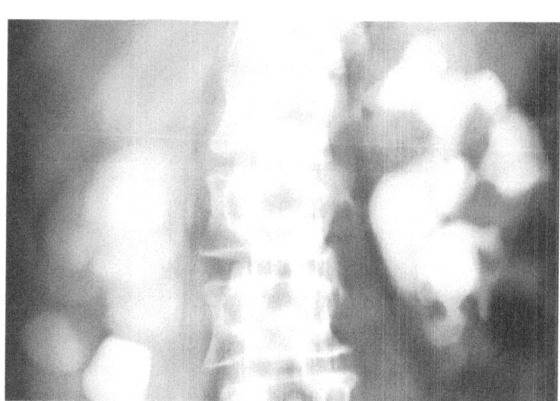

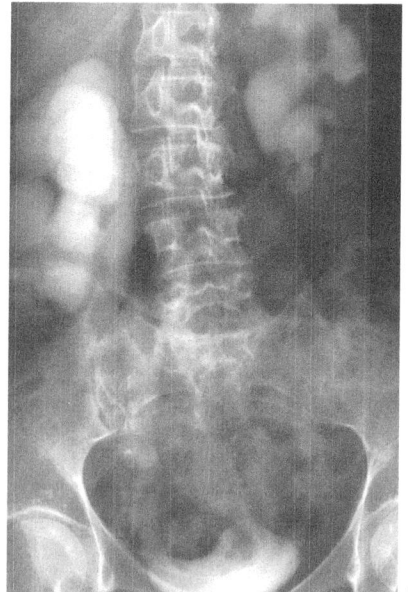

Fig. 4.24. a Early nephrotomogram (1 min post CM injection): Right renal parenchyma is replaced by several "soap bubbles" corresponding to dilated nonopacified calices with important thinning of the opacified parenchyma. **b** 10 min nephrotomogram shows late opacification of the right dilated calices. The left cavities are opacified in time, dilated, but without evident obstruction. Calices are blunted, probably due to post-obstructive atrophy. **c** Late film (1 h) shows right ureterohydronephrosis with pelvic obstruction

cation is delayed and can be improved by a change in position of the patient (prone or erect position), because of the high gravity of CM. The probability of obtaining sufficient opacification of the urinary tract downstream to the level of obstruction is related to the importance of this opacification delay. The CM radiopacity in the obstructed ureter is variable, depending mainly on the degree of obstruction.

4.4.1.2
Morphological Changes

The kidney presents two types of modifications related to its size and structure (Fig. 4.25a–e). The size of the kidney may be normal, increased or decreased. The renal parenchymal opacification is variable in density but most frequently remains normal. The nephrographic phase may show cortical thinning and/or round and bullous lacunar images corresponding to a negative picture of the dilated calices. Depending on the degree of dilation, this "negative pyelogram" can take the form of "soap bubbles" or "rim nephrogram". In some cases, the crescent sign may be observed; it corresponds to the compression of collecting tubes in the medulla collapsed by the obstruction.

Modifications of the excretory tract are variable in function of the degree and the level of obstruction.

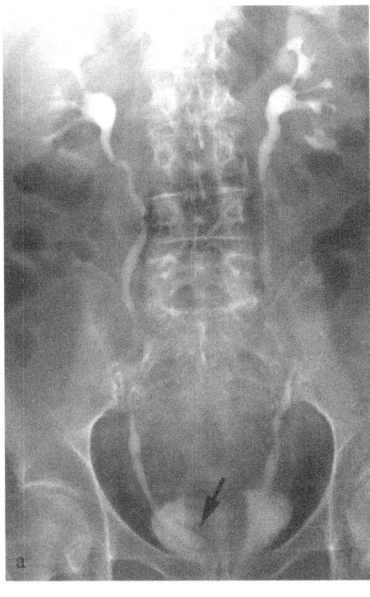
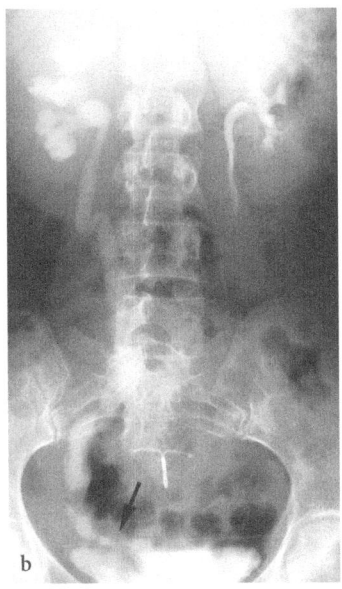

Fig. 4.25-a–e. Several urographic examples of chronic ureteral obstruction. a Discrete obstruction of the right ureter without dilatation related to right ureterocele (*arrow*). b Moderate ureterohydronephrosis secondary to old ureteral stone (*arrow*). c Idiopathic bilateral megaureter with right ureteral dilatation and left ureterohydronephrosis. d Bilateral obstruction due to bladder wall inflammatory thickening: ureterohydronephrosis on the right side and mild ureteral left dilatation. e Mute left kidney with huge left flank mass. Parenchyma is replaced by liquid-dense masses with thin wall, representing the destroyed parenchyma (*arrowheads*)

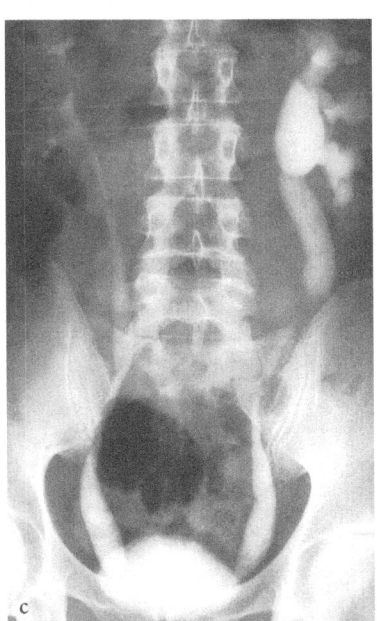
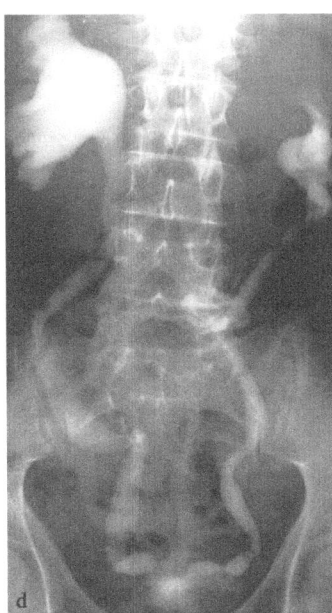
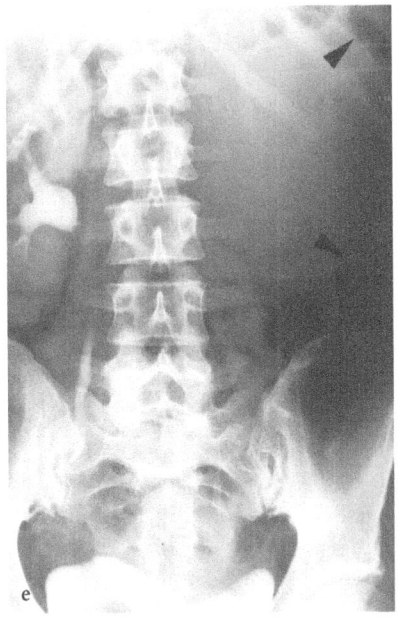

Initially, they are characterized by a denser and per-sistent urinary tract opacification compared with the opposite side, with disappearance of physiological stenoses and external impressions: The expression "too nice image" is often used. As obstruction per-sists, it leads to a convex aspect of the calices, particu-larly at the level of the fornices, and to progressive collapse of the papillae. The excretory urinary tract becomes progressively dilated from the calices down-stream to the site of obstruction with variable dilata-tion and winding, often better demonstrated with delayed prone or erect films. At an advanced stage, the more recumbent dilated calices are opacified first and show the pattern of a "ball pyelogram". Erect films may show a horizontal level between unopaci-fied urine and CM.

Like acute obstruction, chronic obstruction can occasionally lead to urine extravasation secondary to a fornix rupture (Fig. 4.26). A rare consequence is the development of a urinoma in the perirenal space (FRIEDENBERG et al. 1989).

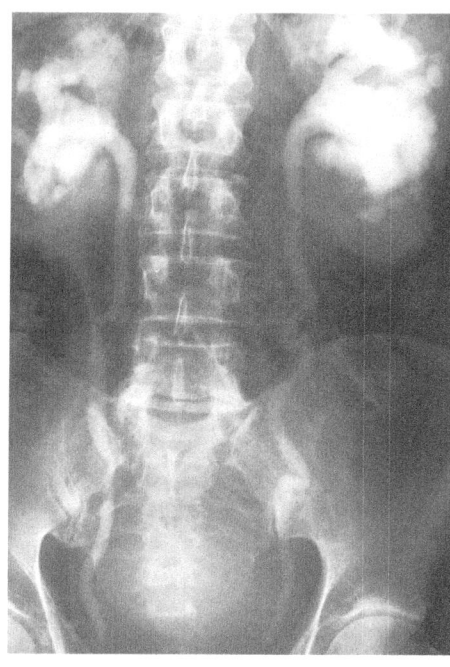

Fig. 4.26. Bilateral sinusal extravasation in a patient with chronic obstruction related to prostatic hypertrophy: moder-ate bilateral ureterohydronephrosis

4.4.2
Ultrasound

As chronic obstruction always leads to dilation of the excretory urinary tract, the diagnostic utility of US in that clinical setting is not discussed. While it permits a confident diagnosis of urinary tract dilatation, it also helps to characterize the degree and even the level and the cause of obstruction. Moreover, it allows direct or indirect needle guidance for interventional procedures.

Ultrasonographic measurement may reveal a small, normal, or enlarged kidney. The thickness of the renal cortex may initially be normal, but in advanced cases the renal parenchyma becomes atro-phic. In severe cases, the renal parenchyma totally disappears and the kidney is replaced by dilated cali-ces separated by thin septa (MOSTBECK et al. 2001).

Early or moderate obstruction is represented by mild splaying of the usually compact central echo complex which is replaced by echo-free tubular structures corresponding to the dilated collecting system. In case of severe obstruction, US shows large fluid-filled rounded areas with septa and disappear-ance of the renal sinus echo complex. Three catego-ries of dilatation were previously described in this chapter (ELLENBOGEN et al. 1978) (Fig. 4.27a–c).

Usually, the collecting system is totally echo free. Echogenic material within the collecting system can be seen in case of hemorrhage or pyonephrosis, but

absence of echoes does not exclude these diagnoses (Fig. 4.28a, b).

Whenever urinary tract obstruction is present an attempt should be made to determine the site and cause of obstruction. Careful examination makes it possible, particularly in thin patients, to follow the dilated ureter downstream in spite of overlying bowel gas. Presence of proximal dilation indicates a down-stream obstruction; visualization of the lumbar por-tion eliminates a UPJ obstruction. Visualization of a dilated ureter beyond the iliac vessels corresponds to a distal obstruction which most often can be stud-ied through a full bladder. In practice, the causes of obstruction are best diagnosed with other imaging modalities.

The limitations of US are well known (AMIS et al. 1982). In chronic obstructions, false-negative find-ings occur in about 2% or 3 % in case of minimal dil-atation (TALNER et al. 1981), which could have great clinical impact, particularly in azotemic patients with renal failure (MAILLET et al. 1986).

Many conditions may simulate obstruction, but the majority of false-positive cases are represented mainly by prominent extra-renal pelvis, peri-pelvic cysts (AMIS and CRONAN 1988), and over-diuresis with distended bladder. These conditions were previ-ously described in this chapter.

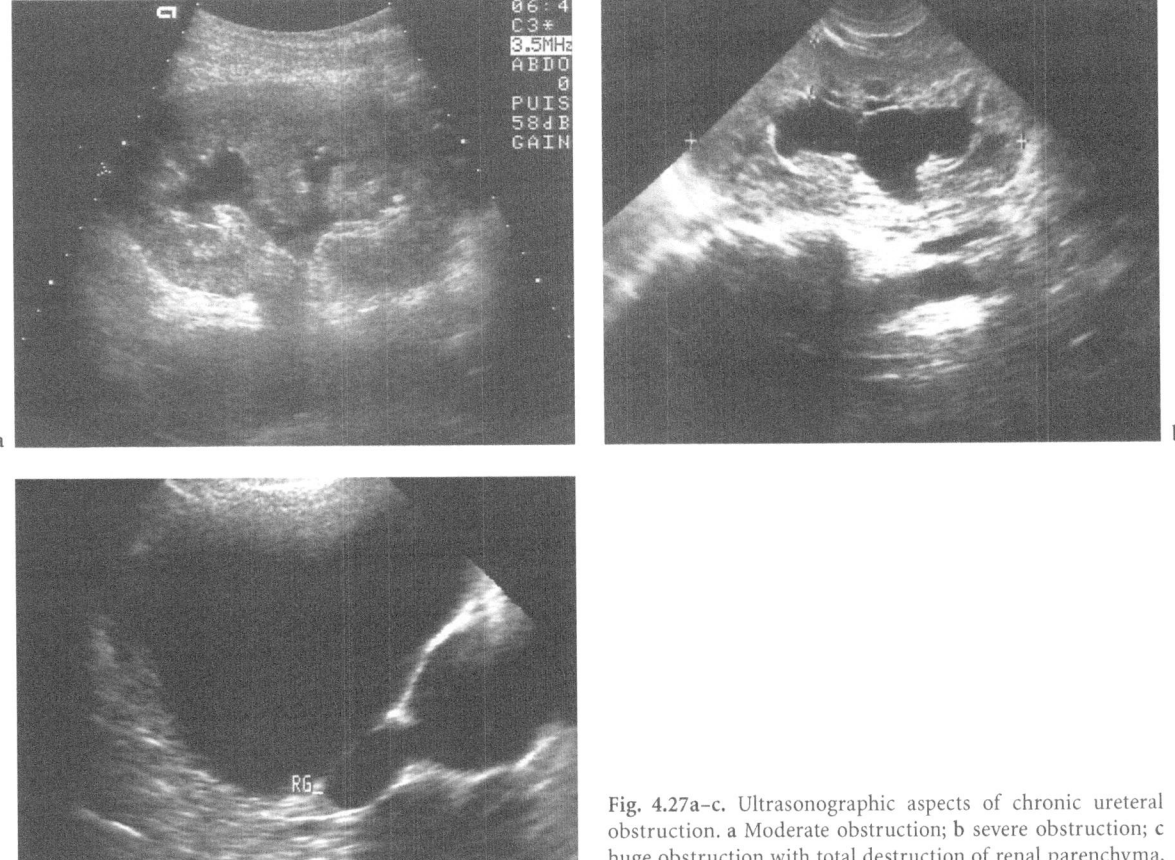

Fig. 4.27a–c. Ultrasonographic aspects of chronic ureteral obstruction. a Moderate obstruction; b severe obstruction; c huge obstruction with total destruction of renal parenchyma, which is replaced by liquid masses

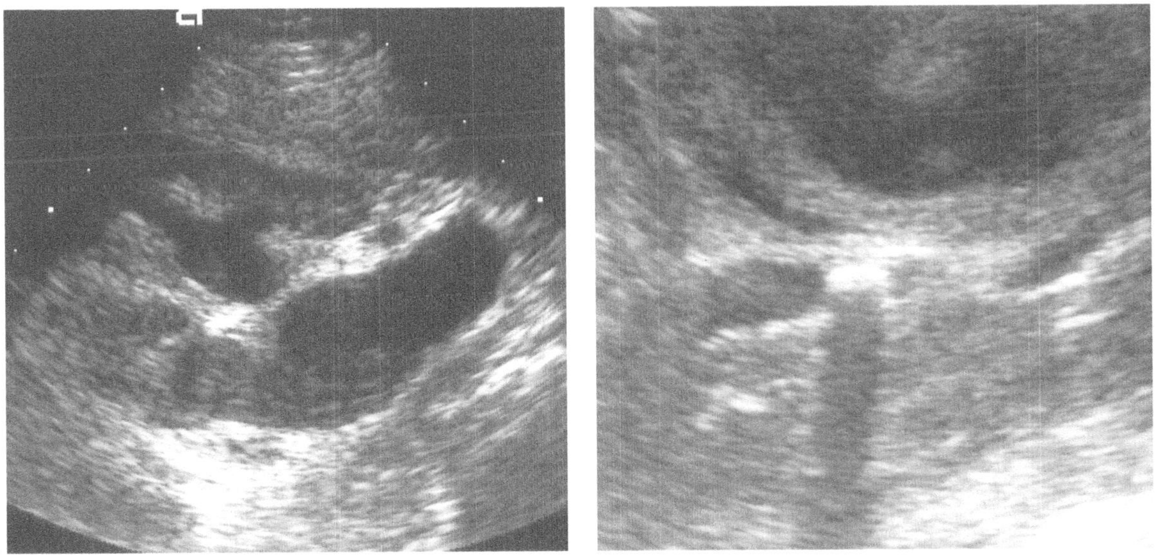

Fig. 4.28a, b. Ultrasonographic aspect of pyonephrosis. a Dilatation of left upper urinary tract with echogenic urine in the pelvis and proximal ureter. b Stone in the left lumbar ureter with ureteral dilatation

4.4.3
Computed Tomography

Computed tomography plays an increasing role in patients with chronic ureteral obstruction (Bosniak et al. 1982; Megibow et al. 1982). Its main role, even in nonfunctioning kidneys, is in determining the cause of obstruction as it permits good depiction of anatomic details of the dilated lumen, the ureteral wall, and the periureteral atmosphere. In difficult cases, CT-guided needle biopsy of the stenotic area may allow the distinction between a benign and a malignant lesion (Barbaric and McIntosh 1981).

Dilated collecting structures may be clearly visualized on unenhanced CT. Calices are seen as rounded fluid-filled defects of water attenuation. The pelvis bulges anteriorly, and the hydroureter can be followed downstream as a water-dense tubular structure until the obstruction area. The distinction between normal aspect, mild dilation, and moderate obstruction may be difficult. In severe obstruction, the kidney is replaced by multiple water-dense masses and CM injection allows good evaluation of renal parenchymal thickness (Fig. 4.29). Delayed scan may show variable opacification of the urinary tract with layering of CM in the dependent portions of calices, pelvis, and ureter. In case of ureterectasis, ureteral wall thickening with CM enhancement is frequently observed, which is associated with inflammatory edema, hypervascularization, and possibly muscle layer proliferation (Fig. 4.30) Finally, CT is

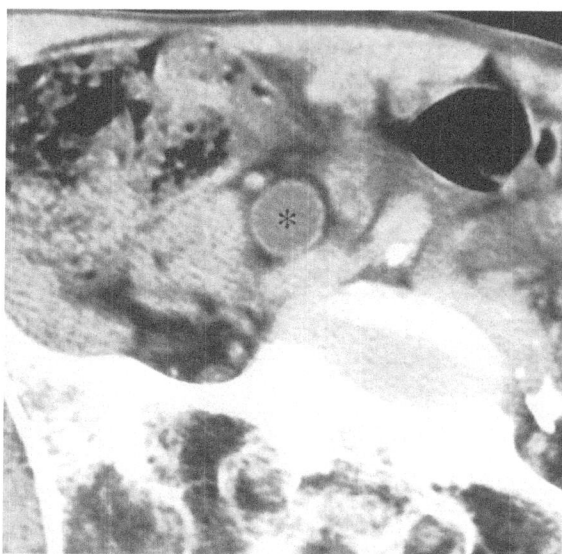

Fig. 4.30. Late CT slice after CM injection showing a dilatation of the lumbar ureter (*asterisk*) and thickened and enhanced ureteral wall

useful to detect some complications of chronic ureteral obstruction such as extravasation or urinoma (Fig. 4.31a–c). CT technical improvements allow 3D urinary tract reconstructions, making it possible to build a true CT-negative urography even in case of contraindication to CM (Fig. 4.32). Thus, excellent frontal, oblique, and profile views of the ureter can be obtained, similar to classical EU (Lemaitre et al. 2000) (Fig. 4.33a–c). Besides positive or negative 3D visualization of the upper urinary tract, post-processing techniques also allow clarification of the cause of obstruction (Figs. 4.34a, b, 4.35a, b).

4.4.4
Retrograde Pyelography (Joffre et al. 1990)

In chronic ureteral obstruction, retrograde pyelography (RUP) was used largely to identify the exact site of obstruction, especially where EU failed. The use of this invasive technique diminished markedly with the improvement of EU and, more recently, the development of new imaging modalities. In fact, the current main use of RUP is the first step of retrograde ureteral catheterization, which allows fast urine drainage, prevents further damage to the kidney, and provides improvement of the patient's condition in preparation for definitive treatment. RUP makes it possible to determine the length of the obstructed segment and the status of the ureter distal to the obstruction, but sometimes it does not give any information

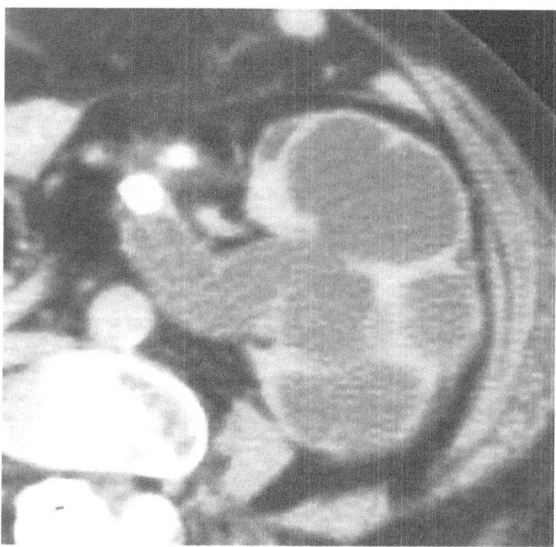

Fig. 4.29. CT slice of a post-lithiasis chronic obstruction of the left kidney: ureterohydronephrosis with pelvicaliceal dilatation, destruction, and important decrease in parenchymal thickness

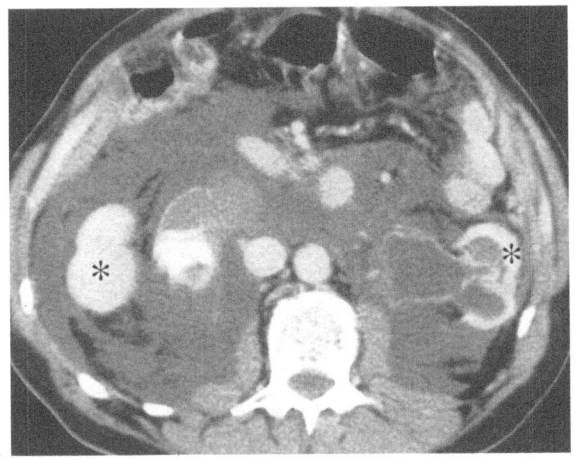

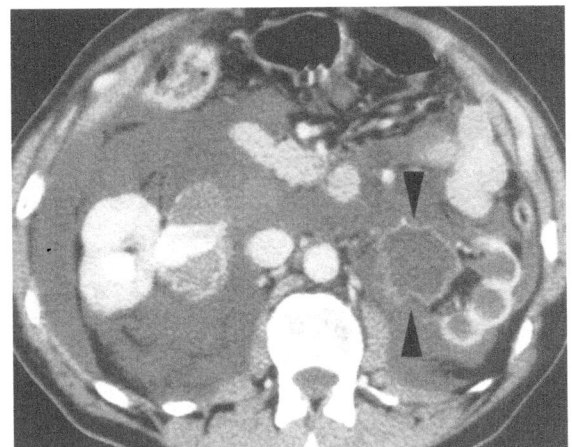

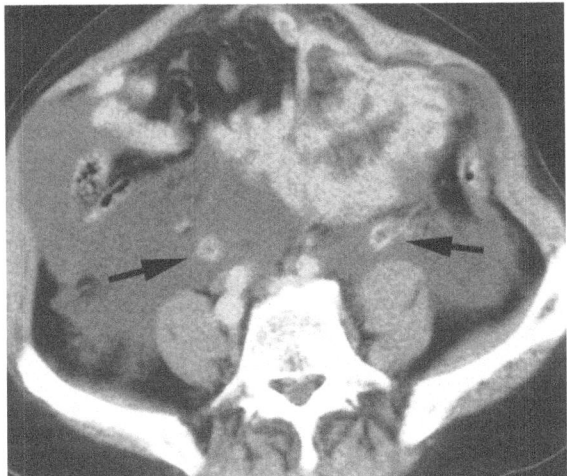

Fig. 4.31a–c. Urinous ascites in a patient with bilateral chronic obstruction. **a, b** Diffuse perirenal and intraperitoneal collection surrounding atrophic, poorly functional kidneys with dilated urinary tract (*asterisks*). On the right side a discrete opacification is noted. The left kidney is mute and the pelvis wall is visible surrounded by urine (*arrowheads*). **c** Both ureters are visible, moderately dilated. The ureteral wall is thickened (*arrows*)

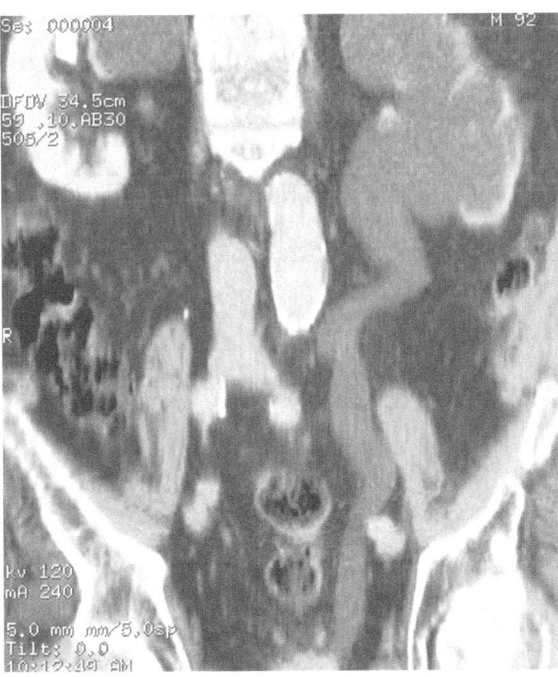

Fig. 4.32. CT frontal reconstruction of the dilated and left urinary tract in a case of left ureterohydronephrosis secondary to bladder tumor

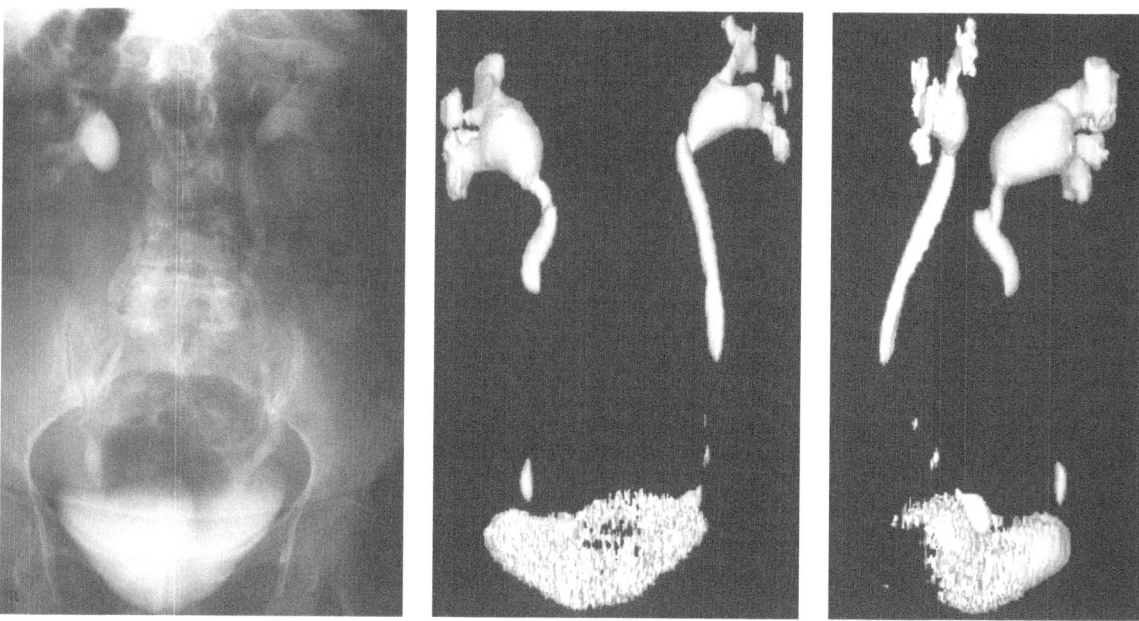

Fig. 4.33a–c. Comparative EU and CT views in a case of bilateral ureterohydronephrosis secondary to a uterine fibroma. **a** EU showing the bilateral obstruction and the uterine mass. **b, c** Frontal and oblique CT views after SSD reconstruction

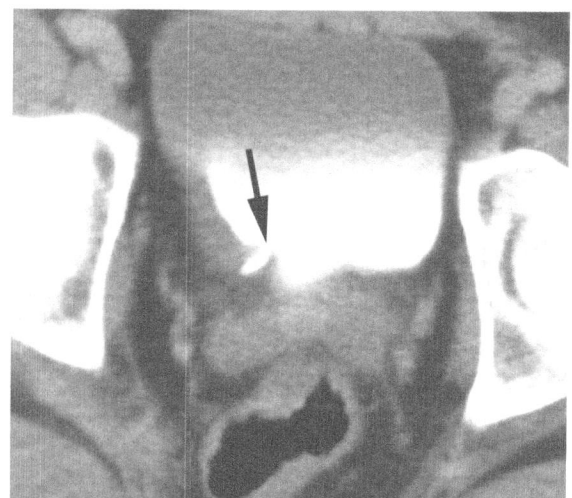

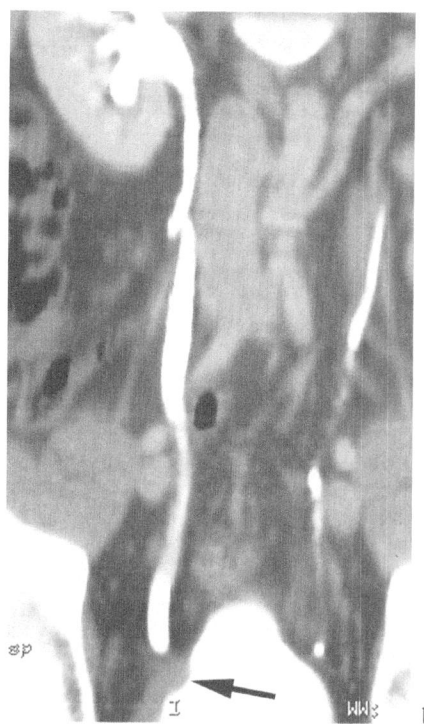

Fig. 4.34a, b. CT aspect of a moderate chronic right ureteral obstruction secondary to a bladder tumor. **a** Axial view showing encasement of the terminal ureter by the thickened tumoral bladder wall (*arrow*). **b** MPR reconstruction giving a urographic view of the dilated ureter up to the bladder tumor (*arrow*)

a 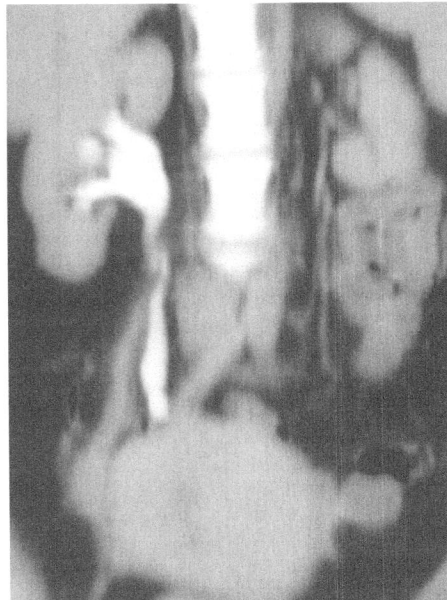 b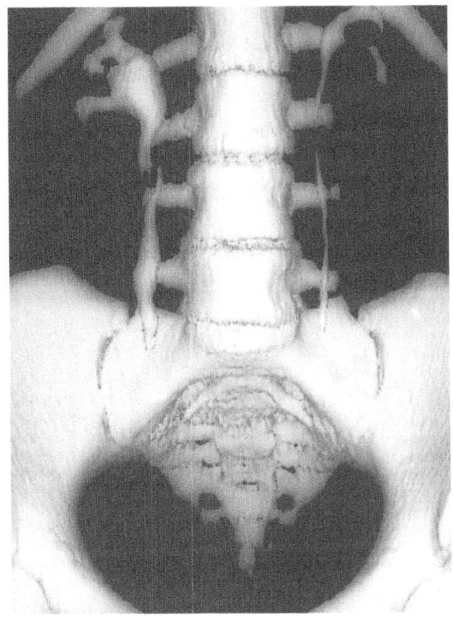

Fig. 4.35a, b. Frontal CT reconstruction in a patient with right moderate ureterohydronephrosis related to a uterine mass. a MIP; b SSD

about the upstream segment of the ureter. Ureteral wall changes in the stenosis area may suggest some specific cause of obstruction (Fig. 4.36a–d). The use of RUP should also be considered for imaging the collecting system in autosomal dominant polycystic kidney disease. EU is not contributive in case of renal failure, and modern imaging modalities are often equivocal in this situation. This technique allows more accurate diagnosis of obstruction, radiolucent lithiasis, and ureteral tumors.

4.4.5
Antegrade Pyelography and Pressure Flow Studies

Antegrade pyelography allows opacification of the collecting system by percutaneous puncture and injection of CM. Like RUP, and for the same reasons, the current main usefulness of antegrade pyelography is to guide any subsequent percutaneous uroradiological procedures and mainly percutaneous nephrostomy (Fig. 4.37a–d).

Antegrade pyelography improves visualization of the site of obstruction and can provide useful anatomic details about the stenosis area (length, edges, aspect of the ureteral wall, presence of fistula) (Fig. 4.38). However, in severe stenosis, antegrade pyelography does not allow opacification of the ureter distal to the stenosis, and retrograde studies are often needed.

Antegrade puncture of the collecting system

allows urine sampling and flow pressure studies. Its use for urodynamic evaluation is considered largely to be a valuable contribution to the investigation of obstructive uropathy, associated, nevertheless, with some drawbacks and pitfalls (O'REILLY and RICKARDS 1986). Some groups consider it practical for differentiating between urinary tract obstruction and dilation without obstruction (DJURRHUS and STAGE 1976). With a perfusion rate of 10 ml/min, obstructive pressure is considered normal if less than 15 cm H_2O and obstructive if above 22 cm H_2O (WHITAKER 1978b). Between 15 and 22 cm H_2O, the results have to be regarded as equivocal (PFISTER et al. 1981). However, the wide use of these flow pressure studies is currently not well accepted by most uroradiologists.

4.4.6
Magnetic Resonance Imaging

Until now, MR Imaging has not been frequently used in cases of ureteral disorder and particularly urinary tract obstruction. However, this technique may easily demonstrate upper urinary tract dilation on conventional sequences: A dilated collecting system may be visualized as low signal intensity on T_1-weighted images and as high signal intensity on T_2-weighted images. 3D acquisition allows easy axial and coronal visualization of the dilated cavities and sometimes of the level and the cause of obstruction

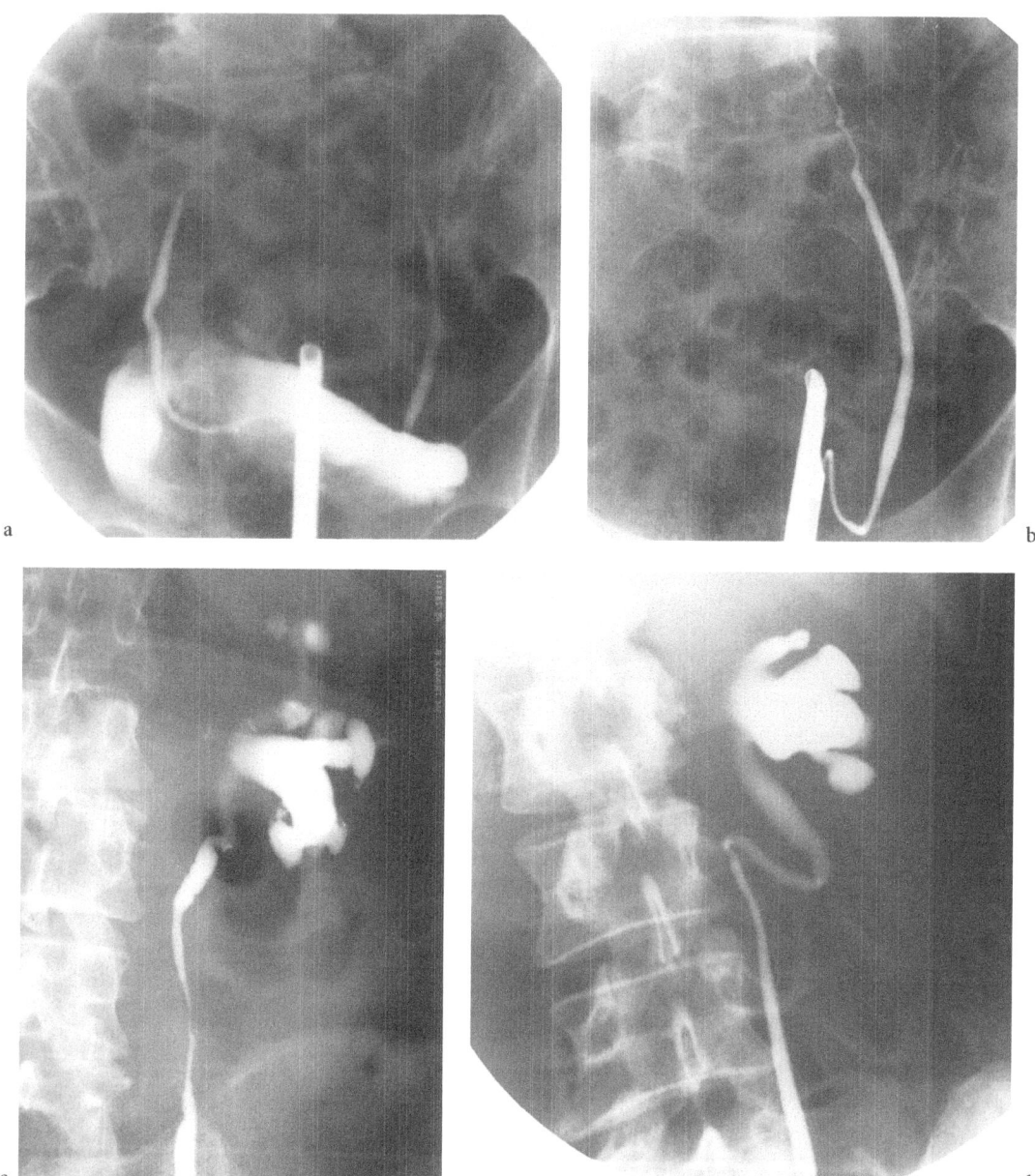

Fig. 4.36a–d. Several examples of ureteral opacification by RUP. **a, b** Bilateral retroperitoneal neoplastic obstruction with absence of opacification beyond the irregular narrowing. **c** Left ureterohydronephrosis related to an extrinsic stenosis of the lumbar ureter due to benign RPF. **d** Left ureterohydronephrosis secondary to an angulated narrowing of the lumbar ureter, attributed to an aberrant left polar renal artery

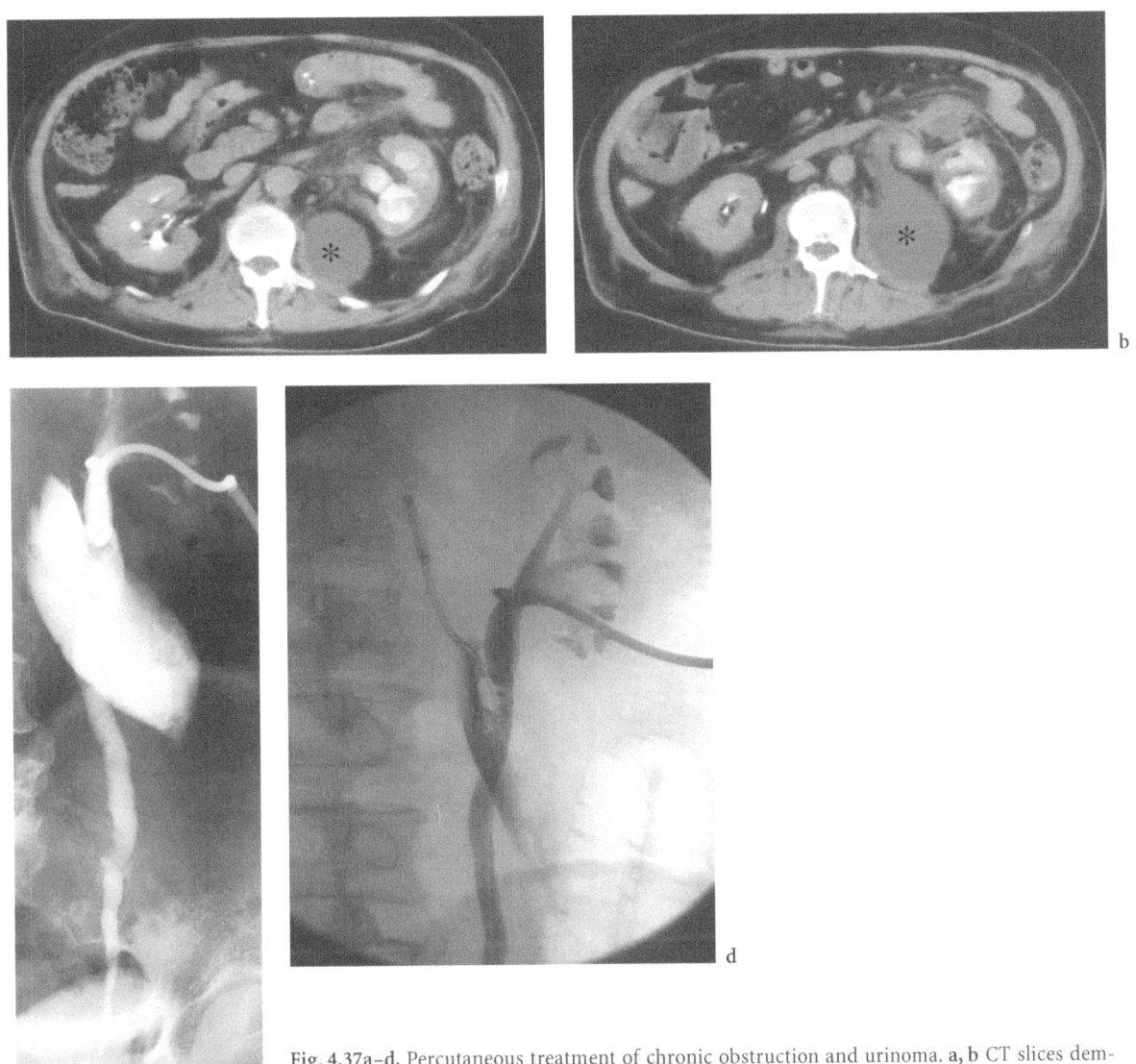

Fig. 4.37a–d. Percutaneous treatment of chronic obstruction and urinoma. **a, b** CT slices demonstrate a left atrophic and obstructive kidney with urinoma in the psoas compartment (*asterisk*). **c** Antegrade pyelography via the nephrostomy catheter shows opacification of the urinoma. **d** Drainage of the upper urinary tract by nephrostomy and 2-J catheter. External drainage of the urinoma

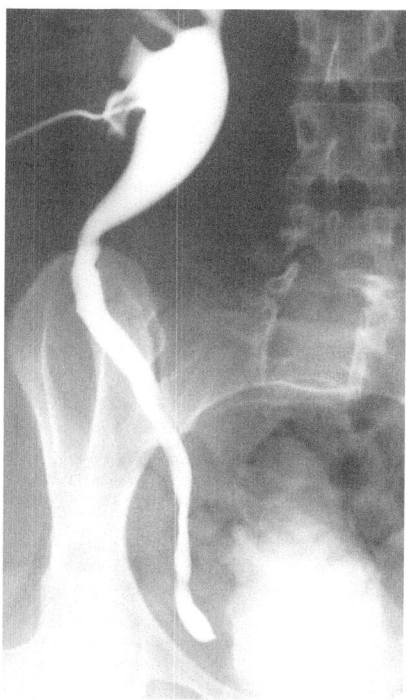

Fig. 4.38. Antegrade pyelography shows right obstruction of the terminal ureter in a patient with thickened bladder wall secondary to neuropathic bladder

(Fig. 4.39a, b) (REUTHER et al. 1997; ROY et al. 1994, 1998). High interobserver agreement in analyzing T_1-weighted images was obtained, with kappa values of 96% (CATALANO et al. 1999). There is also a high degree of agreement with EU in the demonstration of dilation and level of obstruction, with values ranging from 95% to 100% (REUTHER et al. 1997; ROY et al. 1998). MR urography can show anatomic information not visible on EU in patients with dilated urinary tracts that show dilution of CM on delayed images (Fig. 4.40a–d). However, strong T_2-weighted images are unreliable in pyonephrosis and hemorrhagic hydronephrosis because of shorter T_2.

Two types of obstruction can be differentiated by MR imaging. Intrinsic obstruction is characterized by a filling defect, while extrinsic obstruction is suggested by gradual ureteral tapering or stricture (CATALANO et al. 1999). Although MR urography easily shows the level of obstruction, there is still a debate about how accurately it performs in the determination of the cause of the obstruction. In fact, in some situations, MR is limited by lower spatial and/or contrast resolution compared with EU. For example, small calculi may be hidden by the surrounding bright signal of urine, and the same is true for small infiltrative urothelial tumors. Large staghorn calculi that completely fill the

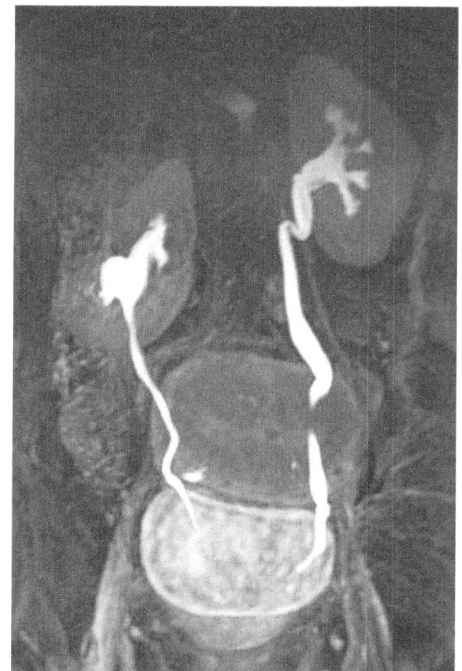

a

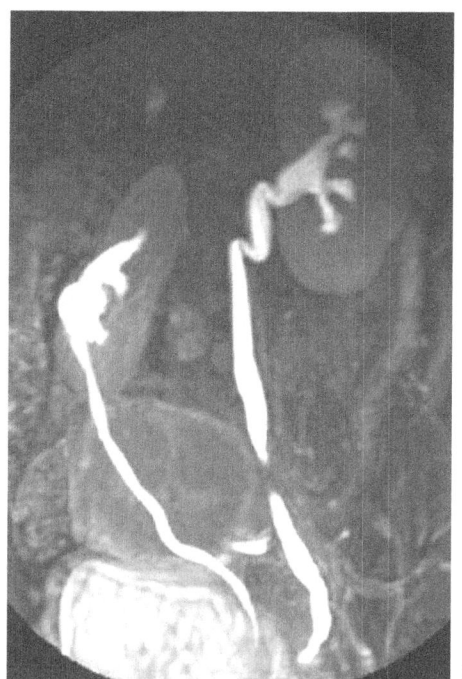

b

Fig. 4.39a, b. Evaluation of the urinary tract in a 60-year-old woman presenting with multiple fibromas of the uterus. 3D T_1-weighted acquisition was performed after administration of 20 mg furosemide and 20 ml gadolinium chelate. Slice thickness is 60 mm, matrix is 512_512, and acquisition time is 21 s. **a** Coronal view shows an anomalous rotation of the right kidney, and a slight compression of the left ureter at the level of the enlarged uterus. **b** Oblique view better demonstrates the course of both ureters

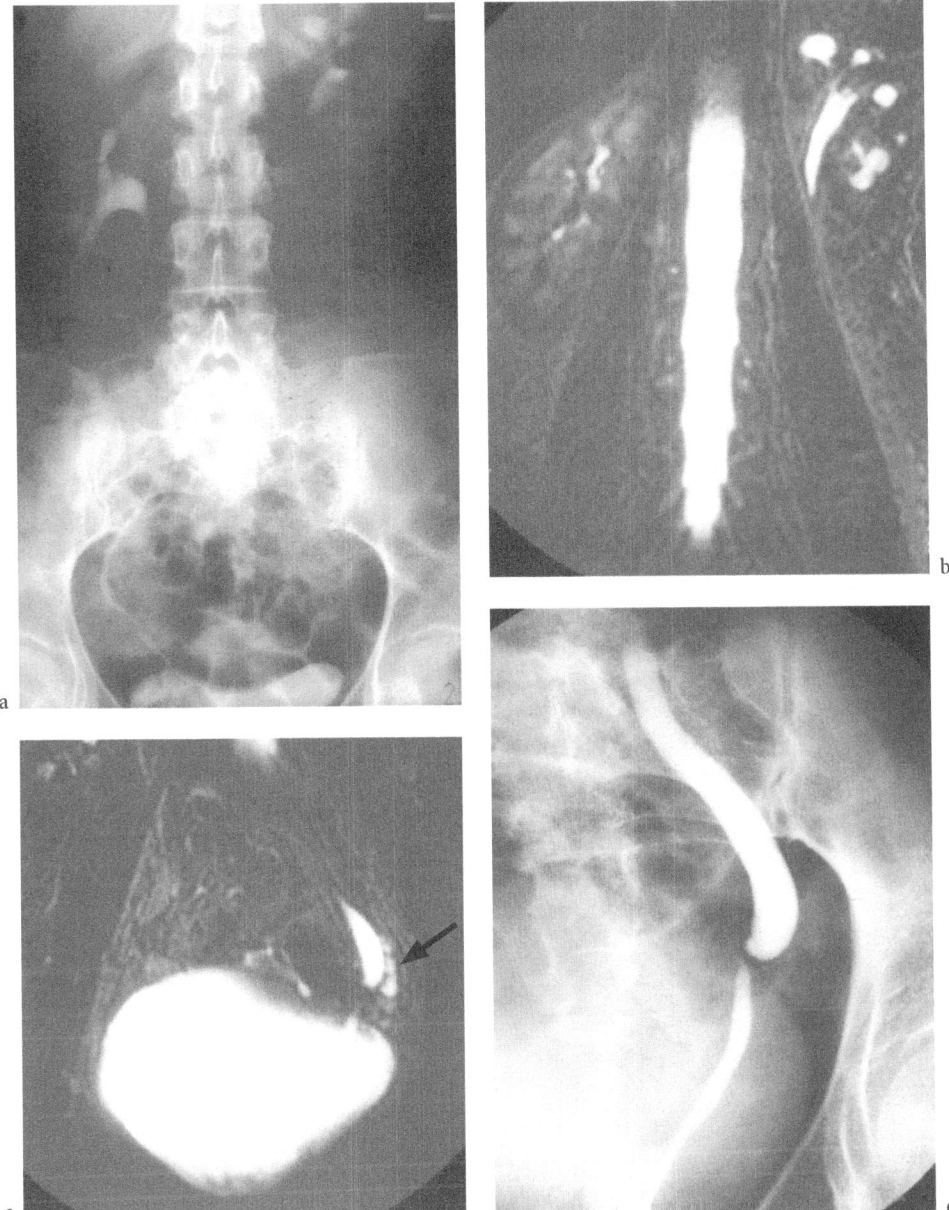

Fig. 4.40-a–d. Extrinsic compression of the lower ureter by endometriosis of the left ovary. **a** EU shows normal right upper urinary tract and reveals a poorly functioning left kidney, with moderate dilatation of the calices. **b, c** Heavily T_2-weighted coronal image better shows the morphology of the calices of the left kidney, which suggests chronic pyelonephritis, and reveals an extrinsic compression of the lower ureter at the level of the left ovary (*arrow*). **d** Subsequent retrograde pyelography confirms the extrinsic compression

renal cavities may not be recognized since they are not outlined by urine (Gaeta et al. 1999). Struvite stones may appear as areas of high signal on T_2-weighted images and be mistaken for normal urine (Gaeta et al. 1999). Ureteral tuberculosis may be mistaken for neoplastic ureteral thickening (Catalano et al. 1999). The use of MIP techniques may also increase the potential for error if careful analysis of source images is not done. Ureteral jets or streams appear as loss of signal, which can mimic polypoid tumors of the bladder at the ureterovesical junction (Gaeta et al. 1999).

The use of dynamic sequences after injection of gadolinium chelate makes it possible to distinguish nonobstructive dilation from obstructive dilation and acute and chronic obstruction (Knesplova and Krestin 1998).

Animal model-based calculations of time-intensity curves from the dynamic sequences allow the determination of single kidney function from renal parenchyma regions of interest, and of urinary excretion using the whole kidney. A good correlation was observed between the functional changes seen on MR and renal scintigraphy data (ROHRSCHNEIDER et al. 2000).

The MR protocol depends first on patient clinical data, and also on the demonstration of renal cavity dilation on ultrasound. The initial study of the urinary tract is usually based on fast T_2-weighted sequences which accurately demonstrate the presence and level of obstruction(Fig. 4.41a, b). However, the cause of obstruction may be more difficult to diagnose. T_2-weighted images using short effective TE permit better analysis of the ureteral contents, wall, and surrounding tissues. Dynamic gadolinium-enhanced T_1-weighted images may demonstrate a vascular cause of obstruction and show early enhancement within urothelial tumors. Excretory MR images seem more accurate in the evaluation of small lesions because of a higher spatial resolution. The administration of furosemide facilitates the diagnosis of partial or intermittent obstruction (KIKINIS et al. 1987) and allows a better evaluation of the contralateral kidney and ureter. When using gadolinium chelate, the appropriate dose

is mandatory to avoid a T_2 effect related to a too high concentration of the contrast agent. The repetition of T_1-weighted sequences in the same plane makes it possible to evaluate renal excretion.

MR urography is now a viable alternative to EU and contrast-enhanced CT in selected patients such as those with severe allergy to iodinated contrast agents, pregnant women, or patients for whom radiation exposure is of great concern (LI et al. 1997). Recent technical improvements show that this technique is able to offer a highly accurate morphological and comprehensive functional diagnostic evaluation of the urinary tract in most conditions (HUSSAIN et al. 1997). It has the potential to become the preferred imaging modality for the diagnosis of suspected ureteral disease, significantly decreasing the need for EU and RUP (NOLTE-ERNSTING et al. 1998).

4.5
The "Dilated Ureter"

"There are few topics in urology that are more confused and confusing than that the wide ureter" (TALNER 1990b). The first question is to precisely determine the normal limit of ureteral diameter: Measurement

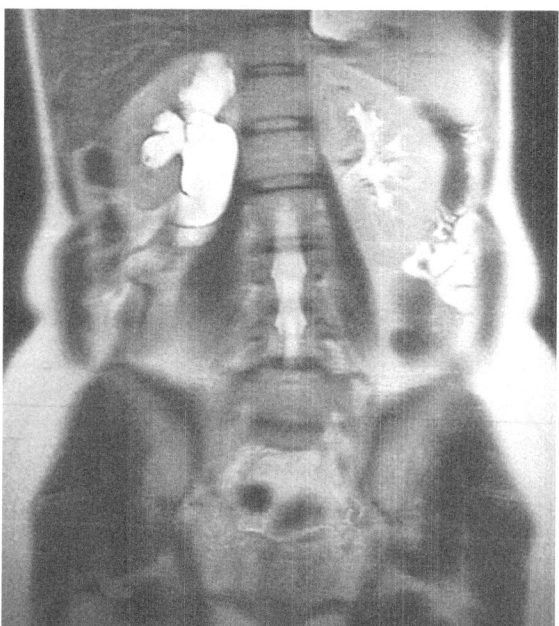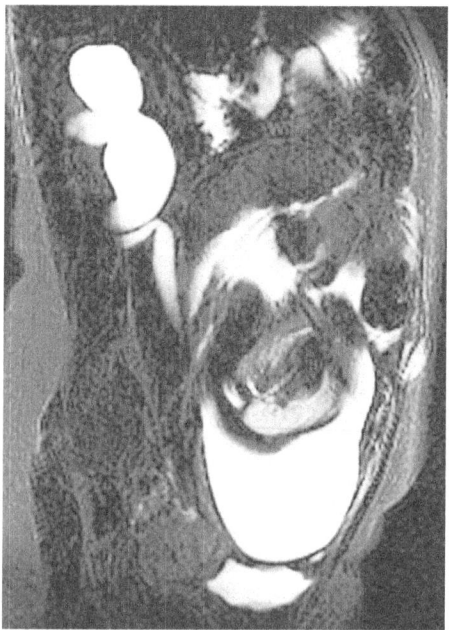

a   b

Fig. 4.41a, b. Woman, 30 weeks pregnant, presenting with right lumbar pain. **a** Short effective TE T_2-weighted coronal image shows asymmetry of kidney size with a marked dilatation of the upper right urinary tract. **b** Oblique, heavily T_2-weighted image demonstrates gradual tapering of the ureter at the level of the uterus without identifiable filling defect, suggesting physiological compression

on EU depends on many factors such as age and sex, level of measurement, peristalsis, degree of hydration and bladder filling, ureteral compression, and technical parameters (magnification). A diameter greater than 5–6 mm is considered abnormal (FLOWER 1977; SHERWOOD 1979; PFISTER et al. 1986). The second question is to determine exactly the origin of dilatation.

Several classifications have been proposed to aid in the diagnosis and treatment of "dilated ureter". These classifications have the advantage of classifying dilated ureter according to the mechanism of obstruction. The term "megaureter" should be used cautiously because it creates some confusion (SMITH et al. 1997). The classification shown in Table 4.3 distinguishes three groups of megaureter and in each group two subgroups, primary and secondary. The association of different mechanisms is possible.

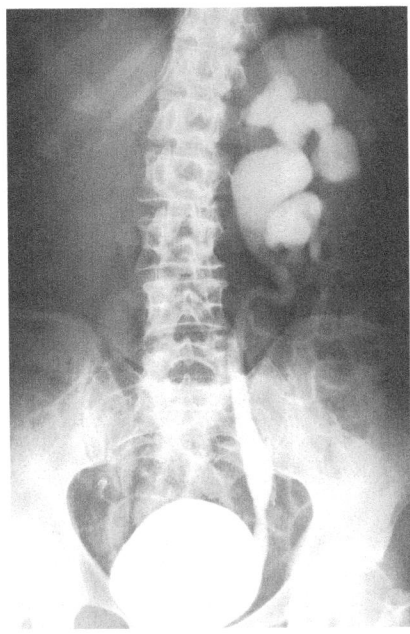

Fig. 4.42. Retrograde cystography: left, passive, total vesicoureteral reflux with ureteral dilatation

Table 4.3. International classification of "megaureters" (From SMITH et al. 1997)

Group	Characteristic
I: Refluxing megaureter	–
Primary	–
Secondary	Abnormality of bladder and/or urethra
II: Obstructed megaureter	
Primary	Stricture, intraluminal lesions, congenital lesions (primary megaureter)
Secondary	Bladder and/or urethra obstruction
III: Nonrefluxing, nonobstructed megaureter	
Primary	Idiopathic (primary megaureter)
Secondary	Infection, postobstructive, increased fluid load

4.5.1
Refluxing "Megaureter"

The presence of unilateral or bilateral upper urinary tract dilation may necessitate a voiding cystogram to detect vesicoureteric reflux, which is a common cause of nonobstructive upper urinary tract dilation.

Primary reflux is usually a pediatric disease and is related to abnormal ureterovesical function with a short and horizontal intramural ureter, or to an ectopic ureteral ending (see Chap. 3). Secondary reflux is generally related to bladder outflow obstruction (Figs. 4.42, 4.43). The role of the voiding cystogram is important, as it also allows a complete examination of the urethra. The main causes are urethral valves, prostatic hypertrophy, neuropathic bladder, and acquired urethral narrowing (Fig. 4.44). In these situ-

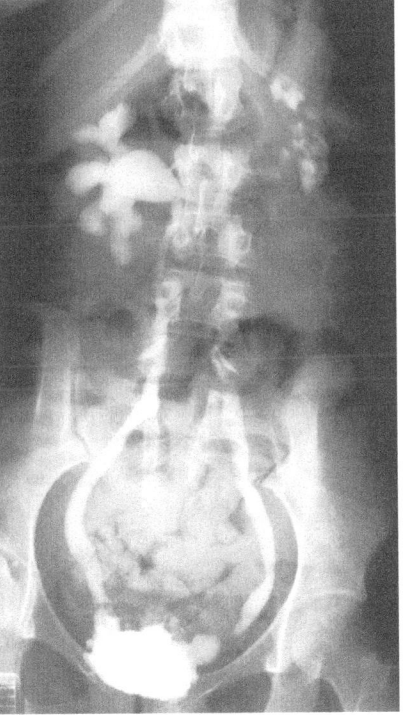

Fig. 4.43. Post-voiding view during retrograde cystography : bilateral, total vesico-ureteral reflux with ureteral dilatation. Signs of bilateral reflux nephropathy with major atrophy of the left kidney. Post-voiding bladder residue with multiple diverticula

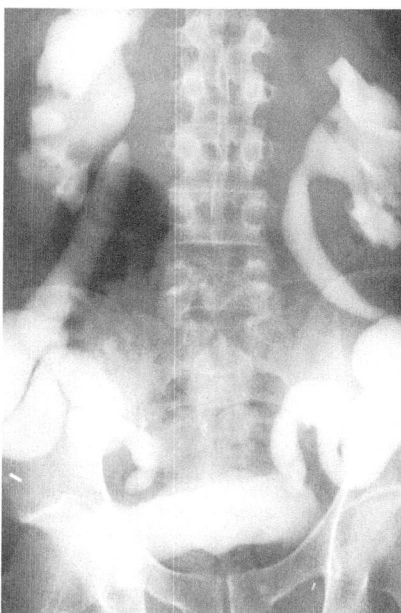

Fig. 4.44. Post-voiding view during retrograde cystography: bilateral vesicoureteral reflux with dilatation and abnormal route of both ureters related to a prune-belly syndrome

ations reflux is secondary to morphological changes of the ureterovesical junction related to increasing intravesical pressure. Inflammatory changes of the bladder wall secondary to tuberculosis, bilharziosis, radiation cystitis, and other causes of cystitis, as well as lower ureteral surgery (all kinds of reimplantation) and bladder surgery near the meatus, may also result in vesicoureteral reflux.

In case of refluxing ureter, the role of the radiologist is to determine the cause and to assess the impact

on the upper collecting system and renal parenchyma. Before treatment it is important to verify the absence of ureterovesical obstruction, which can be associated with reflux mainly in case of infection.

4.5.2
Obstructing "Megaureter"

The causes of obstructing "megaureter", either primary or secondary, are multiple, and the majority of these are developed in other chapters. However, a lot of chronic obstructions, generally bilateral, are secondary to bladder lesions or outflow obstruction (Table 4.4) (TALNER 1990a). Bladder lesions located near ureteral orifices may result in ureteral obstruction. The main causes of bladder outflow obstruction are urethral valves in children and prostatic enlargement, neuropathic bladder, and acquired urethral narrowing in adults. EU and/or US show changes related to chronic retention (Figs. 4.45a–c, 4.46a–d).
- Enlarged bladder with wall thickening and trabeculations related to detrusor hypertrophy
- Significant post-voiding residue
- Acquired bladder diverticula and sometimes stasis lithiasis

Treatment of retention generally suppresses ureteral obstruction but a dilation can persist for a variable period of time.

Ureteral obstruction secondary to bladder lesions is generally related to wall thickening leading to narrowing or anatomic modification of the intramural ureter. This thickening can be diffuse (cystitis, neuropathic bladder, prostatic hypertrophy), and obstruction is

Table 4.4. Main vesical and urethral causes of ureteral obstruction

Site	Cause	
Bladder	Tumoral	Transitional cell carcinoma
		Sarcoma
		Secondary invasion from prostate or gynecological cancer
	Inflammatory	Cystitis
		Tuberculosis
		Schistosomiasis
		Radiation
	Neuropathic	
	Diverticula	Congenital or secondary to bladder neck obstruction
	Bladder surgery or endoscopic endoluminal procedures	
	Bladder neck obstruction	Prostate enlargement (benign, cancer, prostatitis...)
		Large pelvic tumors
		Congenital, functional, or acquired bladder neck strictures
Urethra	Intrinsic lesions	Urethral valves
		Congenital, traumatic, inflammatory stenoses
		Fibroepithelial polyps
	Extrinsic lesions	Pelvic masses, fecal impaction, hydrocolpos

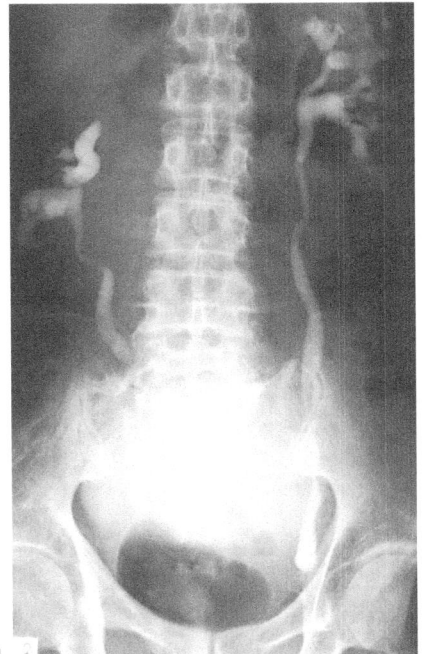

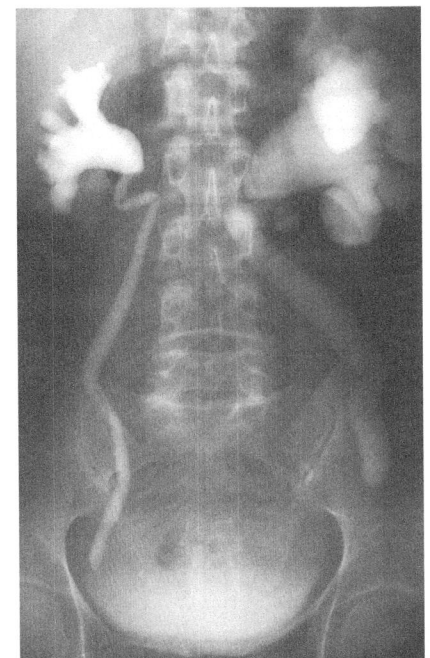

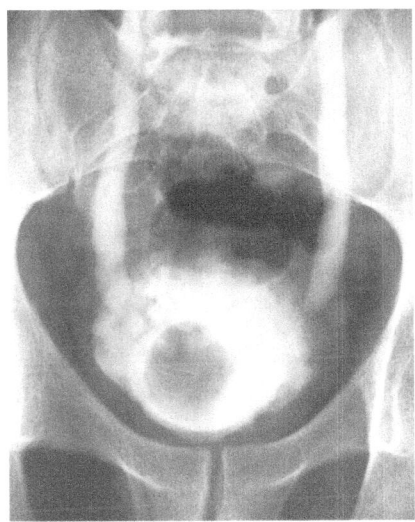

Fig. 4.45a–c. Some urographic examples of bilateral chronic ureterohydrone-phrosis related to bladder outflow obstruction. **a** Moderate bilateral obstruction will enlarged bladder. **b** Important bilateral obstruction with enlarged bladder. **c** Stasis bladder with wall thickening and diverticula

most often bilateral. Unilateral obstruction is rather secondary to a lesion located near the ureteral orifice (tumor, diverticula, iatrogenic trauma) (Fig. 4.47).

4.5.3
Nonrefluxing, Nonobstructed "Megaureter"

This anomaly is frequent, confusing, and easily mistaken for obstruction. The approach to these patients is difficult and depends on the cause (SHERWOOD

1979). The most frequent cause of primary nonrefluxing, nonobstructing "megaureter" is primary mega-ureter or so-called idiopathic megaureter (PFISTER et al. 1971) (Fig. 4.48). This entity is strongly suggested on EU and easily confirmed by the absence of reflux after voiding cystography, but the main problem is to demonstrate the presence or absence of obstruction (HAMILTON and FITZPATRICK 1987). Primary mega-ureter is discussed in Chap. 3.

Other causes of nonrefluxing, nonobstructed ureteral dilatation may be discussed after providing objective evidence for the absence of any obstruction

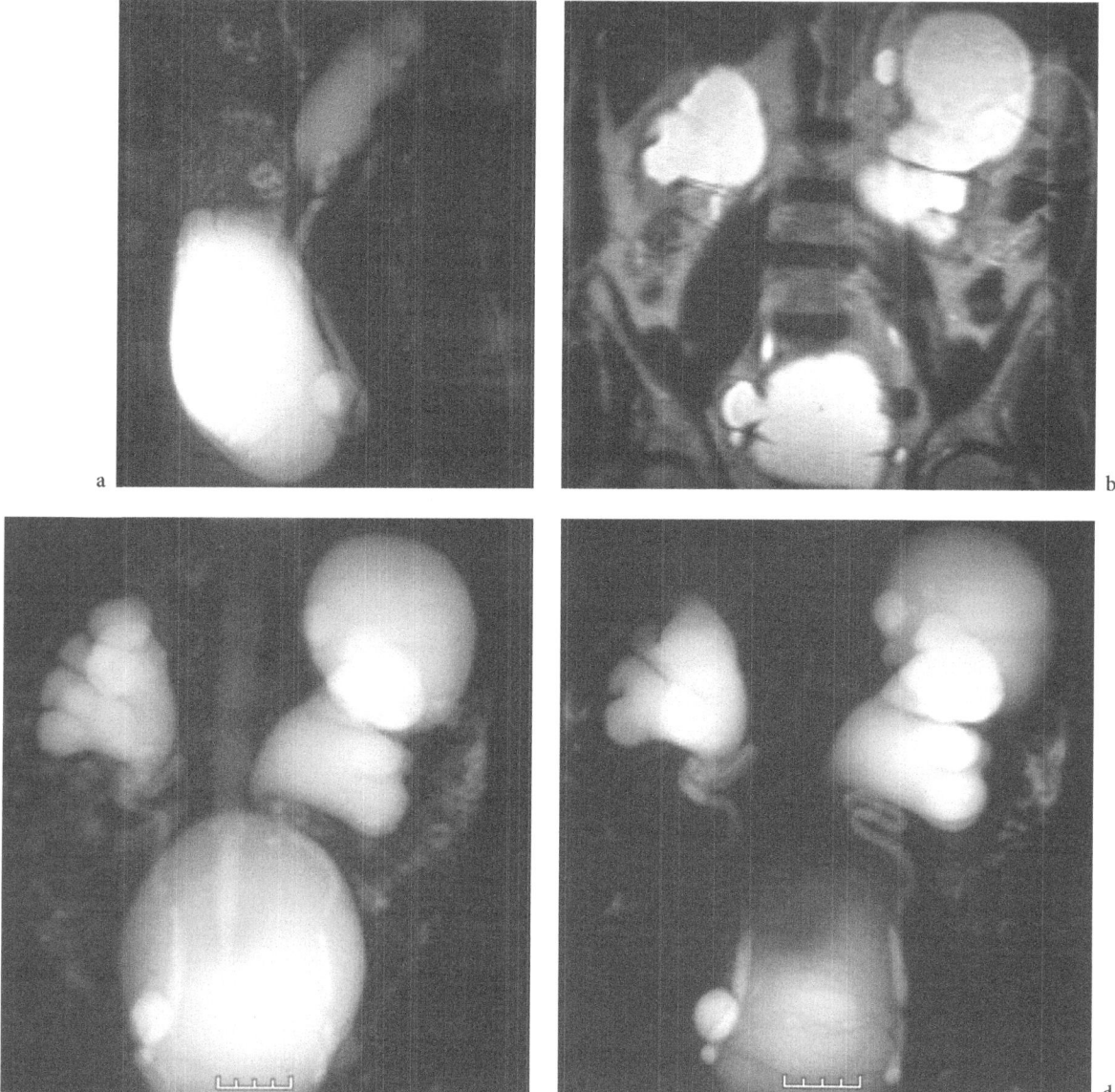

Fig. 4.46a–d. Bilateral chronic obstruction secondary to bladder outflow obstruction: MR urography aspects. **a** Frontal view on HASTE sequence: bilateral ureterohydronephrosis, stasis bladder with multiple diverticula. **b–d** Frontal and oblique views on RARE sequence

(Pfister and Newhouse 1978):

1. Urinary infection: It is well known that urinary tract infection (Fig. 4.49) is frequently associated with segmental or global ureteral dilatation and diminished peristalsis. Dilatation results from a hypotonic effect of bacterial endotoxins on ureteral smooth muscles. It usually disappears after antibiotic treatment (Shopfner 1966).

2. Postobstructive dilatation: With long-term ureteral obstruction, residual dilation is common and remains to a variable extent (Fig. 4.50). Without

knowing the prior medical history of the patient it may be difficult to make a diagnosis.

3. Hyperdiuresis states: Diabetes insipidus (Shapiro et al. 1978) and psychogenic polydipsia are causes of nonobstructive nonrefluxing ureteral dilation (Harrison et al. 1979) (Fig. 4.51). High doses of HOCM could lead to moderate ureteral dilation, but the use of these CM is steadily diminishing.

4. Ureteral dilation: Ureteral dilation during pregnancy is covered in Chap. 8.

In these different clinical situations, it is impor-

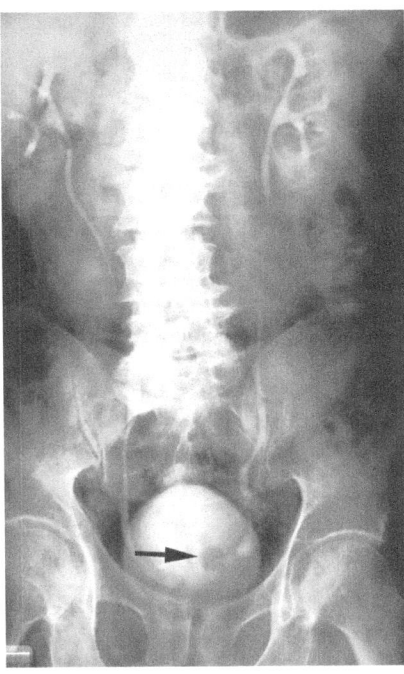

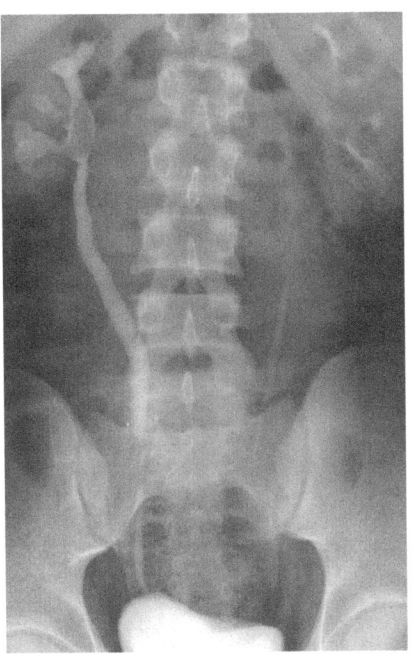

Fig. 4.47. Moderate left pelvic ureteral obstruction related to a TCC located near the ureteral orifice (*arrow*)

Fig. 4.49. Urographic aspect of a wide, nonrefluxing ureter in a patient with urinary infection and uratic pelvicaliceal stone: probable ureteral hypotonia secondary to infection

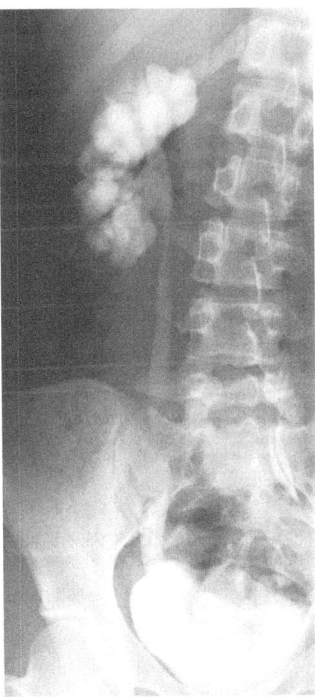

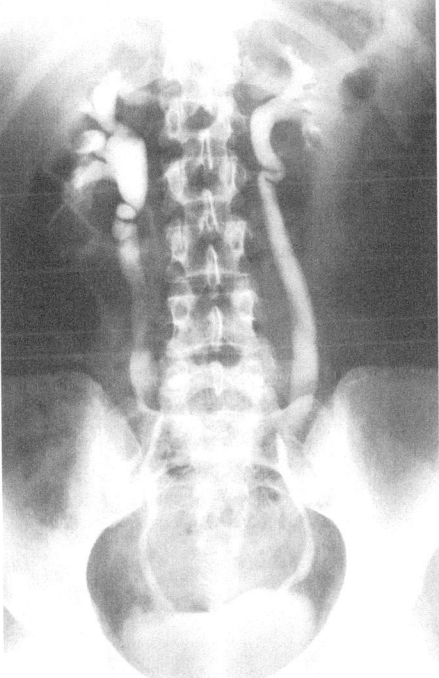

Fig. 4.48. Urographic aspects of a wide, nonrefluxing, right primary megaureter associated with megacalycosis

Fig. 4.50. Urographic aspect of a post-obstructive dilatation of both ureters and upper urinary tract in a previously pregnant woman

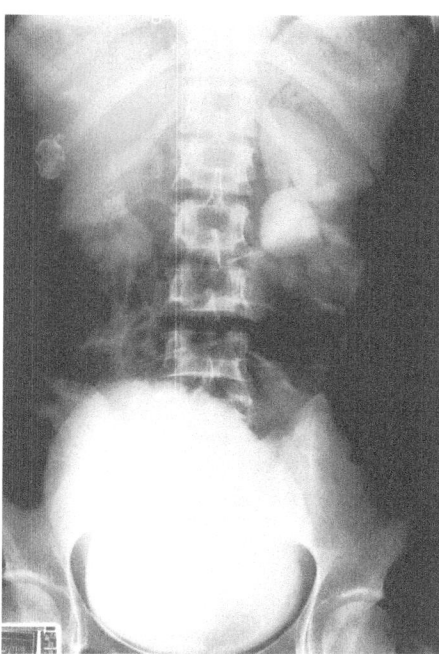

Fig. 4.51. Bilateral ureterohydronephrosis with enlarged bladder in a patient with psychogenic polydipsia

tant to realize that the dilation is not secondary to obstruction and/or reflux, so that needless surgery can be avoided (PFISTER et al 1986). When there are doubts about the presence of obstruction, the current strategy is not clear. Some groups promote pressure flow studies during antegrade pyelography, but this requires skill and specialized equipment and is a relatively invasive technique (WHITAKER 1973).

Radioisotope renal scintigraphy is an alternative method for other groups. More recently, diuresis duplex Doppler ultrasonography was proposed as a substitute for diuresis renal scintigraphy. It is based on measurement of the intrarenal resistive index before and after administration of furosemide (MALLEK et al. 1996). In a series of 48 kidneys with doubtful chronic obstructions, the accuracy rate in diagnosis obstruction was 95%. In each case it is important to have precise information about the clinical history of the patient. Good knowledge of these various problems on the part of the uroradiologist and close cooperation between the concerned medical specialties are mandatory.

References

Abramson S, Walders N, Applegate KE, et al (2000) Impact in the emergency department of unenhanced CT on diagnostic confidence and therapeutic efficacy in patients with suspected renal colic: a prospective survey. AJR Am J Roentgenol 175:1689–1695

Al-Hassan HK, Sabha MN, Taleb HH, et al (1991) Value of ultrasound in persistent flank pain. Int Surg 76:264–265

Amis ES Jr, Cronan JJ (1988) The renal sinus: an imaging review and proposed nomenclature for sinus cysts. J Urol 139:1151–1154

Amis ES Jr, Cronan JJ, Pfister RC, et al (1982) Ultrasonic inaccuracies in diagnosing renal obstruction. Urology 19:101

Barbaric ZI, McIntosh PK (1981) Periureteral thin-needle aspiration biopsy. Urol Radiol 2:181–185

Bateman GA, Cuganesan R (2002) Renal vein Doppler sonography of obstructive uropathy. AJR Am J Roentgenol 178: 921–925

Bell TV, Fenlon HM, Davison BD, et al (1998) Unenhanced helical CT criteria to differentiate distal ureteral calculi from pelvic phleboliths. Radiology 207:363–367

Blake SP, McNicholas MMJ, Raptopoulos V (1998) Nonopaque crystal deposition causing ureteric obstruction in patients with HIV undergoing indinavir therapy. AJR Am J Roentgenol 171:717–720

Boridy IC, Kawashima A, Goldman SM, et al (1999a) Acute ureterolithiasis: nonenhanced helical CT findings of perinephric edema for prediction of degree of ureteral obstruction. Radiology 21:663–667

Boridy IC, Nikolaidis P, Kawashima A, et al (1999b) Ureterolithiasis: value of the tail sign in differentiating phleboliths from ureteral calculi at nonenhanced helical CT. Radiology 211:619–621

Bosniak MA, Megibow AJ, Ambos MA, et al (1982) Computed tomography of ureteral obstruction. AJR Am J Roentgenol 138:1107–1113

Burge HJ, Middleton WD, McClennan BL, et al (1991) Ureteral jets in healthy subjects and in patients with unilateral calculi: comparison with color Doppler US. Radiology 180:437–442

Catalano C, Papone P, Laghi A, et al (1999) MR pyelography and conventional MR imaging in urinary tract obstruction. Acta Radiol 40:198–200

Catalano O, Nunziata A, Altei F, et al (2002) Suspected ureteral colic: primary helical CT versus selective helical CT after unenhanced radiography and sonography. AJR Am J Roentgenol 178:379–387

Chelfouh N, Grenier N, Migueret D, et al (1998) Characterization of urinary calculi: in vitro study of "twinkling artifact" revealed by color-flow sonography. AJR Am J Roentgenol 171:1055–1060

Chen MYM, Zagoria R, Saunders HS, et al (1999) Trends in the use of unenhanced helical CT for acute urinary colic. AJR Am J Roentgenol 173:1447–1450

Chu G, Rosenfield AT, Anderson K, et al (1999) Sensitivity and value of digital scout radiography for detecting ureteral stones in patients with ureterolithiasis diagnosed on unenhanced CT. AJR Am J Roentgenol 173:417–423

Dalla Palma L, Stacul F, Bazzocchi M, et al (1993) Ultrasonography and plain film versus intravenous urography in ureteric colic. Clin Radiol 47:333–336

Dalla Palma L, Pozzi-Mucelli R, Stacul F, et al (2001) Present-day imaging of patients with renal colic. Eur Radiol 11:4–17

Djurrhus JC, Stage P (1976) Percutaneous intra-pelvic pressure registration in hydronephrosis during diuresis. Acta Chir Scan [Suppl] 472:49–53

Ellenbogen PH, Scheible FW, Talner LB, et al (1978) Sensitivity of gray-sale ultrasound in detecting urinary tract obstruction. AJR Am J Roentgenol 130:731–733

Flower CDR (1977) Wide ureters, a dilemma in diagnosis. Br J Radiol 50:539–540

Freed KS, Paulson EK, Frederick MG et al (1998) Interobserver variability in the interpretation of unenhanced helical CT for the diagnosis of ureteral stone disease. J Comput Assist Tomogr 22:732–737

Friedenberg RM, Moorehouse H, Gade M (1989) Urinomas secondary to pyelosinus backflow. Urol Radiol 5:23–29

Gaeta M, Blandino A, Scribano E, et al (1999) Diagnostic pitfalls of breath-hold MR urography in obstructive uropathy. J Comput Assist Tomogr 23:891–897

Gillenwater JY (1986) The pathophysiology of urinary obstruction. In: Walsh PC, Gittes R, Perlmutter AD, Stamey TA (eds) Campbell's urology 5th edn., Saunders, Philadelphia pp 542

Grenier N, Pariente JL, Trillaud H, et al (2000) Dilatation of the collecting system during pregnancy: physiologic vs obstructive dilatation. Eur Radiol 10:271–279

Guest AR, Cohan RH, Korobkin M, et al (2001) Assessment of the clinical utility of the rim and comet-tail signs in differentiating ureteral stones from phleboliths. AJR Am J Roentgenol 177:1285–1291

Haddad MC, Sharif HS, Shahed MS, et al. (1992) Renal colic: diagnosis and outcome. Radiology 184:83–88

Hamilton S, Fitzpatrick JM (1987) Primary nonobstructive megaureter in adults: Clin Radiol 38:181–185

Harrison BR, Ramchandani P, Allen JT (1979) Psychogenic polydipsia: unusual cause for hydronephrosis. AJR Am J Roentgenol 133:327–328

Heneghan JP, Dalrymple NC, Verga M, et al (1997) Soft-tissue „rim" sign in the diagnosis of ureteral calculi with use of unenhanced helical CT. Radiology 202:709–711

Herring LC (1962) Observations on the analysis of ten thousand urinary calculi. J Urol 88:545–562

Hill MC, Rich JI, Mardiaty JG, et al (1985) Sonography vs. excretory urography in acute flank pain. AJR Am J Roentgenol 144:1235–1238

Hodson CJ, Craven JD, Lewis DG, et al (1969) Experimental obstructive nephropathy in the pig. Br J Urol [Suppl] 41:5

Hussain S, O'Malley M, Jara H, et al (1997) MR urography. MRI Clin North Am 1:95-106

Joffre F, Plante P, Tregant P (1990) Techniques d'opacification des voies excrétrices supérieures. Editions techniques. Encycl Med Chir, Paris, France. Radiodiagnostic V 34015 BIO 12; 1–6

Katz DS, Lane MJ, Sommer FG (1994) Unenhanced helical CT of ureteral stones: incidences of associated urinary tract findings. AJR Am J Roentgenol 166:1319–1322

Kawashima A, Sandler CM, Boridy IC, et al (1997) Unenhanced helical CT of ureterolithiasis: value of the tissue rim sign. AJR Am J Roentgenol 168:997–1000

Kerr WS Jr (1956) Effects of complete ureteral obstruction in dogs on kidney function. Am J Physiol 184:521

Kikinis R, von Schulthess GK, Jager P, et al. (1987) Normal and hydronephrosis kidney: evaluation of renal function with contrast-enhanced MR imaging. Radiology 165:837

Klahr S (1991) Pathophysiology of obstructive nephropathy: a 1991 update. Semin Nephrol 11:156–168

Knesplova L, Krestin GP (1998) Magnetic resonance in the assessment of renal function. Eur Radiol 8:201–211

Laing FC, Jeffrey B Jr, Wing VW (1985) Ultrasound versus excretory urography in evaluating acute flank plain. Radiology 154:613–616

Laing FC, Benson CB, Disalvo DN, et al (1994) Distal ureteral calculi: detection with vaginal US. Radiology 192:545–548

Lemaitre L, Ala Edine C, Dubrulle F, et al (2000) Retroperitoneum and ureters. In: Terrier Grossholz M, Becker CD (eds) Spiral CT of the abdomen. Springer-Verlag, Berlin Heidelberg New York

Lerner RM, Rubens D (1986) Distal ureteral calculi: diagnosis by transrectal sonography. AJR Am J Roentgenol 147: 1189–1191

Levine JA, Nietlich J, Verga M, et al (1997) Ureteral calculi in patients with flank pain: correlation of plain film radiography with unenhanced helical CT. Radiology 204:27–31

Levine J, Neitlich J, Smith RC (1999) The value of prone scanning to distinguish ureterovesical junction stones from ureteral stones that have passed into the bladder: leave no stone unturned. AJR Am J Roentgenol 172:977–981

Li W, Chavez D, Edelman PR, et al (1997) Magnetic resonance urography by breath-hold contrast three-dimensional FISP. J Magn Reson Imaging 7:309–311

Maillet PS, Pelle-Francoz DP, Laville M, et al (1986) Nondilated obstructive acute renal failure: diagnostic procedures and therapeutic management. Radiology 160:659

Mallek P, Bankier AA, Etele-Hainz A, et al (1996) Distinction between obstructive and nonobstructive hydronephrosis: value of diuresis duplex Doppler sonography. AJR Am J Roentgenol 66:113–117

Megibow AJ, Mitnick JS, Bosniak MA (1982) The contribution of computed tomography to the evaluation of the obstructed ureter. Urol Radiol 4:95

Morse RM, Resnick MI (1991) Ureteral calculi: natural history and treatment in an era of advanced technology. J Urol 145:263–265

Mostafavy MR, Ernst RD, Saltzman B (1998) Accurate determination of chemical composition of urinary calculi by spiral computerized tomography. J Urol 159:673–675

Mostbeck GH, Zontsich T, Turetschek K (2001) Ultrasound of the kidney: obstruction and medical diseases. Eur Radiol 11:1878–1889

Nolte-Ernsting CC, Bucker A, Adam GB, et al (1998) Gadolinium-enhanced excretory MR urography after low-dose diuretic injection: comparison with conventional excretory urography. Radiology 209:147–157

Olcott EW, Sommer FG, Napel S (1997) Accuracy of detection and measurement of renal calculi: in vitro comparison of three-dimensional spiral CT, radiography, and nephrotomography. Radiology 204:19–25

Onishi K, Watanabe H, Ohe H, et al (1986) Ultrasound finding is urolithiasis in the lower ureter. Ultrasound Med Biol 12: 577–579

O'Reilly P, Rickards D (1986) Radiology. In: O'Reilly P (ed) Obstructive uropathy. Springer-Verlag, Berlin Heidelberg New York, pp 31–57

Otal P, Irsutti M, Chabbert V, et al (2001) Exploration radiologique de la colique néphrétique. J Radiol 82:27–33

Pfister RC, Newhouse JH (1978) Radiology of the ureter. Urology 12:15–39

Pfister RC, McLoughlin AP, Leadbetter WF (1971) Radiological evaluation of primary megaureter. Radiology 99:503–510

Pfister RC, Yoder IL, Newhouse JH (1981) Percutaneous uroradiological procedures. Semin Roentgenol 16:135–151

Pfister RC, Papanicolaou N, Yoder IC (1986) The dilated ureter. Semin Roentgenol 21:224–235

Platt JF (1996) Urinary obstruction. Radiol Clin North Am 34: 1113–1129

Platt JF, Rubin JM, Ellis JH (1993) Acute renal obstruction: evaluation with intrarenal duplex Doppler and conventional US. Radiology 186:685–688

Regan F, Bohlman ME, Khazan R, et al (1996) MR urography using HASTE imaging in the assessment of ureteric obstruction. AJR Am J Roentgenol 67:1115–1120

Regan F, Petronis J, Bohlman ME, et al (1997) Perirenal MR high signal. A new and sensitive indicator of acute ureteric obstruction. Clin Radiol 52:445–450

Reuther G, Kiefer B, Wandl E (1997) Visualization of urinary tract dilatation: value of single-shot MR urography. Eur Radiol 7 1266–1281

Rohrschneider WK, Becker K, Hoffend J, et al (2000) Combined static-dynamic MR urography for the simultaneous evaluation of morphology and function in urinary tract obstruction. II. Findings in experimentally induced ureteric stenosis (in process citation). Pediatr Radiol 30: 523–532

Roy C, Saussine C, Jahn C, et al (1994) Evaluation of RARE-MR urography in the assessment of uretero-hydronephrosis. J Comput Assist Tomog 18:601–608

Roy C, Saussine C, Guth S, et al (1998) MR urography in the evaluation of the urinary tract obstruction. Abdom Imaging 23:27–34

Shapiro SR, Woerner S, Adelman RD, et al (1978) Diabetes insipidus and hydronephrosis. J Urol 119:715–719

Sheley RC, Semonsen KG, Quinn SF (1999) Helical CT in the evaluation of renal colic. Am J Emerg Med 17:279–282

Sherwood T (1979) The dilated upper urinary tract. Radiol Clin North Am 17:333–340

Shopfner CE (1966) Nonobstructive hydronephrosis and hydroureter. AJR Am J Roentgenol 98:172–180

Smith ED, et al (1977) Report of working party to establish an international nomenclature for the large ureter. In: Bergsma D, Duckett JW (eds) Birth defects: original article series vol 13, no 5. Alan R. Liss, New York, for the National Foundation March of Dimes, pp 3–8

Smith RC, Rosenfield AT, Choe KA, et al (1995) Acute flank pain: comparison of non-contrast-enhanced CT and intravenous urography. Radiology 194:789–794

Smith RC, Verga M, Dalrymple N, et al (1996) Acute ureteral obstruction: value of secondary signs on helical unenhanced CT. AJR Am J Roentgenol 167:1109–1113

Soyer P, Levesque M, Lecloirec A, et al (1990) Évaluation du rôle de l'échographie dans le diagnostic positif de colique néphrétique d'origine lithiasique. J Radiol 71:445–450

Sourtzis S, Thibeau JF, Damry N, et al (1999) Radiologic investigation of renal colic: unenhanced helical CT compared with excretory urography. AJR Am J Roentgenol 172: 1491–1494

Sudah M, Vanninen R, Partanen R, et al (2001) MR Urography in evaluation of acute flank pain: T_2-weighted sequences and gadolinium-enhanced three-dimensional FLASH compared with urography. AJR Am J Roentgenol 176:105–112

Sudah M, Vanninen R, Partanen R, et al (2002) Patients with acute flank pain: comparison of MR urography with unenhanced helical CT. Radiology 223:98–105

Takahashi N, Kawashima A, Ernst RD, et al (1998) Ureterolithiasias: can clinical outcome be predicted with unenhanced helical CT? Radiology 208:97–102

Talner LB (1990a) Specific causes of obstruction. In: Pollack HW (ed) Clinical urography. Saunders, Philadelphia, pp 16--29

Talner LB (1990b) Urinary obstruction. In: Pollack HW (ed) Clinical urography. Saunders, Philadelphia pp 15--35

Talner LB, Scheible W, Ellenbogen PH, et al (1981) How accurate is ultrasonography in detecting hydronephrosis is azotemic patients? Urol Radiol 3:1--6

Traubici J, Neitlich JD, Smith RC (1999) Distinguishing pelvic phleboliths from distal uretral stones on routine unenhanced helical CT: is there a radiolucent center? AJR Am J Roentgenol 172:13–17

Tublin ME, Dodd III GD, Verdile VP (1994) Acute renal colic: diagnosis with duplex Doppler US. Radiology 193: 697–701

Veno A, Kawamura T, Ogawa A, et al (1977) Relation of spontaneous passage of ureteral calculi to size. Urology 10: 544–546

Whitaker RH (1973) Methods of assessing obstruction in dilated ureters. Br J Urol 45:15–22

Whitaker RH (1978a) Clinical assessment of pelvic and ureteral function. Urology 12:146–150

Whitaker RH (1978b) Pathophysiology of ureteric obstruction. In: Williams DI, Chisholm GD (eds) Scientific foundations of urology, vol 2, chap 3. Heinemann, London

Yilmaz S, Sindel T, Arslan G, et al (1998) Renal colic: comparison of spiral CT, US and IVU in the detection of ureteral calculi. Eur Radiol 8:212–217

Zagoria RJ, Khatod EG, Chen MY (2001) Abdominal radiography after CT reveals urinary calculi: a method to predict usefulness of radiography on the basis of size and CT attenuation of calculi. AJR Am J Roentgenol 176:1117–1122

5 Ureteral Lithiasis and Other Intraluminal Diseases

M. Soulie, Ph. Otal, L. Bouchard, F. Joffre, P. Chemla, V. Chabbert

CONTENTS

Intraluminal ureteral abnormalities not related to the ureteral wall are a frequent pathology, the most frequent specific etiology being lithiasis. The diagnosis of these intraluminal defects is usually unproblematic, but sometimes the use of new diagnostic techniques such as CT is necessary. Newly developed ureteral endoscopic techniques, interventional radiology, and extracorporeal shock-wave lithotripsy (ESWL) provide new diagnostic and therapeutic approaches.

M. Soulie;
Service d'Urologie, CHU Rangueil, 1, avenue Jean-Poulhès, 31403 Toulouse Cédex 4, France
Ph. Otal; L. Bouchard; F. Joffre; P. Chemla; V. Chabbert
Service de Radiologie, Hôpital de Rangueil, 1, avenue Jean-Poulhès, 31403 Toulouse Cédex 4, France

5.1 Ureteral Lithiasis

Imaging techniques have an important role in the diagnosis, evaluation, treatment, and follow-up of urinary lithiasis, especially in cases of ureteral calculus, which is the most common urologic problem in the young male adult.

Ureteral lithiasis is the most common cause of ureteral obstruction (Dufour 1973) and almost 3% of the occidental population will experience renal colic at least once in their lifetime (Williams 1963). Ureteral calculi are almost always secondary to migration of a pyelocaliceal lithiasis. Exceptionally, a primary stone may develop in a ureteral segment that is dilated due to malformation (idiopathic megaureter, ureterocele, diverticula, blind-ending ureter) (Drach 1986).

Ureteral calculi are identical in structure to other urinary stones, having a protein matrix with different crystals (oxalate, phosphate, ammoniac, magnesium, urate) (Table 5.1). Radiolucent calculi account for about 10%–20% of all calculi. Special attention should be given to urolithiasis in HIV patients, in whom lithiasis is secondary to systemic infection (Sundaram and Saltzman 1999). It is important to make a specific diagnosis, because conservative treatment with hydration is efficient in the majority of cases.

The spontaneous evolution of a ureteral calculus depends on several factors: stone size, level of obstruction, ureteral diameter, and status of diuresis.

Stone size is an important element in stone migration (Thornbury and Parker 1982). It generally varies between 1 and 10 mm, but a stone can exceptionally reach 20 mm (O'Reilly 1986).

Smaller stones, with a diameter of less than 4 mm are the most frequent. Most of them are spontaneously eliminated within 6 weeks (81% of proximal and 85% of distal stones). Stones smaller than 5 mm may be blocked at the different physiological strictures (pyeloureteral junction, crossing of the iliac vessels, broad ligament, bladder ligaments, vas

Table 5.1. Main characteristics of ureteral stones

Chemical composition	Radiopacity	Morphology	Frequency (%)
Calcium phosphate	Densely opaque	Smooth, homogeneous	10
Calcium oxalate	Moderately opaque	Spiculated	50–80
Magnesium ammonium phosphate (struvite)	Faintly opaque	Heterogeneous, stratified	10
Cystine	Radiolucent	Smooth	5
Urates	Radiolucent	Smooth	10
Xanthine	Radiolucent	Smooth	5
Matrix	Radiolucent	Smooth	10

deferens). The ureterovesical junction is the most common location (70%–80%)of ureteral calculi (DRACH 1986). Larger stones (more than 6 mm) are less frequently spontaneously evacuated and carry a higher risk of complications.

Migration is spontaneous, helped by ureteral peristalsis and diuresis. Hyperhydratation or osmotic diuresis caused by the injection of contrast medium can increase the pain but can also aid stone migration. The presence of an impacted stone produces spasms and edema that make stone progression more difficult. These phenomena are more important if calculus blockage has been present for a long time or is associated with a urinary tract infection. This "ureteritis" may extend to the periureteral region ("periureteritis"). The mucosa becomes hyperemic and may ulcerate because of the stone friction, thus explaining the hematuria. This inflammatory phenomenon may result in ureteral fibrosis in a case of long-standing calculus. In some cases, migration of the stone into the ureteral submucosa may be responsible for the failure of ESWL and endoscopic stone extraction (YOUNG et al. 1990). This type of migration is common in chronic cases because of the important inflammatory reaction and is also related to the repeated endoscopic maneuvers and/or ESWL sessions. The fibrosis may be responsible for the radiological and macroscopic pseudotumoral aspect (DUFOUR 1973). Sometimes, the stone itself may cause rupture of the ureteral wall.

The classical clinical presentation of ureteral lithiasis is renal colic. In 10%–15% of cases, stones remain asymptomatic and are discovered incidentally on KUB or other imaging performed for other reasons. Lithiasis may be diagnosed on a radiological examination of the urinary tract because of recurrent urinary infection, macroscopic hematuria, proteinuria, pollakiuria, or abdominal pain. Exceptionally, the diagnosis is made in a patient with a severe clinical presentation such as septicemia, acute renal insufficiency, or pyonephrosis.

Ureteral lithiasis is the most common cause of lumbar pain requiring hospitalization in pregnant women. The rate of lithiasis during pregnancy is about one in every 1500 patients (BORIDY et al. 1996). A discussion of urinary tract lithiasis in pregnant women is presented in Chap. 8.

5.1.1
Radiological Findings

The radiologist must be able to answer three questions when a patient with suspicion of ureteral calculus is examined (VAN ARSDELEN et al. 1990).
1. Is a stone present in the radiological study?
2. Is treatment needed? This decision depends on the patient's clinical status, the radiological characteristics of the stone, and the degree of obstruction.
3. What is the best treatment strategy? Because of the multiple treatment alternatives, the radiological findings can be very helpful in making an appropriate choice.

The evolution in imaging techniques in recent years has changed the radiological approach to ureteral lithiasis. Helical CT is responsible for most of these changes. The radiological diagnostic strategy depends on the clinical presentation, and the radiological management of acute ureteral obstruction is discussed in Chap. 4. Here we will focus on the diagnostic problems associated with ureteral calculus.

5.1.1.1
KUB

Historically, the main role of kidney, ureter, and bladder (KUB) film was the detection of ureteral stones, which are spontaneously radiopaque in about 90%, and often obscured by contrast medium after excretory urography (EU) or direct opacification.

The increasing use of HCT has changed the diagnostic strategy for ureteral calculi and modified the usefulness of KUB. For many authors, CT has become the first examination for patients with renal colic (SMITH et al. 1995). Due to the chemical composition (uric acid) or the small size of most ureteral calculi, the management is mainly conservative. Serial CT is impractical for following the stone progression, however, and KUB is always needed every 1–2 weeks to follow the patient until spontaneous passage of the calculus occurs. In addition, KUB can be useful to predict the detectability of the stone prior to ESWL.

Its efficacy depends on its technical qualities and particularly on the kilovoltage of the X-ray beam (SINGH and MALEK 1982). Visualization of a stone depends on its size, its topography, and its chemical composition, which influences its density. The superimposition of bony structures (sacrum, transverse processes) (Fig. 5.1) and the presence of a paralytic ileus make the examination for stone diagnosis more challenging (ROTH et al. 1985; ZANGERLE et al. 1983). The film must be made while the patient is supine with abdominal compression, or prone if needed. Multiple planes (oblique, lateral) and in rare cases tomography are useful to determine the ureteral topography of the stone and to suppress superimposed structures. Digital radiography, currently using storage phosphorus plate technology, is progressively replacing conventional radiology with comparable accuracy (FAJARDO and HILLMAN 1988).

All stones have a certain degree of radiopacity that usually allows identification on KUB (JOFFRE and PORTALEZ 1983). Banner proposes classifying stones as densely opaque, moderately opaque, faintly opaque, and nonopaque (BANNER 1990a). However, the term nonopaque must be replaced by nonvisible. Even radiotransparent stones (urate) can be visualized on linear tomography, but the tomography level must pass through the stone (Fig. 5.2) (AMBOS and BOSNIAK 1975). It is difficult to precisely determine the relation between the chemical composition of a stone and its radiopacity, because it is very subjective and dependent on the stone size. Moreover, it is exceptional to find a stone that is completely pure (PRIEN 1974). Calcium phosphate stones, rare in the ureter, have very high radiopacity, whereas calcium oxalate stones are the most frequent in the ureter but are less radiopaque. Ammoniac-magnesium phosphate (struvite) stones have very faint radiopacity. Stones with a matrix of cystine, urate, and xanthine are usually not visualized on KUB, but they may be visible if they are impure (SINGH and MALEK 1982). Stratified ureteral calculi, with concentric layers

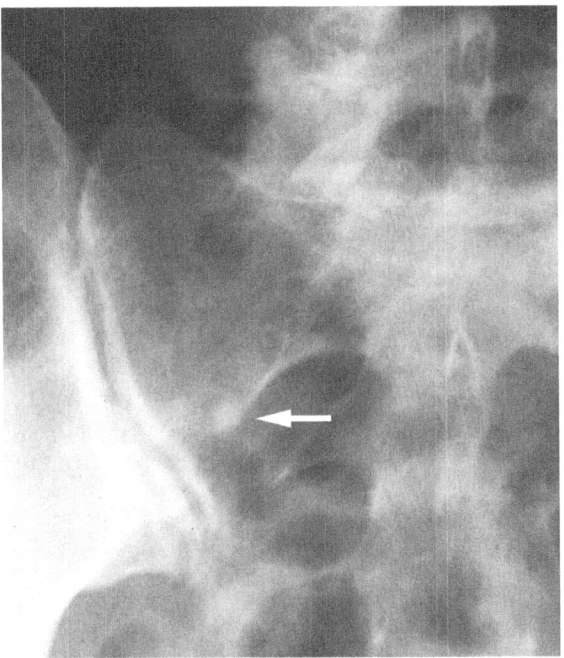

Fig. 5.1. Faintly opaque ureteral stone with superimposition of sacrum (*arrow*)

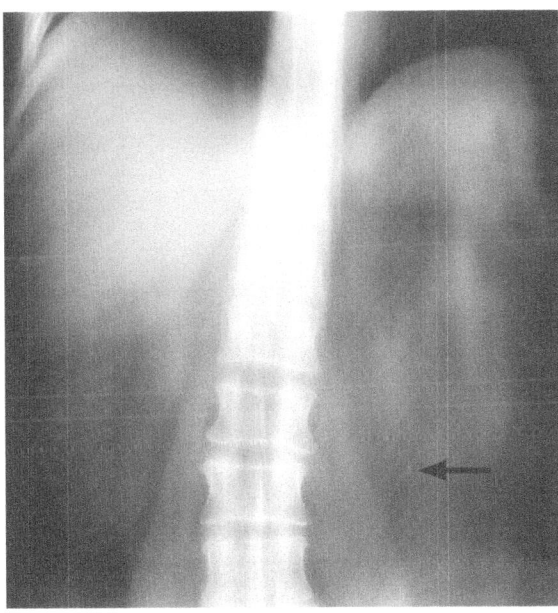

Fig. 5.2. So-called radiotransparent stone, visualized only on linear tomography (*arrow*)

secondary to successive accumulation of different crystals, are uncommon.

The sensitivity of KUB for detecting ureteral stones is low, particularly in patients with acute flank pain. The diagnosis of ureteral lithiasis is accomplished in about 45%–58% of such cases (MUTGI et al. 1991; Jackman et al. 2000). Some authors propose interpreting KUB in combination with CT, especially multislice CT with coronal MIP reconstruction (Van Beers et al. 2001).

Usually, ureteral calculi are small – less than 10 mm in diameter and frequently even less than 4 mm – round or oval, and in the same axis as the ureter (Fig. 5.3a–d). Some calculi have an inverted pyramidal shape. Described by Bloom, who named it "the tooth root sign", this morphology is seen in about 20% of intraureteral radiopaque calculi (Bloom et al. 1988). The stone contours are usually regular but are frequently spiculated in oxalic lithiasis.

Some lithiasis, like pyelocaliceal stones, are secondary to urinary stasis and infection. In this situation, stone casting in a dilated ureteral lumen or "milk of calcium" appearance can be observed (Becker and Pollack 1981; Garcia-Cuerpo 1985; Mac-Millian and Fritzhand 1978) (Figs. 5.4, 5.5). These stones are usually formed in an abnormally dilated ureter, secondary to inflammatory or tumoral obstruction, congenital anomalies (Fig. 5.6a–c) (idiopathic megaureter, ureterocele), post nephrectomy ureteral stump, or a real "stone nest" (Baro and Julia 1989). A particular aspect of ureteral stone was described after ESWL: Fragmentation of lithiasis of the upper collecting system leads to ureteral migration, producing a cast of the lumen, a so-called *Steinstrasse* (Fig. 5.7a, b) (Banner 1990a).

Ureteral stone topography usually corresponds to

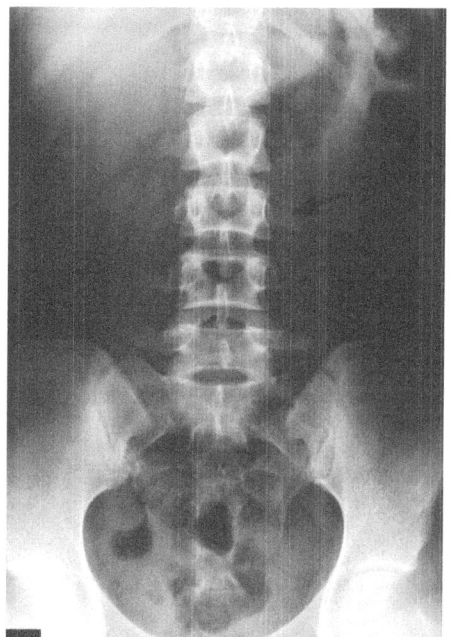

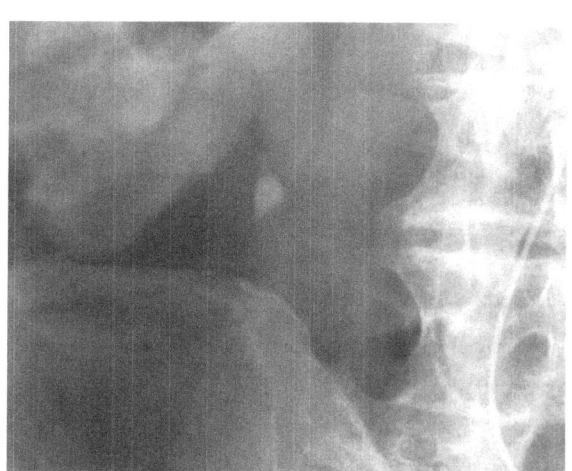

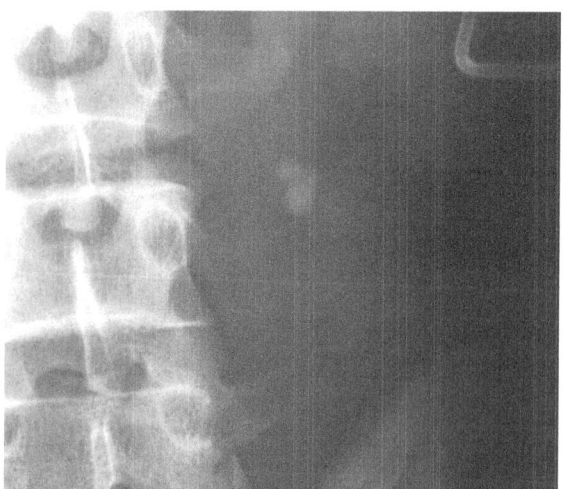

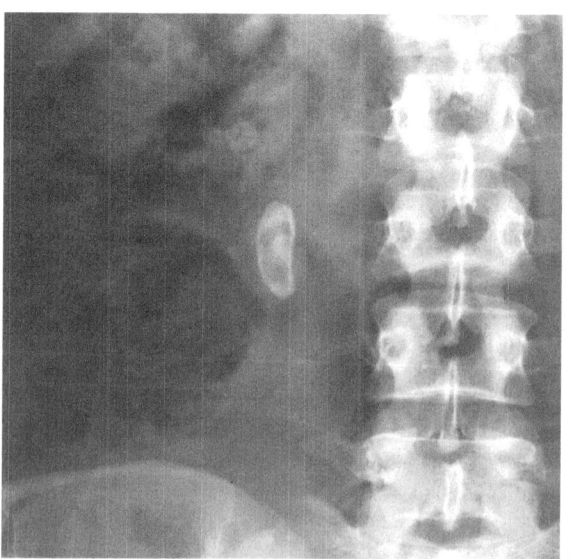

Fig. 5.3a–d. Some examples of radiopaque stones: **a** Faintly opaque lithiasis of left lumbar ureter (*arrow*). **b, c** Two examples of "tooth root" stones. **d** Stratified ureteral stone

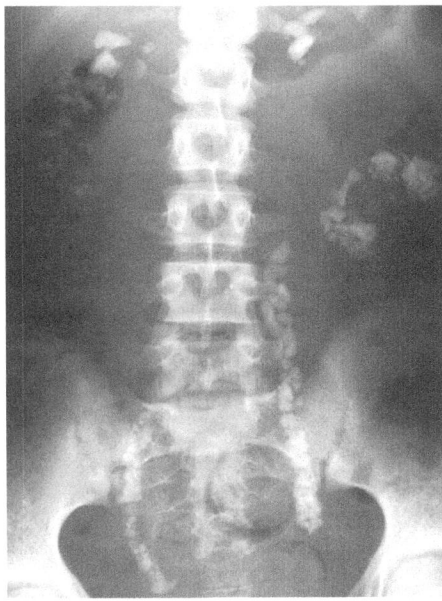

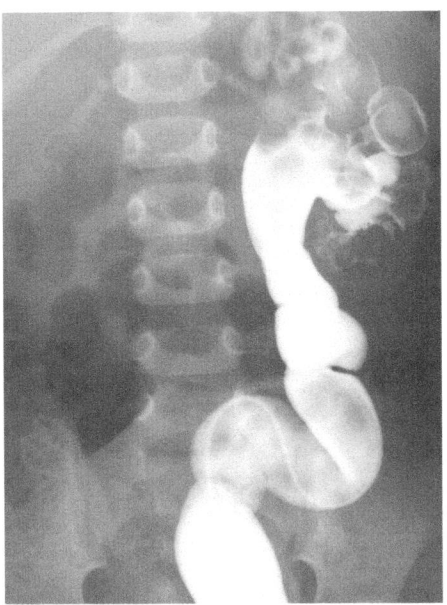

Fig. 5.4. Casting of both ureters with multiple calculi in a patient with bilateral congenital ureterohydronephrosis probably related to idiopathic bilateral megaureter

Fig. 5.5. Casting of left pelvicaliceal cavities and ureter by a struvite stone in a young patient with congenital ureterohydronephrosis

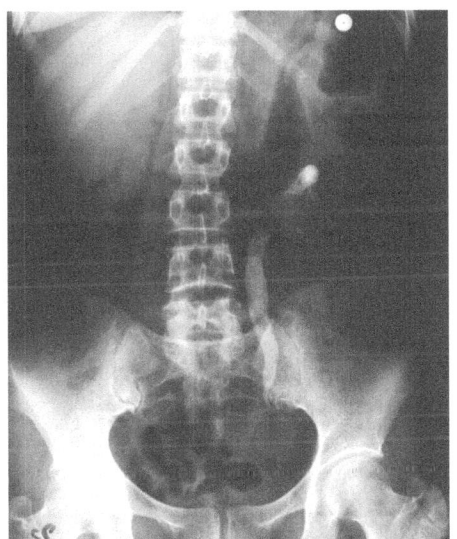

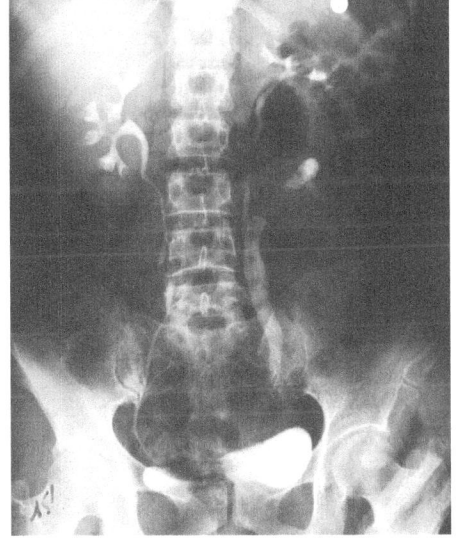

a

b

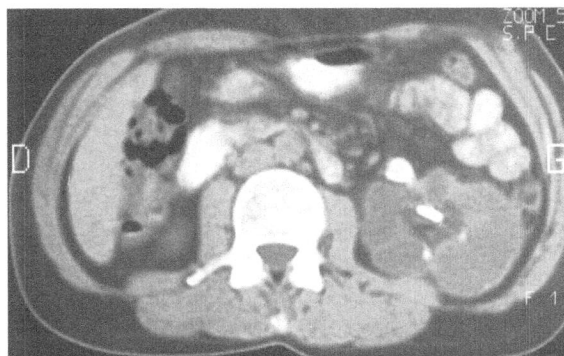

c

Fig. 5.6a–c. Pelvicaliceal and ureteral casting of the lower moiety of duplicated left cavities. **a** KUB: densely opaque calculus of the ureter. **b** EU: nonfunctioning of the lower moiety of the urinary tract. **c** Unenhanced CT: ureteral and caliceal stones with hydronephrosis

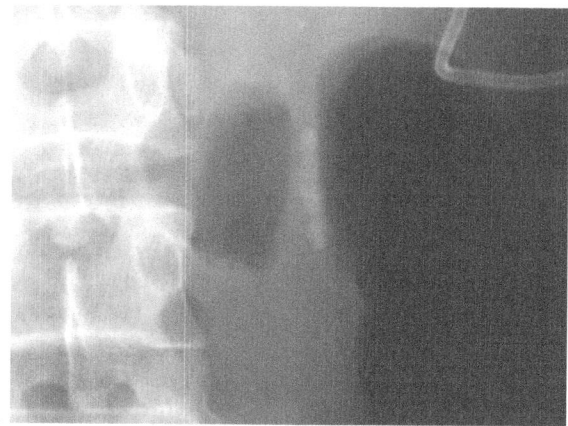

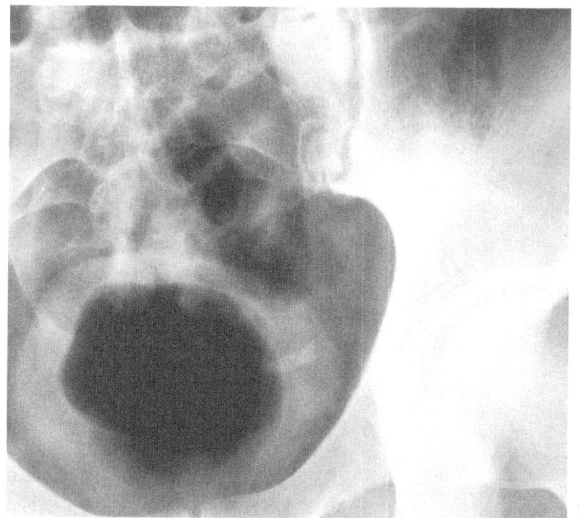

Fig. 5.7a, b. Two examples of post-ESWL ureteral stone migration, so-called *Steinstrasse*

the presumed position of ureters, but aberrant locations may exist in dilated urinary tract or abnormal ureteral topography (genitourinary prolapse, for example). Some stones can move inside the ureter, thus appearing in different locations on KUB, depending on the position of the patient.

Ureteral lithiasis must be distinguished from extraurinary calcifications (SINGH and MALEK 1982). The differential diagnosis comprises calcified mesenteric nodes (that have the appearance of a bunch of grapes and are mobile from film to film), psoas muscle calcifications (that are oblique following the muscle orientation), iliac vessel calcifications

(straight or curved), appendicoliths (more lateral), and pelvic phleboliths which have regular contours and a clear center, and are usually multiple and bilateral). Gonadal vein phleboliths and some devices used for fallopian tube occlusion are very difficult to differentiate from ureteral stones, but these situations are exceptional (BERLOW 1979; SPRING 1982). Certain tumoral calcifications (ovarian dermoid cyst, urothelial calcified tumor) may be mistaken for ureteral calculi but are also associated with other anatomical modifications. In most of these situations opacification of the ureter allows the diagnosis (Figs. 5.8a, b; 5.9a, b).

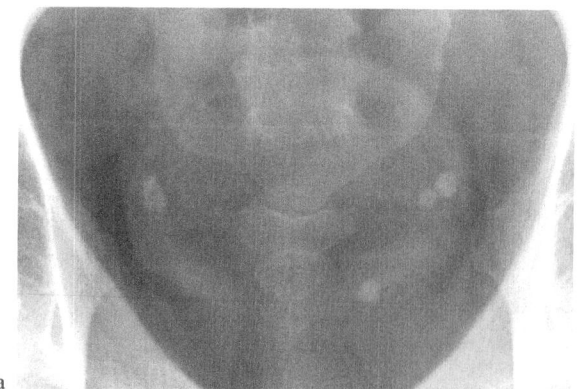

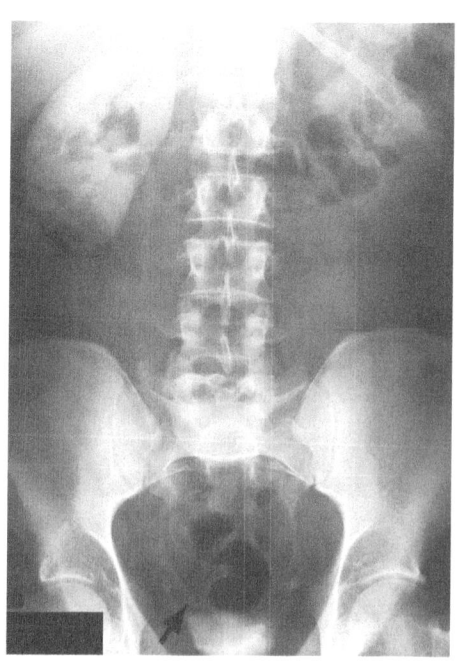

Fig. 5.8a, b. Role of EU in the differential diagnosis between phleboliths and pelvic lithiasis: **a** KUB: Presence of several pelvic calcifications in a patient with right renal colic. **b** EU: late film identifies the ureteral stone among the multiple phleboliths (*arrow*)

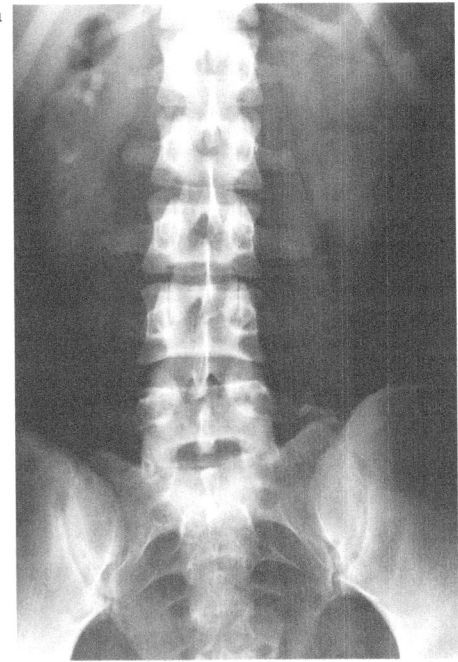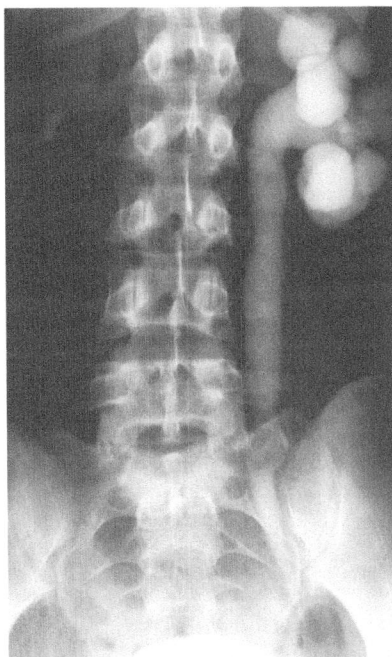

Fig. 5.9a, b. Role of EU in the diagnosis of undetermined abdominal calcification: a KUB shows an egg-shell calcification in the left paravertebral area. b EU allows the diagnosis of large left ureteral stone with a radiotransparent central area and peripheral calcification

5.1.1.2
Excretory Urography

For many years, EU and KUB were considered the gold standard for diagnosing ureteral lithiasis. Their indications are nowadays challenged because of the development of new diagnostic techniques and risks associated with the use of contrast media.

The presence of a ureteral calculus may reduce the urinary flow or result in an acute or, more rarely, chronic obstructive syndrome associated with variable ureterohydronephrosis (Fig. 5.10a, b). Pyeloureteral dilatation is present in about 12% of cases, usually in connection with an extrasinusal renal pelvis (WOLFMAN et al. 1979; THORNBURY and PARKER 1982).

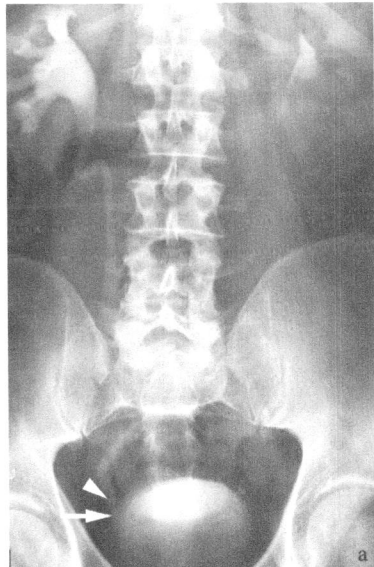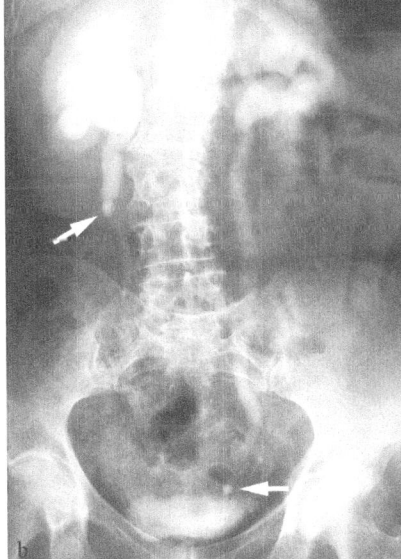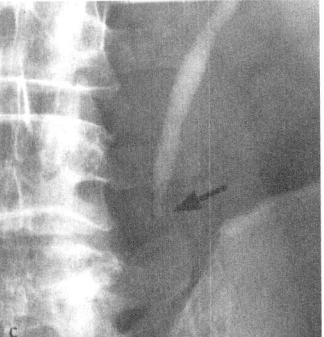

Fig. 5.10a, b. Three examples of obstructive ureteral stone: a Right moderate ureterohydronephrosis secondary to a small calculus in the pelvic ureter (*arrow*). Note the surimposition of a phlebolith on right pelvic ureter (*arrowhead*) b Bilateral severe and chronic ureterohydronephrosis related to ureteral stones (*arrows*). The right stone is stratified and incompletely obstructive. c Small calculi of the terminal lumbar ureter (*arrow*)

In the majority of cases, the ureteral opacification is sufficient and makes it possible to follow the opaque column to the level of the calculus, confirming the intraureteral topography. However, urinary excretion is sometimes so delayed that late (up to 24 h) films have to be done. More than one film is usually necessary: oblique, prone, post-voiding to avoid bladder and distal end of the ureter superposition, and late films if the opacification is insufficient or delayed. Usually, the calculus is not completely obstructive because of its contour irregularities and roughness that allow the urine to pass through. Decreased early nephrogram followed by prolonged and increased nephrogram on the same side of the ureteral calculus has been described as an indirect obstructive sign (Korobkin et al. 1978). Decreasing pyeloureteral opacification is also the rule (Fig. 5.11). Urine filtration after post-voiding films is mandatory, because the contrast medium used for EU causes a hyperdiuresis state that could help calculus migration and expulsion.

Faintly radiopaque stones can be concealed within the opacified ureter, particularly with LOCM, or may appear as an intraluminal filling defect (Fig. 5.12a–c). Radiolucent stones can also appear as an intraluminal defect or may be totally invisible but suspected because of the constant difference in ureteral size (Fig. 5.13).

The morphology of the ureteral opacification at the calculus level is variable (Fig. 5.14a–d). Usually, there is a dilatation of the proximal ureter with spasmodic narrowing over and below the calculus area.

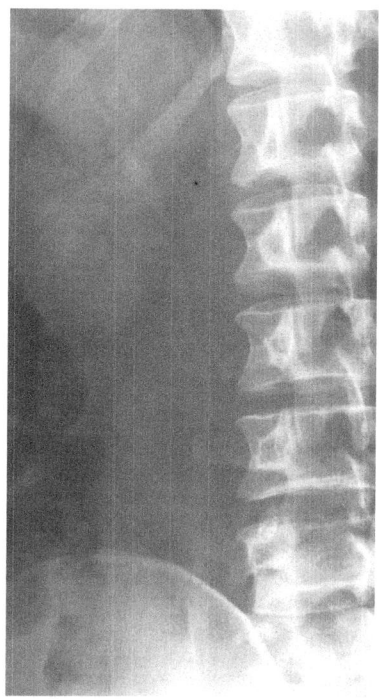

Fig. 5.11. Decreasing pyeloureteral opacification without dilatation of the collecting system in a post-lithiasis acute ureteral obstruction

Sometimes the distal ureter is threadlike. In case of pre-existing urinary tract obstruction, the ureter usually has a cylindrical or tube-like aspect, and a diameter which does not change at the calculus area.

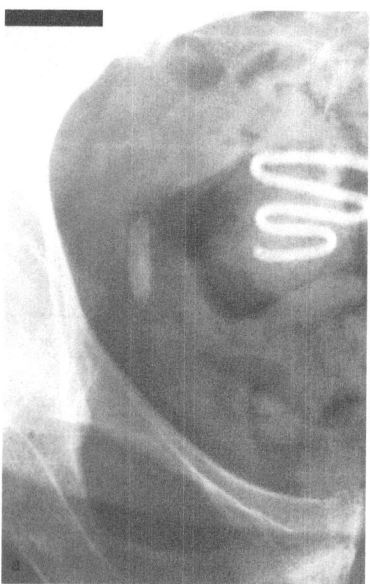 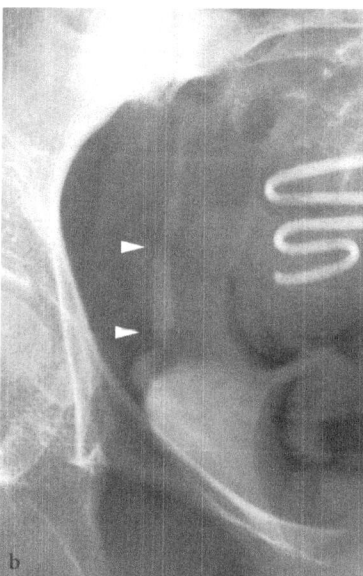 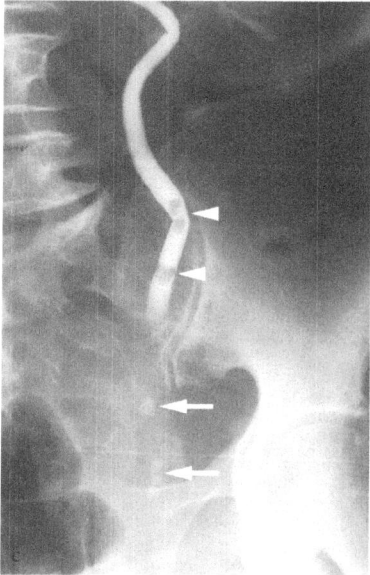

Fig. 5.12a–c. Different aspects of ureteral lithiasis: **a, b** Spontaneously opaque stone on KUB hidden after ureteral opacification (*arrowheads*). **c** Faintly opaque ureteral stones (*arrows*) giving a filling defect aspect after opacification (*arrowheads*)

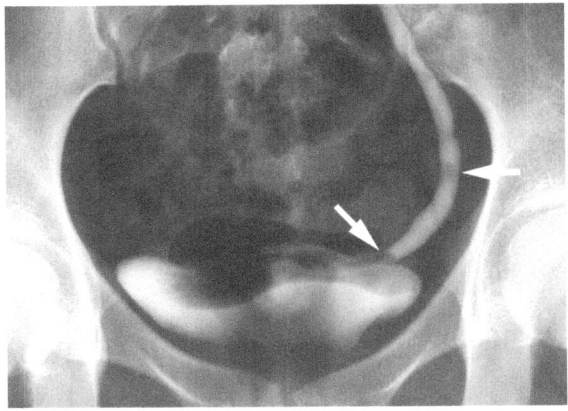

Fig. 5.13. EU for left renal colic. Two weakly obstructive radiolucent uratic stones of the left pelvic ureter (*arrows*)

The stone can be mobile inside the ureter and can change its position from film to film. In case of ureteral duplication, the calculus inside an unopacified ureter may be mistaken for an extraureteral calcification (Fig. 5.15a, b).

The most frequent location for a ureteral calculus is at the ureterovesical junction. There, it has a particular aspect in early opacification or in the post-voiding film. The morphology of the bladder horn and interureteral ridge is frequently modified and thickened by 3 mm or more (CHEN et al. 1995). VESPIGNANI describes ureteral meatus edema as an image of intravesical defect lateral to the interureteral ridge and sometimes having the aspect of a pseudo-ureterocele (VESPIGNANI 1962) (Fig. 5.16a–c). The blurred contours of this image precludes the diagnosis of ureterocele. A spastic deformation of the bladder horn may also be present and may persist

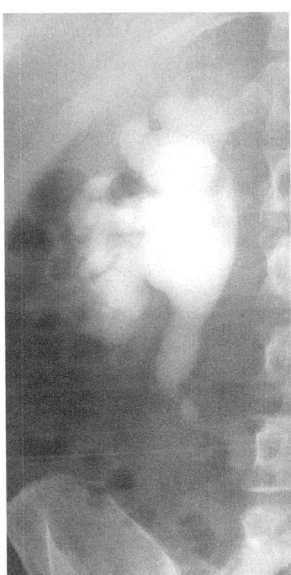

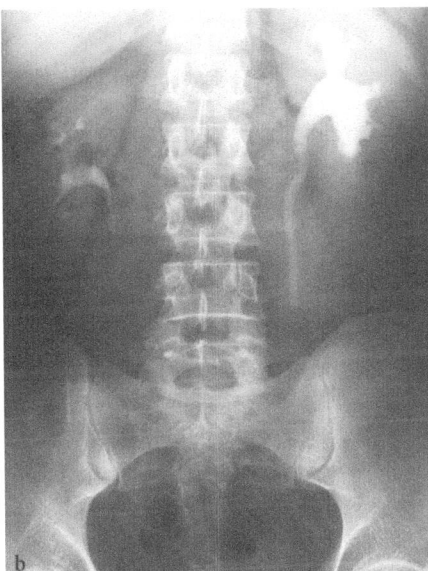

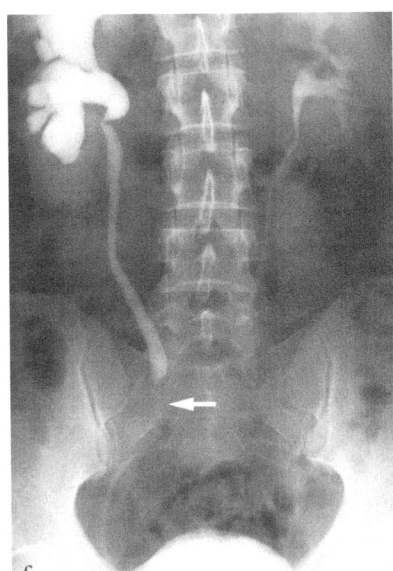

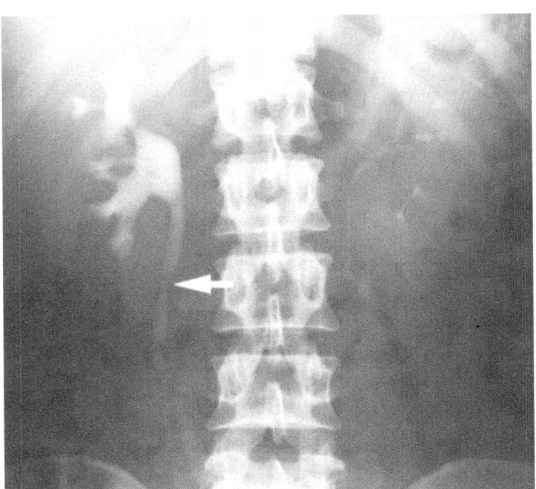

Fig. 5.14a–d. Some examples of changes induced by a ureteral calculus: a Total obstruction by a large spiculated oxalic stone. b Total lithiasic obstruction of the mid-lumbar ureter without change of the diameter. c, d Spasmodic narrowing of the ureter over and below a small and faintly visible calculus (*arrows*)

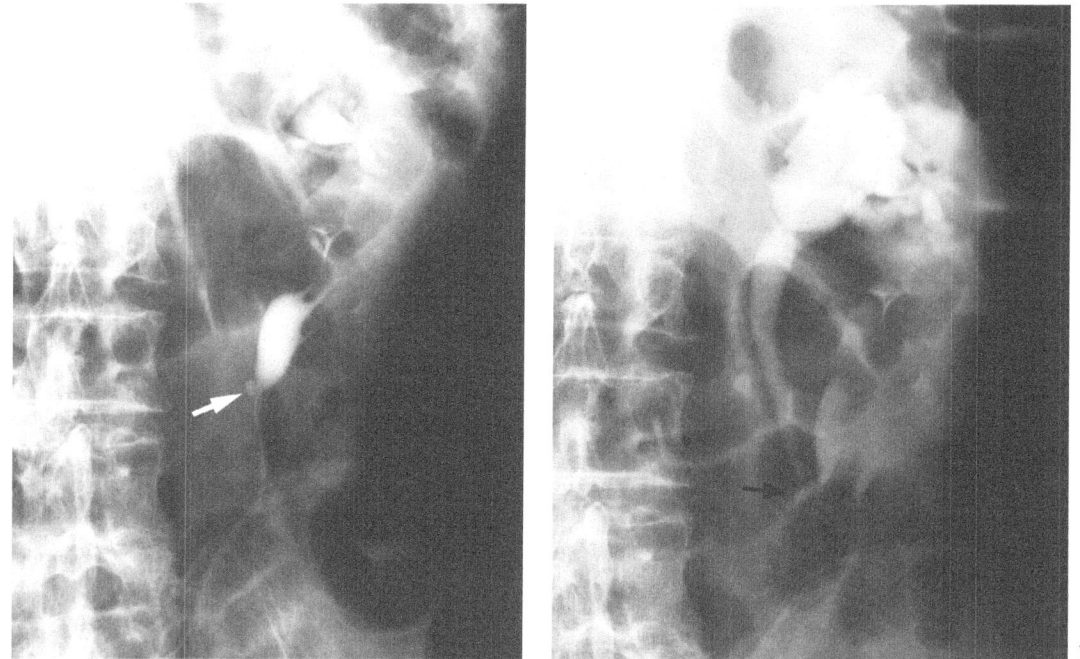

Fig. 5.15a, b. Ureteral stone with duplication. **a** Opacification of the lower excretory cavities of a duplication. Presence of a rounded extraureteral calcification (*arrow*). Delayed opacification of the upper calices. **b** Delayed film shows obstruction of the upper collecting system secondary to a ureteral stone which corresponds to the previously considered extraureteral calcification (*arrow*)

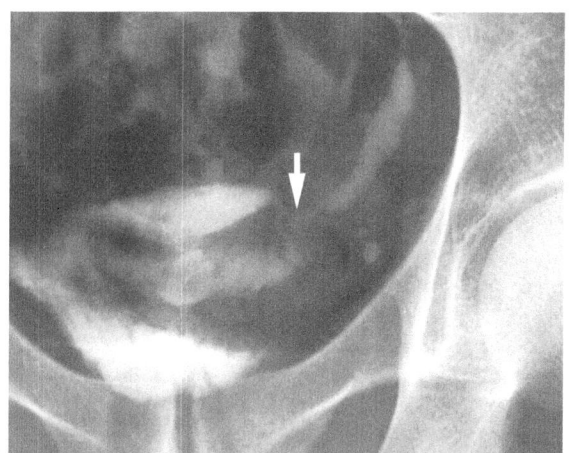

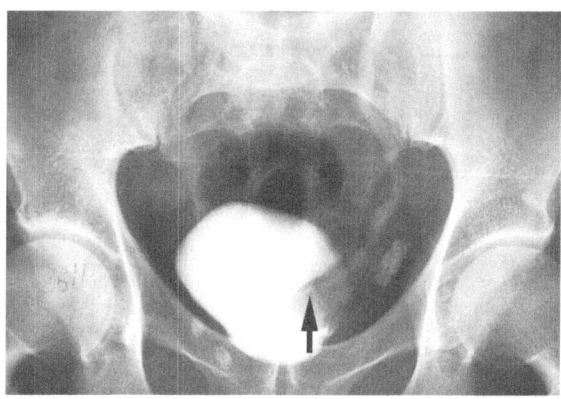

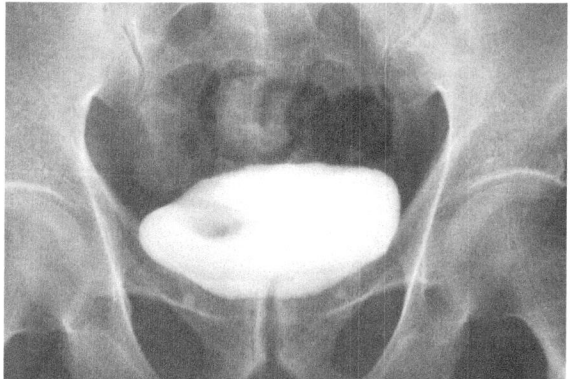

Fig. 5.16a–c. Some examples of Vespignani's sign. Edematous changes of the ureteral meatus area around the stone (**a, b**) (*arrow*), sometimes giving the aspect of a pseudo-ureterocele (**c**)

for some hours after calculus expulsion, allowing a retrospective diagnosis (BANNER 1990)

EU permits the diagnosis of stones not seen on KUB because of their characteristics (size, density) or because of the technical limitations of KUB. On EU, stones appear as intraluminal defects, round or oval, with regular contours which make an acute angle with the ureteral wall. If the stone is not totally occlusive, the defect is surrounded by contrast medium in all views. In some cases, an inverted cupula-shaped interruption of the contrast column can be visualized. The differential diagnosis includes papillary sloughs, mycotic and caseous fragments, a fibroepithelial polyp, and urothelial tumors (FEIN and McCLENNAN 1986). Ureteral clots are usually mobile, deformable, and associated with macroscopic hematuria. The ureteral fibroepithelial polyp is also mobile but has a characteristic long pedicle. Papillary sloughs and mycotic and caseous fragments occur in specific clinical conditions and can be associated with urinary tract morphological abnormalities. In urothelial tumors, the ureteral dilatation beyond the tumor (goblet sign) is not always present (BERGMAN et al. 1961). In difficult cases, direct opacification or computed tomography can be helpful.

In certain circumstances, a urinary calculus may not be radiologically detectable. A normal EU makes it possible to eliminate the diagnosis of renal colic only if performed during the acute crisis, but in this clinical setting, if it demonstrates an obstructive syndrome without detectable calculus, the diagnosis of renal colic secondary to radiolucent calculus or other causes of obstructive uropathy must be suspected.

5.1.1.3
Ultrasonography

US is considered as a limited method for visualizing intraureteral calculus. Its limitations for the diagnosis of obstruction are also well known (see Chap. 4). Detection of calculus is favored by demonstration of ureteral dilatation.

Ureteral dilatation must be looked for carefully using the appropriate ultrasonographic techniques. The proximal end of the ureter can be seen through the lower pole of the kidney. Using a coronal approach it is possible to follow the lumbar ureter until it courses over the common iliac vessel. Color Doppler is very helpful to differentiate a dilated ureter from iliac vessels (MACNEILY et al. 1991).

The transabdominal approach with bladder repletion allows identification of a dilated pelvic ureter. The same approach may allow the detection of a

ureteral stone which is characterized by an intraluminal hyperechogenic area with posterior shadowing (POLLACK et al. 1978). This classical pattern is observed mainly at the level of the pelvic ureter (THORNBURY and PARKER 1982). Edema of the ureteral meatus around the stone can also be seen, corresponding to the urographic sign of VESPIGNANI (Fig. 5.17a–c).

These ultrasonographic signs are very useful when the calculus is radiolucent, small, or concealed because of the presence of fecal opacities or gas on KUB. However, considerable differences in the sensitivity and specificity of ultrasonography for detecting ureteral lithiasis are found in the literature.

The sensitivity varies from about 10% in the lumbar ureter to 100% in the pelvic ureter (HADDAD et al. 1992; ONISHI et al. 1986). The transrectal or transvaginal approach can increase the ultrasonographic sensitivity for small calculus at the ureterovesical junction (LAING et al. 1994; LERNER and RUBENS 1986).

"Twinkling artifacts" on color Doppler US can also help to identify small pelvic urinary stones (Fig. 5.18a, b). These artifacts, related to complex interactions between ultrasonographic beams and the stone surface, are characterized by an area of aliasing color Doppler echoes around the stone location; they are useful in difficult or equivocal cases when a hyperechogenic image is seen without visible acoustic shadowing (CHELFOUH et al. 1998; LEE et al. 2001). A relationship between the stone composition and the "twinkling artifact" has been demonstrated: This artifact is significantly more important for calcium oxalate monohydrate stones. This type of calculus is more resistant to treatment by ESWL, and the "twinkling artifact" makes it possible to predict fragmentability (CHELFOUH et al. 1998).

5.1.1.4
Antegrade and Retrograde Explorations

Direct urinary tract opacification techniques are used for two main reasons: as a diagnostic tool in difficult or equivocal cases, and to provide guidance for the therapeutic procedure by means of endoscopy and/or interventional uroradiological methods.

In most cases, direct ureteral opacification allows the confirmation of intraureteral topography of the calcification seen on KUB. There is no strong difference in urographic imaging characteristics whether the ureteral opacification is antegrade, retrograde, or intravenous (Figs. 5.19a, b, 5.20a, b, 5.21). Most of the intraluminal defects correspond to lithiasis (MALEK et al. 1975). The problem of air bubbles is easily avoided with a careful technique. Intraureteral clots

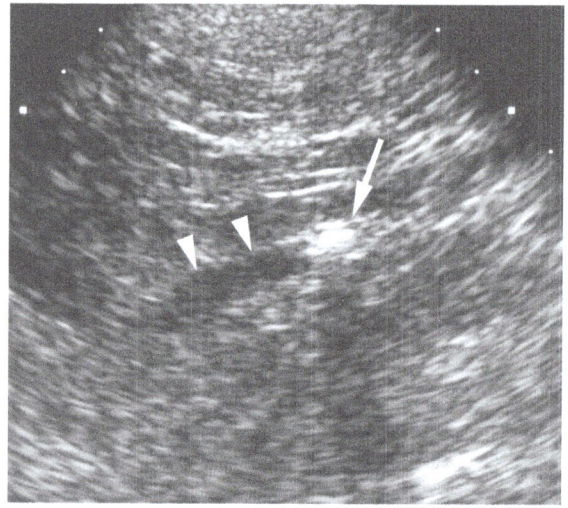

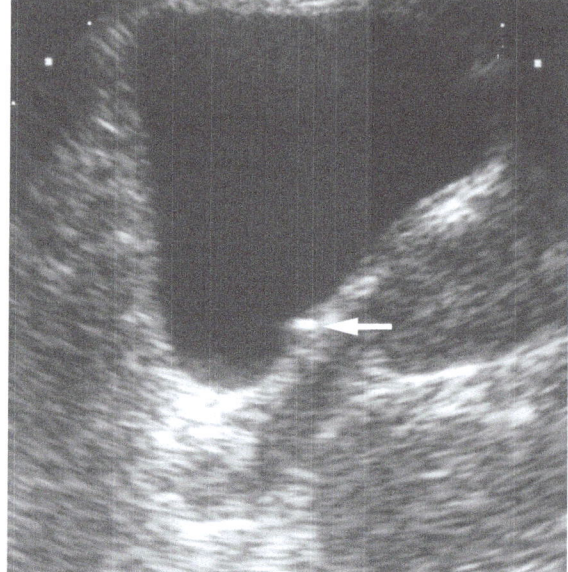

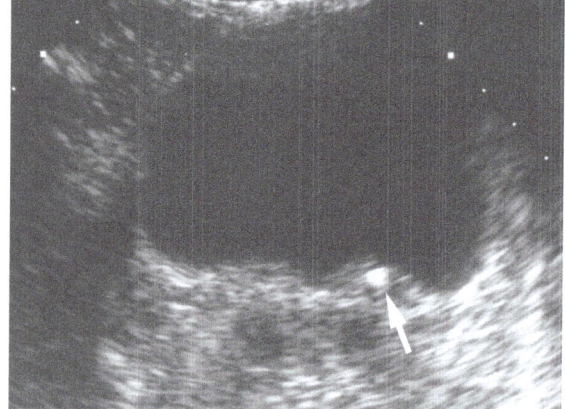

Fig. 5.17a–c. Ultrasonographic aspects of ureteral lithiasis: a Lithiasis of the lumbar ureter: hyperechoic area with posterior shadowing (*arrow*) below a dilated ureter (*arrowheads*). b Lithiasis of the left ureteral meatus without posterior shadowing (*arrow*). c Lithiasis of the left ureteral meatus with perilithiasic edema (*arrow*)

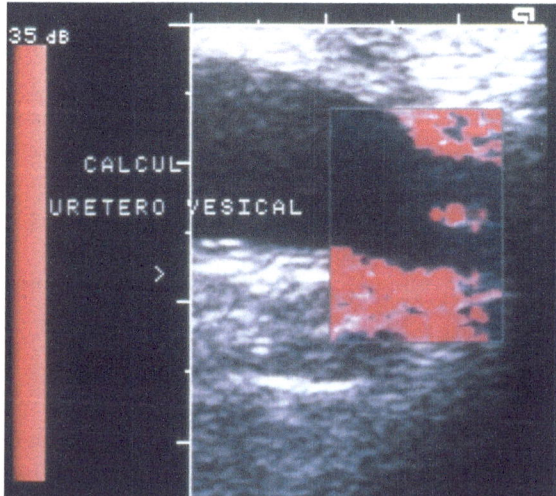

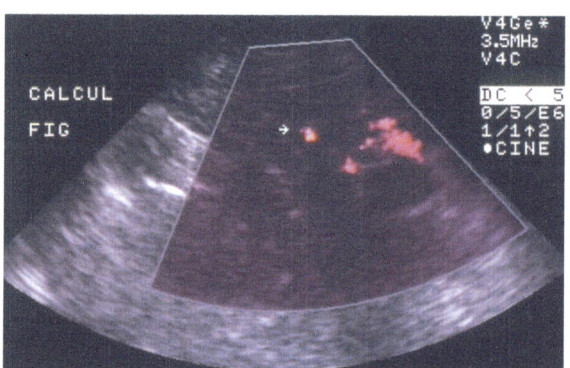

Fig. 5.18a, b. Two examples of "twinkling artifact": a Power Doppler ultrasonography showing a stone in a dilated pelvic ureter with artifact. b In this case the twinkling artifact allows identification of a left pelvic ureteral stone (*arrow*)

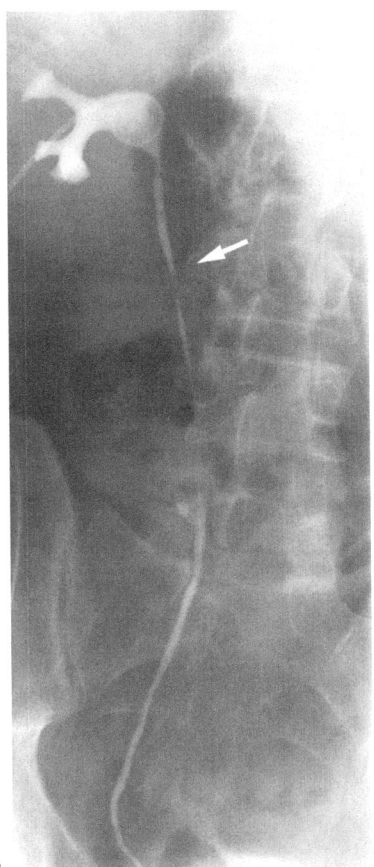
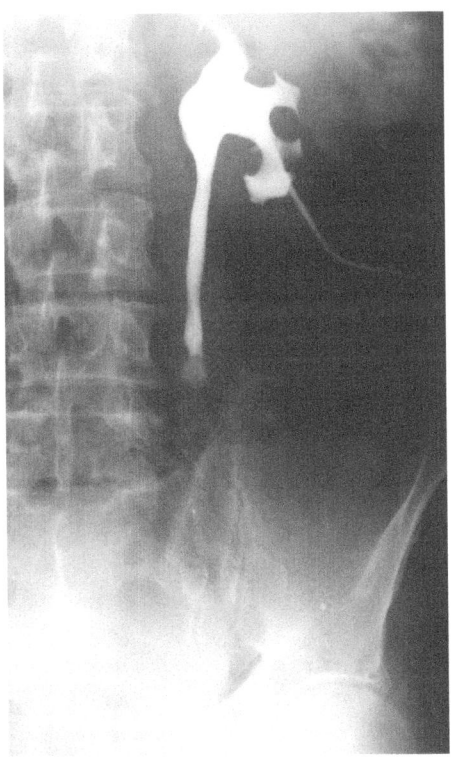

a

b

Fig. 5.19a, b. Two examples of ureteral stone on antegrade pyelography. **a** Small radiolucent calculus of the right lumbar ureter (*arrow*). **b** Larger ureteral radiopaque stone with absence of opacification of the lower ureter

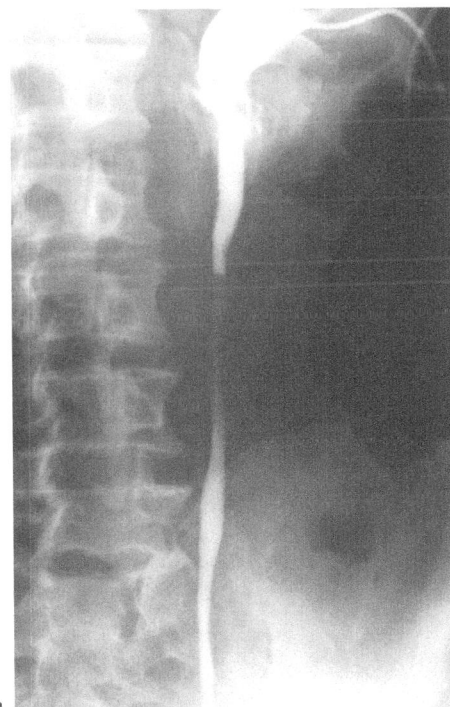
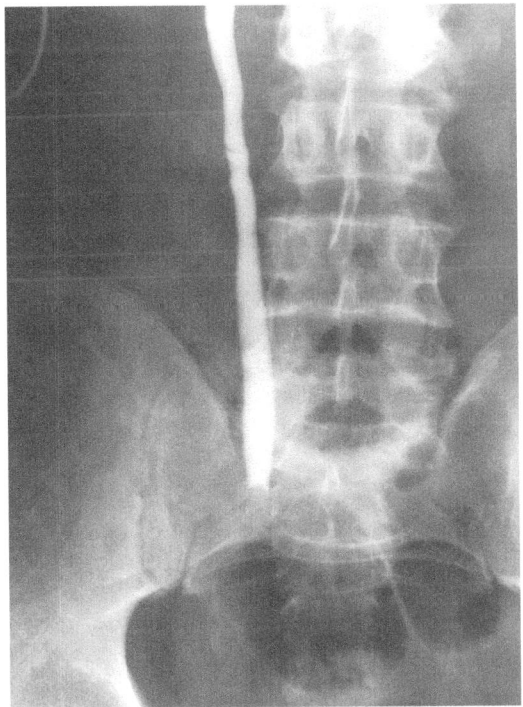

a

b

Fig. 5.20a, b. Migration of a radiolucent ureteral stone during antegrade pyelography

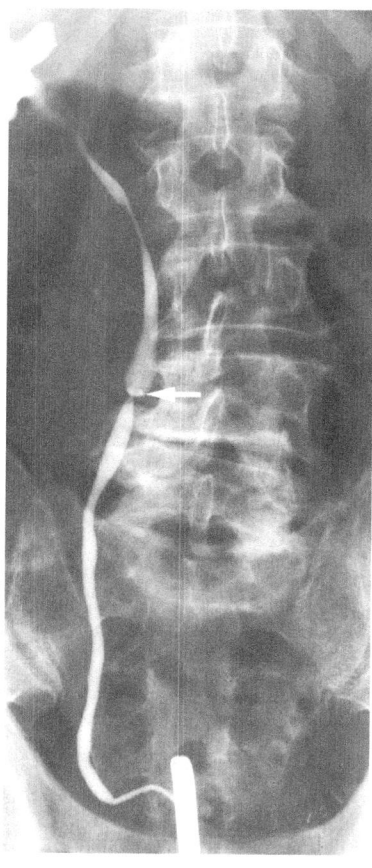

Fig. 5.21. Retrograde ureteropyelography shows a tight diaphragm-like stenosis of the right lumbar ureter with a small radiopaque stone just at the stenosis (*arrow*)

are easy to recognize because of their mobility and morphological modifications. Papillary sloughs may be difficult to differentiate if they are not associated with caliceal changes. The most difficult diagnostic problem is to differentiate between ureteral tumors and pseudo-tumoral changes secondary to the ureteral lithiasis (DUFOUR 1973). Indeed, prolonged calculus wedging produces a chronic ureteritis that may be impossible to differentiate from tumor-induced irregular stenosis or lacunar images (Fig. 5.22a, b). CT can be helpful in these difficult cases.

5.1.1.5
Computed Tomography

CT plays an increasing role and has changed the diagnostic approach to ureteral lithiasis, especially since the arrival of helical scanning technology (SMITH et al. 1995). Ureteral lithiasis signs and their appearance on CT are described in depth in Chap. 4 (Fig. 5.23a, b). Unenhanced CT should demonstrate all ureteral stones except in patients with HIV infection (BLAKE et al. 1998). CT sensitivity and specificity are estimated to be around 97%–98% and 95%–98%, respectively. CT is now considered to have the capacity to detect calculi as small as 1 mm, that may be missed on EU (Figs. 5.24a–f, 5.25a–c). Calculi in HIV patients are totally radiolucent and require intravenous contrast medium to be visualized (Fig. 5.26a–e). However, partially calcified stones can occur in these patients and may then be detected

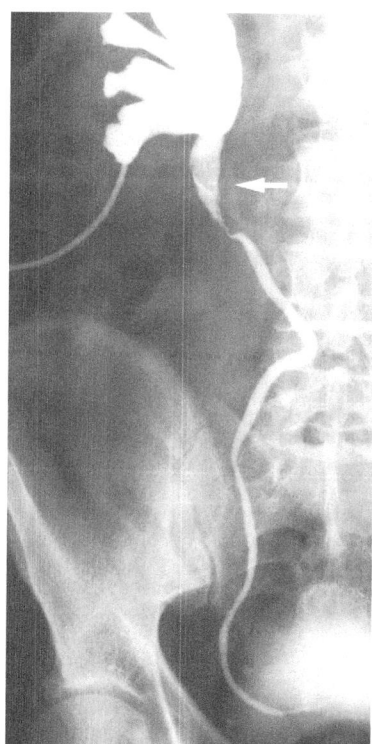

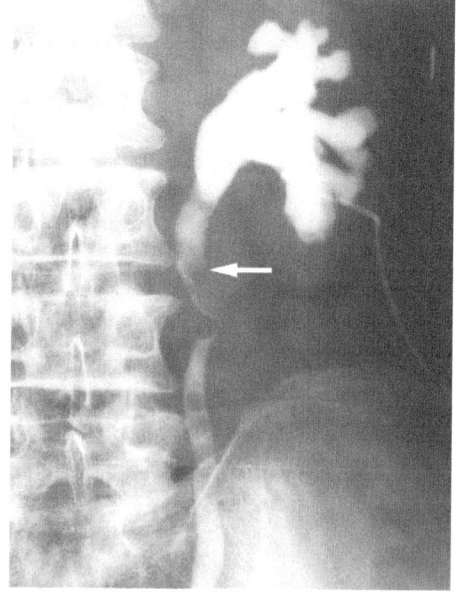

Fig. 5.22a, b. Two examples of pseudotumoral changes of the ureter immediately underneath the stone (*arrows*)

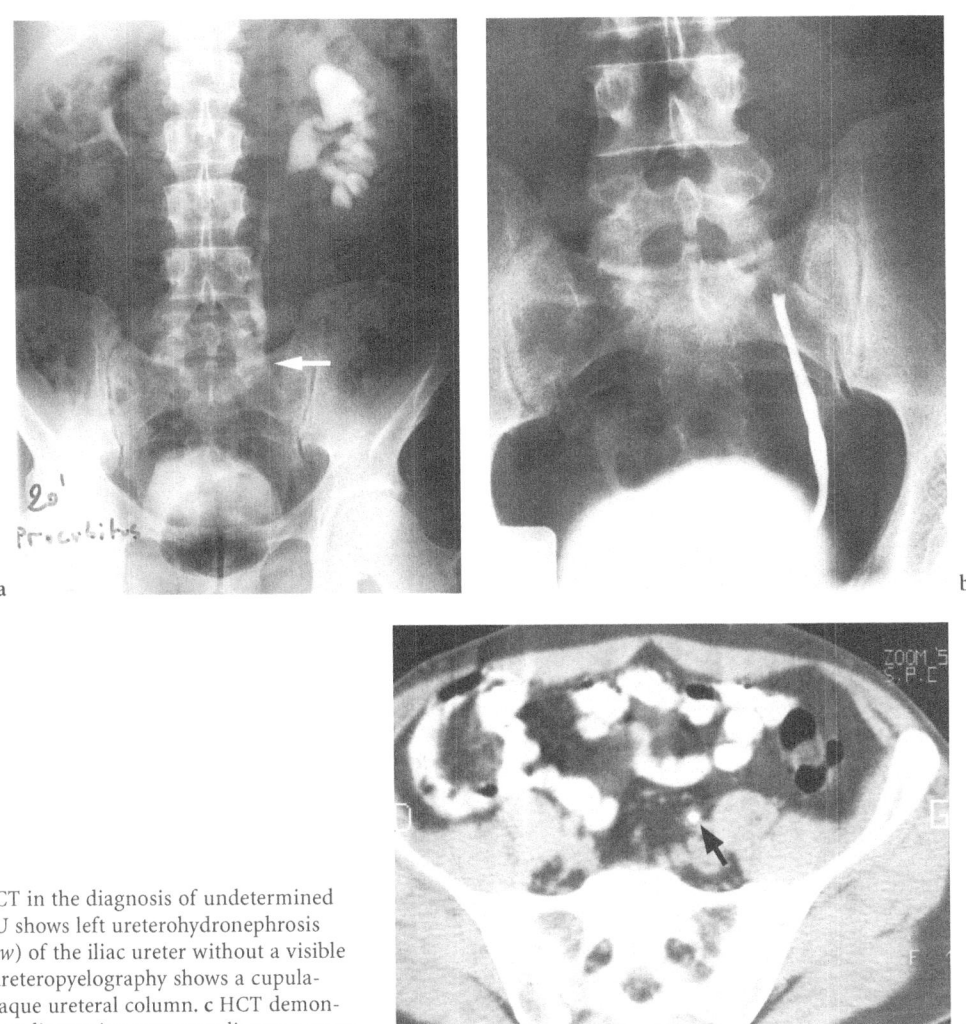

Fig. 5.23a–c. Role of CT in the diagnosis of undetermined ureteral stenosis. **a** EU shows left ureterohydronephrosis with narrowing (*arrow*) of the iliac ureter without a visible stone. **b** Retrograde ureteropyelography shows a cupula-shaped end of the opaque ureteral column. **c** HCT demonstrates a spontaneous radioopacity corresponding to a stone and sourrounded by a rim sign (*arrow*)

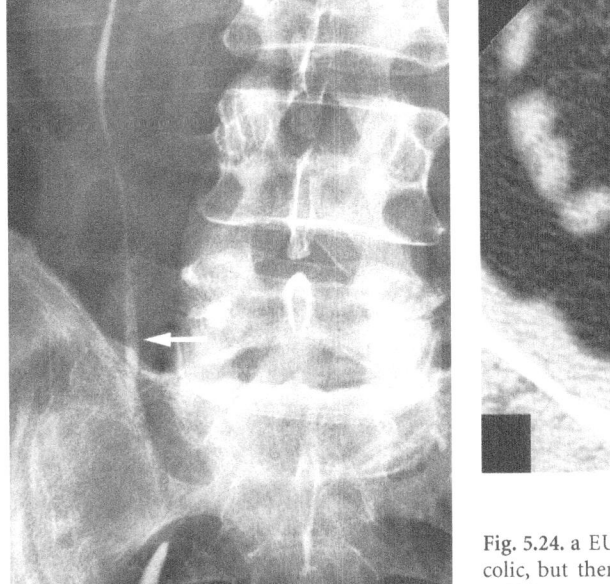

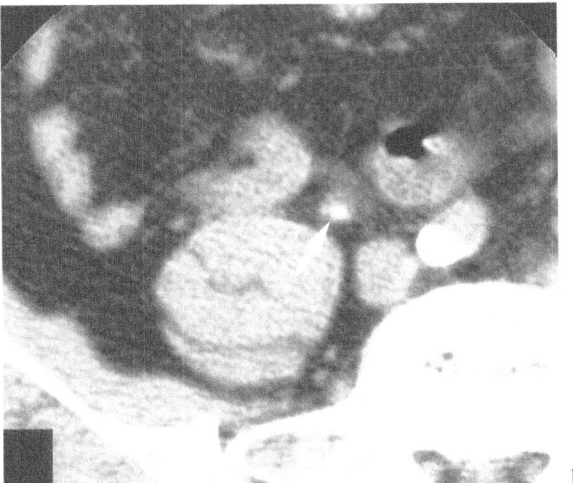

Fig. 5.24. **a** EU performed with the patient prone is positive for left renal colic, but there is no clear demonstration of acute obstruction. A small radiolucent stone is suspected at end of lumbar ureter (*arrow*). **b** CT demonstrates a small stone with rim sign (*arrow*)

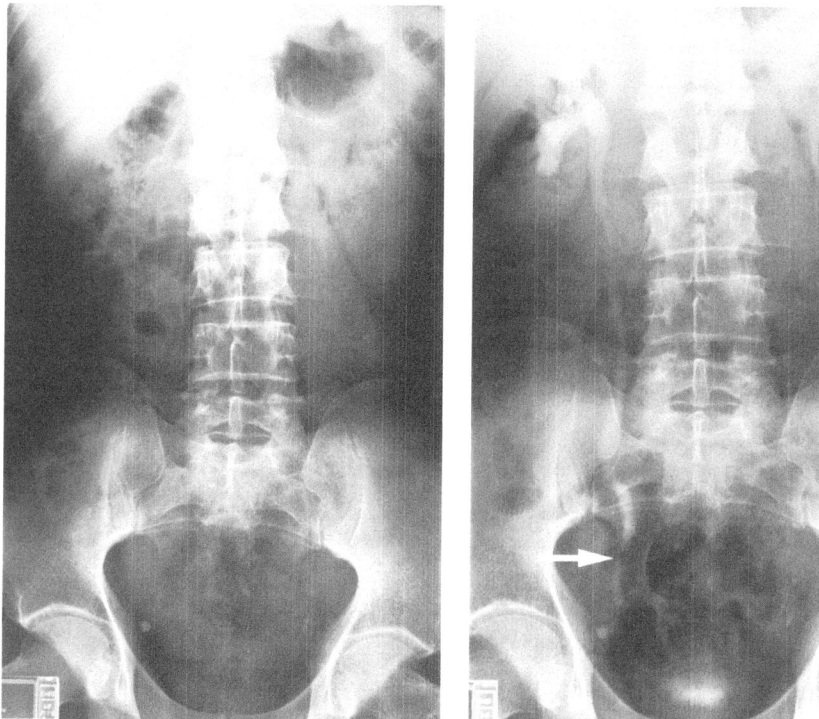

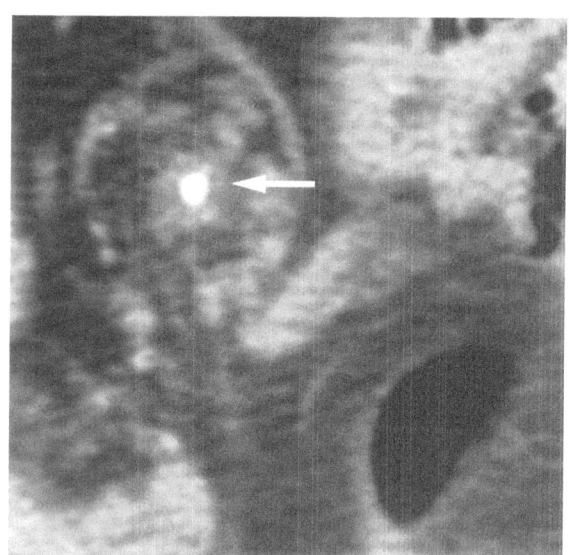

Fig. 5.25. a KUB: absence of visible lithiasis. **b** EU: discrete right ureterohydronephrosis with a stenosis of the pelvic ureter without clear identification of a stone (*arrow*). **c** CT: presence of radiopaque stone with rim sign (*arrow*)

(SUNDARAM and SALTZMAN 1999).

Usually, density measurements are useful only for the differential diagnosis of ureteral tumors or radiolucent lithiasis. Technically, thin slices over the calculus before ureteral opacification and correct cursor positioning over the measured area are mandatory for a correct measurement. All ureteral calculi have a high density, usually of more than 300 HU (PARIENTY et al. 1982). Uric acid stones have a lower density than calcium stones, but this is not statistically significant and does not allow precise determination of the com-

position of the stone (NEWHOUSE et al. 1984; HILLMAN et al. 1984). However, when the calculus is more than 10 mm in diameter, density measurements are more precise. Indeed, uric acid and oxalate calculi usually have a density of less than 500 HU and more than 1600 HU, respectively (KUWAHARA et al. 1984). Uric acid calculi are radiolucent on KUB but have a high CT density because of their high physical density and possible deposits of contrast medium from preceding radiological examinations (RESNICK et al. 1984; SEGAL et al. 1978).

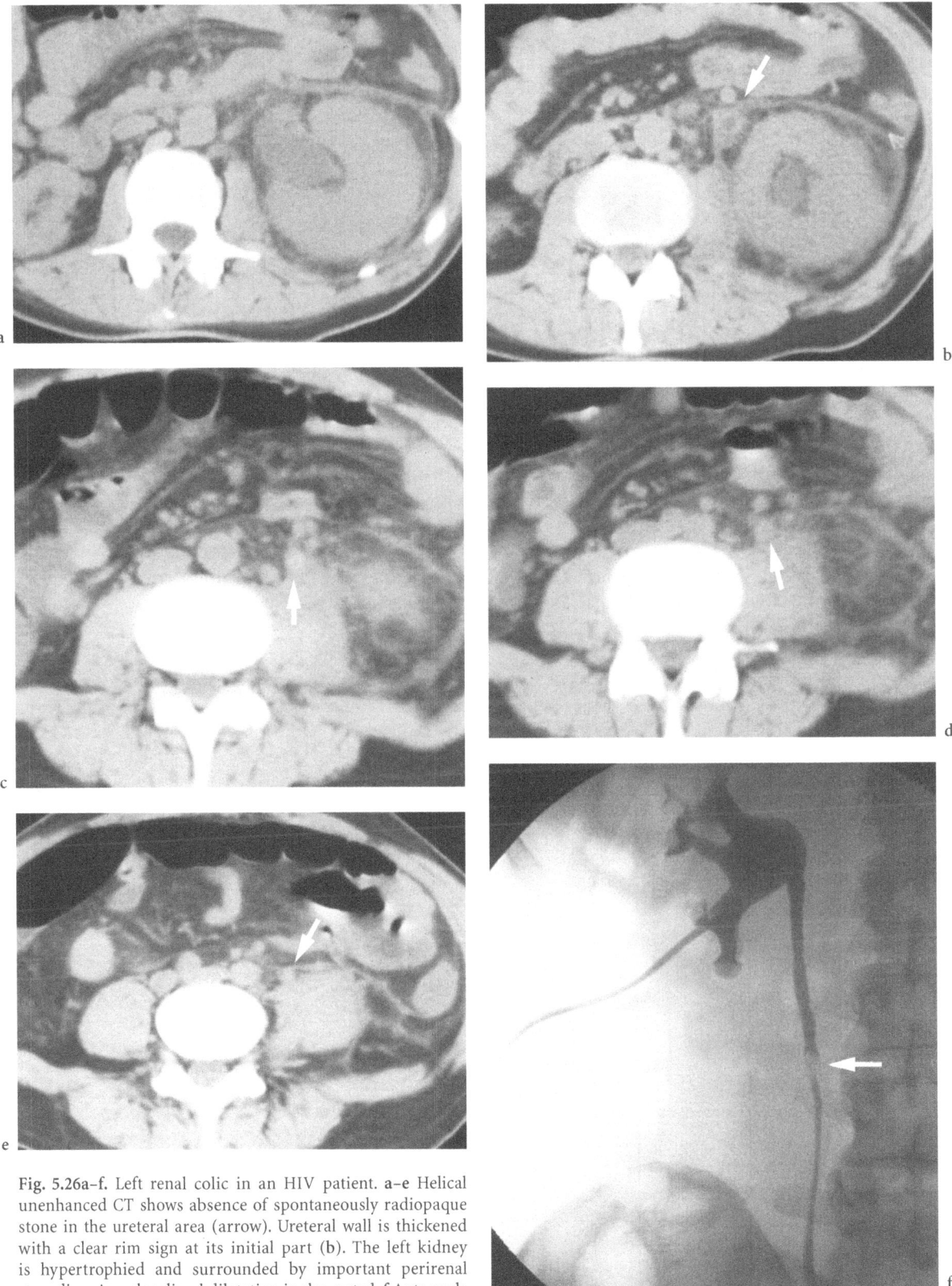

Fig. 5.26a–f. Left renal colic in an HIV patient. **a–e** Helical unenhanced CT shows absence of spontaneously radiopaque stone in the ureteral area (arrow). Ureteral wall is thickened with a clear rim sign at its initial part (**b**). The left kidney is hypertrophied and surrounded by important perirenal stranding. A pyelocaliceal dilatation is also noted. **f** Antegrade pyelography is performed because of the presence of fever. Opacification shows a radiolucent obstructive lacuna at the middle part of lumbar ureter (*arrow*)

CT is more accurate than KUB for stone size measurement; this is of great clinical importance for patient management in terms of outcome and therapeutic strategy. In addition to stone size, indirect signs of acute obstruction (perirenal stranding) are well correlated with the likelihood of spontaneous stone passage (TAKAHASHI et al. 1998). Vespignani's sign may also be noted (Fig. 5.27a, b).

Both CT attenuation and size appear useful for determining which patients require KUB, thus avoiding unnecessary radiography (ZAGORIA et al. 2001). For patients with CT attenuation lower than 200 HU, a stone will not be visible on KUB. For patients with attenuation higher than 300 HU the chance of KUB detection is very high. Between 200 and 300 HU, KUB is useful if the calculus measured on CT is greater than 5 mm. A calculus larger than 5 mm not visible on KUB is probably a uric acid or xanthine stone.

The main diagnostic problem is still to differentiate distal ureteral calculi from pelvic phleboliths on unenhanced helical CT (HENEGHAN et al. 1997). Some authors have reported an interest in analyzing the geometric configuration, the presence of central lucency, the mean attenuation, the profile attenuation analysis, and the periureteral changes (BELL et al. 1998) (Fig. 5.28a–d). The different characteristics of each item are summarized in Table 5.2. However, the rim and comet-tail signs until now considered helpful for the differential diagnosis are currently under debate, because they are rarely isolated signs (GUEST et al. 2001). The best way to confirm the diagnosis of ureteral stone is to demonstrate the exact position of the stone in the ureteral site by careful analysis of the different slices and multiplanar reconstruction (DALRYMPLE et al. 2000) (Fig. 5.29a, b).

Most urinary tract calculi do not have a significant MRI signal. The uro-MRI sequences show the obstructed slowness of the urinary flow and sometimes an intraluminal signal void. The role of MRI in urinary tract lithiasis is indeed still very limited (ROTHPEARL et al. 1995).

5.1.2
The Role of the Radiologist in the Therapeutic Strategy

In the past 10 years the therapeutic approach to ureteral lithiasis has changed. Formerly, only two therapeutic alternatives were available: (a) a conservative approach using medical treatment and radiological follow-up in the majority of cases, and (b) a surgical approach which was reserved for large calculi (more than 7 mm in diameter) associated with hematuria or infection, or with very painful crises with repetitive and persistent symptoms lasting 6 weeks or more (DUFOUR 1973).

Other effective and less invasive methods have been developed, the more significant ones being the ureteral approach from retrograde (ureteroscopy) or the antegrade approach (nephroscopy) and ESWL (BARR et al. 1990; DRACH 1983; JORION et al. 1989). The therapeutic decision involves two steps:

1. Is there a need for direct treatment?
2. Which method should be selected if direct treatment is mandatory?

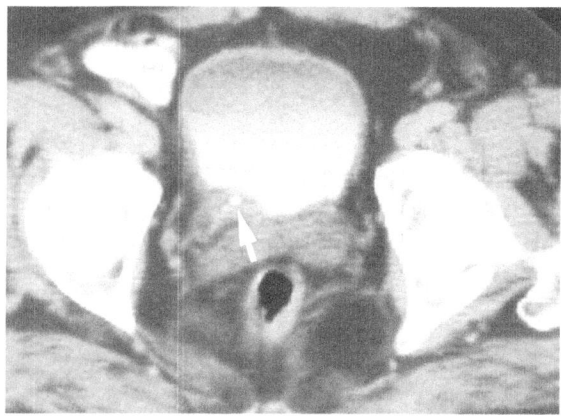
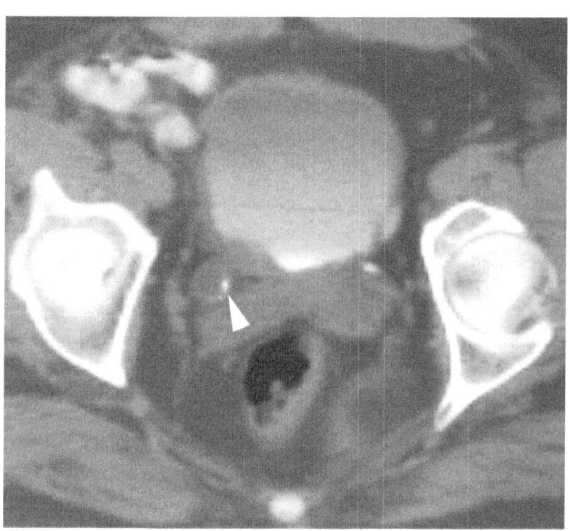

Fig. 5.27. a Post-contrast CT with presence of a small stone at the right meatus with edema (*arrow*). **b** The pelvic ureter is not opacified and is dilated with another small stone (*arrowhead*)

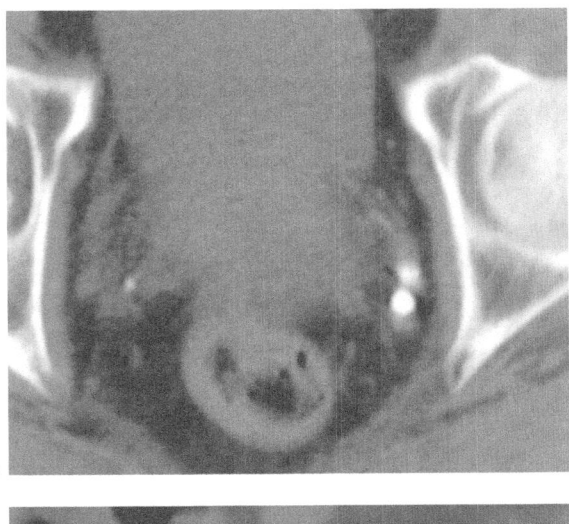

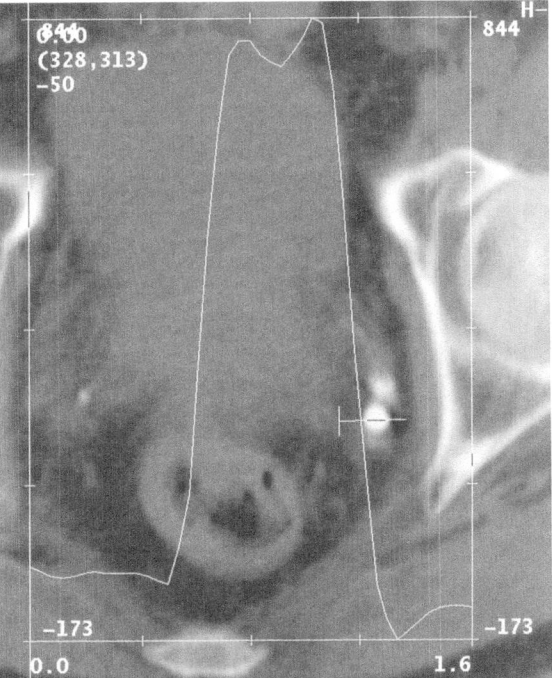

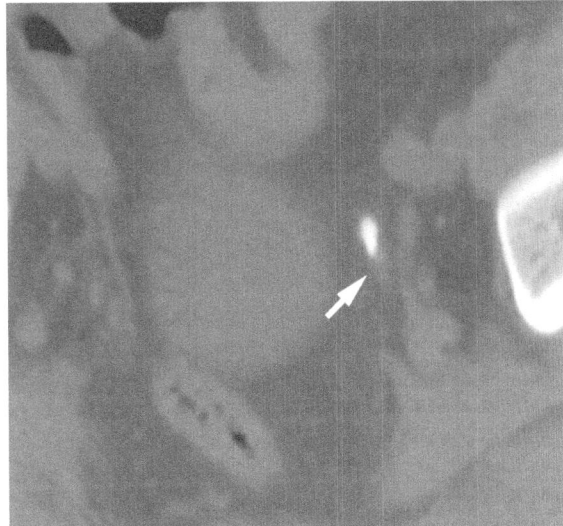

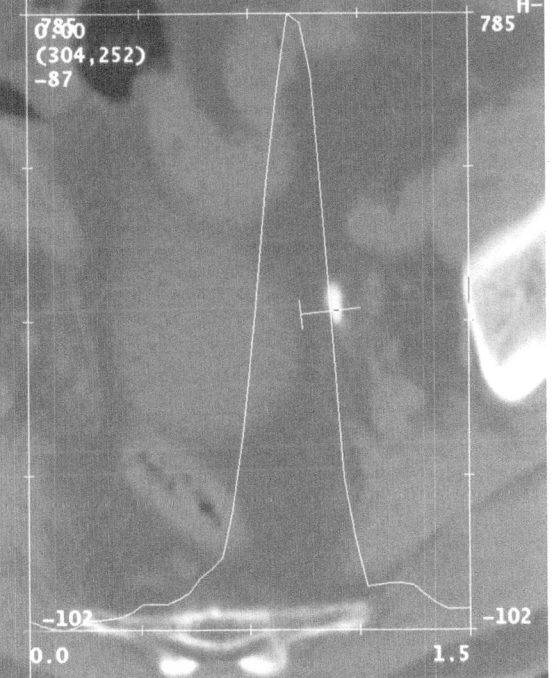

Fig. 5.28a–d. CT analysis of the profile attenuation of a phlebolith and a calculus in a patient with left renal colic. **a, b** Left pelvic calcification with radiolucent center. The histogram shows a bifid shape which confirms the diagnosis of phlebolith. **c, d** Slice at an upper level shows another calcification with a comet sign (*arrow*). The histogram does not present a bifid profile; this is in favor of stone despite the comet sign, which is not reliable

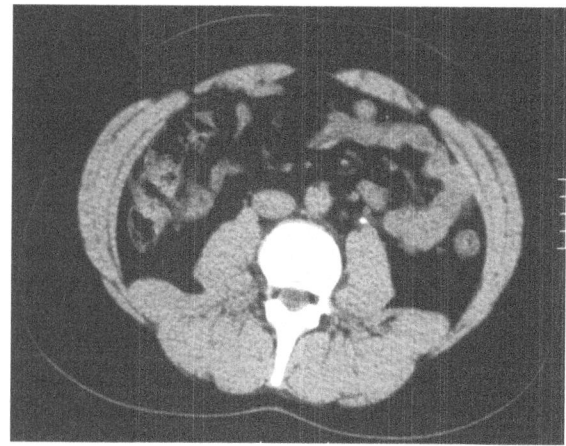

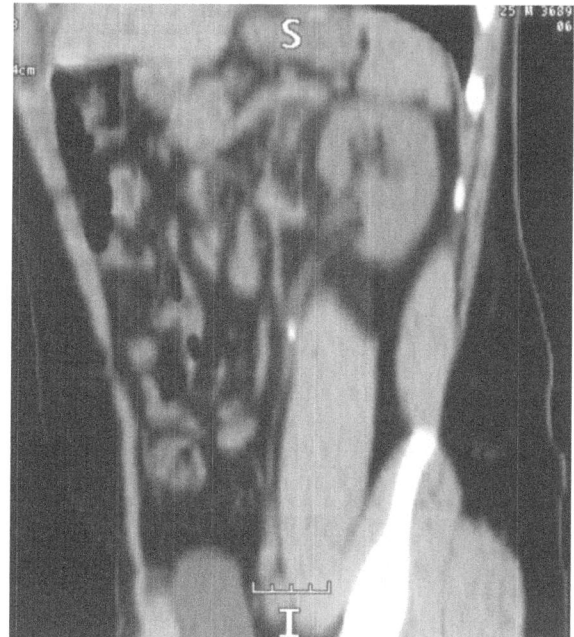

Fig. 5.29a, b. Multiplanar reconstruction of a left ureteral stone: **a** axial view, **b** sagittal view

Table 5.2. Differential diagnosis between pelvic ureteral stone and phlebolith. (Modified from BELL et al. 1998)

	Stone	Phlebolith
Mean attenuation	>300 HU	<278 HU
Central lucency	No	Yes (PPV=100%)
Bifid peak at profile analysis	No	Yes
"Comet" sign	No	Yes (?)
Soft tissue rim sign	Yes (PPV 91%)	No (?)
Shape	Geometric	Rounded

PPV, Positive predictive value.

5.1.2.1
Is There a Need for Direct Treatment?

This question is essential in view of the associated risks and because medical treatment alone may often be sufficient. This is why clinical and radiological information is crucial. The radiologist has to provide sufficient information regarding the characteristics of the stone(s) and urinary tract status:

- Size and volume of the calculus. Indeed, 90% of stones with a diameter of 5 mm or less usually migrate spontaneously, aided by antispasmodic anti-inflammatory medication and also diuresis. In contrast, stones larger than 20 mm are resistant to ESWL.
- The exact stone topography.
- If possible, the suspected chemical composition

of the stone, because certain types of calculi are resistant to ESWL (BANNER et al.1990).
- The functional and morphological status of the kidney, in terms not only of urinary tract dilatation but also of the consequences of obstruction for the affected kidney, because this plays an important role in the therapeutic decision. Indeed, painful and resistant renal colic in a patient with a silent kidney is an indication for emergency surgery. Conversely, obstructive uropathy can occur in patients who become asymptomatic (COE et al. 1992). Disappearance of pain does not always signify calculus migration but might correspond to interrupted diuresis (DRACH 1986; VAN ARSDALEN 1990). The anatomical and functional characteristics of the opposite kidney are also important to know.
- The anatomical and morphological characteristics of the ureter are also very important. Ureteral sinuosities and post-surgical anomalies must be known prior to ureteroscopy.
- The imaging techniques provide other information essential to the therapeutic approach: the existence of kyphoscoliosis, coxarthrosis, aortoiliac atherosclerosis, and calcified lesions must be documented prior to ureteroscopy, just as kidney ectopia, malformations, duplications, expansive lesions (renal cysts or polycystic kidneys), and caliceal anatomy must be known about before a percutaneous approach is taken.

5.1.2.2
Which Method if Direct Treatment Is Necessary?

Calculus topography is the major factor influencing which technique should be used. DRETLER proposes the following algorithm (DRETLER et al. 1986): If the kidney is in good condition, a middle- or upper-third ureteral calculus can be treated by ESWL, either directly or following a pushback technique using a retrograde endoluminal approach, which allows the calculus to be treated in the renal pelvis with a ureteral 2 J protection (Fig. 5.31a, b). In difficult cases, ureteroscopy, percuta-

neous stone extraction, or chemical stone dissolution (uric acid or struvite calculus) can be attempted.

For inferior-third ureteral lithiasis, ESWL or ureteroscopy extractions are usually performed. Ureteroscopy has the advantage of usually being technically successful, but it carries a relatively high morbidity. ESWL has a very low morbidity and a technical efficacy of about 85%, which depends on the chemical composition of the stone. It is important to remember that the majority of ureteral calculi resolve spontaneously, without direct intervention (KINDER et al. 1987; PREMINGER 1994).

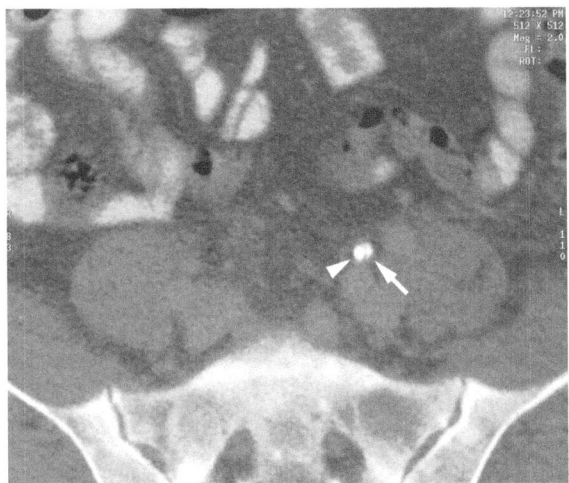

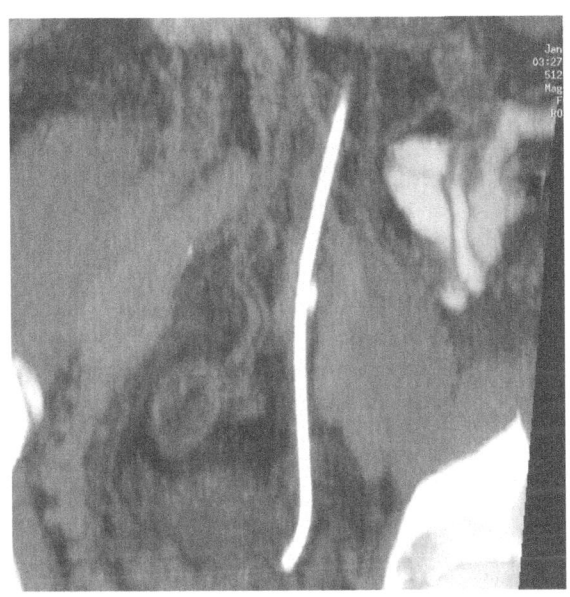

Fig. 5.30. a Axial view of a ureteral calculus (*arrow*) with a 2-J catheter (*arrowhead*). **b** MIP reconstruction of the same patient

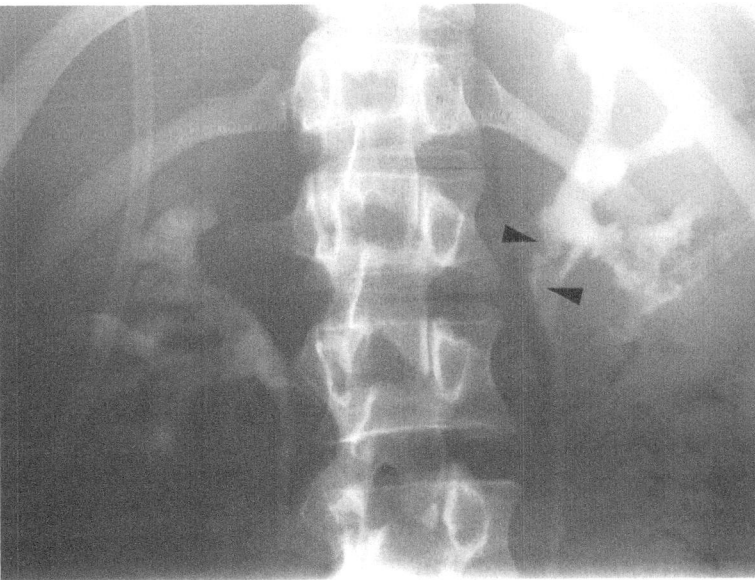

Fig. 5.31. Ureteral candidiasis. EU shows multiple filling defects, mainly on both sides of the renal pelvis and also in the initial portion of the left ureter (*arrowheads*)

5.2
Other Intraureteral Diseases

Although the most frequent etiology of acute ureteral obstruction is ureteral lithiasis, other rarer causes should be considered in certain clinical circumstances. These intraureteral "foreign bodies" may be associated with symptoms of variable seriousness, or they may be totally silent clinically. The most frequent etiologies are ureteral candidiasis, clots, papillary sloughs, and caseous debris (MALEK et al. 1975).

5.2.1
Ureteral Candidiasis

The urinary system is one of the most frequent targets of *Candida albicans* infections. Rarely, it is also affected by other mycoses (torulosis, cryptococcosis, aspergillosis). The infection may be bloodborne as in systemic candidiasis or retrograde as in vesicoureteral reflux. Many factors can explain the increasing frequency of severe urinary tract candidiasis observed nowadays.

General: Broad-spectrum antibiotherapy and/or corticotherapy, immunocompromised patients, immunosuppressive treatment or chemotherapy, radiotherapy, malignant hematological diseases or neoplasms, diabetes, drug addiction, organ transplantation, and invasive surgery

Local: Urinary tract foreign bodies (lithiasis), bladder or ureteral catheters

Urinary tract candidiasis may be isolated or part of a systemic infection. Usually, an initial pyelocaliceal infection characterized by diffuse abscess formation, papillary necrosis, and proliferation of mycelium filaments into the urinary tract leads to the formation of a "fungus ball" that can migrate to the ureter, which is then secondarily infected (MINDELL and POLLACK 1983) and can even contain a solitary myotik fragment (DOMART et al. 1986).

The clinical presentation is variable, associating signs of septicemia with back pain and a progressive renal insufficiency secondary to urinary tract obstruction (MELCHIOR et al. 1972). The infection may also be clinically silent or disappear when the factors favoring it are suppressed (SCHONEBECK 1986).

Sometimes, US or EU shows suggestive abnormalities in the renal pelvis, such as filling defects, but the initial diagnosis of ureteral candidiasis based on these diagnostic methods is exceptional (GERLE 1973) (Fig. 5.32). In some cases, US shows a hyperechoic mass without acoustic shadowing (BARTONE et al. 1982). The diagnosis can be made by direct retrograde or antegrade opacification techniques (DEMBNER and PFISTER 1977; MAZER and BARTONE 1982). The radiological findings are characterized by an intraluminal defect with irregular contours which casts the pyelocaliceal cavities and often has an elongated "rat-tail" appearance (MINDELL and POLLACK 1983) (Fig. 5.33a, b). The lesions may be mobile and have a changeable morphology. The association with ureteral emphysema is possible (MARGOLIN 1971).

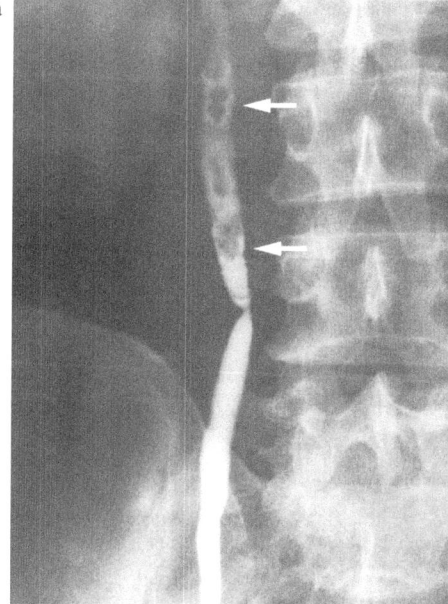 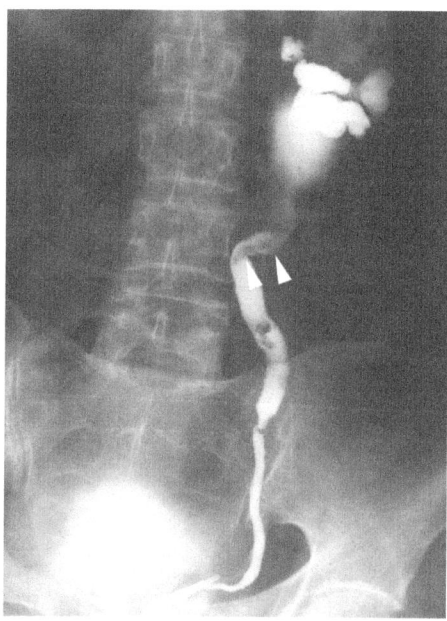

Fig. 5.32a, b. Ureteral candidiasis. **a** Right RUP demonstrates multiple endoluminal lacunae with irregular contours in the lumbar ureter (*arrows*). **b** On the left side, presence of an intraluminal filling defect with a rat-tail appearance (*arrowheads*)

Others causes of intraureteral filling defects have to be discussed (WILLIAMSON et al. 1986). The fibroepithelial polyp can have a similar aspect but its clinical presentation is different. Other exceptional diagnoses such as cholesteatoma and leukoplasia are possible (WILLIS et al. 1981). Sometimes the defect has no particular radiological characteristic. In this case the diagnosis depends on the histological and microbiological examination of debris.

Percutaneous nephrostomy has a important role in the diagnostic and therapeutic strategy (DOMART et al. 1986), because it allows urine sampling for microbiological analysis, urinary tract opacification, and drainage (DEMBNER and PFISTER 1977), and also in situ antimycotic treatment (amphotericin B) and followup. The endoluminal manipulation of guidewires and catheters allows lesion fragmentation and facilitates the treatment. The catheter must be removed as soon as possible because of the high reinfection rate, usually after 1 week of sterile urine samples associated with a normal EU (DOMART et al. 1986).

5.2.2
Ureteral Clots

Macroscopic hematuria associated with an intraureteral defect is very common. Usually, it does not represent a diagnostic problem because of the clinical context (NAVANI et al. 1968).

EU is usually sufficient for diagnostic purposes: radiological signs are a smooth, homogeneous, intraluminal defect, entirely delimited by contrast medium, with variable topography and morphology. The defect usually disappears spontaneously in a few days because of migration or enzymatic destruction by in situ urinary tract thrombolysis. When bleeding is severe blood can fill the entire urinary tract (spaghetti-like filling defects) (Fig. 5.34). Clots may be responsible for a moderate obstructive uropathy with urinary tract dilation. Sometimes, there is an acute severe obstruction with secondary insufficient urinary tract opacification on EU, necessitating direct opacification or CT (Fig. 5.35a–d). Radiological signs on direct opacification are similar, and unenhanced CT shows a spontaneous slightly hyperdense ureter (POLLACK et al. 1981).

The diagnostic workup of a patient with hematuria comprises US, EU, and cystoscopy. Usually, the search for the responsible lesion is postponed until the patient is free of symptoms. On EU, although the radiological appearance of clots is generally characteristic and different from that of other intraureteral

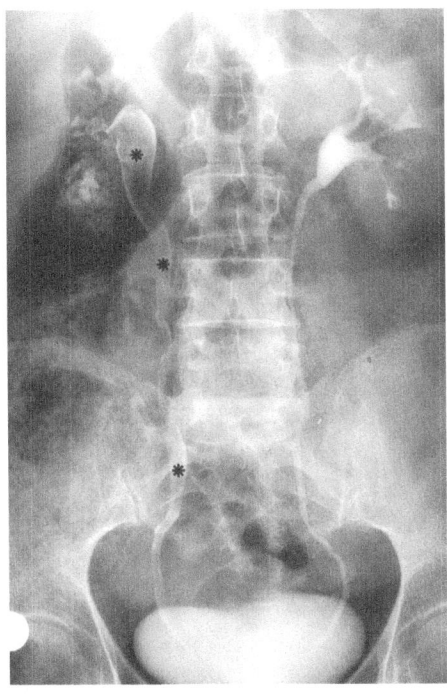

Fig. 5.33. Clotting of the right pyelocaliceal cavities and ureter in a patient with macroscopic hematuria (*asterisks*). EU makes it possible to determine the origin of bleeding on the right kidney, but the etiology cannot be established precisely

defects, it is desirable to postpone the examination while the patient has an active hematuria. Indeed, even if EU were able to determine the renal origin of the hematuria and the bleeding side, the clots could conceal the responsible lesion. Instead, it is preferable to perform cystoscopy during active hematuria to eliminate a bladder origin and, in case of an upper urinary tract origin, to determine the site of bleeding.

In exceptional circumstances, the clot may persist. The use of in situ thrombolytic agents has been described to dissolve the clots in case of acute obstruction (BERGMAN et al. 1990).

5.2.3
Other Causes of Intraluminal Defects

There are several other causes of intraluminal defects that should be considered (FEIN and MCCLENNAN 1986). Intraureteral air is rare, but can be spontaneously found after a uretero-intestinal anastomosis or secondary to a uretero-digestive fistula (Fig. 5.36a, b). Rarely, it is produced by anaerobic germs or mycotic infection. On KUB, the presence in ureteral topography of multiples gas bubbles with variable morphol-

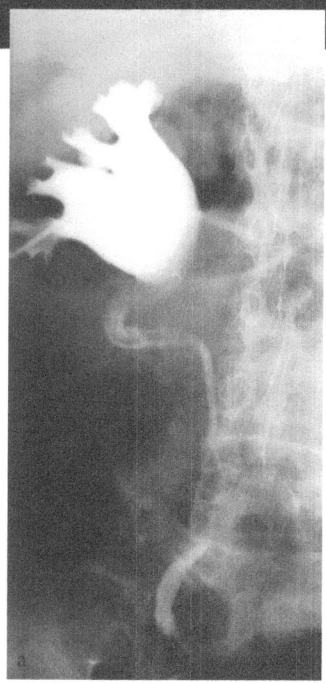 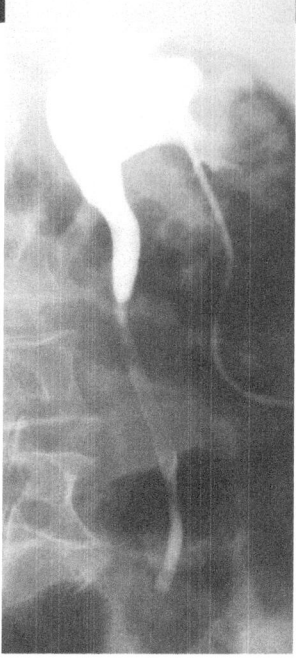 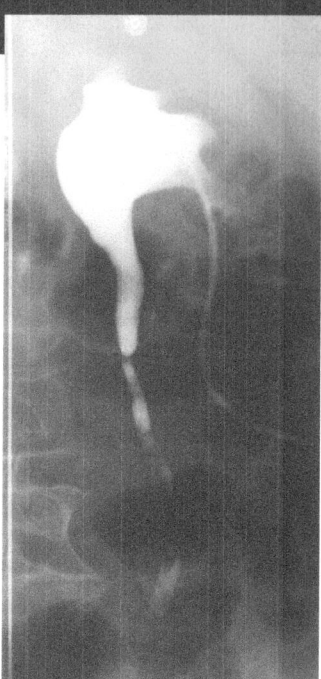

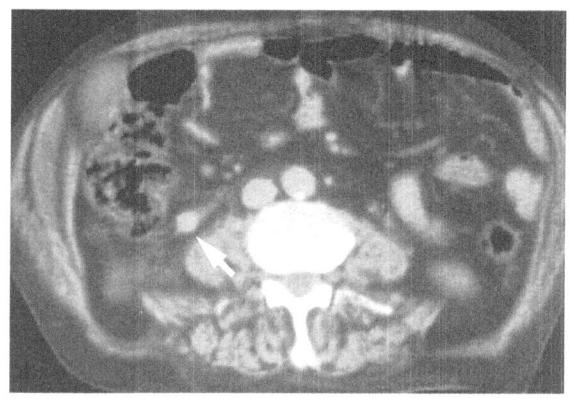

Fig. 5.34 a Right antegrade pyelography in a patient with renal colic and macroscopic hematuria. Multiple "spaghetti-like" filling defects in the lumbar ureter with obstructive uropathy. **b, c** Same pattern in prone position. **d** Unenhanced CT showing spontaneous hyperdensity of the right lumbar ureter (*arrow*)

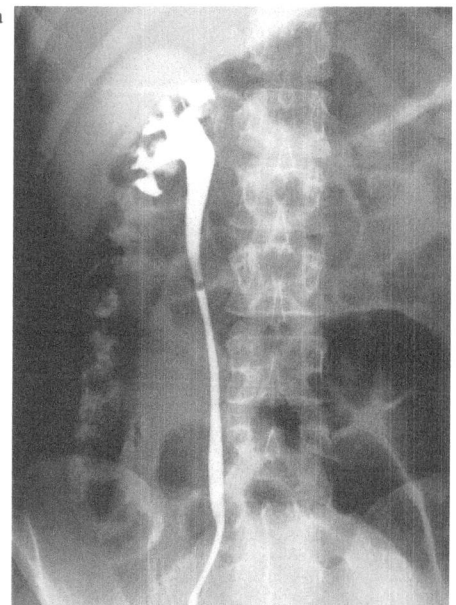 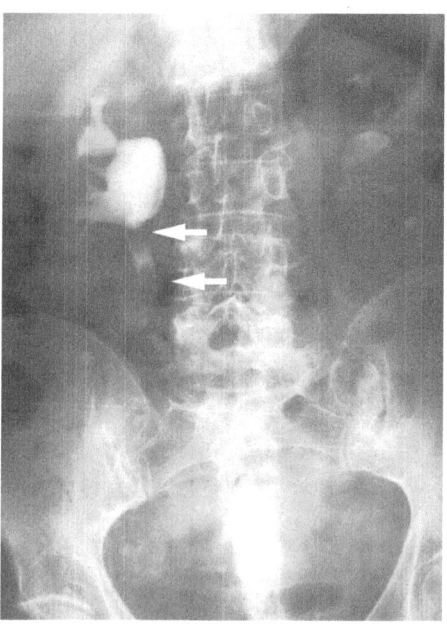

Fig. 5.36a, b. Examples of ureteral air bubbles. **a** Air bubbles in the right lumbar ureter after unfortunate injection of contrast medium during RUP. **b** Air bubbles in the right lumbar ureter after uretero-rectal fistula (*arrows*)

ogy and mobility indicates the diagnosis. In doubtful cases, CT can be very useful.

Papillary necrosis can result in papillary slough migration, which may also be responsible for acute or subacute ureteral obstruction (ANDRIONE and BAHNSON 1987). This diagnosis can be made with EU or direct pyelography. An intraluminal ureteral defect with central calcification and associated caliceal anomalies can sometimes be demonstrated. However, these anomalies might be concealed by pyelocaliceal distension. A ureteral mass with central microcalcifications can be identified on CT, but the intraluminal location is difficult to establish. The definitive diagnosis is made by histological examination of urinary papillary fragments.

Theoretically, urinary tract tuberculosis can result in the migration of caseous fragments, leading to obstructive uropathy. This is currently exceptional.

Renal colic secondary to the presence of a bullet in the ureter after a war injury has been described (bullet colic). The presence of an intraluminal foreign body with a metallic density and specific morphology is characteristic (GUTMAN et al. 1984; LEVINE et al. 1985).

References

Ambos MA, Bosniak MA (1975) Tomography of the kidney bed as an aid in differentiating renal pelvic tumor and stone. AJR Am J Roentgenol 125:331–336

Andriole GL, Bahnson RR (1987) Computed tomographic diagnosis of ureteral obstruction caused by a sloughed papilla. Urol Radiol 9:45–46

Banner MC (1990a) Roentgen evaluation of upper urinary tract urolithiasis. In: Pollack HM (ed) Clinical urography: an atlas and text book of uroradiological imaging, vol 2. Saunders, Philadelphia, pp 1805–1884

Banner MC (1990b) The recently passed ureteral calculus. In: Pollack HM (ed) Clinical urography: an atlas and textbook of urological imaging, vol 2. Saunders, Philadelphia, pp 1884–1886

Banner MP, Van Arsdalen KN, Pollack HM(1990) Extracorporeal shock wave lithotripsy of ureteral calculi. Radiology 174:12–14

Baro PR, Julia CL (1989) Lithiasis inside a blind-ending branch of a trifid ureter. Urol Radiol 11:42–44

Barr JD, Tegtmeyer CJ, Jenkins AD (1990) In situ lithotripsy of ureteral calculi. Review of 261 cases. Radiology 174:103–108

Bartone FF, Hurwitz RS, Rojas EL, et al (1988) The role of percutaneous nephrostomy in the management of obstructing candidiasis of the urinary tract in infants. J Urol 140:338–341

Becker JM, Pollack HM (1981) Milk of calcium and ureterocele. Urol Radiol 3:31–33

Bell TV, Fenlon HM, Davison BD, et al (1998) Unenhanced helical CT criteria to differentiate distal ureteral calculi from pelvic phleboliths. Radiology 207:363–367

Bergman H, Friedenberg RM, Sayegh V (1961) New roentgenologic signs of carcinoma of the ureter. AJR Am J Roentgenol 86:707–717

Bergman SM, Frentz GD, Wallin JD (1990) Ureteral obstruction due to blood clot following percutaneous renal biopsy: resolution with intraureteral streptokinase. J Urol 143:113–115

Berlow ME (1979) Gonadal vein phleboliths simulating a mid ureteral stone. AJR Am J Roentgenol 133:919–920

Blake SP, McNicholas MMJ, Raptopoulos V (1998) Nonopaque crystal deposition causing ureteric obstruction in patients with HIV undergoing indinavir therapy. AJR Am J Roentgenol 171:717–720

Bloom RA, Libson E, Verstandig A, Rackow M (1988) The tooth-root sign; a characteristic appearance of distal ureteral calculi. Clin Radiol 39:212–213

Boridy IC, Maklad N, Sandler CM (1996) Suspected urolithiasis in pregnant women: imaging algorithm and literature review. AJR Am J Roentgenol 167:869–875

Chelfouh N, Grenier N, Higueret D, et al (1998) Characterization of urinary calculi: in vitro study of "twinkling artifact" revealed by color-flow sonography. AJR Am J Roentgenol 171:1055–1060

Chen MYM, Zagorlia RZ, Dyer RB (1995) Inter-ureteric ridge edema: incidence and etiology Abdom Imaging 20:368–370

Dalrymple NC, Casford B, Raiken DP, et al (2000) Pearls and pitfalls in the diagnosis of ureterolithasis with unenhanced helical CT. Radiographics 20:439–447

Dembner AG, Pfister RC (1977) Fungal infection of the urinary tract: demonstration by antegrade pyelography and drainage by percutaneous nephrostomy. AJR Am J Roentgenol 129:415–418

Domart Y, Delmas V, Cornud F, et al (1986) Obstruction des voies urinaires par des Bezoards candidosiques ou „fungus ball". Presse Med 15:153–156

Drach GW (1983) Transurethral ureteral stone manipulation. Urol Clin North Am 10:709

Drach GW (1986) Urinary lithiasis. In: Walsh PC, Gittes RF, Perlmutter AD, Stamey TA (eds) Campbell's urology, vol 1, 51st edn. Saunders, Philadelphia, pp 1094–1187

Dretler SP, Keating MA, Riley J (1986) An algorithm for the management of ureteral calculi. J Urol 136:1190–1193

Dufour B (1973) Les obstructions de l'uretère lombo-iliaque. Association Française d'Urologie Edition, Paris, pp 71–84

Fein AB, McClennan BL (1986) Solitary filling defects of the ureter. Semin Roentgenol 21:201–213

Garcia-Cuerpo E, Martinez F, Llorente C, et al (1985) New location of milk of calcium. Urology 25:425–427

Gerle RD (1973) Roentgenographic features of primary renal candidiasis. "Fungus ball" of the renal pelvis and ureter. AJR Am J Roentgenol 119:731–738

Guest AR, Cohan RH, Korobkin M (2001) Assessment of the clinical utility of the rim and comet-tail in differentiating ureteral stones from phlebolithes. AJR Am J Roentgenol 177:1285–1291

Gutman H, Rothberg M, Johanson KE (1984) Ureteral obstruction by shotgun pellet seven years after injury. Urology 23:170–172

Heneghan JP, Dalrymple NC, Verga M, et al (1997) Soft tissue "rim" sign in the diagnosis of ureteral calculi with use of unenhanced helical CT. Radiology 202:709–711

Hillman BJ, Drach GW, Tracey P, et al (1984) Computed tomographic analysis of renal calculi. AJR 142:549–552

Joffre F, Portalez D (1983) Radiologie de la lithiase urinaire. Enc Med Chir, Paris Radiodiagnostic V 34173, C10 et C20, 9

Jorion JL, Lorge F, Hennebert PN, et al (1989) Lithiases uré-térales. Evolution de la stratégie thérapeutique et place du traitement endoscopique. Ann Urol 23:17–22

Kinder RB, Osborn DE, Flynn JT, et al (1987) Ureteroscopy and ureteral calculi: how useful? Br J Urol 60:506–508

Korobkin M, Jacobs RP, Clark RE (1978) Diminished radio-opacity of contrast material: a urographic sign of ureteral calculus. AJR Am J Roentgenol 131:847–850

Kuwahara M, Kageyama S, Kurosu S (1984) Computed tomography and composition of renal calculi. Urol Res 12:111–113

Laing FL, Benson CB, Disalvo DN, et al (1994) Distal ureteral calculis: detection with vaginal US. Radiology 192: 545–548

Lee JY, Kim SH, Cho JY, et al (2001) Color and power Doppler twinkling artifacts from urinary stones: clinical observations and phantom studies. AJR Am J Roentgenol 176:1441–1445

Lerner RM, Rubens D (1986) Distal ureteral calculi: diagnosis by transrectal sonography. AJR 147:1189–1191

Levine RS, Abramowicz CJ, Pollack HM, et al (1985) Bullet colic. Urol Radiol 7:16–18

Malek RS (1977) Calculous diseases of the genito-urinary tract. In: Witten DM, Myers GH, Utz DC (eds) Emmet's clinical urography, 4th edn, vol 2. Saunders, Philadelphia, pp 1294–1338

Malek RS, Aguilo JJ, Hattery RR (1975) Radiolucent filling defects of the renal pelvis. Classification and report of unusual cases. J Urol 114:508–513

Margolin HN (1971) Fungus infection of the urinary tract. Semin Roentgenol 6:323–330

Mazer MJ, Bartone FF (1982) Percutaneous antegrade diagnosis and management of candidiasis of the upper urinary tract. Urol Clin North Am 9:157

Mac-Millian BG, Fritzhand MD (1978) Milk of calcium in the ureter. Radiology 127:376–378

MacNeily AE, Goldenberg SL, Allen EJ, et al (1991) Sonographic visualization of the ureter in pregnancy. J Urol 146:298–301

Melchior J, Mehest WH, Volk WL (1972) Ureteral colic from a fungus ball. Unusual presentation of systemic aspergillosis. J Urol 108:698–699

Mindell HJ, Pollack HM (1983) Fungal diseases of the ureter. Radiology 146:46–50

Navani S, Bosniak MA, Shapiro JH (1968) Varied radiographic manifestations of urinary tract bleeding. J Urol 100: 339–343

Newhouse JH, Prien EL, Amis ES, et al (1984) Computed tomographic analysis of urinary calculi. AJR Am J Roentgenol 142:545–548

Onishi K, Watanabe H, Ohe H, et al (1986) Ultrasound findings in urolithiasis in the lower ureter. Ultrasound Med Biol 12: 577–579

O'Reilly PH (1986) Urinary stone disease. In: O'Reilly PH (ed) Obstructive uropathy. Springer, Berlin Heidelberg New York, pp 93–110

Parienty RA, Duceller R, Pradel J, et al (1982) Diagnostic value of CT numbers in pelvo-calyceal filling defects. Radiology 143:743–747

Pollack HM, Arger PH, Goldberg BB (1978) Ultrasonic detection of nonopaque renal calculi. Radiology 127:233–237

Preminger GM (1994) Technique versus technology: what is the most appropriate method for the removal of ureteral calculi? (editorial). J Urol 132:66–67

Prien EL (1974) The analysis of urinary calculi. Urol Clin North Am 1:229

Resnick MI, Kursh ED, Cohen AM (1984) Use of computerized tomography in the delineation of uric acid calculi. J Urol 131:9–10

Roth CS, Bowyer BA, Berquist TH (1985) Utility of the plain abdominal radiograph for diagnosing ureteral calculi. Ann Emerg Med 14:311–315

Rothpearl A, Frager D, Subramanian A, et al (1995) MR urography: technique and application. Radiology 194:125–130

Schonebeck J (1986) Fungal infections of the urinary tract. In: Walsh PC, Gittes RF, Perlmutter AD, Stamey TA (eds) Campbell's urology, vol 1, 5th edn. Saunders, Philadelphia, pp 1094–1197

Segal AJ, Spataro RF, Linke CA, et al (1978) Diagnosis of nonopaque calculi by computed tomography. Radiology 129: 447–450

Singh EO, Malek RS (1982) Calculus disease in the upper urinary tract. Semin Roentgenol 27:113–132

Smith RC, Rosewfield AT, Choe KA, et al (1995) Acute flank pain: comparison of non-contrast-enhanced CT and intravenous urography. Radiology 194:789–794

Spring DB (1982) Fallopian tube occlusion rings; a consideration in the differential diagnosis of ureteral calculi. Radiology 145:51–52

Sundaram CP, Saltzman B (1999) Urolithiasis associated with protease inhibitors. J Endourol 13:309–312

Takahashi N, Kawashima A, Ernst RD (1998) Ureterolithiasis: can clinical outcome be predicted with unenhanced helical CT? Radiology 208:97–102

Thornbury JR, Parker TW (1982) Ureteral calculi. Semin Roentgenol 17:133–139

Van Arsdalen KN, Banner MP, Pollack HM (1990) Radiographic imaging and urologic decision making in the management of renal and ureteral calculi. Urol Clin North Am 17:171–190

Van Beers BE, Dechambre S, Hulcelle P, et al (2001) Value of multislice helical CT scans and maximum intensity projection images to improve detection of ureteral stone at abdominal radiography. AJR 177:1117–1121

Vespignani L (1962) Signes urographiques de la migration récente d'un calcul urétéral. Radiol Med 48:137–158

Wills JS, Pollack HM, Curtis JA (1981) Cholesteatoma of the upper urinary tract. AJR Am J Roentgenol 136:941–944

Williams RI (1963) Long term survey of 538 patients with upper urinary tract stones. Br J Urol 35:416–437

Williamson B, Hartman GW, Hattery PR (1986) Multiple and diffuse urétéral filling defects. Semin Roentegnol 21: 214–223

Wolfman MG, Thornbury JR, Braunstein EM (1979) Nonobstructing radiopaque ureteral calculi. Urol Radiol 1:97–104

Young MJ, Rubenstein MA, Norris DM, et al (1990) Submucosal ureteral calculi: a new entity? J Urol 143:800–801

Zagoria RJ, Khatod EG, Chen MYM (2001) Abdominal radiography after CT reveals urinary calculi: a method to predict usefulness of abdominal radiography on the basis of size and CT attenuation of calculi. AJR Am J Roentgenol 176: 1117–1122

Zangerle KF, Iserson KV, Bjelland JC (1983) Usefulness of abdominal flat plane radiography in patients with suspected ureteral calculi. Ann Emerg Med 14:316–319

6 Ureteral Tumors

Ph. Plante, T. Smayra, L. Bouchard, F. Joffre, P. Seguin, G. Escourrou, Ph. Otal

CONTENTS

Ureteral tumors are rare and usually of urothelial origin. Urothelial tumors are most frequently malignant, and their prognosis is variable, depending on their degree of differentiation (grading) and their extension through the ureteral wall (staging). Much rarer are tumors of connective tissue origin, which are most frequently benign (Table 6.1).

The development of new radiological (ultrasonography, computed tomography, MRI) and endoscopic (ureteroscopy) techniques has improved diagnostic performance and permits a more precise pretherapeutic investigation. The indications for excretory urography (EU), long the key diagnostic tool, are now challenged in the light of the new urographic techniques using CT and MRI multiplanar reconstructions.

P. Plante, MD; P. Seguin, MD
Service d'Urologie
T. Smayra, MD; L. Bouchard, MD; Ph. Otal, MD; F. Joffre, MD
Service de Radiologie
G. Escourrou, MD
Service d'Anatomo-pathologie, CHU Rangueil, 1, avenue Jean-Poulhès, 31403 Toulouse Cédex 4, France

6.1
Benign Ureteral Tumors

6.1.1
Ureteral Fibroepithelial Polyp

Fibroepithelial polyp is a rare tumor, representing less than 20% of all the primitive ureteral tumors (De Bruyne et al. 1990). Approximately 150 cases are reported in the literature (Bellin et al. 2002). However, it is by far the most frequent benign tumor of the ureter, the benign nature of papillomas not being definitely established. Ureteral fibroepithelial polyp is not a real tumor, but consists of hyperplasia of fibroconnective tissue proliferation covered by normal epithelium (Abeshouse 1956; Corkill et al.

Table 6.1. Classification of ureteral tumors, according to Bennington and Beckwith (1975) and Richie (1988)

Primitive tumors
Epithelial tumors
Benign
Papilloma
Inverted papilloma
Malignant
Transitional cell carcinoma
Transitional cell carcinoma with differentiation
squamous differentiation
glandular differentiation
mixed
Squamous cell carcinoma
Adenocarcinoma
Undifferentiated carcinoma
Mesodermal tumors (nonepithelial)
Benign tumors
Fibroepithelial polyp
Leiomyoma
Hemangioma
Neurinoma
Malignant tumors
Leiomyosarcoma
Secondary tumors
Seeding from renal adenocarcinoma
or pelvic urothelial tumor
Direct extension from adjacent tumors
True metastasis

1987). The stroma is swollen and richly vascularized, which explains the frequent occurrence of hematuria (Van Poppel et al. 1986). There is no malignant transformation. Macroscopically, it is characterized by a pedunculated polypoid mass, mobile in the lumen and sometimes responsible for ureteral intussusception (Maindenberg et al. 1990). In some cases, this polypoid formation shows multiple digitiform extensions; these extensions can implant themselves in a group, directly on the ureter wall, as multiple tentacles (Ledor et al. 1982).

Fibroepithelial polyp is found mainly in persons between the ages of 20 and 40 years but can be seen in children and older people. It predominates in men and involves mostly the upper third of the left ureter. It is rarely multiple and bilateral (Hugues and David 1976). It may be associated with Peutz-Jeghers syndrome. First clinical signs are often intermittent lumbar pain, and sometimes recurrent renal colic in connection with transitory intussusception phenomena (Vogelzang et al. 1981). Hematuria is frequent and can be isolated or associated with pain.

Diagnosis is the responsibility of radiology (Banner and Pollack 1979; Naucler et al. 1983) and must be made preoperatively to avoid nephroureterectomy. It is most frequently made on EU because the polyp is usually incompletely obstructive. Even in case of a large polyp, the kidney remains functional unless EU is performed during a period of acute obstruction by transitory intussusception (Fig. 6.1a–c). The most frequent pattern is a regular pedunculated lacuna of variable shape and length, progressively enlarging and dilating the ureteral lumen ("bell-tongue" aspect). It is surrounded by contrast medium and sometimes presents in a corkscrew pattern (Banner and Pollack 1979). The implantation zone of the peduncle is normal. This formation is very mobile and, from one image to the other, is capable of moving from the renal pelvis to the ureteral meatus, depending on its length (Fig. 6.2a, b).

The other causes of intraureteral lacunae are easily eliminated: malignant tumor, pyeloureteritis cystica or pyelitis striata, radiolucent lithiasis. The

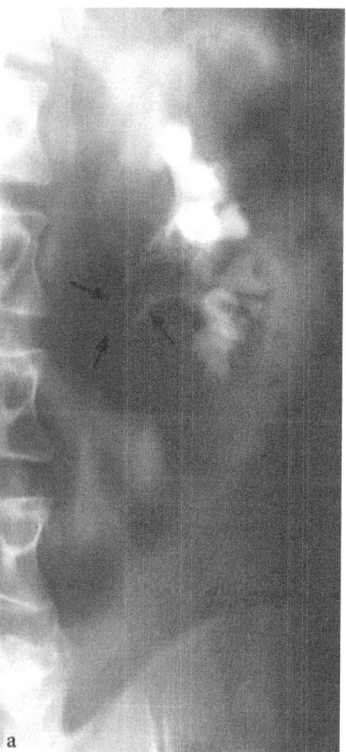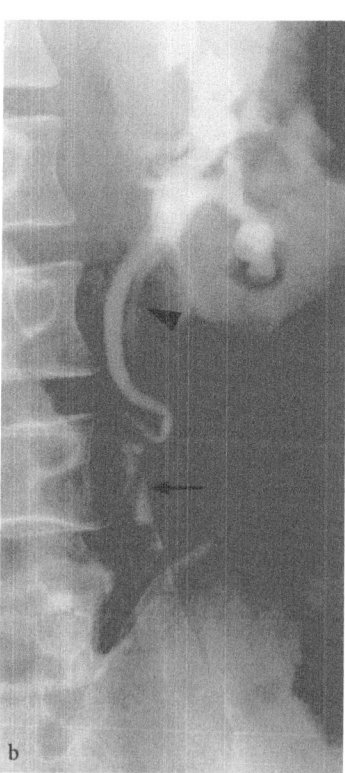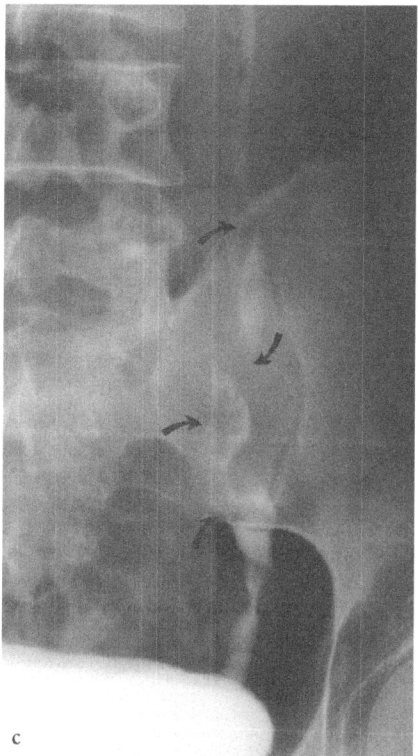

Fig. 6.1a–c. EU in a 20-year-old patient with hematuria and left renal colic. a 5-min X-ray: slight excretion delay with moderate dilatation of left calices. Presence of a lacunar image inside the left pelvis (*arrows*). b 20-min X-ray: opacification of the left ureter with moderate obstruction. Enlargement of the lower part of the lumbar ureter which presents an irregular intraluminal lacuna with possible peduncle (*arrow*). Peripelvic extravasation of contrast medium (*arrowhead*). c 25-min X-ray: this picture shows the variable shape and pattern of the lacuna. This pattern associated with intraluminal mobility is characteristic of fibroepithelial ureteral polyp

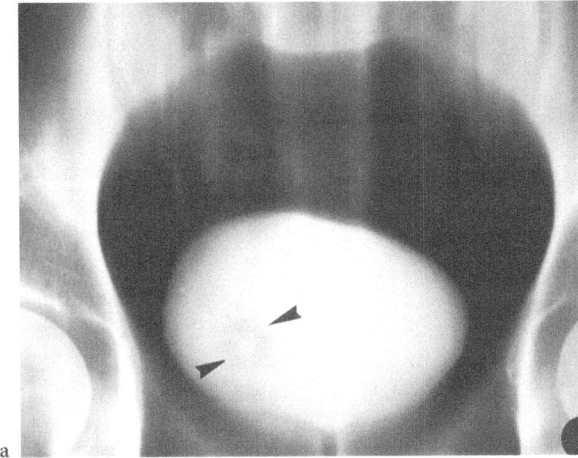

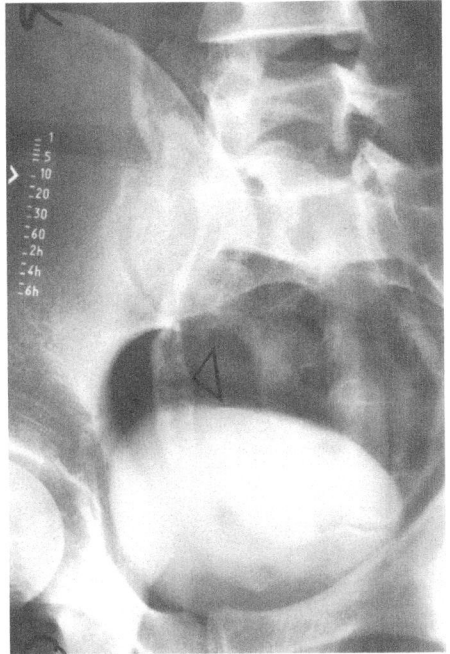

Fig. 6.2. a Tomographic view of the opacified bladder during EU shows a rounded lacuna which could simulate a bladder tumor (*arrowheads*). **b** This EU view shows enlargement of the right lower ureter by a pedunculated irregular lacuna which corresponds to a fibroepithelial polyp growing out of the ureteral meatus (*arrowhead*)

differential diagnosis may be difficult when there is a associated clot.

In case of an incomplete EU, retrograde or antegrade pyelography can be performed. The radiological aspect is identical, but the intraluminal mass and its peduncle are somewhat better demonstrated. Contrast medium injection under fluoroscopic guidance allows real-time assessment of the intraluminal mobility of the lesion.

Until now, the role of CT has been largely underestimated (BELLIN et al. 2002). This technique allows the demonstration of a tissular ureteral mass which enhances after CM administration. The presence of a continuous rim of CM surrounding the mass corresponding to the length of the lesion can suggest the diagnosis (OESTERLING et al. 1989).

Cystoscopy sometimes allows direct visualization of a tumor extending from the ureteral meatus with urine ejection (EMMET and WITTEN 1971). Brush biopsy has little clinical value in this type of tumor. Urinary cytology is negative as a rule. The classic error is to ignore this diagnosis in the differential diagnosis of a bladder tumor.

Treatment is required in order to alleviate the symptoms. Localized ureterectomy with excision of the polyp and its implantation base is the procedure of choice. Nephroureterectomy is reserved for extensive or multiple lesions, where the polyps are responsible for important destruction of the renal parenchyma, and when the diagnosis is uncertain (VAN POPPEL et al. 1986).

Ureteroscopy is becoming the therapeutic method of choice, allowing the diagnosis and possibly treatment of this tumor by endoureteral resection, often facilitated by its pedunculated aspect (OESTERLING et al. 1989).

6.1.2
Other Benign Tumors of the Ureter

Real benign tumors of the ureter are of epithelial or mesenchymal origin. Benign epithelial tumors are a very controversial subject. They have the same histology as malignant urothelial tumors. They are characterized by their frequent ureteral and also renal pelvis and bladder locations. These multiple locations can sometimes produce a real ureteral papillomatosis (KYUNG et al. 1972; LANG and NOURSE 1969). The radiological pattern is characterized by multiple filling defects of parietal origin (WILLIAMSON et al. 1986) (Fig. 6.3). Their malignant potential is uncertain. All these factors make it very difficult, even impossible, to confirm their benignity, and most authors consider them to be in situ or low-grade (WHO grade A or I) carcinomas (BENNINGTON and BECKWITH 1975; BATATA et al. 1975).

The inverted papilloma of the ureter is a peculiar type of tumor. It is mostly reported in the bladder and its first description goes back to 1963 (POTTS and HIRST 1963). Its location in the ureter is exceptional (about 20 cases reported; CORKILL et al. 1987). It is a

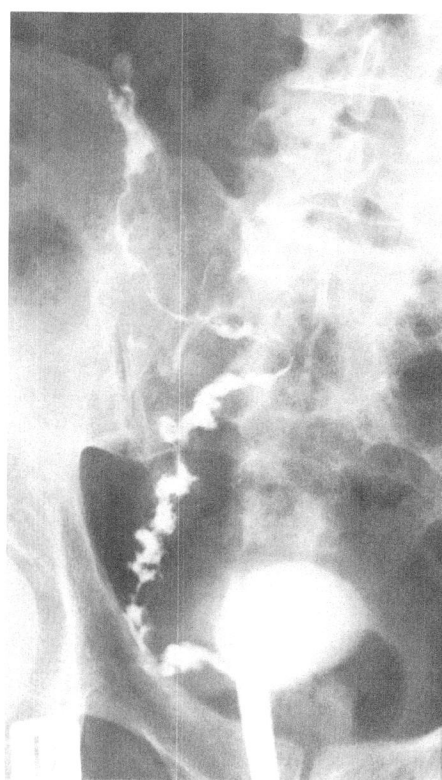

Fig. 6.3. RUP shows multiple filling defects of right ureter with a "corkscrew" pattern corresponding to papillomatosis of the ureter

papilloma, identical to the preceding one, consisting of transitional cell epithelium, without cellular atypia, which proliferates into the ureteral wall instead of growing intraluminally (GEISLER et al. 1980). There are usually multiple locations (KYRIAKOS and ROYCE 1989). The possibility of malignant degeneration is considered exceptional. However, a few cases of urothelial tumors that developed into this kind of tumor, more frequently in the ureter than in other locations (18% vs 6%), have been reported (GRAINGER et al. 1990). The radiological aspect is nonspecific (AJRAWAT et al. 1982). We must consider this diagnosis, however, in the presence of a sessile lacuna in the distal ureter with smooth, slightly scalloped margins, in a man aged approximately 50 years (CORKILL et al. 1987). Ureteral intussusception is possible (DUCHEK et al. 1987). Preoperative diagnosis by excision biopsy through ureteroscopy, along with close postoperative monitoring by EU and urinary cytology, is essential to avoid nephroureterectomy, given the fact that malignant degeneration or the association with urothelial carcinoma is possible (SCHULTZ and BOYLE 1988). The prognosis is identical to that for other papillary tumors of the ureter.

Mesenchymal benign tumors are very rare observations, with nonspecific radiological aspects. Hemangioma of the ureter seems to be the most frequent of these tumors (ABRAMS et al. 1977; JANSEN et al. 1982). Several cases of ureteral hemangiomas were recently reported (BIYANI et al. 1998): One case involved a cavernous type in a 10-year-old child, presenting a 30-mm ureteral mass of soft-tissue density without specific CT characteristics (OGATA et al. 1985). Another case involved a hemangiomatous granuloma with vascular and inflammatory components, simulating a fibroepithelial polyp (KAWABE 1987). Congenital cysts of the ureter were also reported. These cysts are most frequently located at the ureterovesical junction, simulating a ureterocele or a malignant tumor of the ureter (ORR and McGREGOR 1978).

6.2
Primary Malignant Tumors of the Ureter

Described for the first time by RAYER, malignant tumors of the ureter represent about 1% of malignant urinary tract tumors (RAYER 1941; BATATA et al. 1975; CANCELMO et al. 1973). It is possible, however, that the frequency of these tumors is greater, because some ureteral tumors can be mistaken for others in the bladder or renal pelvis. They are essentially epithelial tumors with characteristics identical to those of bladder tumors. They are much rarer than pelvis or bladder locations, representing only 5%–6% of all urothelial tumors (MILLS and VAUGHAN 1983). The relative frequency of bladder, renal pelvis, and ureteral urothelial tumors is about 50 to 3 to 1 (BENNINGTON and BECKWITH 1975). This distribution can be explained by the larger endothelial surface of the bladder and by the longer contact of urine with the bladder mucosa (DROLLER 1986). However, even if their malignant potential is identical, the aggressiveness of ureteral tumors is greater, given the local anatomy, particularly the smaller size of the ureter and its thinner wall. Malignant connective tumors are exceptional. They are represented essentially by leiomyosarcoma of the ureter, of which only a few cases have been reported (ABESHOUSE 1956).

6.2.1
Pathophysiology

Ureteral tumors arise most frequently between the ages of 60 and 80 years with a clear male predominance (3 M:1 F). They are exceptional in persons younger than 30 years (KYUNG et al. 1972).

The risk factors for ureteral tumors development are the same as for all urothelial tumors: smoking takes first place (found in 80% of cases), followed by chronic obstruction, lithiasis, or chronic infection (GITTES 1979). On the other hand, no ureteral tumor secondary to bilharziasis has ever been reported. Some toxic substances are also implicated (aniline and other dyes). Other reported risk factors are Balkan nephropathy and analgesic intoxication (DROLLER 1986; HULTERGREN et al. 1965). It is difficult to precisely determine the mode of action of these different factors, to establish how they are behind metaplasia transformation, but the link between metaplasia and cancer occurrence has not been demonstrated (MOSTOFI 1954). Relations with intoxication to analgesics have been the subject of many recent publications, however. STEFFENS reported a series of 57 patients with ureteral tumors, 35 of whom had suffered intoxication with phenacetin or other analgesics. The tumor appeared about 2 years after the beginning of intoxication (STEFFENS and NAGEL 1988). Some urothelial tumors may develop on the ureteral stump of a nephrectomy done for other indications. They may be favored by infection related to vesicoureteral reflux (POLLACK et al. 1982).

6.2.2
Pathology

Two large histological categories are encountered: transitional cell carcinomas and epidermoid carcinomas (squamous cell carcinomas). According to BENNINGTON, 90% of urothelial tumors are transitional cell carcinomas, 8% are epidermoid carcinomas, and less than 1% are undifferentiated adenocarcinomas (BENNINGTON and BECKWITH 1975). Among the transitional cell carcinomas, 20% present with epidermoid or glandular cells. They must then be considered transitional cell carcinomas with squamous or glandular metaplasia (RICHIE 1988). This is closely related to the strong differentiation potential of urothelial cells.

The morphological aspect is important because it influences radiological images and also the prognosis. We distinguish between three categories: papillary, plane and infiltrative tumors. Papillary tumors are polypoid and exophytic lesions with a peduncle. Their prognosis is better because of their moderate potential for local wall infiltration and distant metastasis. They represent about 60%–70% of nodular primitive ureteral tumors. Nonpapillary tumors have a nodular or a stenosing morphology. These are infiltrative tumors, with a greater malignant potential than papillary tumors. They are encountered in about 40% of cases. Transitional cell carcinomas are most frequently of the papillary type (85%). Epidermoid carcinomas are most frequently infiltrative and thus have a more rapid extension towards the periureteral region and a worse prognosis (UTZ and MCDONALD 1957). They are often of higher cellular grade (II or III). However, these epidermoid carcinomas have special features compared with the other ureteral tumors: the absence of a preferential site, the rarity of multiple locations, and the frequent coexistence of lithiasis (50%) or infectious disease. The more rapid evolution to obstruction allows an earlier diagnosis, but it is not possible to statistically evaluate how this fact affects the prognosis, given the rarity of these tumors (DROLLER 1986). For other authors, these tumors are diagnosed late because of the absence of intraluminal lacunae and the tendency of the tumor to extend superficially along the mucosa (WINALSKI et al. 1990).

Mucosecretant adenocarcinomas are very rare and secondary to ureteral metaplasia (GHAZI et al. 1979). Metaplastic changes of the transitional epithelium can be exceptionally associated with signet-ring cell carcinoma of the urinary tract, mainly in the bladder (KUME et al. 2000). Such tumors have not been previously described at the ureteral level.

There are several classifications concerning the grade (degree of anaplasia) and the stage (degree of locoregional extension) (JEWETT and STRONG 1946) (Fig. 6.4, Table 6.2). There is a good correlation between grade and stage, and between local extension and metastatic disease (BATATA et al. 1975). Metastatic disease involves the retroperitoneal nodes, the skeleton, and the lungs. Nodal involvement is encountered in 30% of cases at the time of diagnosis (ABESHOUSE 1956). Nodes are seen in about 75% of autopsy series: this can be explained by the rich lymphatic network in the ureteral wall and by the obstruction that favors lymphatic circulation (RAFLA 1975). The presence of metastatic disease is well correlated with local extension, since invasive tumors beyond the muscularis and the adventitia (stages 3 and 4 or stages C and D) have distant metastasis in 40%–75% of cases (DROLLER 1986).

The prognosis is well correlated with both the stage and the grade. The survival of patients with tumors that do not extend to the muscularis is 90% at 5 years (DROLLER 1986; BLOOM et al. 1970). Tumor locations

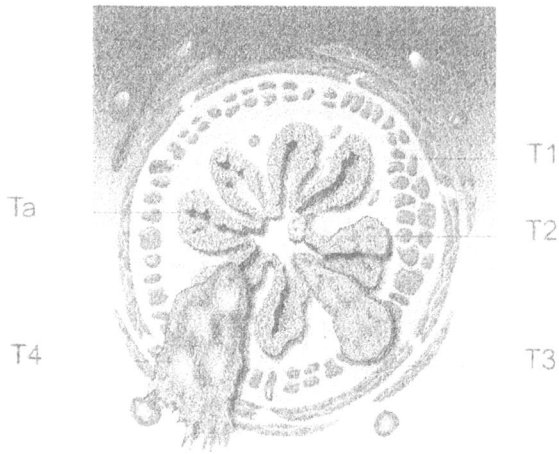

Fig. 6.4. Schematic illustration of intramural extension of ureteral tumor

Table 6.2. Pathological classification of ureteral tumors

Jewett	TNM	Locoregional extension
0	Tis	Cancer in situ
0	Ta	Epithelial, noninvasive, papillary
A	T_1	Subepithelial connective tissue
B	T_2	Muscularis
C	T_3	Adventitia
D1	T_4	Periureteral tissue
	N+	Lymph nodes
D2	M	Distant metastasis

predominate in the inferior third (65%–70%) as well as in the left ureter (63%, according to LEDER), but the fundamental characteristic is multiplicity (SCOTT and MCDONALD 1970; LEDER and DUNNICK 1990). In fact, multiple locations are frequent, whether on the same ureter or in association with the pelvis or the bladder (14% according to KYUNG et al. 1972, 40% according to HUIDT and FELDT-RASMUSSEN 1973 and YOUSSEN et al. 1988). Tumors of different grades can coexist, particularly cancers and "benign papillomas". This multiplicity can also be synchronous or sequential. The chance of finding another location at the same time as a ureteral tumor is 32% at the renal pelvis, 6% at the bladder (YOUSSEM et al. 1988). Also, a renal pelvis or a vesical tumor appears metachronous to a ureteral tumor in 10%–30% of cases. On the other hand, a ureteral tumor discovered after the diagnosis of a renal pelvis tumor is found in 25% of cases (RICHES et al. 1951).

While multiple ureteral tumors are frequent, bilateral synchronous or metachronous locations are more exceptional and found in about 1% of cases (BERGMAN and HOTCHKISS 1967). Only 22 cases of bilateral simultaneous locations have been

found in the literature (DALY et al. 1988). Some of these percentages might in fact be higher because bilaterality has not been systematically studied (MCDONALD et al. 1982). The explanation for this multiplicity is not quite clear. Is it an antegrade or retrograde dissemination or a simultaneous and similar stimulation of the whole urothelium by a cancerous agent? In other words, are there multiple primary tumors, or are some of them metastases of a primary one by intraluminal or submucosal lymphatic extension?

Distant metastases are proportionally more frequent than bladder tumors because of the thinner wall and the richer ureteral and periureteral lymphatic network (MARINCEK et al. 1993). Metastases are found in 10% of cases at the first examination. The most frequent sites are the retroperitoneal lymphatics, liver, lung, and spine.

The association between transitional cell carcinoma (TCC) and ureteral pseudodiverticula is described in Chap. 10. Its frequency, approaching 50%, should lead to the consideration of ureteral pseudodiverticula as a sign of potential malignancy (WASSERMAN et al. 1991).

6.2.3
Clinical Symptoms

Macroscopic hematuria is the chief symptom, encountered in 85% of cases (KYUNG et al. 1972). The presence of microhematuria does not exclude ureteral tumor. Significant lesions of the urinary tract in 19% of patients with microhematuria are reported in the literature (KHADRA et al. 2000). Lumbar pain secondary to urinary tract dilation is found in 40%–50% of patients. Sometimes it is a colicky pain, but it can also present as acute abdominal pain secondary to urinary tract rupture or ureteral intussusception over the tumor (COMPTON and DRUMMOND 1986). A painless hematuria is encountered in 15% of cases, while 20% of patients can be totally asymptomatic. Obstructive uropathy with acute renal insufficiency can occur in case of bilateral ureteral involvement, or with unilateral involvement in the case of congenital or acquired single kidney (BERGMAN 1983; WU et al. 1986). Finding a lumbar mass is exceptional and corresponds most frequently to the perception of an obstructed kidney. Cystoscopy is frequently the first diagnostic test done, particularly in case of persistent macroscopic hematuria. It can sometimes detect a ureteral tumor protruding from the meatus, which must not be taken for a bladder tumor (GRAHAM

1973). Endoscopic examination must also verify the absence of an associated bladder tumor. Urinary cytology has a sensitivity that varies from 70% to 90% depending on whether or not bladder flushing is performed. False negatives are not uncommon, particularly in the case of obstruction (DROLLER 1986; YOUSSEM et al. 1988).

6.2.4
Imaging

Radiological investigation most frequently allows an easy diagnosis owing to progress in opacification techniques. EU always plays a key role in the screening of patients for ureteral tumors. Recent technical improvements of helical CT and MRI have shown interesting results that could mean an increasing role of these techniques for the diagnosis of ureteral tumor (LEMAITRE et al. 2000). New imaging techniques are also essential for the staging of ureteral tumors. Imaging is needed in case of symptoms pointing at the possibility of a urothelial tumor of the upper urinary tract or in the settings of tumor staging or post-treatment monitoring.

6.2.4.1
Excretory Urography

EU is classically the first-line test (LANTZ and HATTERY 1984). It is very effective when opacification is adequate and has the advantage of exploring in one single test the whole urinary tract, allowing the detection of other tumor locations. The presence of a tumor may alter the homolateral kidney function and thus decrease the quality of the opacification, secondary to the obstructive phenomena. The diagnostic efficiency of EU varies, according to the literature. The detection of ureteral tumors requires adequate opacification of all portions of the urinary tract and optimal technical quality. For KYUNG, the sensitivity of EU is 16%, whereas more recent series had better results, up to 50% (KYUNG et al. 1972; BOOTH and KELLETT 1981; VAN POPPEL et al. 1987). The higher frequency of nonfunctioning kidney compared with other locations should also be noted, estimated at more than 50%, which implies that RUP must be performed (ARGER and STOLE 1972; CANCELMO et al. 1973). In about 30% of cases EU can also show ureterohydronephrosis of variable importance without specific findings, helping to determine the cause of this obstruction (DROLLER 1986). In some exceptional cases, obstruction may appear in an acute or a rapidly progressive manner and be responsible for contrast medium extravasation due to fornix rupture, resulting in formation of a urinoma (BRYNIAK and AWAD 1982; MURAI et al. 1989; TWERSKY et al. 1976).

Two types of radiological lesions can be encountered. The most frequent is the intraluminal lacuna (Fig. 6.5a, b). This lacuna is of variable size, about 10–20 mm in diameter, and almost totally surrounded by contrast medium. It is located most frequently at

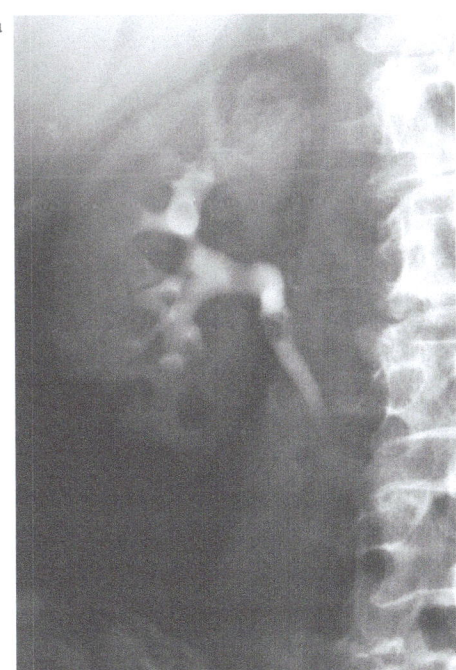

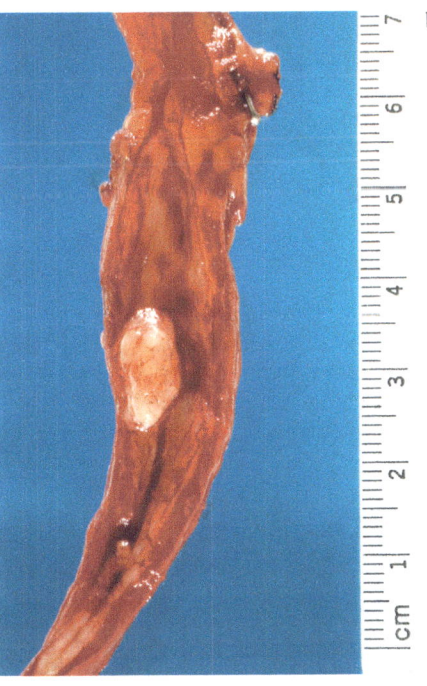

Fig. 6.5. a EU shows a rounded lacuna of the proximal part of right ureter corresponding to a transitional cell carcinoma (TCC). The lacuna dilates the ureter and is totally surrounded by CM, with moderate obstructive effect. b specimen of the nephroureterectomy showing the tumor

the level of the pelvic ureter (Fig. 6.6a–d). It generally has a wide base and is most frequently sessile. The base of implantation can be shown by multiple views, but it frequently remains difficult to demonstrate. The lacuna structure is most frequently heterogeneous and mulberry-shaped (Fig. 6.7a, b). At the level of the lacuna the ureter is always dilated. Upstream, there is a dilation in case of obstruction to urinary evacuation. Downstream the ureter presents classical modifications described by BERGMAN: The portion immediately underneath the tumor presents a cupula-shaped dilation ("Bordeaux" glass sign, goblet sign) (BERGMAN et al. 1961). These signs show the ureter adaptation to the presence of an intraluminal mass,

this mass frequently hanging downstream under ureteral peristalsis (DANIELS 1999; LEDER and DUNNICK 1990). In the majority of cases, the tumor leads to an impassable cupula-shaped blockage of the contrast column. It is particularly in these situations that lithiasis may be considered. The sign of BERGMAN would be rarely encountered in case of ureteral calculus, which causes rather a spasmodic stenosis upstream and downstream of the lacuna. However, the sign of BERGMAN is not specific, and exceptions may be seen. Some tumors of the distal ureter can protrude through the meatus and simulate a bladder tumor (Fig. 6.8).

The differential diagnosis includes the other intraluminal lacunae and particularly the images of clot,

Fig. 6.6a–d. Ureteral TCC. **a** EU shows slight dilatation of the lower part of the right ureter with a cupula-shaped blockage of the CM by a lacuna. **b–d** CT slices upstream (**b**) and at the level of the lacuna, which narrows the ureteral lumen (*arrow*)

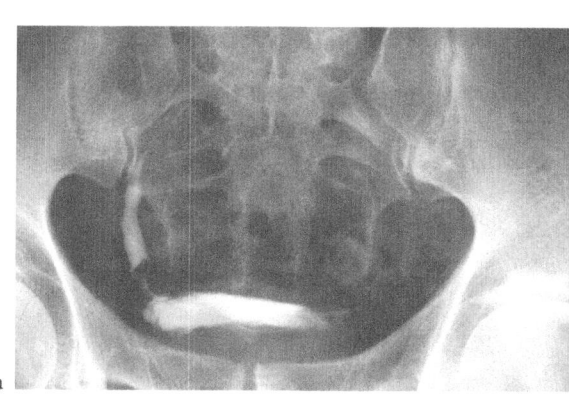

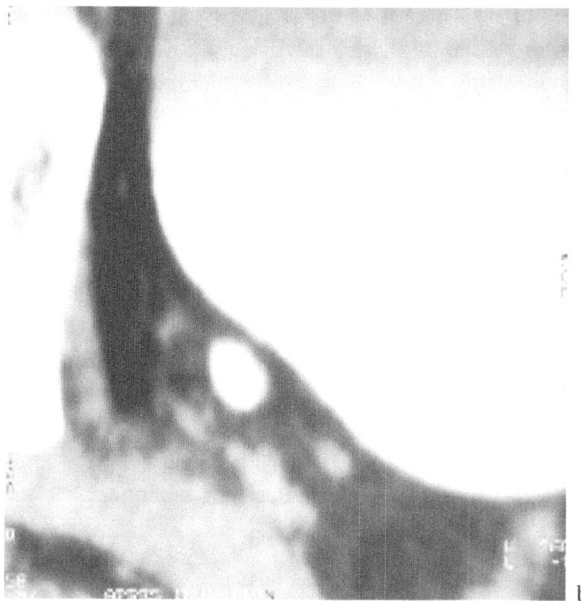

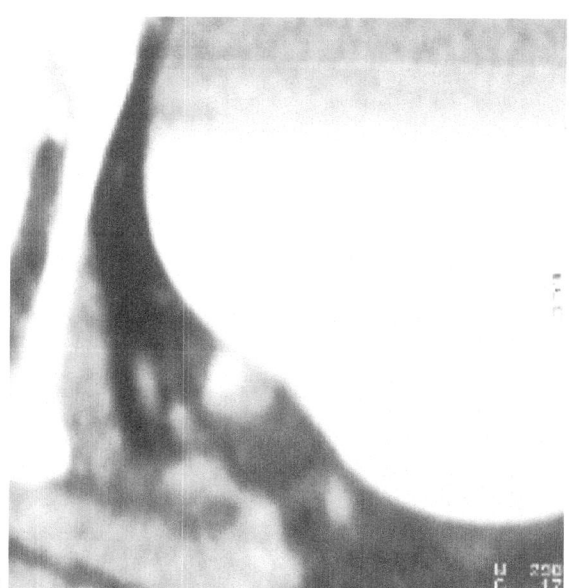

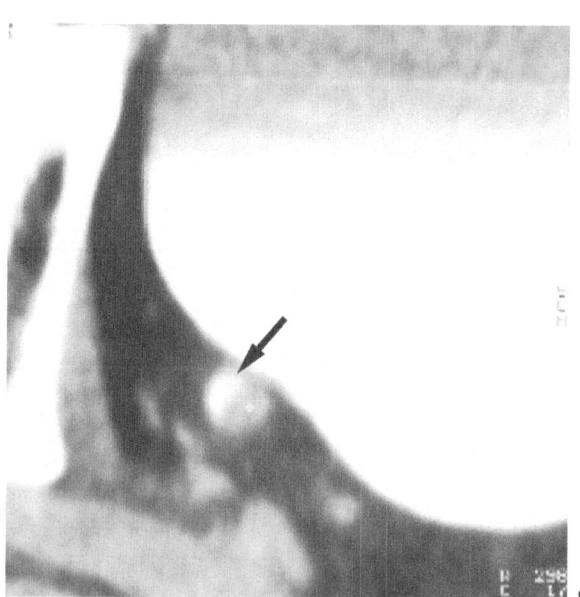

a

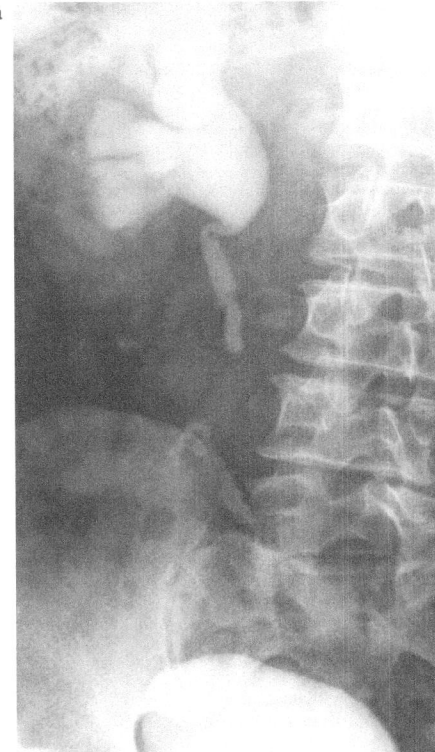

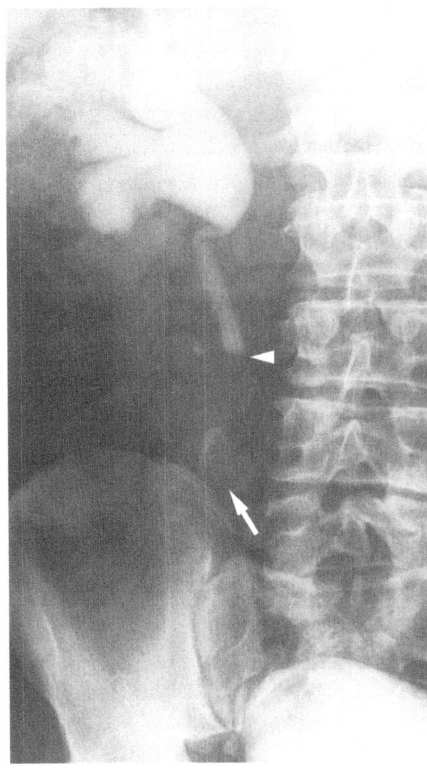

b

Fig. 6.7. a EU shows right ureterohydronephrosis secondary to a transitional cell carcinoma of the midpart of the lumbar ureter. The proximal ureter has multiple pseudodiverticula which are often associated with TCC. b The tumor has a complex morphology with a stenotic nonopacified area (*arrowhead*) and a dilation of the distal part by a mulberry-shaped lacuna (*arrow*). The lower ureter is not visualized

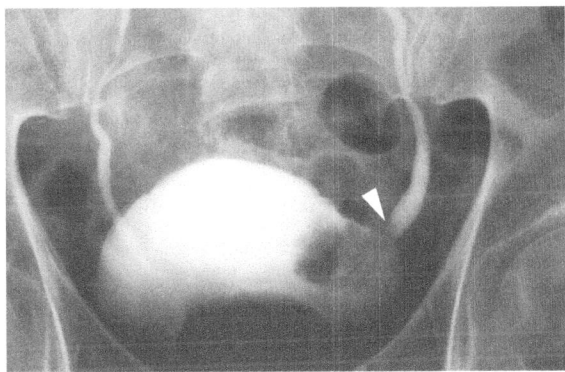

Fig. 6.8. Left pedunculated ureteral TCC (*arrowhead*) protruding through the meatus and simulating a bladder cancer

papillary fragments, and ureteropyelitis cystica. In case of doubt, retrograde opacification is the classical diagnostic method used (FEIN and MCCLENNAN 1986).

The second radiological type of lesion is more rarely encountered in the course of an EU. It is characterized by a ureter stenosis that leads most frequently to functional disturbance with no ureteral opacification. In this situation, direct opacification of the urinary tract is also needed. This type of stenotic lesion is more often described for squamous cell carcinoma and uncommon adenocarcinoma (Fig. 6.9).

Besides the diagnostic information it gives about morphological anomalies, EU also shows the importance of the urinary tract dilation and the functional impact above the tumoral obstruction. However, it provides no information about the tumoral extension. Nevertheless, it must be noted that 70% of tumors accompanied by a mute kidney or ureterohydronephrosis are invasive tumors extending to the perirenal region (LEDER and DUNNICK 1990).

In case of a normal EU, it is insufficient to exclude this diagnosis in a patient with hematuria: the false-negative rate is about 15% for EU (ARGER and STOLZ 1972).

6.2.4.2
Retrograde Ureteropyelography

RUP is the classic second diagnostic step. It is done using an occlusive catheter, placed at the meatus. Most frequently it produces images sufficiently explicit to confirm the diagnosis. The study of the whole upper and lower urinary tract can be realized in the course of the same examination, as well as cytology specimens, brush biopsy (GITTES 1984), and endosonographic views (BAGLEY et al. 1998). It is preferable to perform the urinary cytology before opacification, which gives a more reliable cytology test.

However, retrograde ureteral catheterization for RUP is not always possible, particularly in the juxtameatal locations protruding into the bladder. Antegrade pyelography is then indicated, a procedure that provides images similar to those obtained with RUP. Antegrade pyelography and RUP give no information about extraluminal tumoral extension (Baron et al. 1982), but they do permit temporary treatment of the obstruction by implementing percutaneous nephrostomy (Fig. 6.10) and/or a ureteral 2-J catheter. However, retrograde implantation of a 2-J catheter can be responsible for tumoral dissemination in the upper urinary tract.

The diagnostic contribution of RUP is undeniable. It allows better delineation of the tumor and a complete study of the upper urinary tract. However, for the diagnosis itself, it often only makes more evident the images already seen on EU. In fact, Van Poppel showed in 54 pyeloureteral tumors that RUP gave information essential to diagnosis in only 13 cases (Van Poppel et al. 1987b). The diagnosis was confirmed on RUP in 75% of cases for Kyung and 95% of cases for Geersden. Images of lacunae are identical but more clearly delineated (Geersden 1979; Kyung et al. 1972). The implantation base and the heterogeneous aspect are better shown (Fig. 6.11). Bergman's sign is also usually present, and twisting of the ureteral catheter in the dilated zone under the tumor is frequently noted (Bergman and Hotchkiss 1967). Images of stenosis can be more precisely analyzed:

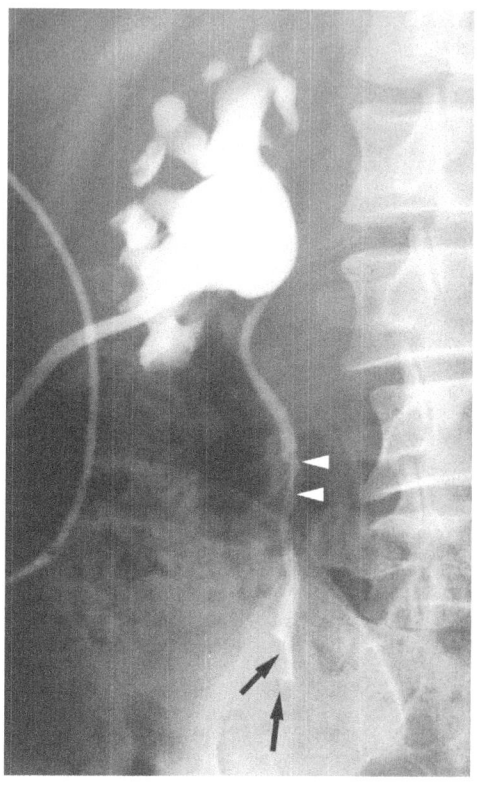

Fig. 6.10. Antegrade pyelography performed via the nephrostomy catheter. Drainage by nephrostomy was preferred because of probable pyonephrosis. Delayed opacification allows a good display of two TCC of the right lumbar ureter: the upper one is moderately stenosing and irregular (*arrowheads*). The lower results in a total cupola-shaped obstruction (*arrows*)

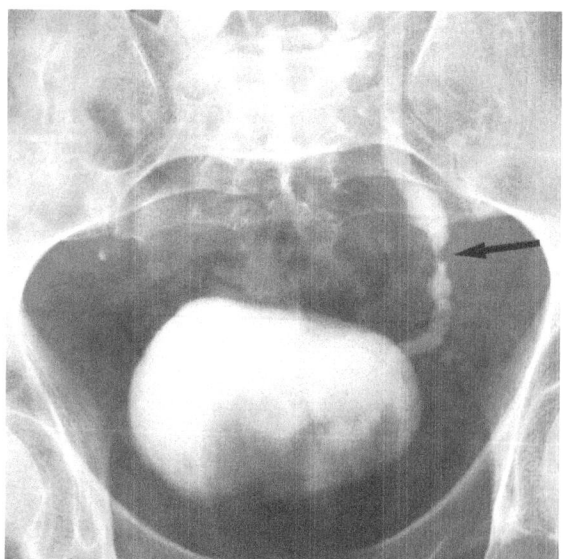

Fig. 6.9. Left pelvic ureteral stenosis corresponding to squamous cell carcinoma (*arrow*)

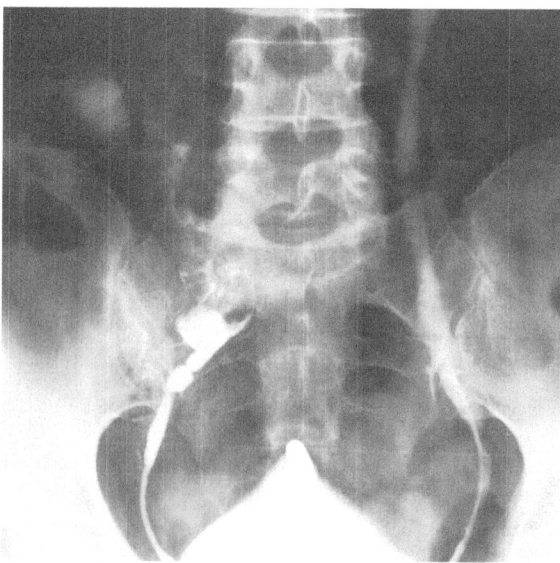

Fig. 6.11. RUP shows a cupula-shaped dilatation immediately beneath a irregular mulberry-shaped lacuna of the right ureter with absence of proximal opacification

most commonly, the stenosis is irregular and multi-lacunar with irregular, ill-defined edges (Fig. 6.12). The diagnosis is then confirmed without much discussion. On the other hand, a short stenosis, localized anywhere on the ureter, regular and centered, tubular or diaphragm-like, is more difficult to diagnose. Some ureteral tumors, even microscopic ones, can be associated with a periureteral fibrous reaction with ureteral stenosis images of extrinsic origin (MIEZA et al. 1982; MURRAY and WOO-MING 1966). The lesions with a budding tendency correspond most frequently to transitional cell carcinomas. The rather stenosing lesions must raise the possibility of epidermoid carcinoma.

Many diseases must be considered in the differential diagnosis, notably benign retroperitoneal fibrosis, retroperitoneal neoplastic invasion, inflammatory stenosis, or endometriosis. As noted by ABESHOUSE, a stenosis of the lower third of the ureter must be considered malignant until proven otherwise in a patient who is at an age where urinary tract neoplasms are common. It is then necessary to pursue investigations, first performing a brush biopsy coupled with

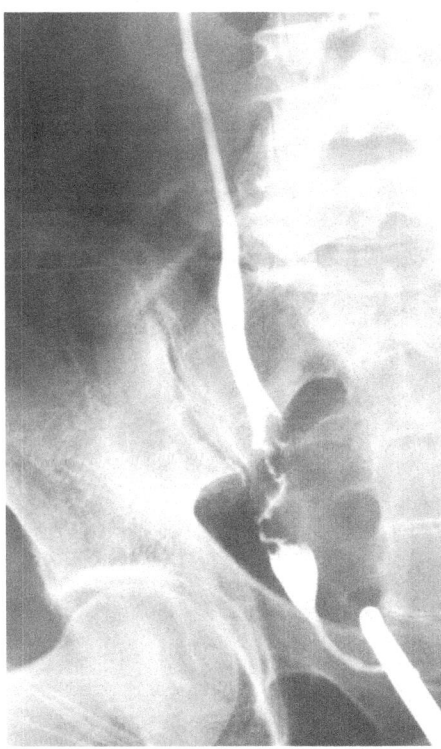

Fig. 6.12. RUP performed after EU, which showed a right mute kidney, demonstrates a large TCC of the right distal ureter. The distal ureter is dilated and shows a goblet sign. The tumor is characterized by an irregular multilacunar stenotic area with dilation of the proximal ureter

cytology (ABESHOUSE 1956). The performance of fine-needle biopsy oriented toward the ureteral lesion was proposed in order to determine the nature of ureteral obstruction in difficult cases (FREIMAN et al. 1978). It is rarely useful in case of ureteral tumors. The progress made with ureteroscopy has resolved these difficult diagnostic problems, at least at the level of the inferior third of the ureter (PEREZ-CASTRO et al. 1982; PAPADOPOULOS et al. 1987). The diagnosis of ureteral tumor is given in 90% of cases, with a complication rate of 7% (BLUTE et al. 1989). In some favorable cases, such as with small pedunculated lesions localized in a large and expansive ureter, endoscopic treatment can be contemplated. Finally, RUP is an essential tool to demonstrate a urothelial tumor that has developed in the ureteral stump after nephrectomy (POLLACK et al. 1982).

6.2.4.3
New Imaging Techniques

New imaging techniques classically have a limited place in ureteral tumors diagnosis. Ultrasonography may be useful in case of a mute kidney on EU, in that it shows signs of urinary tract obstruction. Careful examination of the ureter by an experienced ultrasonographer might show a hypoechoic intraluminal soft tissue mass, and also permits the elimination of calculus disease in the proximal or distal ureter (HADAS-HALPERN et al. 1999). However, ultrasonography cannot differentiate a tumor from a clot or a papillary fragment (EGENDER and FURTSCHEGGER 1987). Endoureteral ultrasonography using endovascular US probes has been proposed (Fig. 6.13a–e). This method allows a precise analysis of the ureteral wall and could be an interesting adjunct to RUP for the evaluation of tumor extension to the ureteral wall and periureteral soft tissues, but its use is limited by the cost of the ultrasonography equipment and the expensive single-use probes (BAGLEY and LIV 1998; GRASSO et al. 1999).

Computed tomography has a double role: It can be helpful in some difficult diagnostic cases, but is also invaluable for locoregional extension analysis (RAMCHANDANI and POLLACK 1995). Concerning the diagnosis, uncertainties may persist even after EU, RUP and brush biopsies have been performed. The diagnostic efficiency of RUP is about 80% (GEERDSEN 1979), and ureteral brushing has a 30% false-negative and a 16% false-positive rate (GITTES 1984). To be efficient, CT exploration must be centered on the occlusion zone, previously identified by opacification techniques. It must include an unenhanced study

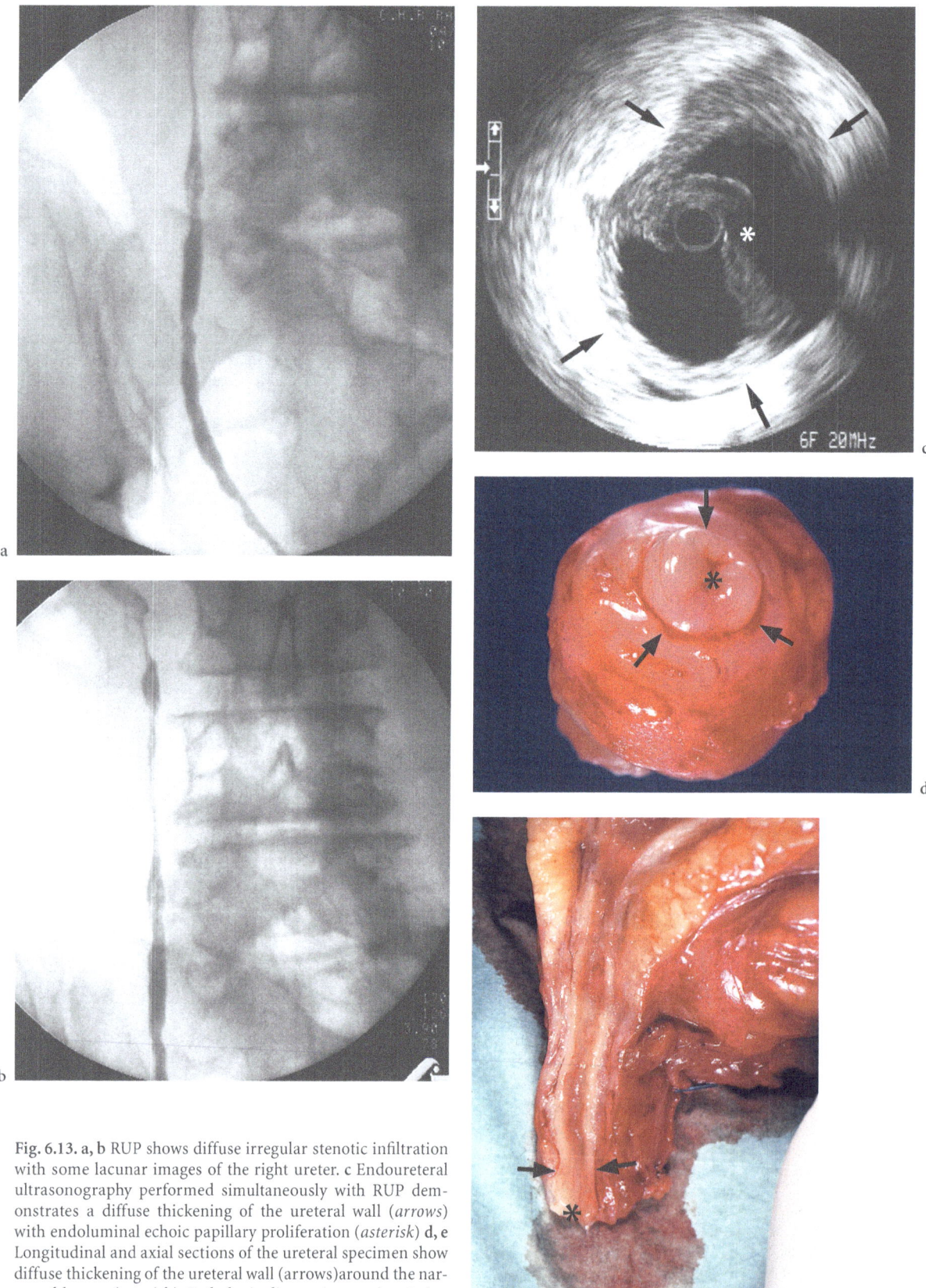

Fig. 6.13. a, b RUP shows diffuse irregular stenotic infiltration with some lacunar images of the right ureter. **c** Endoureteral ultrasonography performed simultaneously with RUP demonstrates a diffuse thickening of the ureteral wall (*arrows*) with endoluminal echoic papillary proliferation (*asterisk*) **d, e** Longitudinal and axial sections of the ureteral specimen show diffuse thickening of the ureteral wall (arrows) around the narrowed lumen (asterisk). Pathologic diagnosis was signet-ring cell carcinoma of the ureter

to eliminate calculus disease and a high-resolution enhanced study searching for an intraluminal abnormality or a soft tissue mass (PARIENTY et al. 1982) (Fig. 6.14a, b). The presence of a hyperdense intraluminal image does not totally eliminate the diagnosis of tumor, however: in fact, 2% of ureteral tumors bear calcifications and can simulate a calculus (BARON et al. 1982). In rare cases, there is an intraluminal lacuna surrounded by contrast medium, which can be ignored if the viewing window is inadequate (BARON et al. 1982). Thus, it is important to change the window width and use high-level windows (between 1500 and 2000 HU). Most frequently, CT demonstrates a soft tissue mass, generally rounded and of variable size (5 mm to 3 cm). The mass is located at the level of the presumed position of the ureter, this position being easily identifiable by following the appearance of the upstream opacified or dilated ureter on the upper images. Helical CT with multiplanar reconstruction allows easier diagnosis with coronal visualization of the unenhanced or enhanced ureter above the tumor (LEMAITRE et al. 2000) (Fig. 6.15a–e). The mass is of soft tissue density and moderately enhances after contrast medium injection. In a series of ten patients, the mean density was 48 HU after CM administration (KENNEY and STANLEY 1987). Its contours are usually regular but can sometimes be hazy with spiculated margins toward the periureteral fat, representing tumor extension beyond the adventitia (WONG-YOU-

CHEONG et al. 1998) (Fig. 6.16). It is generally easy to eliminate an intestinal loop, a vascular structure, or an adenopathy. On the other hand, it may be difficult to identify a small mass (less than 5 mm) and to differentiate it from a collapsed ureter (RYAN et al. 1979). In the series of KENNEY, the diagnosis was made in seven of ten cases and, in a retrospective manner, in two additional cases (KENNEY and STANLEY 1987). One small tumor less than 5 mm in diameter was missed. The presence of a localized thickening of the ureter wall or of a nodular intraluminal mass is not specific. The differential diagnosis includes: parietal inflammatory disease, papillary fragments, radiolucent lithiasis in case of HIV, mycelia or purulent fragments, and ureteral intussusception (BOSNIAK et al. 1982). Demonstration of contrast enhancement may help to differentiate a tumor from other filling defects, but such enhancement can be undetectable because the tumor might be small and poorly vascularized (HELENON et al. 1991). The diagnostic performance, though limited when the technique was introduced (10% of cases in the series of VAN POPPEL, b) has improved with helical acquisition, which allows multiplanar views of the urinary tract. Coronal views are particularly useful to distinguish a distal pedunculated ureteral tumor protruding through the meatus from bladder cancer near the ureteral orifice (LEMAITRE et al. 2000). Ureteral virtual endoscopy is feasible, but its clinical usefulness has still not been demonstrated (Fig. 6.17a–d).

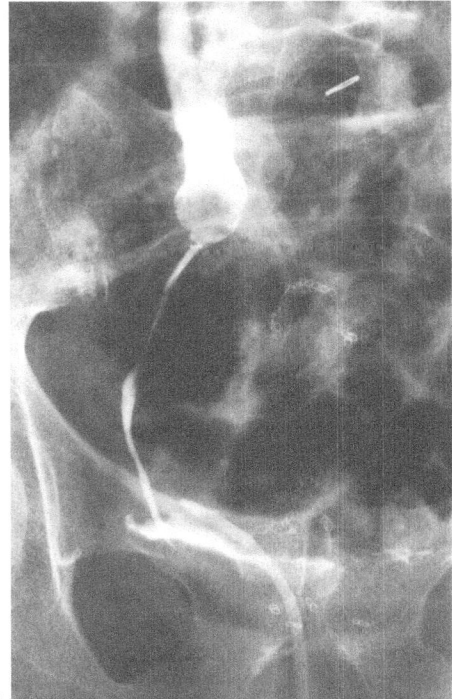

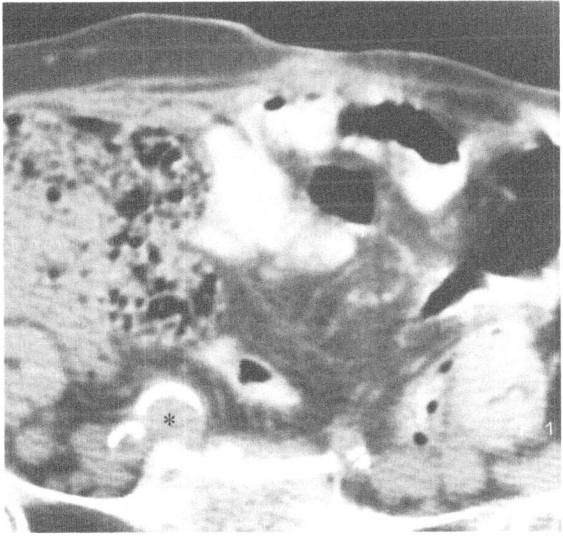

Fig. 6.14. a Antegrade pyelography shows obstructive endoluminal lacuna of the iliac right ureter. **b** CT slice at the lacunar level demonstrates a soft tissue mass (*asterisk*) surrounded anteriorly by a crescent-like opacification of the ureteral lumen, which is compressed by the mass situated near the calcified right iliac artery. Diagnosis of TCC was confirmed at surgery

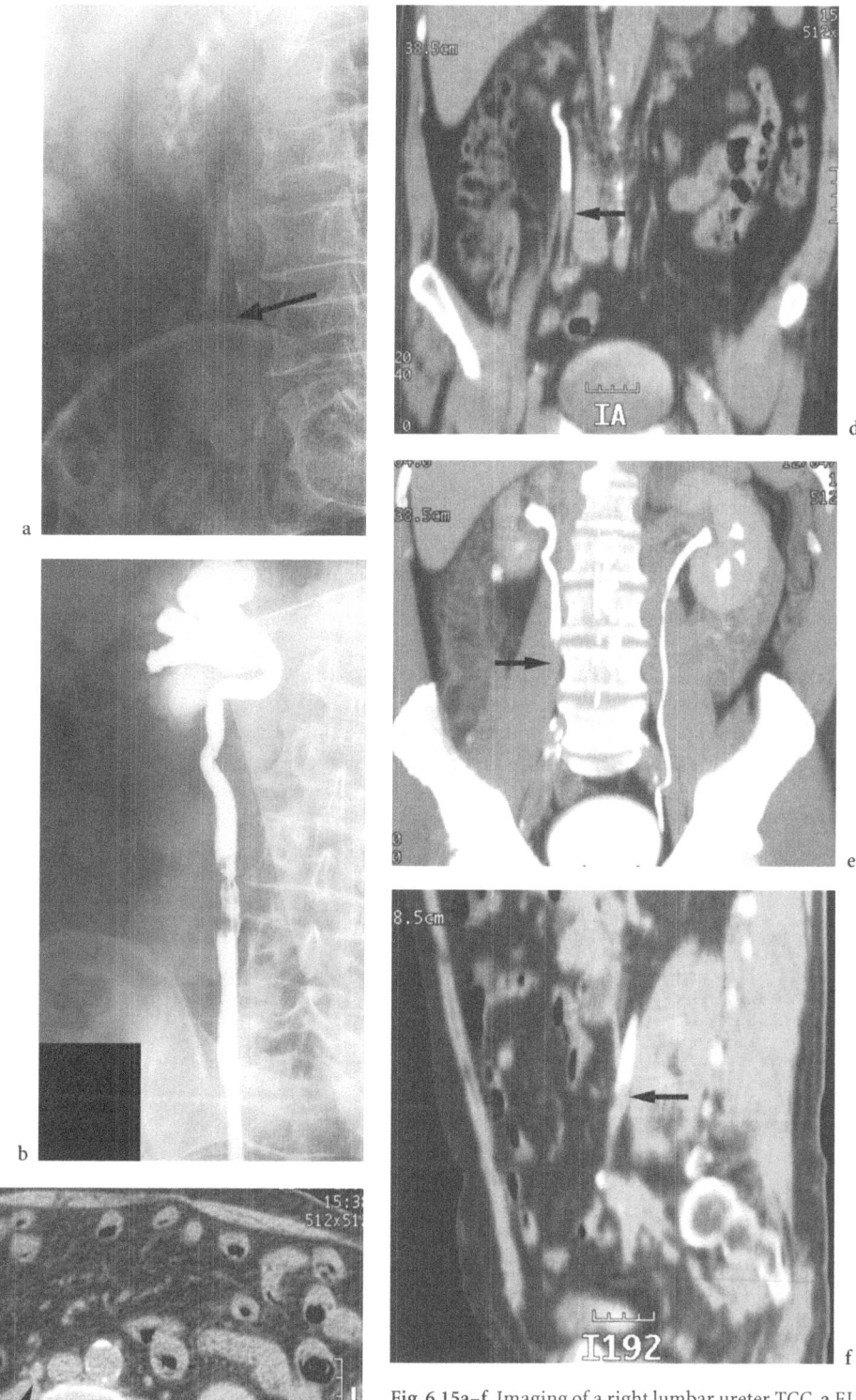

Fig. 6.15a–f. Imaging of a right lumbar ureter TCC. **a** EU shows faint opacification of the right lumbar ureter with a nonobstructive lacuna (*arrow*). **b** RUP confirms the presence of an irregular, eccentric lacunar image developed from the ureteral wall. **c** CT, axial view, showing a soft tissue mass in place ,of the ureter (*arrowhead*). **d–f** Coronal and sagittal views after MPR and MIP reconstruction demonstrating the tumor (*arrows*) and the ureter above it

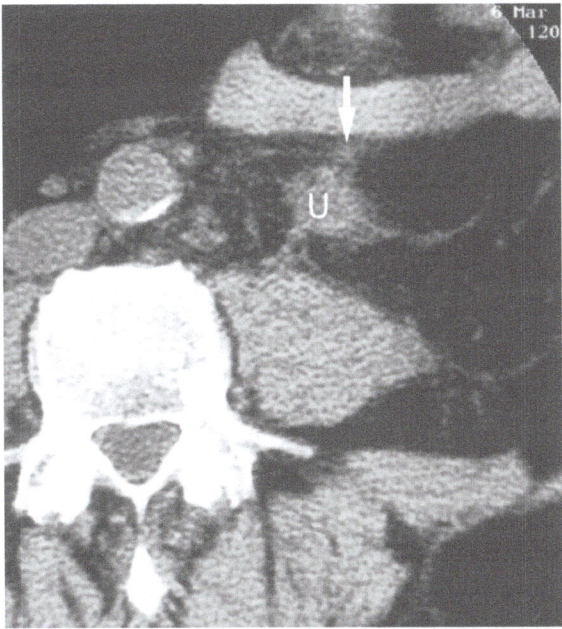

Fig. 6.16. CT slice at the level of a left ureter TCC (*u*) shows periureteral infiltration with spiculated margins and thickening of periureteral fascias (*arrows*)

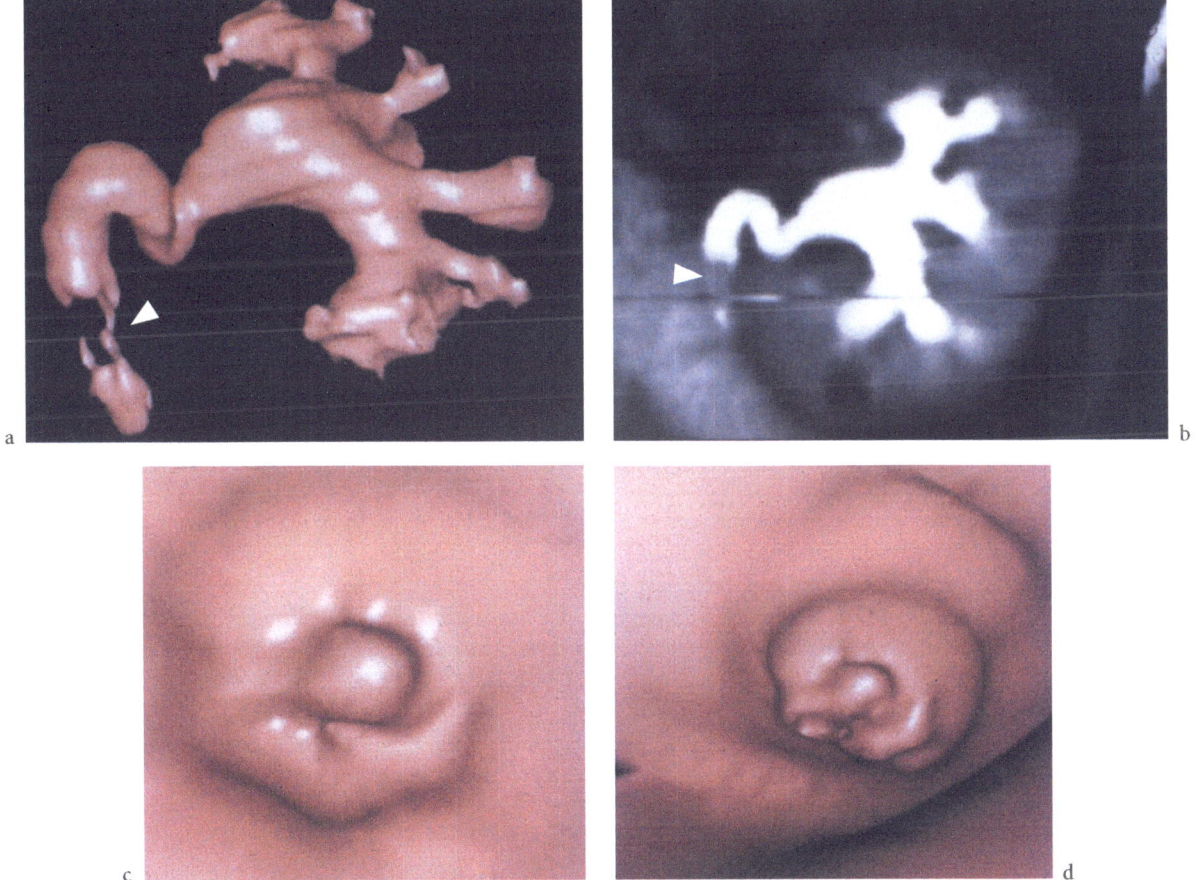

Fig. 6.17a–d. CT imaging of a TCC of the left proximal ureter (Courtesy of Dr. S. Merran). **a, b** SSD and MIP reconstructions: presence of a lacunar stenotic image of the beginning of the left lumbar ureter (*arrowhead*). **c, d** Antegrade and retrograde views after virtual endoscopic intraureteral navigation

Locoregional staging is reliably accomplished by CT, whether periureteral infiltration or retroperitoneal adenopathy is present. CT is unable to differentiate T_1 from T_2 lesions, while T_3 and T_4 lesions are easily characterized by periureteral fat infiltration and/or retroperitoneal lymph nodes. In fact, CT correlates well with surgical findings (KENNEY and STANLEY 1987). However, it cannot differentiate tumor infiltration from a reactive periureteral fibrosis (MURRAY and WOO-MING 1966). Finally, CT can be useful for diagnosing a urothelial tumor in the ureteral stump (JAFFE et al. 1987).

More and more, CT is proving useful in the investigation of malignant ureteral tumors. Even if the impact on the diagnosis is limited, CT patterns must be known in case of incidental ureteral tumor detection while staging a bladder or, more rarely, a renal pelvis tumor.

Radiological descriptions of urothelial tumors studied by MRI are rarely reported in the literature. MRI has roughly the same advantages as helical CT, also allowing pseudo-EU information. Visualization of the tumor is possible, but MRI gives no other supplementary information for tumor diagnosis and, like CT, does not permit the elimination of other causes of localized thickening of the ureteral wall. The better tolerance of gadolinium derivatives as contrast media may make this technique an alternative in case of renal insufficiency (ROFSKY et al. 1991; ROY et al. 1998) (Fig. 6.18a–e). Owing to its possibility of providing urographic images, MRI will become more and more important in the future (Fig. 6.19a, b).

6.2.5
Treatment

The treatment of ureteral urothelial tumor is surgical. It is only in the case of local or general surgical contraindications that interventional radiology techniques are needed, such as antegrade or retrograde ureteral interventions. The classical strategy is to perform a wide nephroureterectomy, often completed by excision of the perimeatal vesical region. However, tumor locations and grading may also be considered. Grade 1 tumors (papilloma or papillary carcinoma T_1) can be treated by partial ureterectomy. For some tumors of the inferior third as well, when the risk of upper recurrence is negligible, a partial resection can be done with ureteral replacement or ureterovesical reimplantation if the removed portion is less than or equal to 7–8 cm, given that the whole inferior portion of the ureter is removed. Partial resection

can also be considered in cases of solitary kidney, bilateral tumors, or severe renal failure. Endoscopic resection can be proposed as an alternative palliative treatment, but is still rarely feasible (WEBB et al. 1985). The arguments in favor of a large resection are the following:
1. A homolateral recurrence is seen in 10%–40% of partial resections.
2. It is difficult to define the tumor extension peroperatively. However, the cellular grade, identified by biopsy and/or urinary cytology, is usually indicative of tumor aggressiveness (grade 3 is very frequently associated with infiltrative tumors).

Those in favor of partial resection rely on the lack of a difference in 5-year survival rates between radical and conservative surgery (MAZEMAN 1976; DROLLER 1986). Proximal tumors with a high rate of recurrence after conservative surgery must be treated by nephroureterectomy.

Radiological, endoscopic, and cytological surveillance is essential whatever the type of surgery is performed (HATCH et al. 1988). Cystoscopy, associated with urinary cytology, must be done every 3–6 months for 2 years. Thereafter, EU or even contralateral RUP must also be done every year.

6.2.6
Mesenchymatous Malignant Tumors

Connective malignant tumors are exceptional (BENNINGTON and BECKWITH 1975). Since the first case reported by ROEMER (ROEMER et al. 1940), only 13 other cases have been described. These tumors do not have any specific radiological pattern, either on EU or with newer imaging techniques (GRIFFIN and WATERS 1996).

6.3
Secondary Malignant Tumors of the Ureter

There are four types of secondary ureteral tumors (MARINCEK et al. 1993):
- Ureteral locations secondary to a urothelial pelvicaliceal or ureteral tumor
- Renal tumors with ureteral extension
- Direct extension from an adjacent retroperitoneal or pelvic tumor
- True ureteral and/or periureteral metastasis

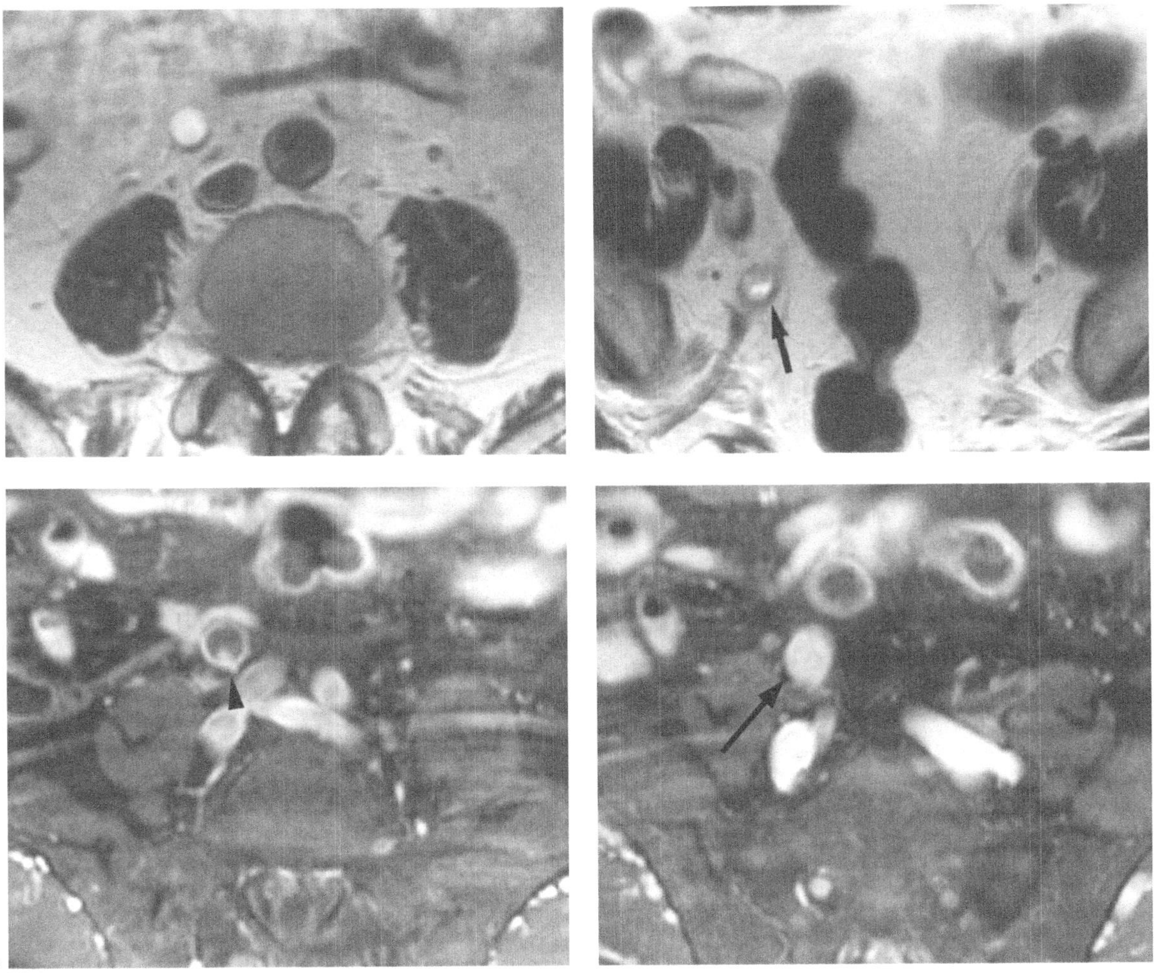

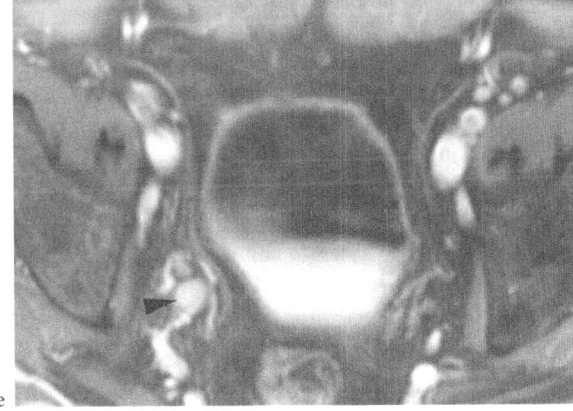

Fig. 6.18a–e. MRI of a TCC with double localization of the right ureter in a patient with renal failure. **a** Spin-echo T_2 weighted sequence: axial slice shows dilatation of the right lumbar ureter. **b** Spin-echo T_2 weighted sequence: Thickening of the ureteral wall with narrowed and irregular lumen (*arrow*). **c** Spin-echo T_1 post-gadolinium sequence with fat saturation: right ureteral dilatation with enhancement of the wall and a lacunar enhanced intraluminal mass (*arrowhead*). **d, e** Same sequence: The second tumor site is characterized by a soft tissue enhanced mass in place of the right ureter (*arrowheads*)

6.3.1
Ureteral Involvement Secondary to Urothelial Tumor

Ureteral involvement secondary to a urothelial tumor was largely covered in the preceding sections. These locations are difficult to differentiate from primary synchronous multiple urothelial tumors but, in fact, this has a poor clinical impact (YOUSSEM et al. 1988). This distant involvement has the same histology and can evolve afterwards or simultaneously. When there are multiple locations, the uppermost lesion is considered the primary one, with seeding along the urinary stream. However, secondary ureteral foci after

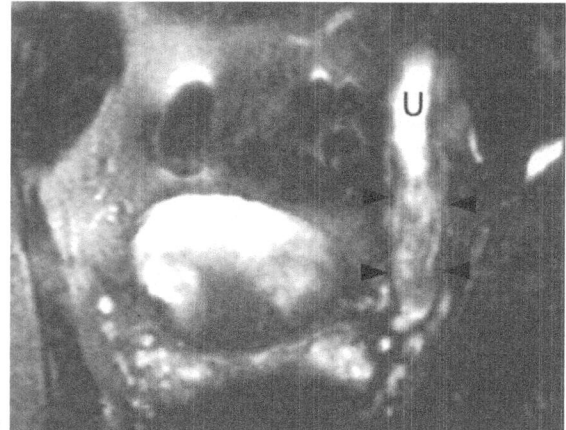

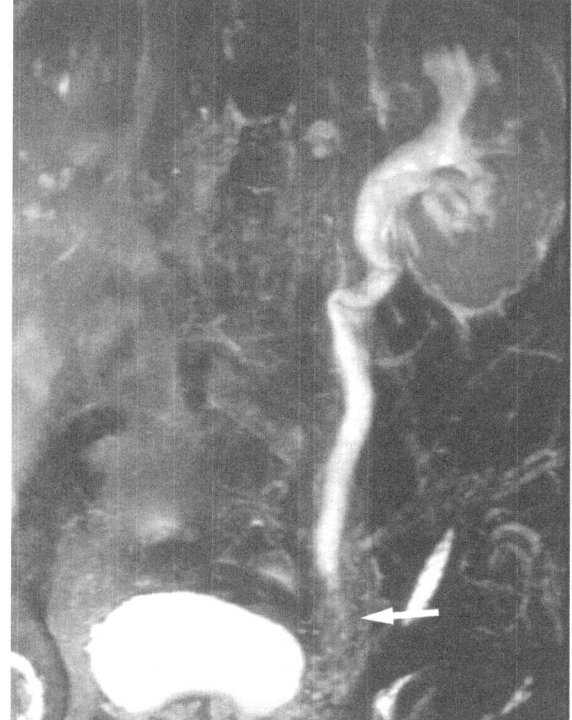

Fig. 6.19a, b. MRI of a left ureteral TCC in a patient with renal failure. **a** TSE T$_2$ weighted coronal acquisition with 4-mm-thick slices: dilatation of pelvic ureter (*U*) upstream and ureteral polypoid filling defects with moderate hypersignal (*arrowheads*). **b** MIP coronal reconstruction showing obstruction of the upper urinary tract upstream of the ureteral TCC (*arrow*)

surgical excision of bladder tumors are also encountered. This upstream involvement can be explained by the presence of a homolateral vesicoureteral reflux or as a result of retrograde intervention such as RUP or ureteral intubation and/or ureteroscopy.

6.3.2
Renal Tumors with Ureteral Extension

These tumors mostly grow on the ureteral stump after wide nephrectomy (KENNEY and STANLEY 1962). These ureteral stump recurrences are usually found in cases of urothelial tumors, mostly of the papillary type (JAFFE et al. 1987) (Fig. 6.20a, b). However, they can be encountered after surgery for adenocarcinoma of the renal parenchyma (MITTY et al. 1987). They might correspond to a new tumoral involvement, to a local extension, or to an undetected lesion left in place after surgery (STRONG et al. 1976). Conservative surgery that leaves a ureteral stump in place, whether on purpose or due to the clinical status of the patient, has a major risk of recurrence (50%), and thus strict follow-up is indicated (JAFFE et al. 1987). This surveillance relies on RUP but can also benefit from CT and MRI (POLLACK et al. 1982). Mitty's report on four cases of

renal adenocarcinomas with ureteral stump involvement points out a left predominance and in all cases renal vein involvement (MITTY et al. 1987). A literature review showed that about 6% of renal adenocarcinomas with renal vein thrombosis metastasize to the ureteral stump. This percentage was verified by SAITOH in an autopsy series, whereas the percentage of stump recurrence is 1% when the renal vein is not invaded (SAITOH 1982). Thus, it is possible that the presence of a venous collateral circulation network may facilitate recurrence. This has surgical implications, as ureterectomy should be done to the lowest possible level, with particular attention given to the postoperative development of these patients. In fact, therapeutic possibilities exist if the diagnosis of recurrence is done in time. This screening benefits, of course, from CT, particularly when RUP is not possible.

6.3.3
Direct Extension from an Adjacent Retroperitoneal or Pelvic Tumor Process

Ureteral involvement by an external neighboring process does not represent, in proper terms, a ureteral metastasis. In the majority of cases, these are neigh-

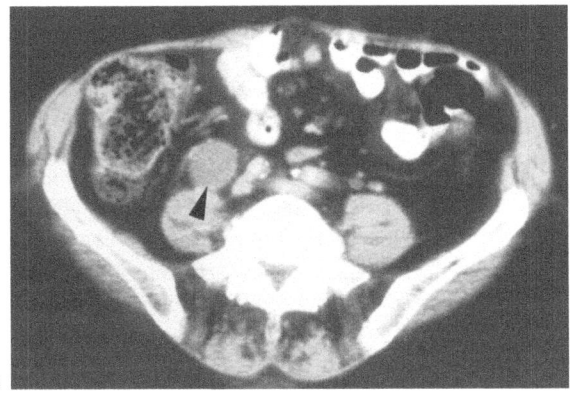 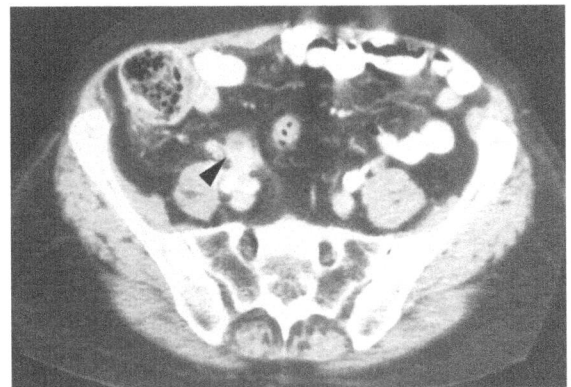

Fig. 6.20a, b. CT performed on a patient with a bladder TCC previously treated by nephrectomy for UPJ obstruction. Slices show soft tissue mass in the ureteral topography (*arrowheads*): TCC involvement of the ureteral stump

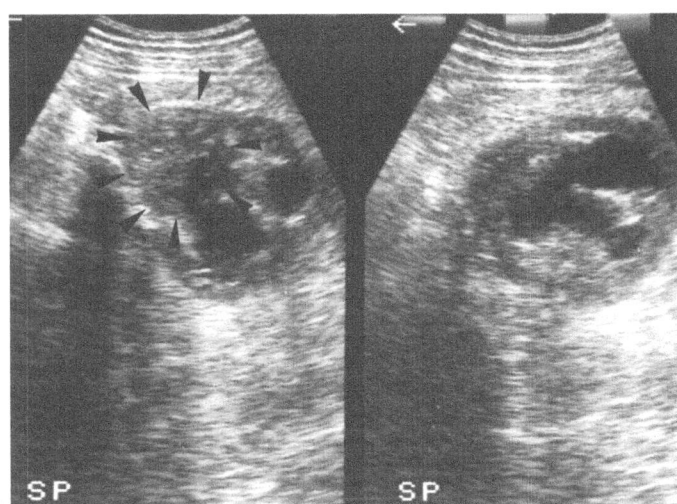

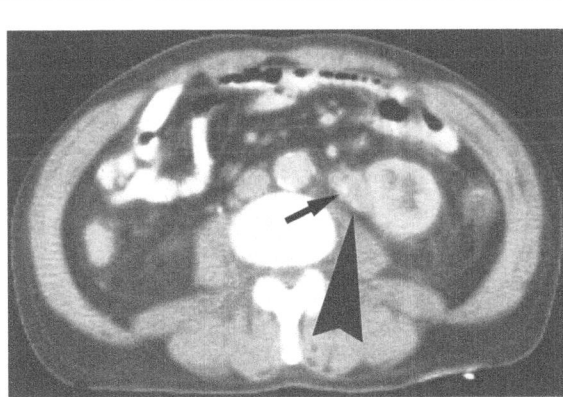

Fig. 6.21a–c. Encasement of proximal lumbar ureter by a lower pole left RCC. **a** Ultrasonographic demonstration of an echoic mass of the lower pole of the left kidney (*arrowheads*) with dilatation of calices. **b** CT shows the ureter (*arrow*) inside the mass (*arrowhead*). **c** RUP shows hydrocalicosis of the left kidney with stenotic and irregular left lumbar ureter (*arrows*)

boring tumors compressing the ureter or directly invading it (uterine, vesical, prostate, rectal, lower pole RCC, primary retroperitoneal tumors, and also retroperitoneal or pelvic nodes) (Fig. 6.21a–c). The retroperitoneal space or the pelvic cavity can also be the site of metastatic disease secondary to a distant pri-mary tumor. These metastases create a desmoplastic reaction, leading to a situation similar to retroperito-neal fibrosis (MIEZA et al. 1982). The most frequently responsible primary tumors are breast, stomach, pan-creas, colon, and prostate tumors (AMBOS et al. 1979). These are discussed in detail in Chap. 9.

6.3.4
True Ureteral and Periureteral Metastasis

The rich vascular and lymphatic network of the ureteral wall and periureteral fat explains the frequent metastatic involvement of the ureteral wall and periureteral region (MARINCEK et al. 1993). It also explains the frequency of longitudinal metastatic extension along the ureteral wall. According to MARINCEK, this metastatic involvement can occur via four mechanisms (MARINCEK et al. 1993) (Fig. 6.22):

1. Hematogenous involvement of the ureteral mucosa and submucosa. These are the true ureteral metastases and appear to be the rarest form.
2. Metastatic extension to the adventitia by the periureteral vessels
3. Scirrhous periureteral metastatic extension by the periureteral vessels

4. Metastatic extension in the periureteral lymphatics with desmoplastic reaction

Besides their different physiopathologic mechanisms, these ureteral and periureteral metastatic lesions result in clinical and radiological problems identical to those presented by primitive tumor. Practically speaking, it is very difficult to obtain histological proof of the exact parietal or periureteral location of the metastasis, and so to individualize a true ureteral metastasis (PRESMAN and ERLICH 1948). These true ureteral metastases are a poorly known entity. Their frequency is around 1%–4% in autopsy series and in people with cancer (WASSERMAN 1994); this is probably underestimated (SONG et al. 1983; PUECH et al. 1987). They might be the first sign of primary neoplastic disease and cause diagnosis and treatment problems. The uroradiological methods of treatment

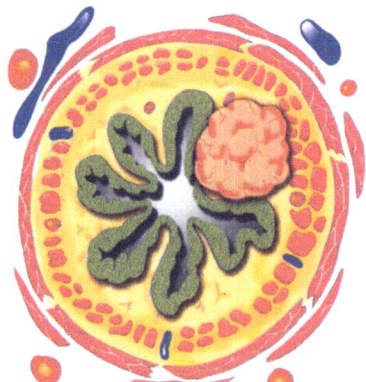

Type 1: Hematogenous submucosal / mucosal

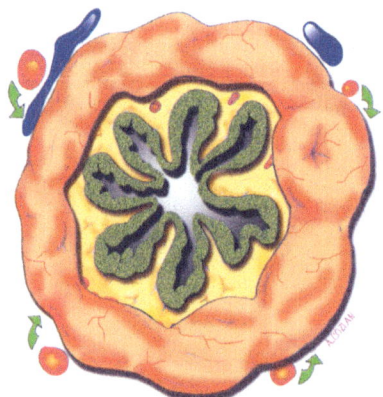

Type 2: Hematogenous adventitia metastasis from peri-ureteral vessels

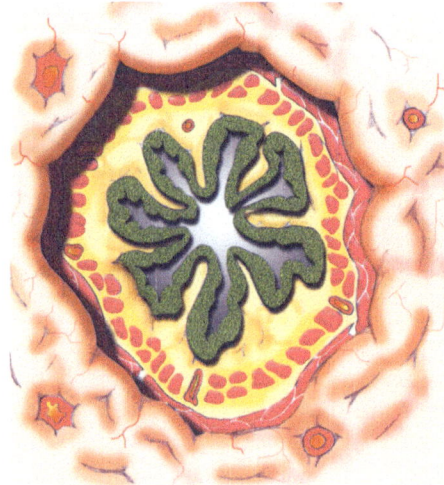

Type 3: Scirrhous metastatic spread along peri-ureteral vessels

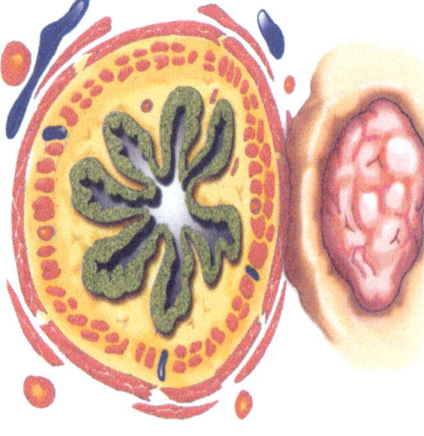

Type 4: Peri-ureteral lymph nodes metastasis with perinodal desmoplastic reaction

Fig. 6.22. Schematic representation of ureteral and periureteral metastasis. (Modified from MARINCEK et al. 1993)

allow the control of clinical consequences of obstruction and the improvement of mid-term prognosis in a certain number of patients.

Ureteral metastases can be localized and unilateral, or bilateral and diffuse in 30% of cases. Anatomical evaluation shows a more or less diffuse parietal thickening, sometimes nodular, sometimes infiltrating, involving the different layers of the wall and/or the periureteral fat. The mucosa is rarely involved, which explains the frequent negative result of intraluminal brush biopsy.

The most frequent primitive tumors are breast and stomach cancer (Ambos et al. 1979). About 8% of ureteral metastases are secondary to breast cancer (Grabstald and Kaufman 1969; Geller and Lin 1975). The other primary sites are the prostate (Benejam et al. 1987), uterine cervix, ovary, colon, melanomas, and pulmonary cancer (Goldstein et al. 1974). Ureteral metastases were also reported in non-Hodgkin's lymphoma (NHL) (Braun et al. 1972; Bruneton et al. 1987; Caro 1985). These lesions must be differentiated from retroperitoneal lymphomatous nodes compressing the ureter. They are found in about 10% of NHL autopsies (Scharifker and Chalasani 1978). They are rarely primitive and isolated and appear most frequently in the setting of advanced disease (Gosnani 1977). Only one case of ureteral involvement in Hodgkin's disease was reported (Tozzini et al. 1999).

Ureteral metastatic disease preceding the diagnosis of a primary cancer is an uncommon clinical situation. This is most frequently the case in patients with gastric cancers (Puech et al. 1987). In the majority of cases, patients have a known primary malignancy, and clinical settings are those of a chronic urinary tract obstruction. In some cases, the presence of bilateral lesions is responsible for anuria (Akmal et al. 1986). Hematuria is rarely encountered because the mucosa is generally preserved. EU most frequently shows an obstructive syndrome, uni- or bilateral, secondary to isolated ureteral stenosis, without ureteral deviation or shifting. Frequently, urinary extravasation secondary to obstruction is encountered (Bryniak and Awad 1982).

Ureteral modifications are seen principally on direct antegrade or retrograde opacification; EU is frequently insufficient due to impaired renal function secondary to obstruction.

Four principal types of lesion can be found (Song et al. 1983):

1. Regular, localized, centered, and unilateral stenosis, particularly difficult to diagnose (Fig. 6.23a–c)
2. Diffuse, string-like, slightly irregular stenosis, most frequently bilateral (Fig. 6.24a, b)
3. Diffuse stenosis with multiple parietal lacunae, giving a corkscrew appearance
4. Multiple stenoses, more or less regular, alternating with slightly dilated normal segments

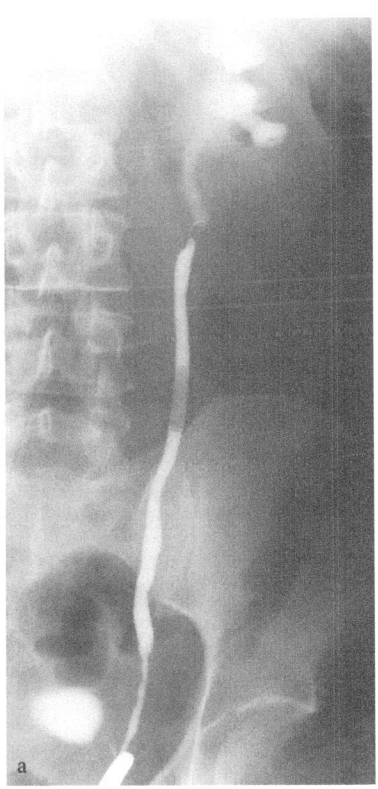

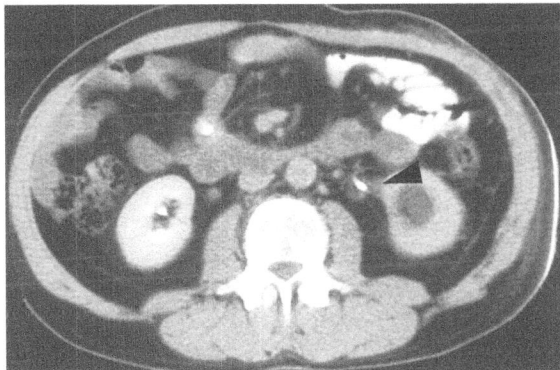

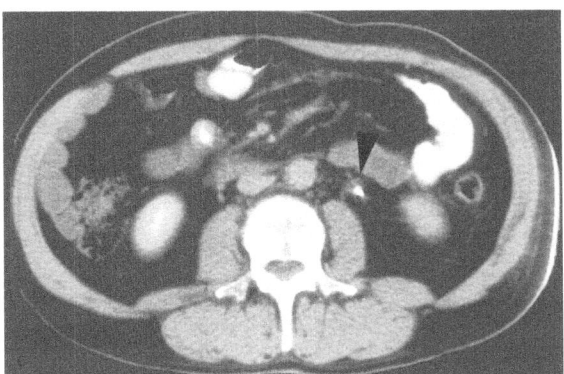

Fig. 6.23a–c. a RUP in a patient with gastric carcinoma and left hydronephrosis: unilateral, regular, and centered stenosis of the left upper lumbar ureter. b, c CT slices at the level of the stenosis demonstrate localized thickening of the ureteral wall around the 2-J catheter. Infiltration of the periureteral fat is also present (*arrowheads*). Surgery confirmed the diagnosis of ureteral metastasis from gastric origin

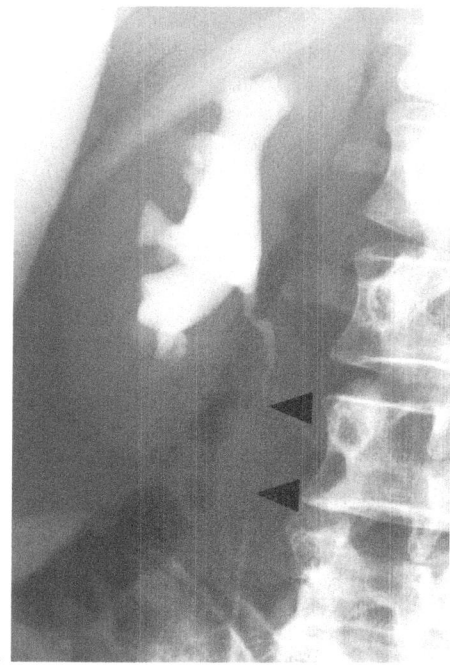

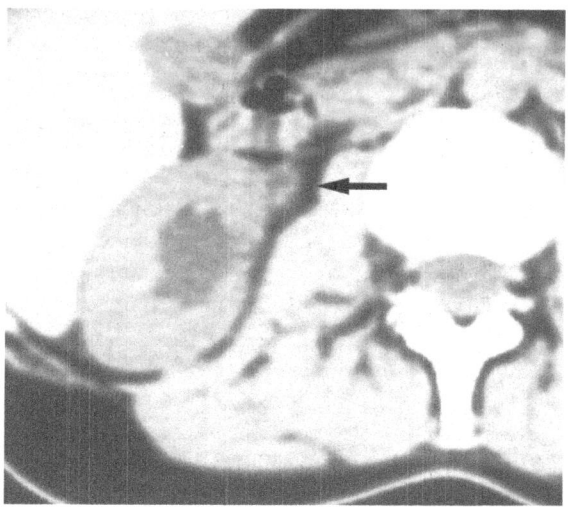

Fig. 6.24a, b. a EU in a 53-year-old woman with a history of breast cancer. Right hydronephrosis secondary to a string-like regular stenosis without displacement of the ureter (*arrowheads*). b CT slice shows diffuse thickening of the wall of the proximal lumbar ureter (*arrow*). Surgery confirmed the diagnosis of ureteral metastatic involvement

More rare patterns have been reported, such as an isolated intraluminal image similar to a urothelial tumor or a pseudodiverticulosis pattern (MARINCEK et al. 1993; WASSERMAN 1994) (Fig. 6.25). This latter aspect could be due to parietal edema secondary to the presence of metastatic involvement and was

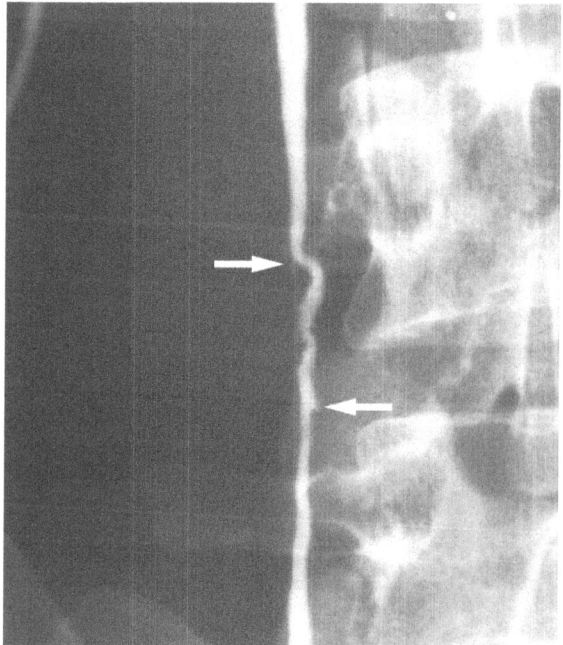

Fig. 6.25. Metastatic involvement of ureter of gastric origin. Antegrade pyelography shows diffuse and irregular stenosis with tiny diverticular images (*arrows*)

encountered on autopsy in four patients who had died of cancer without urinary symptoms. WASSERMAN suggests that urographic evidence of pseudodiverticulosis in a patient without obstruction, lithiasis, or urinary infection must suggest this diagnosis if the images do not regress following anti-inflammatory medication (WASSERMAN 1994). The topography of the different types of lesions is varied and unrelated to the type of primary tumor. Only metastasis from uterine cancer seem to localize preferentially at the crossing of the ureter with the utero-ovarian pedicle (PATOIR et al. 1975).

Direct opacification techniques have the advantage of providing an access for uroradiological techniques performed for palliative relief of obstruction. However, they do not always permit a diagnosis. Ultrasonography can exceptionally show a ureteral wall thickening (BRUNETON et al. 1987; MARINCEK et al. 1993). Endo-ureteral ultrasonography associated with RUP could be a useful diagnostic tool but cannot differentiate primary or secondary tumoral lesions of the ureteral wall (GRASSO et al. 1999) (Figs. 6.26a, b; 6.27a–d).

CT examination allows a discriminative study of the ureteral wall and the periureteral region (BOSNIAK et al. 1982). Images at the level of the stenosis show either a regular parietal thickening or a soft tissue mass centered on the ureter (Fig. 6.27a–d). This mass spreads more or less depending on the lesion extension. An intraluminal lacuna is rarely encountered (MARINCEK et al. 1993). A diffuse periureteral infiltration can be associated, particularly in

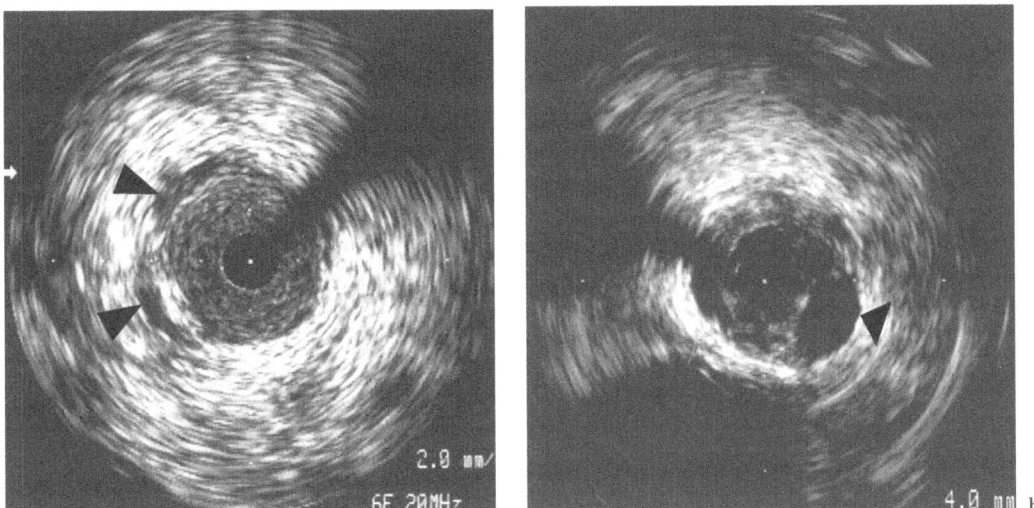

Fig. 6.26a, b. Endoureteral ultrasonography in a patient with ureteral metastatic involvement of the ureter from prostate origin. **a** Diffuse thickening of the ureteral wall with dilated periureteral vessels (*arrowheads*). **b** Heterogeneous infiltration of the ureteral wall with thickening and presence of subadventitial hypoechoic nodules (*arrowhead*)

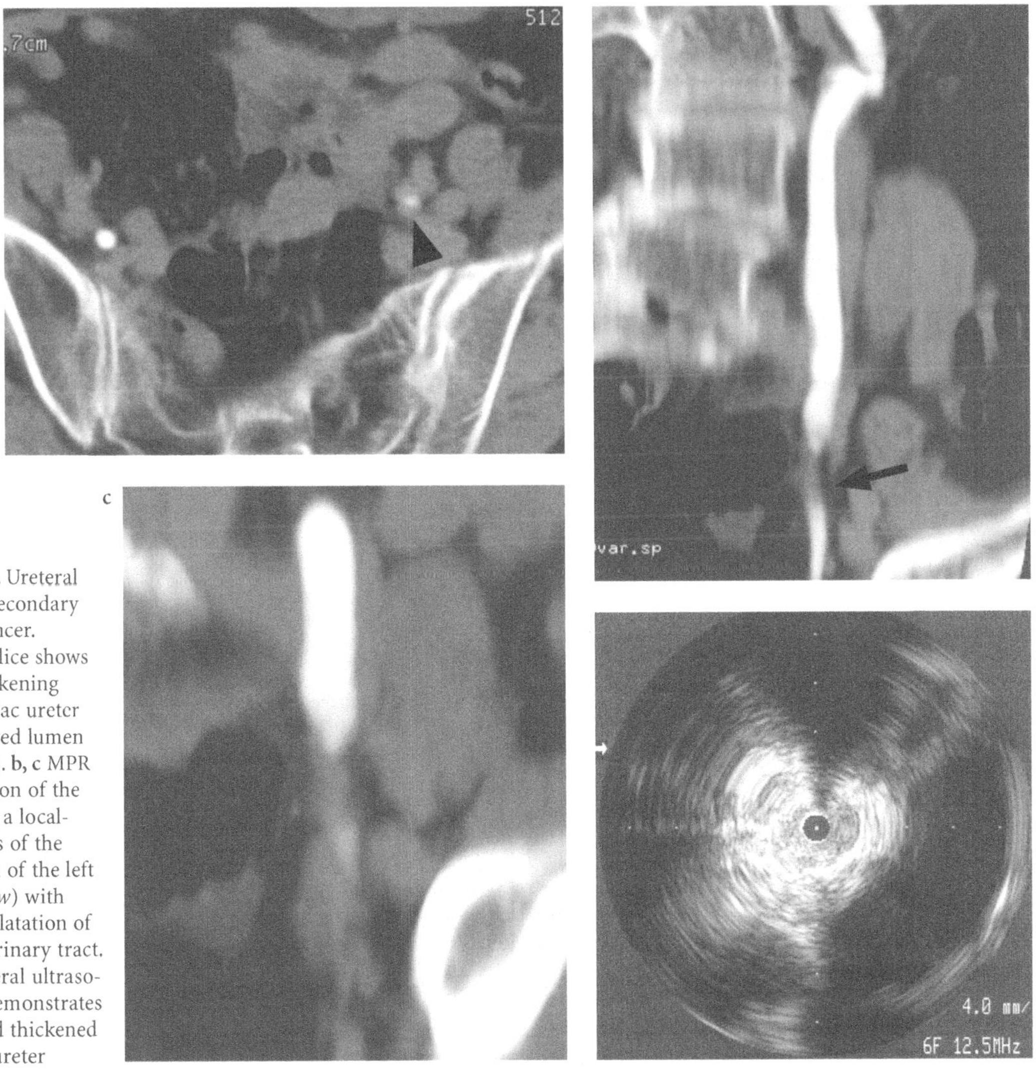

Fig. 6.27a–d. Ureteral metastasis secondary to breast cancer. **a** Axial CT slice shows parietal thickening of the left iliac ureter with narrowed lumen (*arrowhead*). **b, c** MPR reconstruction of the CT showing a localized stenosis of the iliac portion of the left ureter (*arrow*) with moderate dilatation of the upper urinary tract. **d** Endoureteral ultrasonography demonstrates the localized thickened wall of the ureter

prostate tumors with frequent retroperitoneal nodes (CAMPBELL and ALDIS 1980) (Fig. 6.28a, b). Ureteral involvement can be difficult to differentiate from a periureteral lesion. In fact, prostate cancers can have a retroperitoneal nodal extension but also can spread through ureteral and periureteral lymphatics and involve the ureter itself and the periureteral region (CAMPBELL and ALDIS 1980). The pattern seen on CT is not specific and can be seen in primary ureteral tumors or in inflammatory stenosis. However, the presence of multiple lesions is indicative of diffuse disease, and malignant metastatic involvement must then be suspected. The diagnosis is most frequently based on the histological analysis of the surgical specimen or made after endoscopic sampling. The prognosis of ureteral metastasis is very poor, except in prostate tumors (ICARD et al. 1986). Treatment is palliative and consists essentially of ureteral derivation using 2-J catheters. Surgical resection is rarely feasible because of the extensive disease.

The radiological aspects of secondary ureteral involvement in patients with lymphomas are slightly different from those of other metastatic diseases: diffuse involvement with multiple stenosis and nodular lesions giving a corkscrew pattern is seen on EU or RUP. Diffuse thickening of the ureteral wall can also be demonstrated on CT. LEBOWITZ recently described an interesting isolated lymphomatous ureteral involvement, found on MRI as bilateral wall thickening with enhancement after gadolinium injection. The post-chemotherapy regression was also demonstrated on MRI (LEBOWITZ et al. 1995). The diagnosis can be made, however, when there are other disease locations, in particular retroperitoneal adenopathies (TOZZINI et al. 1999).

References

Abeshouse BS (1956) Primary benign and malignant tumor of the ureter. A review of the literature and reports of one benign and 12 malignant tumors. Am J Surg 91:237–271

Abrams HJ, Buchbinder MI, Sutton AP (1977) Benign ureteral lesions. Urology 9:517–520

Ajrawat HS, Skogg DP, Asirwathan JE, et al (1982) Lobulated inverted papilloma of ureter. Urology 20:290–292

Akmal M, Kaptein EM, Bertram J, et al (1986 Acute renal failure due to bilateral ureteral obstruction by metastases from breast cancer. Nephron 42:23–28

Ambos MA, Bosniak MA, Megibow AJ, et al (1979) Ureteral involvement by metastatic disease. Urol Rad 1:105–112

Arger PH, Stolz JL (1972) Ureteral tumours: the radiologic evaluation of a differential diagnosis, "throw-in". AJR Am J Roentgenol 116:812–821

Bagley DH, Liu JB (1998) Three-dimensional endoluminal ultrasonography of the ureter. J Endourol 12:411–416

Bagley DH, Fabrizio M, El-Gabry F (1998) Ureteroscopic and radiographic imaging of the upper urinary tract. J Endourol 12:313–324

Banner MP, Pollack HM (1979) Fibrous ureteral polyp. Radiology 130:73–76

Baron RL, McClennan BL, Lee JK, et al (1982) Computed tomography of transitionnal cell carcinoma of the renal pelvis and ureter. Radiology 144:125–130

Batata MA, Whitmore WF Jr, Hilaris BJ, et al (1975) Primary carcinoma of the ureter: a prognosis study. Cancer 35:1626

Bellin MF, Springer O, Mourey-Gerosa I, et al (2002) CT diagnosis of ureteral fibro-epithelial polyp. Eur Radiol 12: 125–128

Benejam R, Caroll TJ, Loening S (1987) Prostatic carcinoma metastatic to ureter. Urology 29:325–327

Bennington JL, Beckwith JB (1975) Tumors of the renal pelvis and ureter. In: Tumors of the kidney, renal pelvis and ureter. In: Bennington JL, Beckwith JB (eds) Atlas of tumor pathology. Armed Forces Institute of Pathology (AFIP), Washington DC, pp 243–336

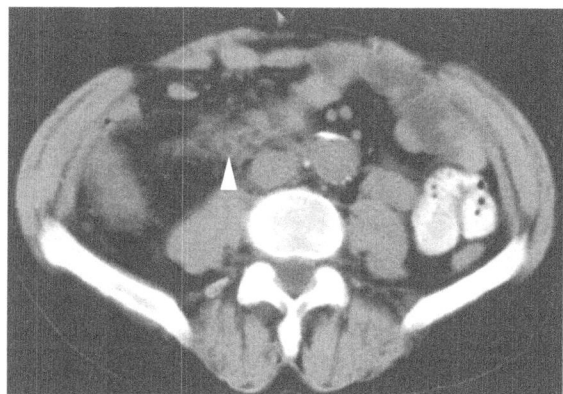

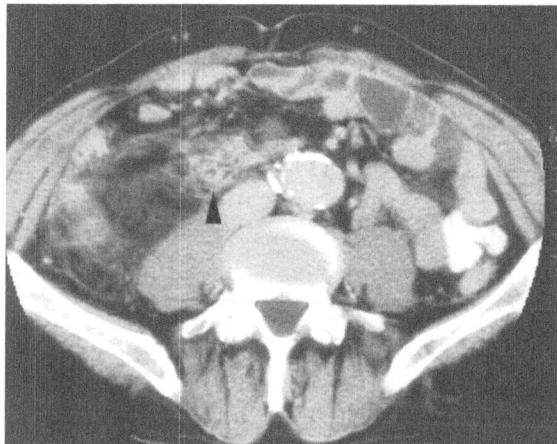

Fig. 6.28a, b. CT in a patient with chronic obstruction of the right upper urinary tract associated with gastric carcinoma. Diffuse infiltration of the periureteral fat by an irregular and heterogeneous soft tissue mass. The lesion is centered by the ureter, which is visible as an oval image with a nonopacified lumen surrounded by the thickened wall (*arrowheads*)

Bergman H (1983) Bilateral ureteral tumors (letter). Urology 21:103

Bergman H, Friedenberg RM, Sayegh V (1961) New roentgenographic signs of carcinoma of the ureter. AJR Am J Roentgenol 86:707–717

Bergman H, Hotchkiss RS (1967) Ureteral tumors. In: Bergman H (ed) The ureter, Harper and Row, New-York, pp 439–457

Biyani CS, MacKay AM, Sissions G, et al (1998) An unusual filling defect in the ureter. Urol Int 61:124–125

Bloom NA, Vidone RA, Lytton B (1970) Primary carcinoma of the ureter: a report of 102 new cases. J Urol 103:590–598

Blute ML, Segura JW, Patterson DE, et al (1989) Impact of endourology on diagnosis and management of upper urinary tract urothelial cancer. J Urol 141:1298–1301

Booth CM, Kellett MJ (1981) Intravenous urography in the follow-up of carcinoma of the bladder. Br J Urol 55:246–249

Bosniak MA, Megibow AJ, Ambos MA, et al (1982) Computed tomography of ureteral obstruction. AJR 138:1107–1115

Braun E, Manley C, Liao K, et al (1972) Intrinsic Hodgkin's disease of the ureter. J Urol 107:952–954

Bruneton JN, Drouillard J, Normand F, et al (1987) Nonrenal urological lymhomas. Fortschr Rontgenstr 146:42–46

Bryniak SR, Awad SA (1982) Spontaneous urinary extravasation secondary to primary ureteric carcinoma. Urology 19:645

Campbell JE, Aldis HW (1980) Lymphangitic ureteral metastases from prostatic carcinoma. J Can Assoc Radiol 31:158–162

Cancelmo JJ, Uhlman RC, Eshleman JL, et al (1973) Tumors of the ureter: problems in diagnosis. AJR Am J Roentgenol 117:132–138

Caro DJ (1985) Clinical presentation of metastatic lymphoma to ureter. Urology 1:53–55

Compton JS, Drummond M (1986) Intussuception of the ureter by a polypoid transitional cell carcinoma. Br J Urol 58:725–726

Corkill M, Srigley J, Graham P, et al (1987) Inverted papilloma: an uncommon benign cause of ureteral filling defect. Urol Radiol 9:164–167

Daly BD, Grainger R, Butler MR (1988) Bilateral ureteric carcinoma. Clin Radiol 39:330–332

Daniels RE (1999) The goblet sign. Radiology 210:737–738

De Bruyne FMJ, Moonen WA, Dafnekindt AA (1990) Fibro-epithelial polyp of ureter. Urology 16:355–359

Droller MJ (1986) Transitional cell cancer of the renal pelvis and ureter. In: Walsh PC, Gittes RF, Pelmutter AD, Stamey A (eds) Campbell's urology, vol 2. Saunders, Philadelphia, pp 1408–1440

Duchek M, Hallmans G, Hietala SO, et al (1987) Inverted papilloma with intussusception of the ureter. Scand J Urol Nephrol 21:147–149

Egender JL, Furtschegger A (1987) Clinical significance of sonography of the ureter. Eur J Radiol 7:42–43

Emmett JL, Witten DM (1971) Tumors of renal pelvis and ureter. In: Emmett JL, Witten DM (eds) Clinical urography: an atlas and text book of roentgenologic diagnosis. Saunders, Philadelphia, pp 1145–1187

Fein AB, McClennan BL (1986) Solitary filling defects of the ureter. Semin Roentgenol 21:201–215

Freiman DB, Ring EJ, Oleaga JA, et al (1978) Thin-needle biopsy in the diagnosis of ureteral obstruction with malignancy. Cancer 42:714–716

Geerdsen J (1979) Tumors of the renal pelvis and ureter. Symptomatology, diagnosis treatment and prognosis. Scand J Urol Nephrol 13:287–290

Geisler CH, Mori K, Leiter E (1980) Lobulated inverted papilloma of the ureter. J Urol 123:270–271

Geller SA, Lin CS (1975) Ureteral obstruction from metastatic breast carcinoma. Arch Pathol 99:476–478

Ghazi MR, Morales PA, Al-Askari S (1979) Primary carcinoma of ureter. Urology 14:18–21

Gittes RF (1979) Tumor of the ureter and renal pelvis. In: Harrison JH, Gittes RF, Perlmutter AD, Stamey TA, Walsh PC (eds) Campbell's urology, 4th edn. Saunders, Philadelphia, pp 1010

Gittes RF (1984) Retrograde brushing and nephroscopy in the diagnostic of upper tract urothelial cancer. Urol Clin North Am 11:617–622

Goldstein HM, Kaminski S, Wallace S (1974) Urographic manifestations of metastatic melanoma. AJR Am J Roentgenol 121:801–805

Goswani AP (1977) Metastatic cancer to ureter and kidney from malignant lymphoma. J Urol 117:381–382

Grabstald H, Kaufman R (1969) Hydronephrosis secondary to ureteral tumors by metastatic breast cancer. J Urol 102:569–576

Graham JB (1973) Delayed recognition of ureteral tumors. J Urol 110:191–194

Grainger R, Gikas PW, Barton Grossman H (1990) Urothelial carcinoma occurring within an inverted papilloma of the ureter. J Urol 143:802–804

Grasso M, Li S, Liu JB et al (1999) Examining the obstructed ureter with intraluminal sonography. J Urol 162:1286–1290

Griffin JH, Waters WB (1996) Primary leiomyosarcoma of the ureter. J Surg Oncol 62:148–152

Hadas-Halpern I, Farkas A, Patlas M, et al (1999) Sonographic diagnosis of ureteral tumors. J Ultrasound Med 18:639–645

Hatch TR, Hefty TR, Barry JM (1988) Time-related recurrence rates in patients with upper tract transitionnal cell carcinoma. J Urol 140:40–41

Helenon O, Rousselin B, Chiche JF, et al (1991) Place de la tomodensitométrie dans l'exploration des tumeurs de la voie excrétrice urinaire haute. Rev Im Med 3:371–375

Hughes FA, David CS (1976) Multiple benign ureteral fibrous polyps. AJR Am J Roentgenol 126:723–727

Huidt V, Feldt-Rasmussen K (1973) Primary tumours in the renal pelvis and ureter with particular attention to the diagnostic problems. Acta Clin Scand [Suppl] 433:91–101

Hultergren N, Lagengren L, Ljunquist A (1965) Carcinoma of the renal pelvis in papillary necrosis. Acta Clin Scand 30:314–320

Icard P, Benoit G, Vieillefond A, et al (1986) Metastase ureterale d'un cancer de la prostate. Ann Urol 10:335–336

Jaffe J, Friedman AC, Seidmon J, et al (1987) Diagnosis of ureteral stump transitional cell carcinoma by CT and MR imaging. AJR Am J Roentgenol 149:741–742

Jansen TTH, van de Weyer FPH, Devries HR (1982) Angiomatous ureteral polyp. Urology 20:426

Jewett HJ, Strong GH (1946) Infiltrating carcinoma of the bladder: relation of the depth of penetration of the bladder to incidence of local extension and metastases. J Urol 55:366–372

Kawabe K (1987) Hemangiomatous granuloma of ureter. Eur Urol 13:138–139

Kenney PJ, Stanley DM (1962) Reccurent carcinoma in the ureteric stump. Br J Surg 50:202–205

Kenney PJ, Stanley DM (1987) Computed tomography of ureteral tumors. J Comput Assist Tomogr 11:102–107

Khadra MH, Pickard RS, Charlton M, et al (2000) A prospective analysis of 1930 patients with hematuria to evaluate current diagnostic practice. J Urol 163:524–527

Kume H, Kanai Y, Tobisu K, et al (2000) Signet-ring cell carcinoma of the urinary bladder associated with transitionnal cell carcinoma of the right ureter. Scand J Urol Nephrol 34:278–279

Kyriakos M, Royce RK (1989) Multiple simultaneous inverted papillomas of the upper urinary tract. Cancer 63:368–380

Kyung HK, Leiter E, Brendler H (1972) Primary tumors of the ureter. J Urol 107:952–954

Lang EK, Nourse M (1969) The roentgenographic diagnosis of obstructive lesion of the ureter. J Urol 101:812–820

Lantz EJ, Hattery RR (1984) Diagnostic imaging of urothelial cancer. Urol Clin North Am 11:567–583

Lebowitz JA, Rofsky NM, Weinreb JC, et al (1995) Ureteral lymphoma: MRI demonstration. Abdom Imaging 20:173–175

Leder RA, Dunnick R (1990) Transitional cell carcinoma of the pelvicalices and ureter. AJR 155:713–722

Ledor K, Mieza M, Ledors S (1982) Multicentric fibroepithelial ureteral polyp. Urol Radiol 4:259–261

Lemaitre L, Ala Edine C, Dubrule F, et al (2000) Retroperitoneum and ureters. In: Terrier F, Grossholz M, Becker CD (eds) Spiral CT of the abdomen. Springer, Berlin Heidelberg New York, pp 277–316

Maidenberg M, Richard F, Conort P, et al (1990) Polypes fibreux de l'appareil urinaire. Ann Urol 24:409–414

Marincek B, Scheideggek JR, Studer UE (1993) Metastatic disease of the ureter: patterns of tumoral spread and radiologic findings. Abdom Imaging 18:88–94

Mazeman E (1976) Tumors of the upper urinary tract, calyces, renal, pelvis and ureter (1118 cases). Eur Urol 2:120–129

McDonald MW, Solomon MH, Konnak JW (1982) Bilateral simultaneous ureteral tumours. Urology 20:168

Mieza M, Rotstein JM, Geffen A (1982) CT demonstration of periureteral fibrosis of malignant etiology. J Comput Assist Tomogr 6:290–293

Mills C, Vaughan ED jr (1983) Carcinoma of the ureter: natural history, management and 5-year survival. J Urol 129: 275–279

Mitty HA, Droller MJ, Dikman SH (1987) Ureteral and renal pelvic metastases from renal cell carcinoma. Urol Radiol 9:16–20

Mostofi FK (1954) Potentialities of bladder epithelium. J Urol 71:701–714

Murai M, Matsuzaki S, Aihara M (1989) Spontaneous peripelvic extravasation due to squamous cell carcinoma of the ureter. Urol Int 44:370–372

Murray SM, Woo-Ming MD (1966) Retroperitoneal "fibrosis" due to carcinoma of the ureter. Br J Urol 38:424–427

Naucler J, Johansson SL, Nilson AE, et al (1983) Fibroepithelial polyp of the ureter. Scand J Urol Nephrol 17:379–383

Oesterling JE, Alexander Liu HY, Fishman EK (1989) Real-time multiphase computerized tomography: a new diagnostic modality used in the detection and endoscopic removal of a distal ureteral fibro-epithelial polyp and adjacent calculi. J Urol 142:1563–1566

Ogata S, Mizoguchi H, Arita M, et al (1985) A case of hemangiomyoma of the ureter in a child. Eur Urol 11:355–356

Orr PS, McGregor CG (1978) Congenital ureteric cyst: a rare anomaly. Urology 12:699–700

Papadopoulos I, Figge M, Weissbach L, et al (1987) Diagnosis of urothelial tumor by ureteroscopy. Eur Urol 13:296–299

Parienty RA, Ducellier R, Pradel J, et al (1982) Diagnosis value of CT numbers in pelvicaliceal filling defects. Radiology 145:743–747

Patoir G, Lemaire G, Mouton Y (1975) Anurie et colique néphrétique révélatrice de métastase urétérale d'un cancer utérin. J Urol Nephrol 81:149–154

Perez-Castro, Ellendt E, Martinez Pineiro JA (1982) Ureteral and renal endoscopy. Eur Urol 117–120

Pollack HM, Banner MP, Popky GL (1982) Radiologic evaluation of the ureteral stump. Radiology 144:225–230

Potts IF, Hirst E (1963) Inverted papilloma of the bladder. J Urol 90:175–179

Presman D, Erlich L (1948) Metastatic tumors of the ureter. J Urol 59:312–325

Puech JL, Joffre F, Song MY, et al (1987) Ureteral metastases. Computed tomographic finding. Eur J Radiol 7:103–106

Rafla S (1975) Tumors of the upper urothelium. AJR Am J Roentgenol 123:540–551

Ramchandani P, Pollack HM (1995) Tumors of the urothelium. Semin Roentgenol 30:149–167

Rayer PFO (1941) Traité des maladies du rein. Balliere, Paris

Riches EW, Griffiths IS, Thackray AC (1951) New growth of kidney and ureter. Br J Urol 23:297

Richie JP (1988) Carcinoma of the renal pelvis and ureter. In: Skinner DG, Liekouski G (eds) Diagnosis and management of genitourinary cancer. Saunders, Philadelphia, pp 323–336

Roemer CE, Pfister RC, Brodsky G, Sacknoff EJ (1940) Primary leiomyosarcoma of ureter. Urology 16:492

Rofsky NM, Weinreb JC, Bosniak MA, et al (1991) Renal lesion characterization with gadolinium-enhanced MR imaging: efficacy and safety in patients with renal insufficiency. Radiology 180:85–89

Roy C, Saussine C, Guth S, et al (1998) MR urography in the evaluation of urinary tract obstruction. Abdom Imaging 23:27–34

Ryan KG, Hoch WH, Craven RM (1979) Intraureteral tumors demonstrated by computed tomography. J Comput Assist Tomogr 3:474–477

Saitoh H (1982) Distant metastatic of renal adenocarcinoma in patients with a tumor thrombus in the renal vein and/or vena cava. J Urol 127:652–653

Scharifker D, Chalasani A (1978) Ureteral involvement by malignant lymphoma: ten years' experience. Arch Pathol Lab Med 102:541–542

Schultz RE, Boyle DE (1988) Inverted papilloma of renal pelvis associated with controlateral ureteral malignancy and bladder recurrence. J Urol 139:111–113

Scott WW, McDonald DF (1970) Tumors of the ureter. In: Harrison JH (ed) Campbell's urology. Saunders, Philadelphia, pp 977–1002

Song MY, Lhez JM, Durand D, et al (1983) Radiologic features of metastatic carcinoma to the ureter. Diagn Imaging 52: 208–223

Steffens J, Nagel R (1988) Tumours of the renal pelvis and ureter. Observations in 170 patients. Br J Urol 61:277–283

Strong DW, Pearse HD, Tank ES, et al (1976) The ureteral stump after nephrectomy. J Urol 115:654–655

Tozzini A, Bulleri A, Orsitto E, et al (1999) Hodgkin's lymphoma: an isolated case of involvement of the ureter. Eur Radiol 9:344–346

Twersky J, Twersky N, Phillips G, et al (1976) Peripelvic extravasation, urinoma formation and tumor obstruction of the ureter. J Urol 116:305

Utz DC, McDonald JR (1957) Squamous cell carcinoma of the kidney. J Urol 78:540–552

Van Poppel H, Nuttin B, Oyen R, et al (1986) Fibro-epithelial polyp of the ureter. Eur.Urol 12:174–179

Van Poppel H, Oyen R, Baert L, et al (1987) Importance de l'urographie intra-veineuse dans le diagnostic des tumeurs des voies excrétrices. Acta Urol Belg 55:31–35

Vogelzang RL, Calenoff L, Buckley GJ (1981) Ureteral intussusseption caused by fibrous ureteral polyp. Urol Radiol 3:47–49

Wasserman NF (1994) Pseudo diverticulosis: unusual appearance for metastases to the ureter. Abdom Imaging 19: 376–378

Wasserman NF, Zhang G, Posalaky IP, et al (1991) Ureteral pseudo-diverticula: frequent association with uroepithelial malignancy. AJR Am J Roentgenol 175:69–72

Webb DR, Crosthawaite A, Angus D, et al (1985) The percutaneous treatment of upper urinary tract urothelial tumor. World J Urol 7:135–137

Williamson B, Hartman GW, Hattery RR (1986) Multiple and diffuse ureteral filling defects. Semin Roentgenol 21:214–223

Winalski CS, Lipman JC, Tumeh SS (1990) Ureteral neoplasms. Radiographics 10:271–285

Wong-You-Cheong JJ, Wagner BJ, Davis CJ jr (1998) Transitional call carcinoma of the urinary tract: radiologic-pathologic correlations. Radiographics 18:123–142

Wu HR, Chang PL, Huang MH (1986) Obstructive uropathy caused by bilateral synchronous ureteral carcinoma: report of a case. Eur Urol 12:287–288

Youssem DM, Gatewood OMB, Goldman SM, et al (1988) Synchronous and metachronous transitional cell carcinoma of the urinary tract: prevalence, incidence and radiographic detection. Radiology 167:613–618

7 Inflammatory Diseases of the Ureter

P. Chemla, T. Smayra, L. Bouchard, M. Mazerolles, Ph. Otal, N. Grenier, F. Joffre

CONTENTS

Inflammatory diseases of the ureter include a wide range of disparate lesions, mainly the result of the presence in the urine of an infectious organism, more rarely by hematogenous spread from a distant site or contiguous organs (kidney, bladder, digestive tract).

Ureteral involvement is mostly a secondary problem related to inflammatory lesions of the kidney or bladder. In some cases the ureteral lesion is the most important lesion, which requires direct treatment to avoid deleterious effects on the renal parenchyma.

P. Chemla, MD; T. Smayra, MD; L. Bouchard, MD;
Ph. Otal, MD; F. Joffre, MD
Service de Radiologie, Hôpital de Rangueil, 1 avenue Jean
Poulhes, F-31403 Toulouse Cedex 4, France
M. Mazerolles, MD
Service d'Anatomo-pathologie, CHU PURPAN, place Baylac,
F-31059 Toulouse Cedex, France
N. Grenier, MD
Service de Radiologie, B.G.H. Pellegrin Tripode, Place Amélie
Raba Léon, F-33076 Bordeaux Cedex, France

The ureter responds to inflammation with some common abnormalities: loss of contraction and hypotonia, mural thickening by edema and cell infiltration, ulceration, pseudo-diverticula, cystic degeneration, and desmoplastic reaction leading to narrowing and obstruction (Wasserman 1996).

Intravenous and retrograde pyelography, cystography, and CT scanning are the main contributory imaging methods.

7.1 Ureteral Tuberculosis

Genitourinary tuberculosis has become relatively rare but remains second in frequency after pulmonary disease. Urinary tract disease is secondary to pulmonary tuberculosis, but pulmonary disease is evident in only about 30% of cases (Elkin 1990). The incidence is currently rising due to the progress of HIV infection.

Finding ureteral involvement is of great clinical importance, as much for the prognosis as for therapeutic choices. It automatically indicates renal disease and must raise the suspicion of bladder involvement. In the course of the disease, ureteral involvement is, together with renal pelvis and bladder lesions, one of the major threats to renal function. Ureteral involvement is of variable extent.

Ureteral localization of tuberculosis is in fact a major step of this disease, almost always secondary to already advanced renal involvement. Less frequently, it is secondary to direct hematogenous spread or to a contiguous lesion such as ovarian disease (Friedenberg 1971). It must be differentiated from ureteral external compression by a paravertebral abscess evolving along the psoas muscle (Dufour 1973). On the other hand, diffuse ureteral dilation can also be found without a ureteral lesion in the presence of inflammatory or sclerotic bladder disease responsible for a stenosis or reflux.

The incidence of ureteral involvement in tuberculosis varies widely, according to the literature, between 5% and 37% (Rees and Hollands 1970; Claridge 1970). Lavasse found 20% ureteral involvement in 1647 cases of urinary tuberculosis (Lavasse 1969). Predominant ureteral lesions are situated in the lower third (70%–85%) (Gow 1986). Pyeloureteral junction involvement is less frequent, but it is more often found when there is renal pelvis disease (O'Reilly 1986). A multifocal lesion is possible in about 27% of cases (Claridge 1970).

Frequently, the ureteral lesion, mainly stenosing, comes within the context of an already known tuberculous disease or of presenting lesions in favor of this diagnosis. In this situation, imaging plays an important part in diagnosis. Microbiological investigation is, however, always essential to confirm the diagnosis.

Sometimes, ureteral involvement is characterized by an isolated stenosis without any specific pattern and no other apparent lesion. Opacification techniques are then insufficient for diagnosis, which can be made by histopathological examination of the surgical specimen (Dufour 1973).

Ureteral disease appears following an "open" papillocaliceal lesion in the excretory system. It spreads essentially throughout the urinary tract. Spreading via the ureteral lymphatic system is not currently accepted by the majority of authors (Caine 1967). The two types of anatomical lesions characteristic of urinary tuberculosis are found in the ureter. Specific lesions, secondary to inflammation, are characterized pathologically by a granulomatous cellular infiltration of the submucosa, associated with important parietal edema and ureteral hypotonia. Ulcerations are frequent, multiple and longitudinal, along the axis of the ureter. They disappear with medical treatment. In fact, during this inflammatory phase, the disease often remains clinically silent and diagnosis is made later when signs of obstruction appear (Wasserman 1996). These inflammatory lesions are in fact reversible but, if medical treatment is delayed, scar fibrosis appears rapidly, evolving on its own even with specific treatment (Wasserman 1996). These lesions end up in more or less diffuse stenosis and longitudinal retraction of the ureter. Ureteral tuberculosis is always associated with renal lesions, whether obvious or not. In exceptional cases, there is diffuse ureteral involvement associated most frequently with a mastic kidney, entirely destroyed and calcified.

7.1.1
Imaging

Classically, intravenous pyelography (EU) is the examination of choice to detect tuberculous ureteral

involvement (Friedenberg et al. 1968). In case of renal dysfunction preventing optimal opacification of the ureter, antegrade and/or retrograde opacification techniques allow better display of the lesion. The current use of CT provides helpful information in difficult cases, particularly with mute kidney.

7.1.1.1
The Abdominal X-ray

The abdominal X-ray (KUB) is most frequently normal. Exceptionally, in "historical" tuberculosis cases, there are linear, vertical, or most frequently patchy or lumpy calcifications in the ureteral topography, mainly in its proximal part (Fig. 7.1). Calcifications indicate, in the majority of cases, quite advanced renal disease. However, Birnbaum et al. (1990) reported on a case of diffuse calcified ureteritis without any underlying major lesion. These calcifications raise essentially the diagnosis of ureteral bilharziosis, where the lesions are more distal and appear as linear calcifications in the dilated wall of the ureter (Hartman et al. 1977). In addition, in tuberculosis the ureter is often stenotic while in bilharziosis it is dilated. More exceptionally, amyloid ureteral disease can be discussed, but there is classi-

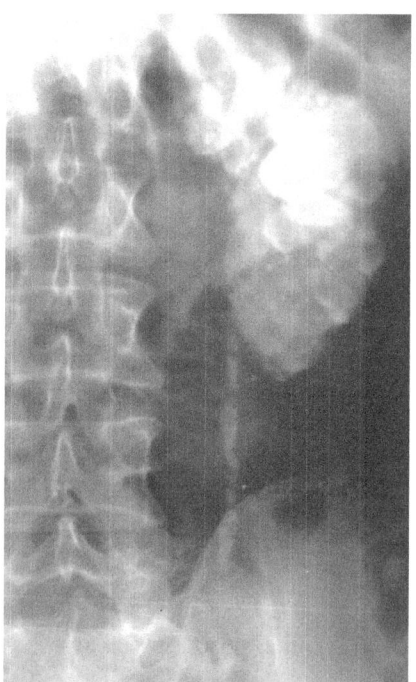

Fig. 7.1. Ureteral calcification in advanced urinary tuberculosis. Large, destroyed left kidney with diffuse calcifications with lobar distribution. No excretion is visible. Diffuse, probably mural, calcifications of the proximal part of the ureter

cally a radiotransparent line between contrast-filled ureteral lumen and calcification. The presence of a calcified ureteral calculus, secondary to an obstruction, can also be noticed but is usually not a diagnostic problem.

7.1.1.2
EU

EU shows abnormalities in almost all cases and shows essentially two kinds of lesions: parietal anomalies and stenotic lesions (KOLLINS et al 1974).

Parietal anomalies correspond to early lesions of the inflammatory type. They are specific to tuberculosis and respond to antituberculous treatment. Ureteral edges can present parietal irregularities such as spiking and notching, giving a jagged "stamp-like" pattern corresponding to ulcerations or a simple parietal haziness due to edema. The ureteral lumen can present longitudinal or transversal striations or round, nodular lacunae. These anomalies are, in general, diffuse and can be accompanied by a moderate dilation without obstruction, secondary to hypotonia or simple ureteral overfilling with contrast material (Fig. 7.2). These lesions are currently rarely seen.

Ureteral stenosis is more frequent. Some of these stenotic lesions have an inflammatory origin and can improve under treatment. They cannot be differentiated from the scar stenoses, by far the most frequent, which do not respond to medical treatment. Ureteral stenosis is often nonspecific, centered, regular and short, either diaphragm-like or tube-like and a few millimeters or centimeters long. Rarely, there are irregular eccentric or angulated stenoses. These can be located anywhere but there are sites of predilection (pyeloureteral junction, inferior part of lumbar ureter, juxtameatal or intraparietal pelvic ureter). These stenoses can be multiple, either bipolar (pyeloureteral junction or lumbar ureter or terminal pelvic ureter) or disseminated in the whole ureter with alternating stenosis and dilation, giving the ureter the appearance of a rosary or a pearl necklace (Fig. 7.3).

Diffuse lesions can also achieve two even more rare patterns (TENCATE 1971). In certain cases, the ureter presents with diffuse retracting lesions, appearing as a straight and short ureter of smaller lumen ("pipe-stem"), sometimes with attraction of the homolateral bladder horn (Fig. 7.4). In other patients, the ureter shows diffuse irregular and nonsymmetrical stenosis creating a corkscrew pattern.

Studying ureteral contractions on fluoroscopy would have, according to HARTMAN et al. (1977), a potential benefit, allowing a better evaluation of lesion extension to the wall and a better appreciation of fibrous lesions. This is rarely done today.

A classification into three stages has been proposed according to the degree of ureteral disease. Early involvement responds to medical treatment without sequelae and corresponds to edematous lesions and ulcerations or dilation lesions due to atonia. Chronic lesions correspond to single or multiple ureteral stenoses. Terminal lesions correspond to diffuse ureteral

a

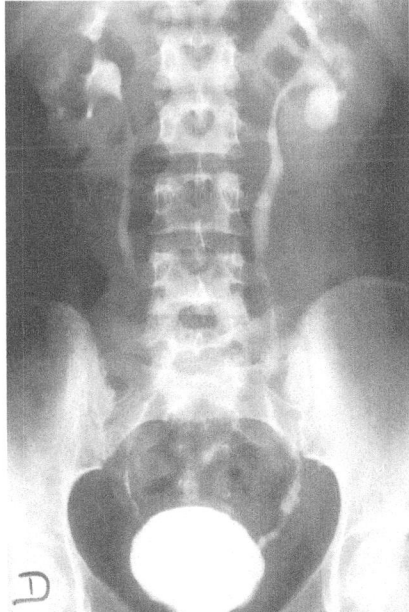

b

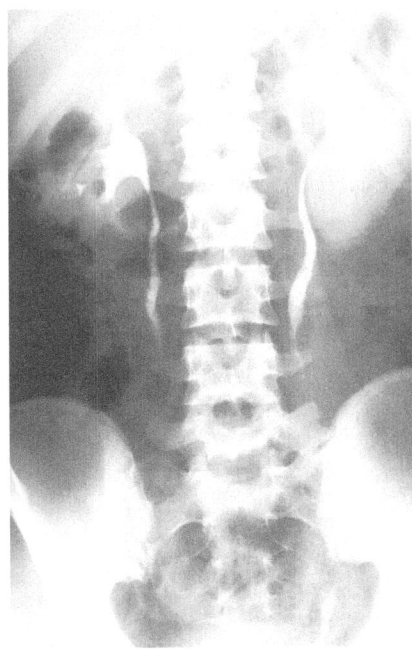

Fig. 7.2a, b. Bilateral ureteral tuberculosis. **a** Presence of diffuse irregularities and multiple lacunar image due to parietal ulcerations and edema of the proximal part of the right ureter. **b** Similar lesions of the lower part of the left ureter. Tuberculosis cavitation of the left lower pole calix

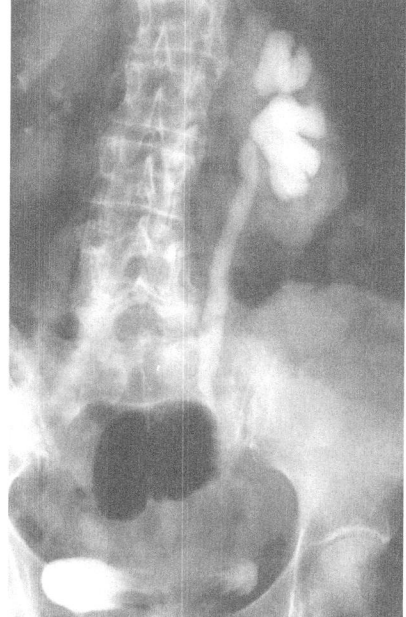
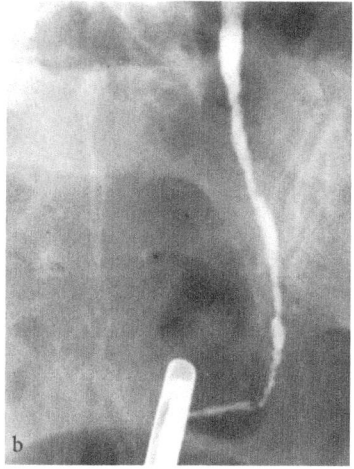
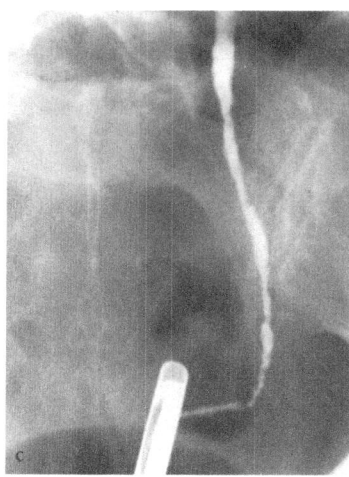

Fig. 7.3a–c. Ureteral tuberculosis strictures. **a** EU showing left hydronephrosis and ureterectasis with short fibrotic strictures at the pelvic level and nonvisualization of the lower part of the left ureter. **b, c** Retrograde opacification shows diffuse and irregular narrowing of the pelvic portion of the ureter. Multiple strictures give the appearance of a "beaded" ureter

involvement with "pipe-like" retraction and calcifications.

7.1.1.3
Direct Opacification Techniques

The lesions described above are properly studied when the urinary tract is well opacified. The presence of severe obstruction or important renal parenchymal lesions does not allow sufficient ureteral opacification. Even if there is opacification of pelvocaliceal cavities, it does not always allow a diagnostic orientation. In such cases a direct opacification technique is necessary.

Retrograde ureteropyelography (RUP) achieves good visualization of ureteral lesions and an accurate appreciation of their importance of these lesions and upstream impact (Fig. 7.5). Direct investigations, antegrade and/or retrograde, must follow certain rules. According to FRIMANN-DAHL, these must be done under specific antimicrobial protection, separating the exploration of one side from the other by an interval of 8 days. Fluoroscopic monitoring and low-pressure injection are essential (FRIMANN-DAHL 1958). Taking into account the progress made in contrast material used today, indications for direct investigations are quite restricted. For Gow, direct investigation must be reserved for poorly or nonfunctioning kidneys on urography, and for low ureter stenoses to assess the length of the lesion and contractility of the underlying ureter (GOW 1986).

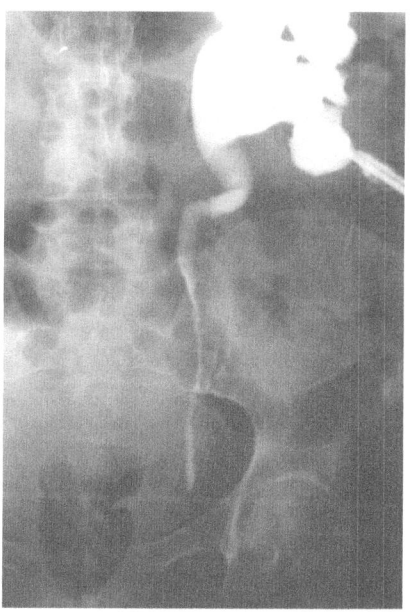

Fig. 7.4. Tuberculosis of the ureter: antegrade pyelography during a percutaneous nephrostomy. Opacification of the left ureter, which is diffusely irregular and stenotic, with association between inflammatory ulcerative lesions and fibrotic narrowing

Ureteral catheterization is also necessary for separate microbiological sampling in case of bilateral lesions.

In case of an entirely dilated ureter without a clearly identifiable obstruction, it is necessary to carry out retrograde cystography to detect a vesi-

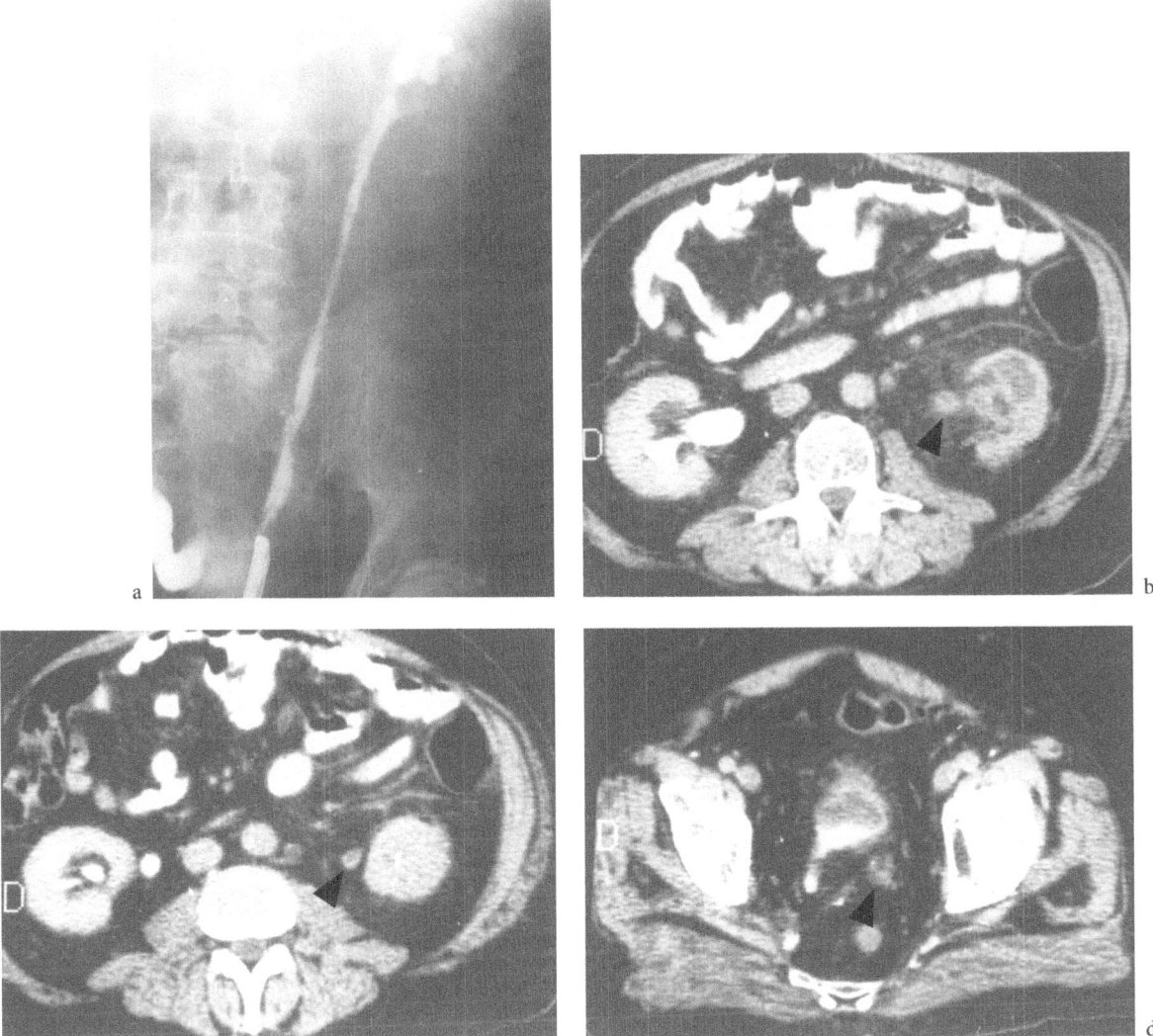

Fig. 7.5a–d. "Pipe-stem" tuberculous ureter. **a** Retrograde pyelogram shows a rigid, straight, and irregular ureter with probably inflammatory and fibrotic lesions of its wall. **b–d** CT scan slices at different levels show diffuse thickening of the ureter wall with a destroyed left kidney (*arrowheads*)

coureteral reflux, frequent in bladder involvement, and to differentiate it from a distal intramural ureter stenosis. In certain circumstances, a patient may present with urinary obstruction secondary to an isolated, centered, and regular stenosis (Fig. 7.6). This stenosis can exist without any radiological lesions suggesting an inflammatory disease and thus isolated urinary tuberculosis can remain unrecognized. This ureteral stenosis, often difficult to diagnose, can extend the discussion to many other diseases: some ureteral tumors in case of an isolated lesion, benign retroperitoneal fibrosis, and retroperitoneal carcinosis in case of an extensive lesion. Bilharzial stenoses can also be discussed, but their topography and the almost constant presence of bladder lesions help in the diagnosis.

An exceptional diagnosis was reported by THOMAS et al. (1980): ureteral involvement by an atypical mycobacterium similar to the Koch bacillus. The reported case shows a stenosis of the entire ureter.

7.1.1.4
CT Scanning

CT scanning can be very useful in difficult cases. It is more sensitive than urography and ultrasonography for the detection of ureteral dilatation (PRENKUMAR et al. 1987). In case of tuberculous stenosis, slices realized at the level of the stenosis show a parietal, regular, and concentric thickening (Fig. 7.5) (GOLDMAN et al. 1985). The periureteral fat is slightly

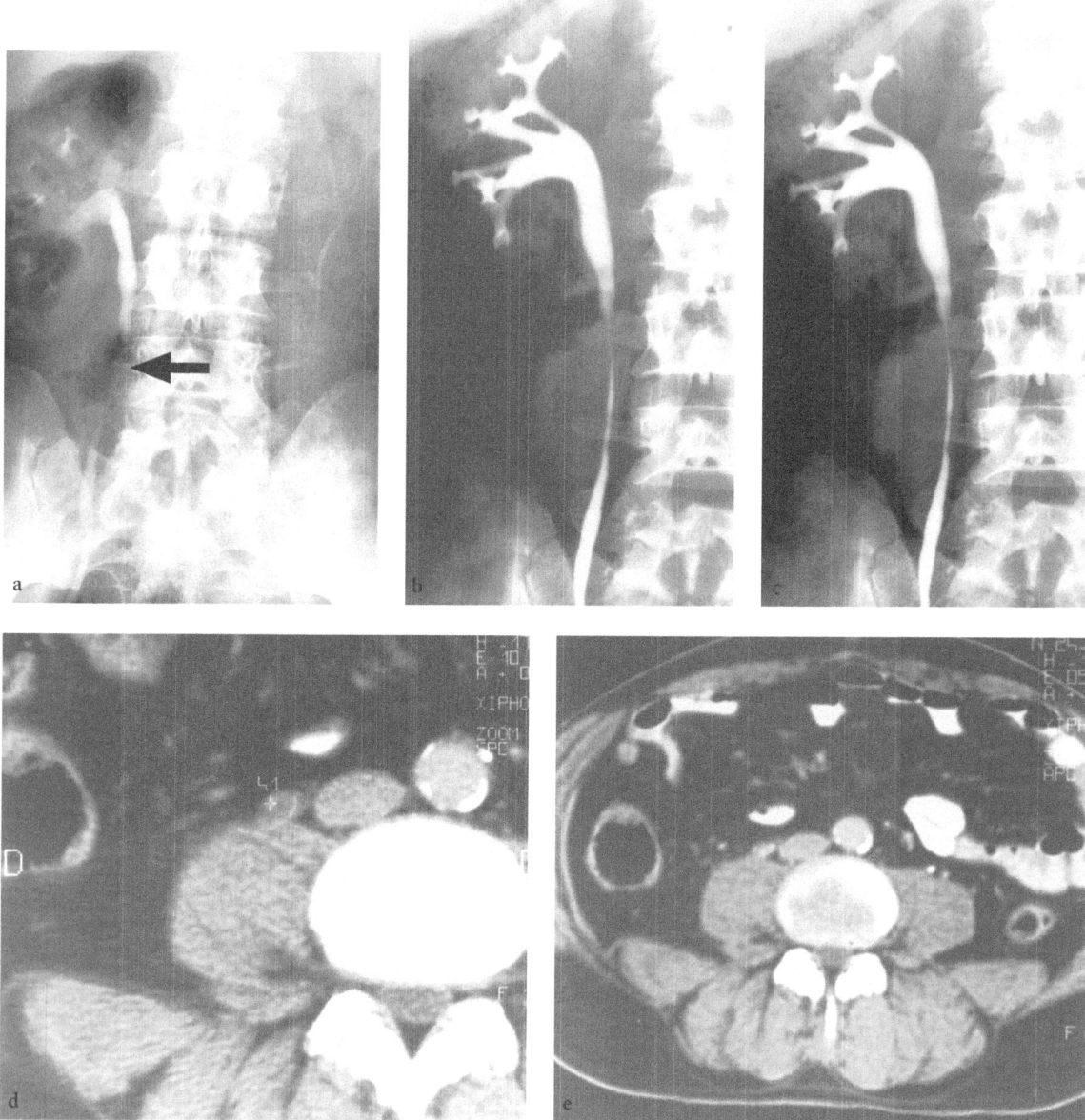

Fig. 7.6a–e. Isolated tuberculous stenosis of the ureter. **a** EU showing a short stricture of the middle part of the lumbar right ureter (*arrow*), without any other lesions of the pyelocaliceal system. **b, c** retrograde pyelography does not demonstrate any particularity of the lesion, which is tubular, smooth, and without a specific pattern. **d, e** CT scan at the stenotic level shows a thickening with contrast enhancement of the ureteral wall. Thus, an extrinsic periureteral disease could be eliminated. Diagnosis of tuberculosis was made only on the basis of the surgical specimen

stranded. Measured densities are in the range of the tissue density and their value is enhanced after intravenous contrast material. These abnormalities are not specific but suggest that the stenosis is probably due to a parietal lesion, thus eliminating the possibility of retroperitoneal disease (BOSNIAK et al. 1982) (Fig. 7.6). Parietal calcifications can be exquisitely shown while remaining undetectable on

KUB (BIRNBAUM et al. 1990; WANG et al. 1997). Helical CT coronal reconstructions of the urinary tract (uro-CT) have not yet demonstrated any superiority to classical EU for depicting and analyzing tuberculous ureteral stenosis. They could be useful in case of nonfunctioning kidney but are probably unable to show inflammatory changes of the ureteral mucosa as precisely as EU.

7.1.2
Role of Radiology

The role of radiology is essential for monitoring the evolution and evaluating the treatment of ureteral tuberculosis. Except for diffuse lesions associated with renal destruction and requiring nephroureterectomy, conservative treatment is preferred, particularly for low ureteral lesions. The finding of a low ureter stenosis with a functioning kidney must be considered as an early specific lesion, still accessible to classical medical treatment. Classically, urographic follow-up must be sequential, using a simplified, frequently repeated EU (every 8 days to every month) (HARTMAN et al. 1977; DUFOUR 1973). The lack of improvement or radiological deterioration must lead to surgery or interventional treatment such as balloon dilation, altogether with the placement of a ureteral 2-J stent, according to the topography of the lesion. This technique gives a positive result in 75% of cases (KIM et al. 1993). If medical treatment is carried out, EU repeated every 3 months for 1 year is necessary. This urographic surveillance concerns all patients with urinary tuberculosis treated with antibiotics, even if there is no apparent ureteral lesion. In fact, a ureteral stenosis can appear in the course of treated renal tuberculosis. Ultrasonographic surveillance must be currently proposed to replace EU, but EU remains useful in any case of doubtful evolution.

In conclusion, a radiological diagnosis of ureteral tuberculosis can generally be made quickly. Associated pelvocaliceal and/or bladder lesions are sufficiently suggestive of the diagnosis, which can then be confirmed by microbiological sampling.

Specifically, radiological investigation permits the evaluation of the extent and impact on the urinary tract of tuberculous ureteral lesions. It allows also their monitoring after medical treatment, given that ureteral lesions are for the most part irreversible. In some cases, an isolated lesion not suggestive of tuberculosis may be demonstrated. A CT scan can then confirm the ureteral origin of the lesion, but in these cases, endoscopic intervention with biopsy or explorative surgery remains essential for diagnosis confirmation.

7.2
Ureteral Bilharziosis

Urinary bilharziosis is an extremely widespread disease in the endemic zones of black Africa, the Middle East, and Egypt. Frequent travel explains the number of observations of this disease in Europe and North America. Bilharziosis is the second among the parasitic diseases worldwide, and the number of people suffering from constitutes about 5% of the world population (JORULF and LINDJTEDT 1985).

Human beings are affected by *Schistosoma haematobium* after exposition in infested water. The parasite, a 12-mm-long worm, enters through the skin and reaches, via the general circulation, the portal system, where it becomes adult. Eggs are laid in the bladder and/or ureteral submucosa veins: armed with a spur, they cross the vessels and locate in the ureteral or vesical wall (NEY and FRIEDENBERG 1981).

Pathologically, urinary involvement is of the inflammatory type, evolving to sclerosis (DANA et al. 1981). Inflammatory lesions are caused by a hyperplastic, nodular or sheet-like cellular proliferation. These specific lesions are accompanied by ulcerations, pre-neoplastic malpighian cell metaplasia, or pseudo-tumoral hypertrophic reactions. These lesions correspond to the bilharziomas and may calcify. Sclerotic reactions appear rapidly and tend to calcify within a few years. Ureteral involvement is found in about 50%–70% of cases. It is most frequently bilateral. Inflammatory lesions are rarely nodular but rather circumferential and lead to narrowing of the terminal portion with upstream dilation. Periureteral tissue is frequently subject to sclerolipomatous modifications. Disease prognosis depends on the parenchymal impact of ureterovesical lesions. There may be pure bladder lesions causing intramural ureteral stenosis or a vesicoureteral reflux due to the meatus remaining open when the bladder is under pressure; a purely ureteral stenosing lesion can also be found. Fatal obstructive uropathy occurs in 5% of cases (CHEEVER et al. 1978).

Radiological investigation is essential for the diagnosis. As logical as this diagnosis is in an African patient with hematuria, it is more difficult in a patient accidentally infested during a trip. In endemic zones, early detection is of major importance to avoid evolution and limit the spread of the disease. The role of radiology in the systematic examination of exposed patients and the importance of early ureteral disease detection which permits an early diagnostic orientation must be emphasized (UMERAH 1977a; HUGOSSON and OLSEN 1986).

In a patient with hematuria who does not live in an affected area, the diagnosis is rarely made by radiology and relies on anamnesis, which may reveal a stay in an endemic zone, and on finding eggs in the urine and during cystoscopy. With radiological investigation one can also evaluate the entire urinary apparatus and estimate the impact on renal parenchyma. Like tuberculosis, bilharziosis is a disease of "the entire urinary apparatus", and the long-term prognosis depends on renal involvement. The monitoring of its evolution relies on radiological examinations.

7.2.1
Imaging

7.2.1.1
KUB, EU, and Retrograde Cystography

Radiological investigation relies nowadays on the KUB, the EU, and retrograde cystography. Retrograde investigations, ultrasonography, and CT scanning are less frequently used. However, the usefulness of ultrasonography for evaluating and monitoring the evolution of lesions has clearly been demonstrated (BURKI et al. 1986). Ureteral modifications are encountered in about 70% of cases (HUGOSSON and OLSEN 1986). Some are classical and depict advanced disease, others correspond to earlier, generally ignored lesions, but these are important to detect, for they allow the implementation of early treatment (HUGOSSON 1987). Ureteral lesions of bilharziosis can be classified into four categories (DANA et al. 1981; LEMAITRE et al. 1966): calcifications, stenoses, and parietal and functional abnormalities. These lesions most frequently involve the terminal ureter and are usually bilateral (Figs. 7.7–7.9).

7.2.1.1.1
Ureteral Calcifications

Ureteral calcifications are quite rare. They are found in about 7%–10% of cases and are quite often associated with bladder calcifications (YOUNG et al. 1974). Their demonstration relies on a good KUB, using localized spots with compression and different angle views. The classical aspect is that of a strip of opacity, hardly visible, ribbon-like, of regular caliber, and with a tortuous course corresponding to the ureter topography (Fig. 7.9). This opacity is limited laterally by denser and thin, grossly parallel lines. It involves the pelvic ureter but may extend to the renal pelvis (HANASH 1971). More frequently, calcifications are more limited, of pelvic topography, linear or punctate, and often hidden by bladder calcifications. Rarely, calculus-like densities can be found. There may be ureteral lithiasis secondary to obstruction or calcified bilharziomas ("melted calculus"), which are essentially radiologically identical (NEY and

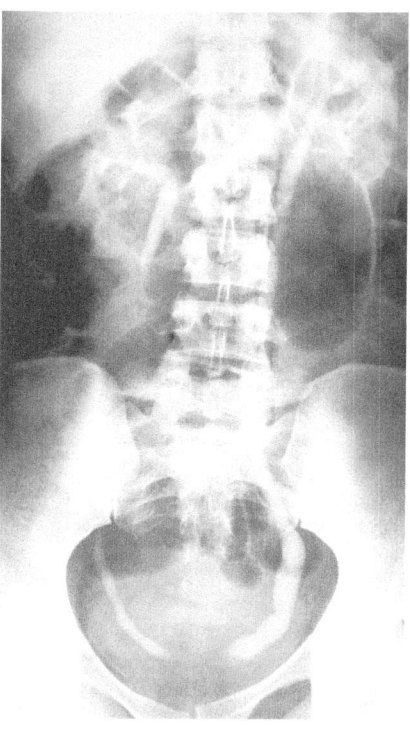

Fig. 7.7. Ureteral bilharziosis. Post-voiding EU X-ray shows persistent filling of the right lower segment and moderate dilatation of the left ureter without dilatation of the pelvocaliceal system. The intramural segment is narrowed by involvement of the bladder wall

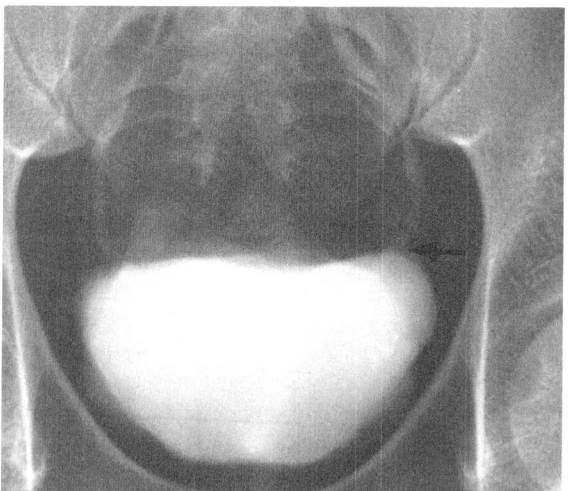

Fig. 7.8. Bilharziomas: IVP shows several nodular filling defects of the pelvic left ureter of parietal origin. Ureteroscopy confirms the presence of bilharzial granulomas (arrow)

a 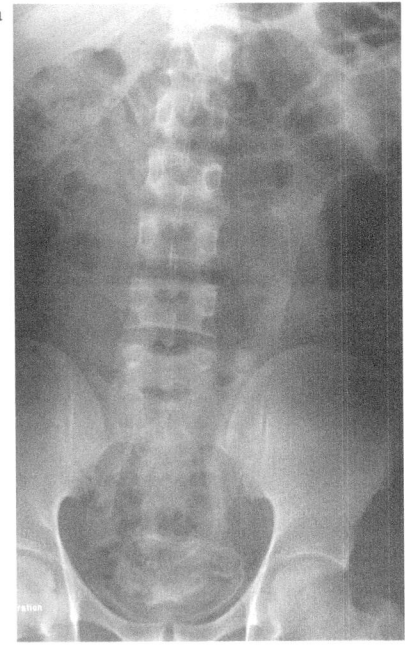 b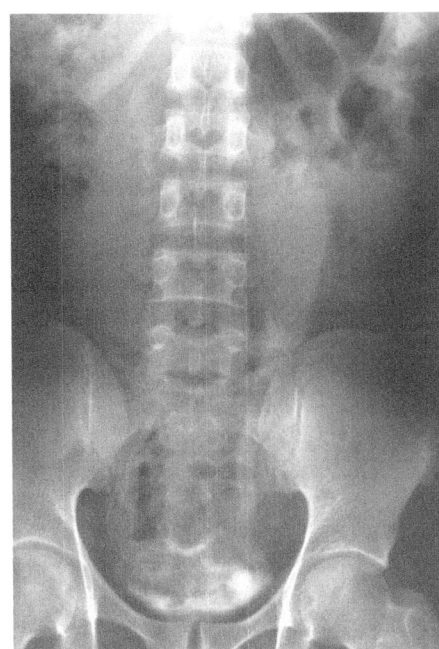

Fig. 7.9a, b. Diffuse and calcified ureterovesical bilharziosis. a KUB: diffuse linear calcifications of the bladder and both ureteral walls. b EU: Bilateral ureterohydronephrosis with poorly functioning kidneys

FRIEDENBERG 1981; HANASH 1971). CT examination would be interesting, according to JORULF (JORULF and LINSTEDT 1985), to detect calcifications invisible on KUB. It reveals a more precise topography thus eliminating calcifications due to ureteral lithiasis or calcification of neighboring structures (rectal wall, vascular structures, or seminal vesicles).

7.2.1.1.2
Stenosis

Stenoses are encountered in about 50% of cases and are the main factor prognosis. However, some authors think that their incidence is less important than is classically reported (UMERAH 1977b). In fact, a dilated ureter can be secondary to hypotonia without any stenosis, and the incidence of stenosis in bilharziosis may be overestimated if this is not taken into account. This type of anomaly is most frequently revealed by EU, except in the case where the renal impact of the obstruction does not permit a sufficient ureteral opacification of the ureter (Fig. 7.9). In these cases, a direct antegrade or retrograde investigation of the urinary tract is necessary. The most frequent type of stenosis corresponds to a regular, tight, localized and short, usually bilateral lesion of the terminal pelvic and intramural portion of the ureter (DANA et al. 1981) (Fig. 7.7). This stenosis is especially well seen in post-voiding views, which show the narrowed area and the resulting stasis of the contrast material in the dilated pelvic ureter. More diffuse, multifocal lesions

can also be found in the lower half of the lumbar and pelvic ureter. These regular, moderately tight stenoses are separated by fusiform dilated portions. In some cases, the lumbar ureter lesions show tubular stenosis that may simulate retroperitoneal fibrosis (AL-GHORAB 1968). CT coronal reconstruction could be useful in case of a poorly functioning kidney.

7.2.1.1.3
Parietal Lesions

Parietal lesions of the ureter are less frequently found. They correspond either to a nonspecific inflammatory lesion or to a pure bilharzial lesion (HANNAFY et al. 1975). Nonspecific inflammatory lesions are of the ureteritis type, i.e., irregularities of the ureteral wall or, more frequently, the presence of lacunar lesions corresponding to ureteritis cystica. A striated pattern of the ureter has also been reported. In about 20% of bilharziosis patients, this sign is noticed precociously as the first radiological manifestation (HUGOSSON 1987). These striations may be associated with a vesicoureteral reflux, which is encountered in about one third of cases (CUTAJAR 1983; HANASH 1971). In an endemic region, this sign should raise suspicion. Bilharziomas (or bilharzial polyps) are rare at the level of the ureter (HANASH 1971) (Fig. 7.8). They have a polypoid aspect with a sharp and polycyclic outline, are frequently multiple with a broad base of implantation, and are grouped in the terminal ureter. They can be obstructing and are easy to differentiate from a pyeloureteritis cystica, which is much more frequent and where the lacunae are smaller and more regular (WILLIAMSON et al. 1987). When the ureter is extensively affected topographic anomalies of pelvic ureters are frequent. These are encountered in about 60% of cases, according to UMERAH (1977b). They are characterized by a median positioning with cranial deviation and straightening of the ureteral course ("ox-horn" aspect). These anomalies are due to retracting fibrosis of the bladder trigone.

7.2.1.1.4
Dilatations and Functional Anomalies

Dilatations and functional anomalies of the ureter are frequently encountered images. Among these anomalies, vesicoureteral reflux secondary to vesical lesions that cause a gaping of the ureterovesical junction is of particular interest (CUTAJAR 1983). Every ureteral dilation, even without any apparently responsible stenosis, imposes a retrograde cystography. The vesicoureteral reflux is most frequently passive. Ureteral dilation can also be due to fibrosis of the vesical wall (UMERAH 1977b). This condition makes ureteral catheterization particularly difficult. The importance of functional ureteral anomalies detected on EU must be emphasized. Indeed, bilharziosis remains asymptomatic for a long time, and it seems that EU performed as a screening test in endemic zones permits the detection of early lesions amenable to efficient treatment before they become irreversible (UMERAH 1977b; ABDEL-HALIM et al. 1985). Fluoroscopic analysis of the ureteral dynamic can demonstrate functional anomalies, particularly in the lower half of the ureter: irritability with increasing peristaltic waves, uncoordinated contractions between the lumbar and pelvic ureter, and finally antiperistalsis. These anomalies correspond to early lesions. On the other hand, the presence of dilation of the low ureter or obstruction without reflux is often associated with more advanced bladder lesions. This already advanced but not stenosing ureteral involvement could explain the failure of some ureterovesical reimplantations.

7.2.1.2
Ultrasonography

When the bladder is full, ultrasonographic examination of the lower ureter can be achieved. This technique also demonstrate the degree of distension of the upper urinary tract and allows characterization of bladder wall involvement. It may also depict thick-ening of the ureter, stenosis, edema of the UVJ, and calcifications (KARDORFF et al. 1994). It could be used to evaluate the efficacy of antimicrobial therapy.

7.2.1.3
CT Scan

CT scanning can detect certain silent or not very symptomatic ureteral anomalies by showing localized or diffuse thickening of the ureter wall (JORULF and LINDSTEDT 1985). However, this type of thickening is nonspecific and can be encountered in cases of pure ureteral dilation, especially if there is an additional urinary infection. CT can also depict tiny ureteral and/or bladder calcifications.

7.2.2
Role of Radiology

Bilharzial ureteral involvement is essential to diagnose because it influences the therapeutic approach. This is generally easy to do because bilharziosis is, in the great majority of cases, associated with bladder lesions (90%). Exclusive ureteral lesions are manifested principally by early functional anomalies (HANASH 1971). These lesions are not pathognomonic and can also result from tuberculous bladder involvement. Ureteral and bladder calcifications are exceptional in tuberculosis. In the absence of calcifications, the diagnosis must rely on clinical elements, such as hematuria or the patient's country of origin, and can then be proven by cystoscopy and a search for eggs in the urine.

There are a few drawbacks to radiological evaluation, however, that must be taken into account when developing therapeutic strategy. The evolution of lesions is difficult to document precisely, and the evaluation of their extension is often optimistic (MAGED 1971). Whichever treatment is selected, medical or surgical, radiological examination with increasing use of US allows monitoring of evolution and therapeutic efficacy. In addition, some related complications can be shown by radiology. Lithiasis is not exceptional, and infectious complications due to stenosis (pyonephrosis) can speed up the disease evolution or sometimes be revealing. Another complication is epidermoid type malignant tumors of the urinary tract, reported in about 15% of cases. The vesical tumor localizations are classical (facilitated by chronic infections). However, the occurrence of ureteral epidermoid tumors has never been reported.

7.3
Other Inflammatory Conditions of the Ureter

The term "nonspecific ureteritis" is imprecise and certainly unsuitable. It is used in the case of multiple lacunar, irregular, hazy images of the ureteral wall suggesting an inflammatory origin. In fact, in a certain number of cases, these images are not due to infectious or inflammatory phenomena, but to a simple parietal edema, most frequently reactive (WASSERMAN 1996).

An inflammatory state of the upper urinary tract can lead to chronic histopathological modifications of the ureteral wall such as ureteritis cystica, malakoplakia, or other infrequent urinary diseases.

Some chronic diseases of the ureteral wall with probable but uncertain inflammatory etiology such as pseudodiverticulosis, leukoplasia, or cholesteatomas will be discussed in Chap. 11.

7.3.1
Primitive Ureteritis

Primitive ureteritis is due to an acute infectious involvement of the mucosa and has some nonspecific radiological manifestations (NEY and FRIEDENBERG 1981). The rare cases surgically verified show the presence of mucosal and submucosal edema, with vascular congestion, lymphocytic reaction, and presence of inflammatory cells (CAPDEVILLE et al. 1973; POOLE et al. 1970). They are found most frequently in the settings of a urinary tract infection, such as acute pyelonephritis. Microscopic and macroscopic hematuria can be associated, due to microulcerations of the mucosa. The offending agent is usually *Escherichia coli*. The most frequent urographic pattern is the presence of ureteral atony with dilation, peristalsis anomalies, and accentuation of vascular imprints (HODSON and EDWARDS 1960; SPATARO 1990). This atony can be encountered even in the absence of vesicoureteral reflux and is seen in about 10% of patients presenting with pyelonephritis (LITTLE et al. 1965; KASS et al. 1976). The release of bacterial endotoxins reduces peristalsis, resulting in a real "ureteral ileus" (SHOPFNER 1970). This phenomenon was also experimentally demonstrated (BOYARSKI et al. 1978). In some cases, radiological signs of ureteral wall edema can be encountered: a hazy aspect of the wall with barely visible, multiple parietal lacunae – sometimes nodular, simulating a ureteritis cystica, sometimes linear, giving a striated

pattern (WILLIAMSON et al. 1987). These modifications are localized mainly in the upper part of the ureter and are frequently associated with identical anomalies at the level of the renal pelvis. These lesions are reversible following adequate treatment of the inflammatory phenomenon. The diagnostic algorithm used nowadays in case of acute pyelonephritis has lead to a restriction in the indications for EU and to a delay in its performance, making the finding of these anomalies exceptional on EU. On the other hand, ultrasonography performed as a first-line examination may reveal the abnormalities described by AVNI et al. (1988) (Figs. 7.10, 7.11). The existence of pyeloureteral wall thickening was observed by these authors on ultrasonography. The systematic and prospective ultrasonographic study of infants suffering from urinary tract infection has shown this anomaly more frequently than urography (NICOLET et al. 1988). A CT scan can also identify ureteral wall thickness sometimes associated with "stranding" of the retroperitoneal fat. Diffuse enhancement after contrast is always shown, but mucosal changes related to inflammation are poorly demonstrated (BOSNIAK et al. 1982; WASSERMAN 1996).

7.3.2
Stenosing Ureteritis

In rare cases, the importance of wall edema may lead to ureteral stenoses, which are a diagnostic dilemma and raise the discussion about the regular and localized stenoses frequently found in the physiological zones of reduced caliber (SPATARO 1990). Infection, instrumentation, inflammation of the contiguous digestive tract, or tubal infection are the most common causes. These lesions are most frequently reversible with antibiotics, but they may sometimes evolve into localized ureteral and periureteral fibrosis (SANO and KITAJIMA 1993; ZAGORA et al. 1993). CT scan examination shows merely a thickened ureteral wall at the level of the stenosis sometimes accompanied by limited periureteral infiltration without a periureteral mass (Fig. 7.12). This aspect cannot be differentiated from primitive or secondary, ureteral or periureteral malignant lesions, but it allows the exclusion of a retroperitoneal disease (Fig. 7.13).

Particular cases must be reported. Some cases of stenosing ureteritis are secondary to a massive eosinophilic infiltration (SPARK et al. 1991). The etiology is unknown but it seems, from most reported observations, that an allergic background or contact with parasites does exist. The radiological aspect is

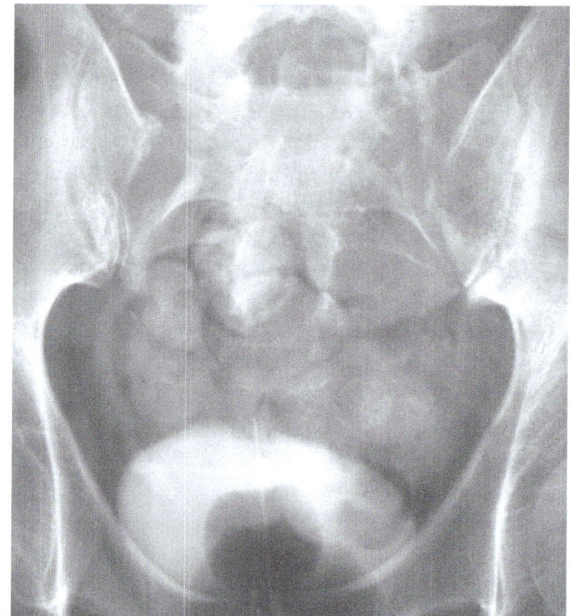

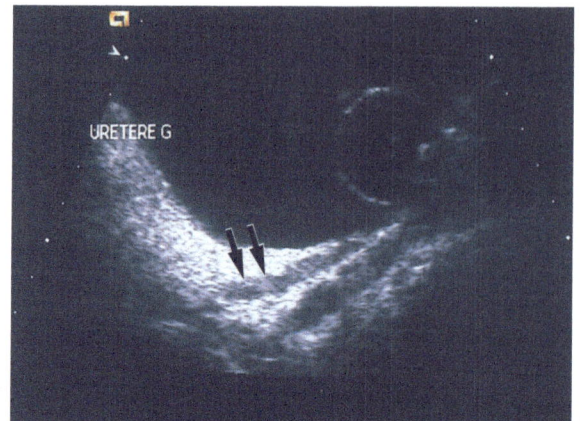

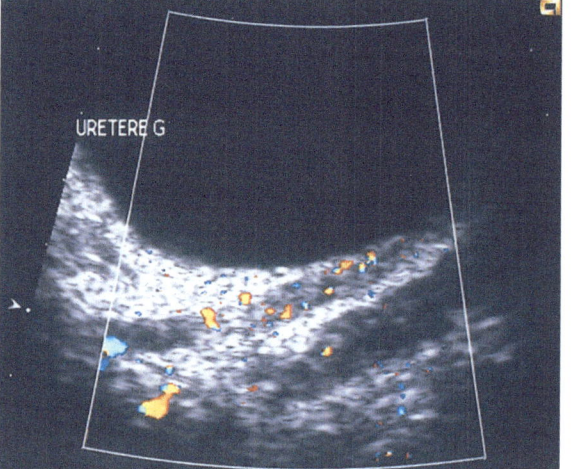

Fig. 7.10a–c. Ureteritis. **a** EU in a 37-year-old woman with acute pyelonephritis. Faint opacification of the left lower ureter without dilatation. **b** Ultrasonographic transvesical examination demonstrates a thickening of the ureteral wall (*arrows*). **c** Doppler color sonography shows hypervascularization of the ureteral wall

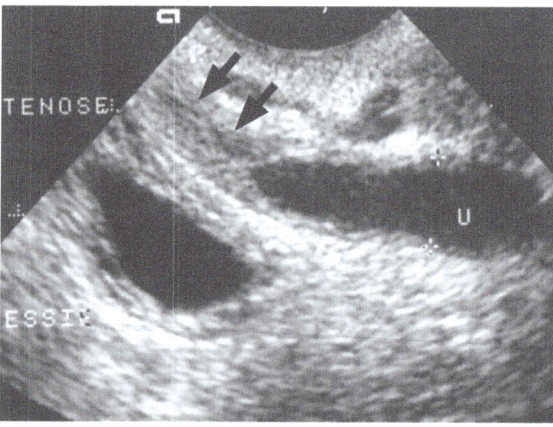

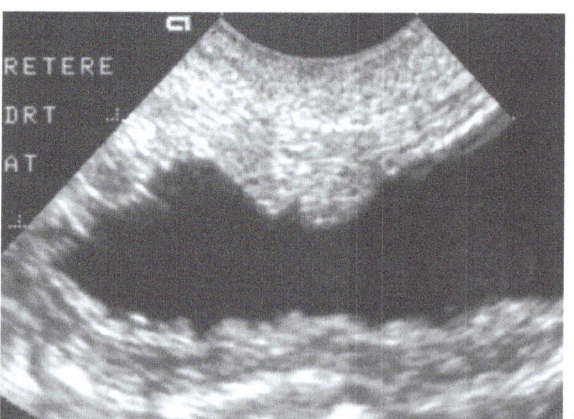

Fig. 7.11a, b. Stenosing ureteritis. **a** Transvaginal examination of the lower portion of the right ureter in a 26-year-old woman with acute pyelonephritis and dilatation of the upper urinary tract. This view shows the dilated ureter (*U*) and the stenotic area (*arrows*) behind the bladder. **b** Magnification illustrates irregular and thickened pattern of the ureteral wall upward of the stenosis

Fig. 7.13a, b. Chronic ureteritis. **a, b** CT scans of a patient with chronic urinary infection secondary to neurogenic bladder disease. The right kidney is hydronephrotic and the ureter is dilated. The wall of the ureter presents massive thickening with hypervascularization and important enhancement after injection of contrast medium (*asterisks*)

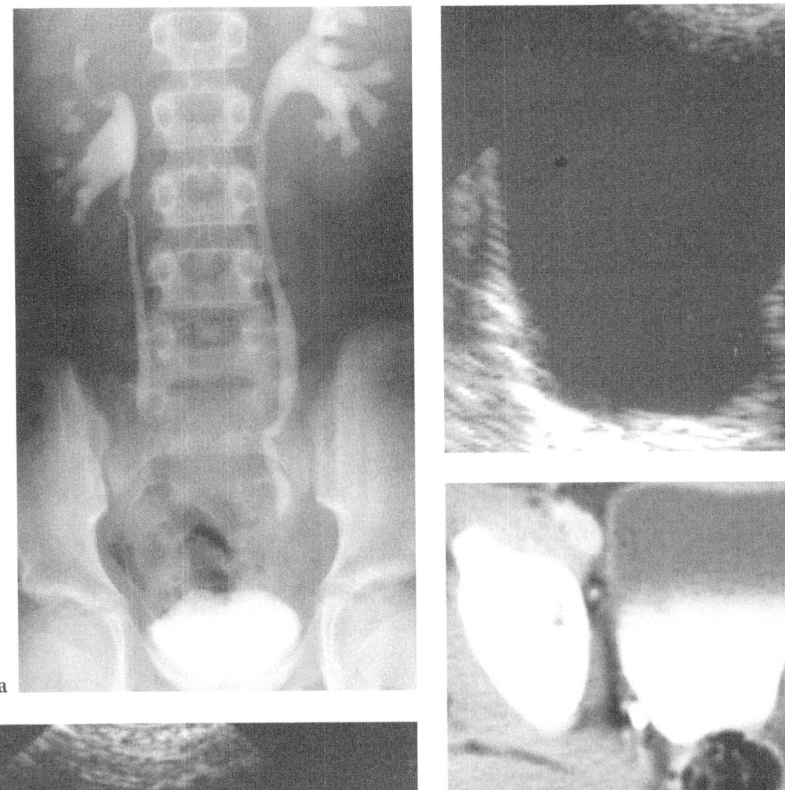

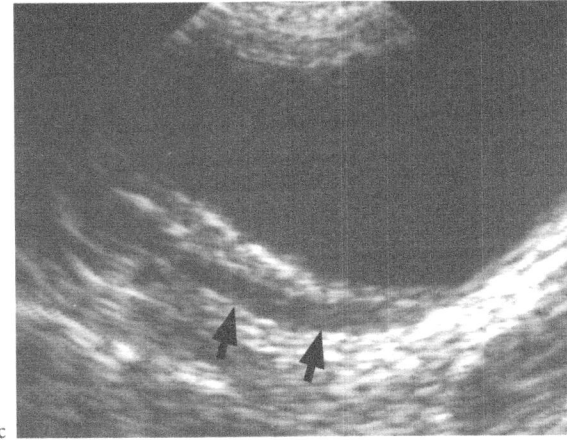

Fig. 7.12a–d. Stenosing ureteritis. a EU in a young boy with acute left pyelonephritis. Moderate ureterohydronephrosis upward of a stenosis of the lower ureter. b, c Ultrasonography demonstrates a thickened left lower pelvic ureter (*lwhite arrows*). d CT scan shows thickening of the ureteral wall (*arrow*) with enhancement after injection of contrast medium. The patient responded favorably to medical treatment

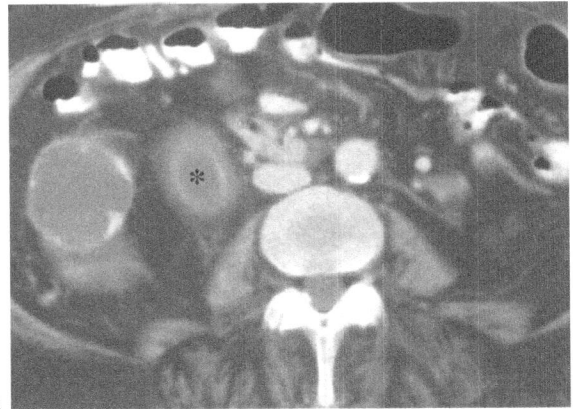

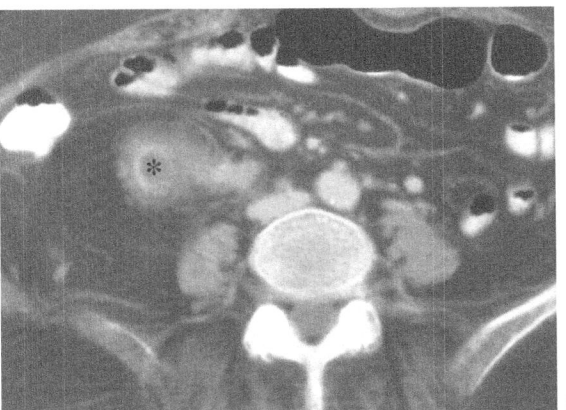

Fig. 7.13a, b.

nonspecific. Inflammatory granulomas, responsible for the ureteral obstruction, were also described but without any precise etiology. Two cases of ureteral localization of sarcoidosis were recently described (MARIANO and SUSSMAN 1998). Genitourinary involvement of the urinary tract is uncommon in this disease, estimated at around 5%. Both cases presented with urinary tract obstruction, and in one case a CT scan showed a soft tissue mass surrounding the ureter. Diagnosis was performed after pathological examination of the resected portion of the ureter.

Cases of xanthogranulomatous ureteritis were also reported, involving the pyeloureteral junction and without xanthogranulomatous pyelonephritis (WADSWORTH and MCCLENNAN 1983). CT scan performed at the level of the stenotic region reveals a ureteral wall thickening with enhancement after i.v. injection of contrast medium. This aspect is nonspecific but allows the exclusion of a retroperitoneal or pelvic disease as possible etiologies of such a stenosis (HARROW et al. 1963).

7.3.3
Emphysematous Ureteritis

An isolated emphysematous ureteritis is exceptional (MICHAELI et al. 1984; HARROW et al. 1963). It is almost always associated with emphysematous cystitis or pyelonephritis. Such a condition is usually the result of an infection by gas-producing organisms and affects mainly diabetic patients with ureteral obstruction or immunocompromised patients. The X-ray diagnosis is difficult, given the superimposed intestinal gases. It is possible to see filamentous, longitudinal, fixed gaseous images in the ureteral course, corresponding to air in the ureteral wall. Air can also be located in the ureteral lumen. This condition can be difficult to differentiate from pneumatosis intestinalis (IMRAY and HUBERTY 1980). Diagnosis is much easier from a CT scan that clearly shows the intraparietal or intraluminal air and its extension, compared with KUB (Fig. 7.14). Given its major clinical importance, prompt treatment is essential. Intravenous antibiotics could be effective in some cases, given a good urinary tract drainage, but urgent nephroureterectomy is often required because it is in fact urinary tract gangrene.

Finally, extrinsic involvement of the ureter by an intestinal inflammatory condition such as Crohn's disease or diverticulitis may rarely be associated with intramural ureteral gas.

7.3.4
Ureteral Striations

A particular problem is raised by the finding of longitudinal ureteral striations, improperly called pyelitis striata or striated ureteritis (HYDE and WASTIE 1971). The first descriptions were made by VEZINA and GWINN, who reported this type of anomaly espe-

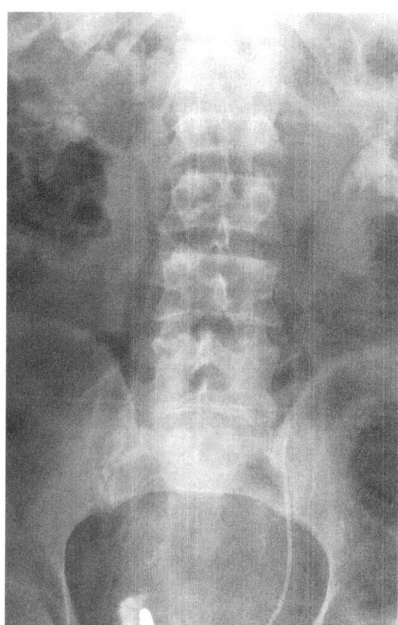

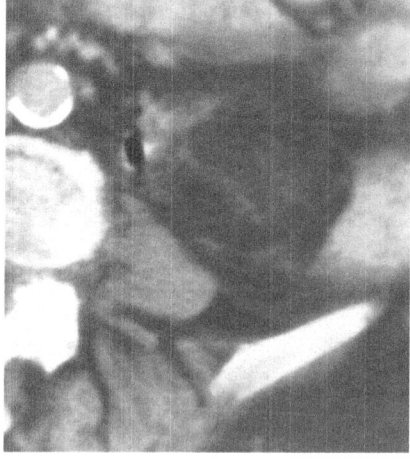

Fig. 7.14a, b. Emphysematous ureteritis. **a** KUB in a 65-year-old diabetic patient with septicemia. Presence of bilateral stag-horn calculi. Ureteral catheter in place on the left side. Presence of air in the lumen of both ureters. Emphysematous cystitis with presence of air in the wall of the bladder. **b** CT scan of the left ureter. Pneumoureter with thickening of the ureteral wall

cially in children suffering from vesicoureteral reflux (VEZINA et al. 1963; GWINN and BARNES 1964). Later, they were described as being associated with reflux, lithiasis, urinary infection, obstruction, and neoplasia. This aspect of pyeloureteral striations is characterized by sharp, regular and isolated longitudinal lacunae, which disappear with ureteral compression and can persist for many months, even under anti-inflammatory treatment (Fig. 7.15). Many hypotheses have been proposed for this entity. For some authors, these anomalies are related to mucosal inflammatory edema secondary to infection (POOLE et al. 1970; WRIGHT 1969). For others, this aspect is a normal variant corresponding to ureteral mucosal foldings, resulting from luminal collapse (DAUGHTRIGE 1969; VEZINA et al. 1963).

These images are exceptionally found on normal EU of patients without a previous urological history. The latter hypothesis is currently appealing: it was demonstrated by comparing two groups of patients in whom EU was performed, one group with high osmolarity contrast medium (HOCM) and the second with low osmolarity contrast medium (LOCM). Striations were significantly much more frequent with the new types of contrast material (15%) than with the classical ones (2%) (PARKER and CLARK 1996). These anomalies were found particularly at the level

of the distal ureter after bladder emptying and could be related to the lesser distension induced by LOCM due to their limited diuretic action. There were no significant disease associations in the 18 patients presenting striations.

However, the association with VUR has been noted by many authors (Fig. 7.16): FRIEDLAND reports that striations are found in about 15% of refluxing patients and never in patients without reflux (FRIEDLAND and FORSBERG 1972). HUGOSSON makes identical statements regarding patients suffering from reflux secondary to bilharziosis (HUGOSSON 1987). Together with others, these authors consider such striations as "mucosal infoldings" resulting from a ureter which has already suffered distension due to reflux or obstruction ("accordion effect") (GWINN and BARNES 1964; WILLIAMSON et al. 1987). However, AVNI et al. were able to find a thickened ureteral wall on ultrasonography, associated with ureter wall striations on EU in patients who did not presented reflux during the examination (AVNI et al. 1988). Moreover, two of these patients had undergone antireflux surgery 5 years earlier.

Whatever the pathogenic hypothesis, finding these anomalies must prompt a search for urinary tract infection or a VUR, particularly if an HOCM was used, even if the patient is asymptomatic.

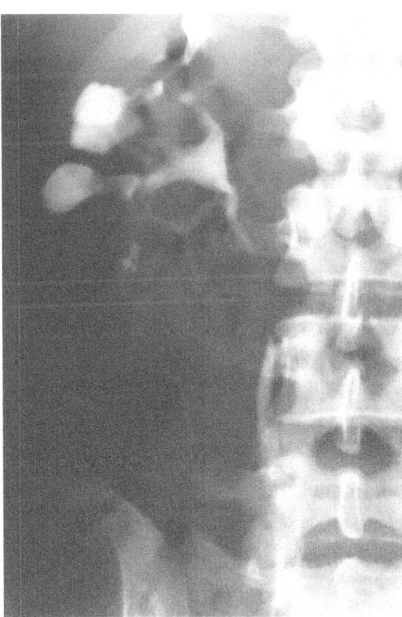

Fig. 7.15. Ureteral striations. Mucosal striations of the renal pelvis and lumbar ureter in a 65-year-old woman presenting with clinical signs of acute pyelonephritis. IVP delineates fine and linear, radiolucent, longitudinal striations and clubbing of several calices

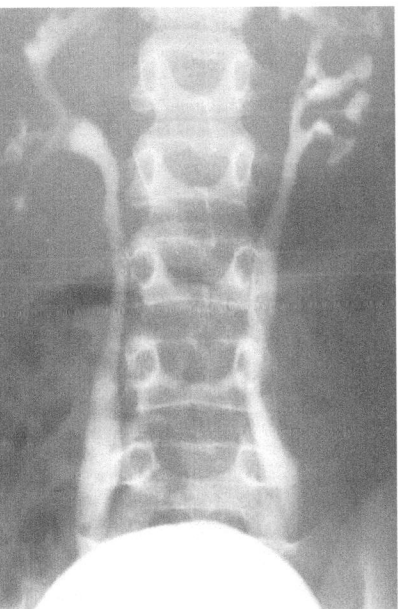

Fig. 7.16. Ureteral striations. Retrograde cystography in a child with bilateral severe reflux and signs of reflux nephropathy on the left side. Dilatation of both ureters with longitudinal, linear, radiolucent striations

7.3.5
Secondary Ureteritis

The term secondary ureteritis is reserved for ureteral caliber reduction secondary to a neighboring inflammatory pathology (appendicitis, salpingitis, Crohn's disease, spondylodiscitis) (SPATARO 1990). In fact, the presence of a neighboring infection can cause a ureteral stenosis, although the exact mechanism cannot be specified. It can be in relation to compressive phenomena, possibly associated with parietal edema. Some of these lesions become chronic, with the appearance of a true ureteral stenosis. All these lesions will be discussed in Chap. 10.

7.3.6
Other Ureteral Thickenings

Ureteral wall anomalies, without any inflammatory context or previous urinary obstruction or reflux, are also encountered. These anomalies have a radiological aspect very close to that of secondary ureteritis and correspond, in general, to parietal edema of noninflammatory and noninfectious origin. They can be encountered in cases of renal vein thrombosis and involve the upper third of the ureter and the renal pelvis (WILLIAMSON et al. 1987). It may be difficult, however, to differentiate between lacunar images that are secondary to edema and those resulting from a periureteral collateral venous system.

The persistent presence of intraluminal foreign objects in the ureter can be responsible for parietal edema without any evidence of infectious phenomena. Around the "foreign object" there is frequently a nodular or spiked wall aspect. These anomalies can be found surrounding a ureteral calculus (THEANDER and WEHLIN 1976). These findings are also encountered also with ureteral percutaneous nephrostomy, double J catheter (Fig. 7.17). Wrong catheter position can sometimes be responsible for this parietal edema and changing position may resolve these anomalies. In other cases, irritation can be attributed to catheter sterilization methods (CORY et al. 1987). As soon as the responsible agent is suppressed these images usually disappear. However, in certain patients, the persistence of a ureteral obstruction for several days was reported (LEVINE et al. 1982). LEVINE et al. recommend leaving a temporary external drainage by percutaneous nephrostomy during the days following ureteral catheter placement, especially if the obstruction is symptomatic.

7.4
Ureteritis Cystica

The multiplicity of designations used to characterize the presence of cystic appearance of ureteral mucosa is due to a misunderstanding of the origin of this

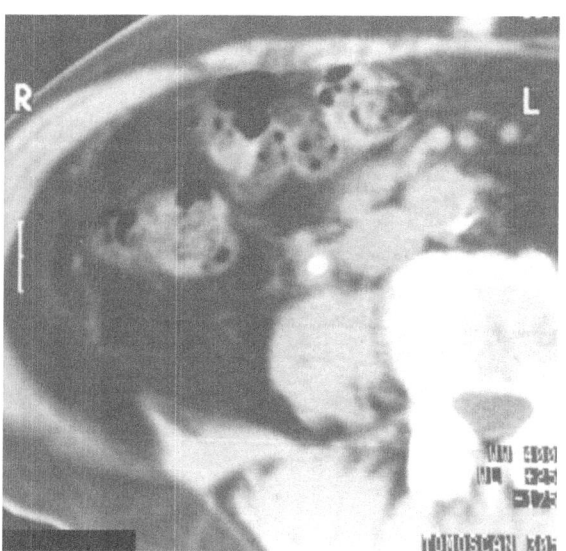
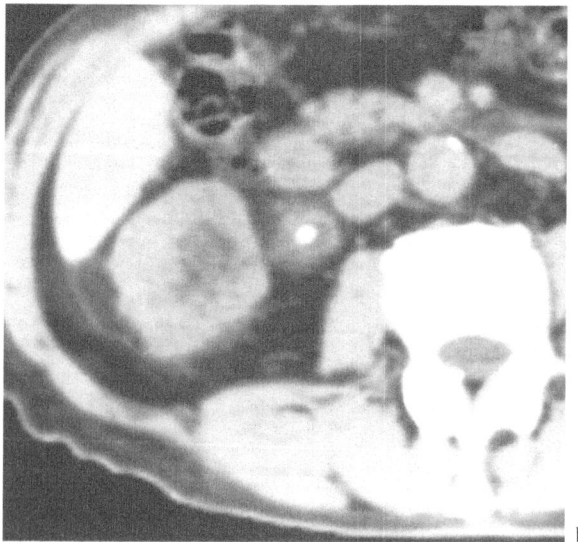

Fig. 7.17a, b. Ureteritis secondary to a foreign body. **a** Pyeloureteral edema secondary to a transcutaneous nephrovesical catheter: parietal thickening of the ureteral wall around the catheter. **b** Parietal thickening of the ureteral wall on a CT scan slice in a patient with a 2-J catheter

anomaly. We speak of "cystic degeneration of ureteral mucosa", of "pyeloureteral bullous dystrophy", or of "pyeloureteritis cystica". This varied terminology testifies to its acquired origin and likely degenerative mechanism, probably facilitated by inflammatory phenomena, leading to urothelial metaplasia, and to its predominantly ureteral location. Cysts are considered to be the result of a dystrophic phenomenon with cavitation of metaplastic urothelium or submucosal cells. This condition was first described by JACOBY (1929), and its incidence is evaluated at between 1/1000 by PUIGVERT (1974) and 2/1000 by GALAKHOFF et al. (1986). It affects particularly women over 50 years of age.

This affection is characterized pathologically by the presence of small cystic submucosal lesions, with epithelial, immature, and macroscopically translucent lining, containing a clear or yellowish mucoproteinous fluid (WILLIAMSON et al. 1987). Cysts are usually surrounded by a lymphoplasmocytic infiltrate.

They are found most frequently when EU is performed, usually in the context of a urinary tract infection, rarely hematuria, or while searching for or monitoring a calculus. Except when there is important functional deterioration, particularly by obstruction, good-quality EU can demonstrate all of their characteristics, even the smallest (Fig. 7.18). The usual image is characterized by a lacuna with sharp edges, round or oval, of varying size, ranging from 2 to 5 mm in diameter. Sometimes cysts can reach a diameter of 20–30 mm and become partially obstructive. In pro-

file, the lacuna has the aspect of an image of parietal origin, thus being arciform, with sharp edges, forming an angle of 90° with the ureter wall.

The disease is bilateral in 50% of cases. The image is variable, ranging from a few lacunae up to a myriad of cysts leaving no normal zone. They are usually found in the lumbar ureter, but a diffuse pyeloureteral involvement may be encountered (BOTHE and CHRISTOL 1942). These anomalies are often associated with signs of an inflammatory urinary tract disease, going from the simple ureteral hypotonia to pelvocaliceal modifications such as atrophic chronic pyelonephritis. Images are most frequently stable and persist indefinitely, but they sometimes disappear with treatment of the associated lesions (calculus) or if an effective anti-infectious treatment is undertaken. Cystic images can be encountered in the Stevens-Johnson syndrome but are generally reversible.

These images are usually not a diagnostic problem. In case of a single lacuna, an intraluminal formation (clot, radiotransparent calculus, air bulla), usually mobile and entirely delineated by contrast material, can be easily eliminated (FEIN and McCLENNAN 1986). Extrinsic compressions, particularly of vascular origin (arterial or venous collateral circulation, for example) make an obtuse angle with the ureteral wall and a linear aspect on the frontal view. Urothelial tumors are larger and usually have irregular and fringed edges. In case of a diffuse form of ureteritis cystica, submucosal hematoma, ureteral papillomatosis, or edematous lesions can be considered (WILLIAMSON et al. 1987). Anticoagulant-related submucosal hematomas are predominant at the level of the renal pelvis and lacunae are transient, have a variable morphology, hazy limits, and a spontaneous hyperdensity on CT scan. Diffuse papillomatosis of the ureter is exceptional, and lacunae have irregular and poorly defined limits. Parietal lacunae of nonspecific edematous ureteritis are most frequently linear, in the longitudinal axis of the ureter. They sometimes present hazy edges (GALAKHOFF et al. 1986). When they are multiple, the ureteral wall can appear spiculated.

The incidence of urinary tract infection associated with the presence of ureteritis cystica suggests an inflammatory origin. The proof was shown experimentally in animals: Lesions strictly identical to those found in the human being were created, by associating the injection of colibacilli with a urinary tract obstruction of the animal (HILL 1971). However, a urinary tract infection is not invariably found. It is possible to find favoring lesions: calculi, particularly coralliform or sponge kidney (Figs. 7.19,

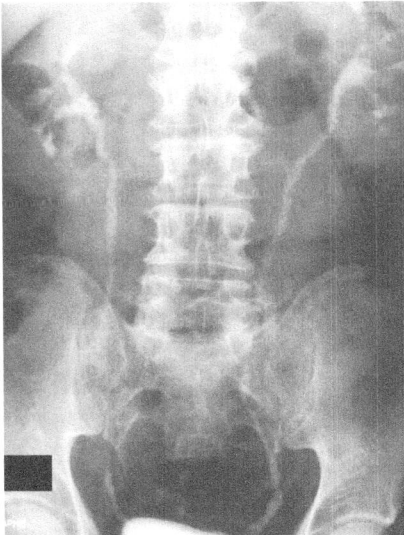

Fig. 7.18. Pyeloureteritis cystica. EU in a 63-year-old woman with history of chronic urinary tract infections: multiple rounded filling defects within both pelvis and ureters

7.20). It is also possible to encounter pyeloureteritis cystica lesions in the course of some bilharziosis (HUGOSSON 1987). On the other hand, associated tumors are fortuitous and these lesions are not considered premalignant.

There is no specific treatment except in the case of secondary ureteral obstruction, where surgery is classically indicated. Even though this has not been reported, percutaneous drainage methods could be useful in this situation.

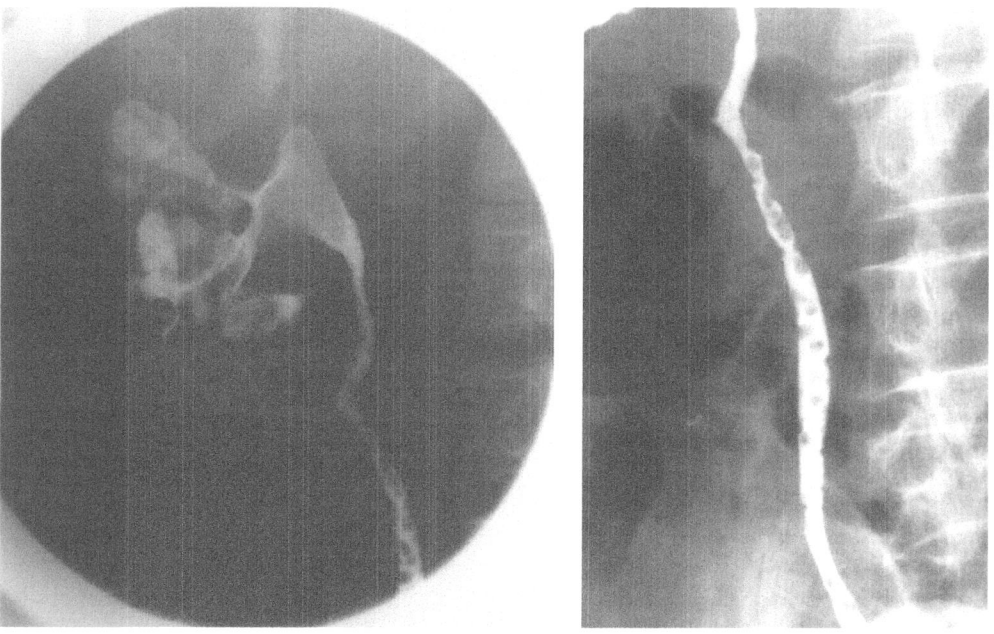

a   b

Fig. 7.19a, b. Ureteris cystica and stag-horn calculi. **a, b** Antegrade opacification of the upper urinary tract via a nephrostomy tube before percutaneous nephrolithotomy: presence of innumerable well-limited, rounded or oval filling defects involving the whole ureter

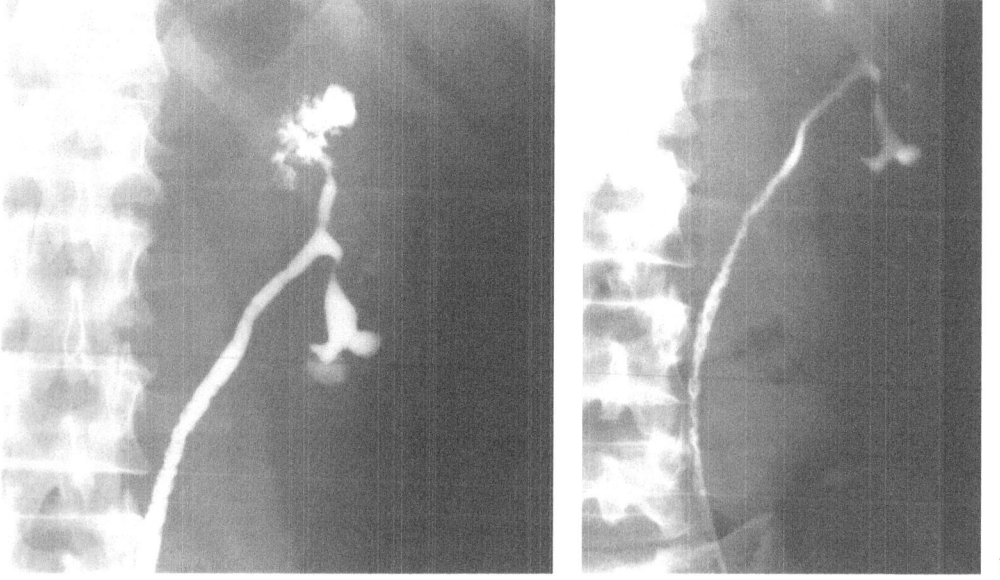

a   b

Fig. 7.20a, b. Ureteritis cystica and urinary tuberculosis. **a** Retrograde opacification of the upper urinary tract in a patient with urine culture positive for tuberculosis. Stricture of the pelvis associated with cavitary lesions of the upper and lower calices and absence of opacification of the middle calix. **b** Presence of multiple rounded filling defects of the ureteral wall considered to be ureteritis cystica secondary to urinary tuberculosis

7.5
Ureteral Malakoplakia

The Greek etymology of malakoplakia explains perfectly the lesional characteristics of this disease described by MICHAELIS and GUTTMAN (1902) (malaco = soft, plaka = plates). The disease corresponds to a tissue reaction of the granulomatous type that is still not well known and is secondary to an inflammatory pathology (Fig. 7.21). It is encountered in association with *E. coli* or *Proteus* infection and found more frequently in diabetic and immunocom-

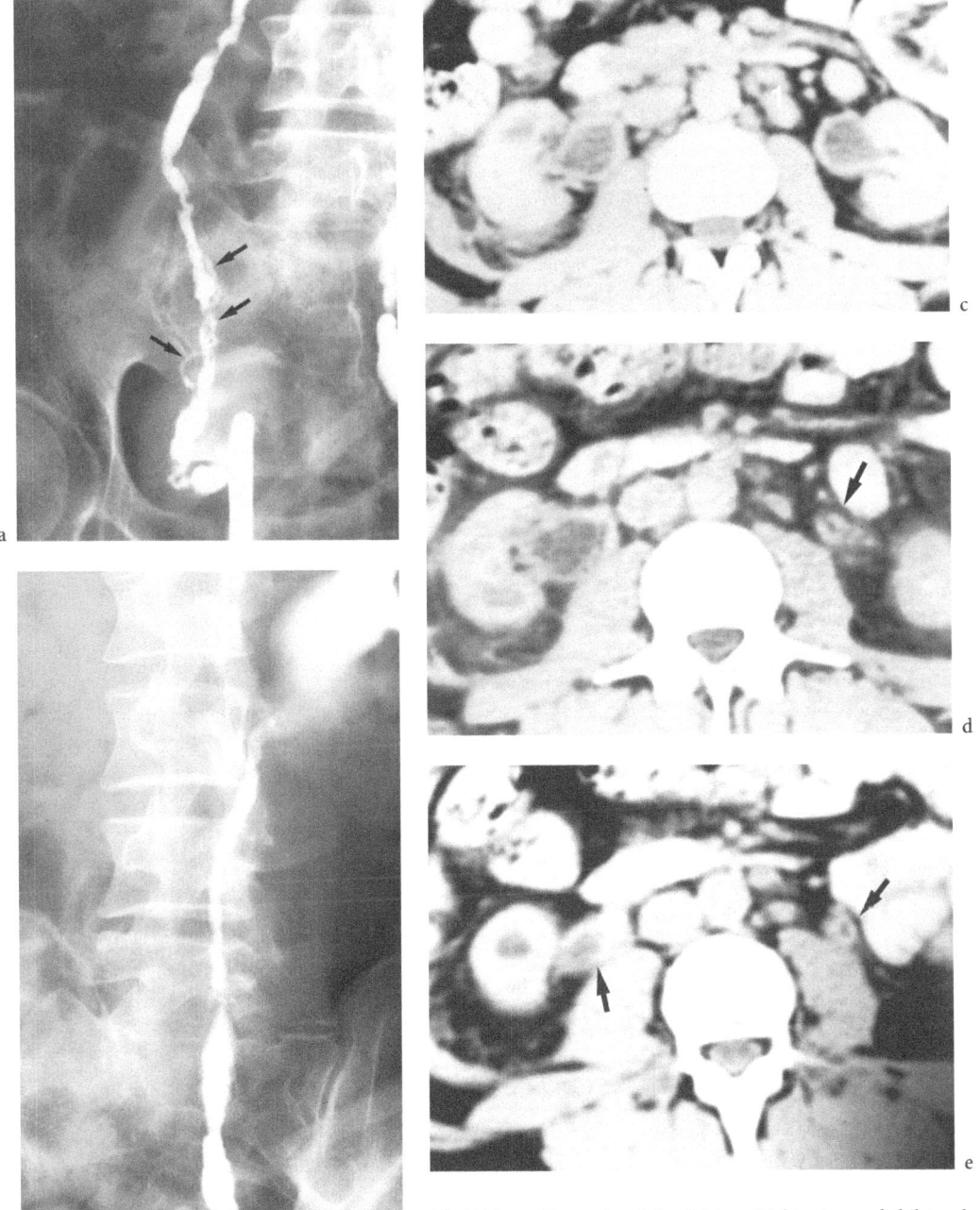

Fig. 7.21a–e. Ureteral malakoplakia. **a** Right retrograde bilateral pyelogram in a 65-year-old man with septicemia and obstructive acute renal failure. Multiple stenotic areas with lacunar and irregular filling defects. Possible opacification of periureteral dilated lymphatic vessels (*arrows*). **b** Similar lesions on the left side. **c–e** CT scan slices at different levels showing bilateral diffuse thickening of the pelvis and ureteral wall (*arrows*)

promised patients. This affection predominates at the level of the urinary tract. It begins at the bladder in 50% of cases and can be multifocal (ureter, pelvis, parenchyma, testis, prostate) (ARAP et al. 1986). There are extraurinary lesions, mostly digestive, and retroperitoneal localizations, most frequently secondary to renal and ureteral involvement. There is no malignant potential. Ureteral involvement is found in 10% of cases, most frequently in the pelvic ureter (STANTON and MAXTED 1981). It can be revealed by a urinary tract obstruction. Bilateral disease can also be encountered. It affects most frequently women (4/1) in their 50s.

Macroscopically, this affection is characterized by the presence of submucosal plate-like lesions. These plates are soft, white or yellowish, sometimes caseous. Underlying mucosa is frequently edematous, sometimes ulcerated. Between the plates, the mucosa remains normal (SMITH 1965). The condition evolves to fibrous stenosis with a possible impact on the upstream excretory tract and renal parenchyma (SEXTON et al. 1982). Histological study shows granulomatous inflammatory lesions which cells of the histiocytic type which contain, in a constant manner, intracytoplasmic polymorphic inclusions: These are the VON HANSEMAN cells (VON HANSEMAN 1983) with the bodies of MICHAELIS and GUTTMAN.

The symptomatology has the multiple aspects of chronic urinary stasis and leads to the performance of EU or to direct exploration of the urinary tract, if the renal function is seriously affected. EU is rarely useful and shows a uni- or bilateral ureteral obstruction. Lesions are well-visualized by antegrade and/or retrograde pyelography. The ureter shows two types of lesions: either filling defects, multiple polymorphic, vaguely rounded and irregular (SCHNEIDERMAN and GUTMANN 1968), disseminated in an anarchic way at the level of the ureter, or staged and regular stenoses (ELLIOT et al. 1972). Stenosing lesions appear at an advanced disease stage. A CT scan shows diffuse thickening of the ureteral wall and allows evaluation of the upper extension of the lesions and of the effect of new therapies currently proposed.

The diagnosis of these lesions is challenging (WILLIAMSON et al. 1987). Pyeloureteritis cystica, which appears in an identical clinical context of urinary tract infection, is characterized by more regular lesions which spread in a more homogeneous manner. Tuberculous ureteritis can have identical lesions but is most frequently associated with pelvocaliceal and parenchymal anomalies. Lesions similar to those of malakoplakia are observed in periarteritis nodosa, or also in diffuse ureteral metastasis and in multiple urothelial tumors. The association of a ureteral anomaly with chronic and/or relapsing *E. coli* urinary infection must suggest the diagnosis of malakoplakia (BAUMGARTNER and ALAGAPPIAN 1990). It is most frequently confirmed by cystoscopy and biopsy of the juxtameatal region, or urinary cytology (FEIN and MCCLENNAN 1986; SPATARO 1990).

Ureteral malakoplakia can benefit from, besides traditional surgical or interventional therapies (internal derivation, percutaneous nephrostomy, ureteral endoprosthesis), medical treatments aimed at suppressing the chronic urinary infection state and fighting the consequences of possible enzymatic deficiencies. Malakoplakia may be due to a bacterial phagocytosis anomaly secondary to lysosomal enzyme deficiencies. The use of cholinergic drugs and vitamin C can achieve the regression of specific plate-like lesions, but it seems ineffective on stenoses, which have a major impact on the long-term prognosis. The role of an immune deficiency was underlined by STANTON and MAXTED (1981), who showed that 40% of patients were carrying a neoplasm or an autoimmune or a systemic disease.

7.6
Ureteral Involvement in Collagenosis

Some forms of collagenosis, particularly polyarteritis nodosa, can be accompanied by ureteral involvement. These diseases, secondary to necrotizing vasculitis lesions, have been reported since the first observation published (FISCHER and HOWARD 1948). Their frequency is possibly underestimated because EU is rarely performed in this type of disease.

These are inflammatory lesions of the ureteral wall, at first edematous then evolving to necrosis and rapidly to parietal sclerosis. The lesions are secondary to obstructive involvement of connective, muscular, and adventitial tissue arteriolae. They must be differentiated from ureteral stenosis secondary to a retroperitoneal fibrosis induced by a polyarteritis nodosa (HOLLINGWORTH et al. 1980). They appear quite early in the course of the disease, as lumbago and sometimes renal insufficiency if the lesions are bilateral. Renal involvement can be associated in some cases (CURET et al. 1980).

EU, or direct opacification techniques in case of renal failure, shows most frequently a tubular or irregular segmental stenosis of the lumbar ureter with a more or less important upstream stasis (COCHRAN and KANTER 1979).

The whole picture of parietal ureteral stenosis can be discussed but quite frequently, the presence of collagenosis (polyarteritis nodosa, more rarely dermatomyositis or scleroderma) is already known, thus facilitating the diagnosis (CURET et al. 1980). A CT scan, if performed, shows a localized parietal thickening.

However, apparently earlier lesions characterized by ureteral hypotonia associated with such parietal irregularities as nodules or indentations, giving the ureter the aspect of a pearl necklace, have been described (GLANZ and GRUNEBAUM 1976). These lesions involve mostly the lumbar ureter and correspond to parietal edema secondary to a disorder of peristalsis (NEY and FRIEDENBERG 1981). These anomalies raise the discussion about ureteral vascular imprints by arterial or venous collateral circulation. These early lesions would be accessible to corticotherapy, and control EU shows their disappearance. Reversible ureterohydronephrosis without obstruction has also been described (CASSERLY et al. 1999). In case of stenosing lesions, an aggressive medical treatment combining corticosteroids with immunosuppressants must be tried, with surgery being reserved for medical treatment failures.

Some cases of ureteral stenosis in the setting of Wegener's granulomatosis have also been described (METSELAAR et al. 1985). Six cases were recently found (LE THI et al. 1988). The mechanism is variable: ureteral localization of angiitis-type lesions or retroperitoneal granuloma (Fig. 7.22). Some of these lesions can be predominating and revealing and sometimes accessible to corticotherapy alone. Some cases of ureteral stenosis in the course of disseminated lupus erythematosus were also reported, as well as ureteral compressions secondary to retroperitoneal rheumatoid nodules (ADELSON et al. 1982; BASKIN et al. 1989).

Rheumatoid purpura, though not a collagenosis, is also responsible for necrotizing vasculitis lesions and its evolution may be troubled by identical ureteral stenoses (MOUGENOT et al. 1978).

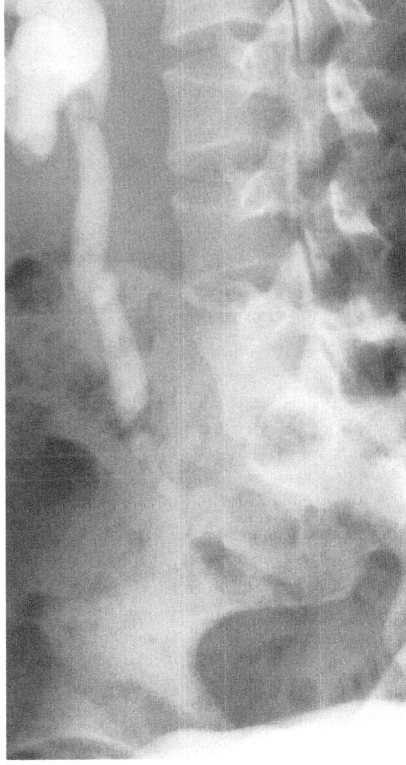

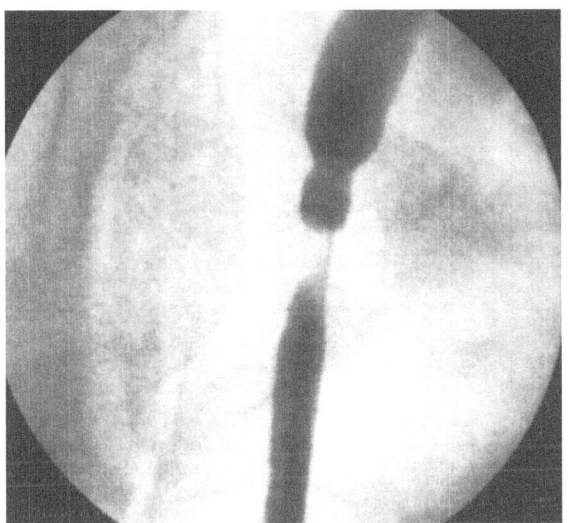

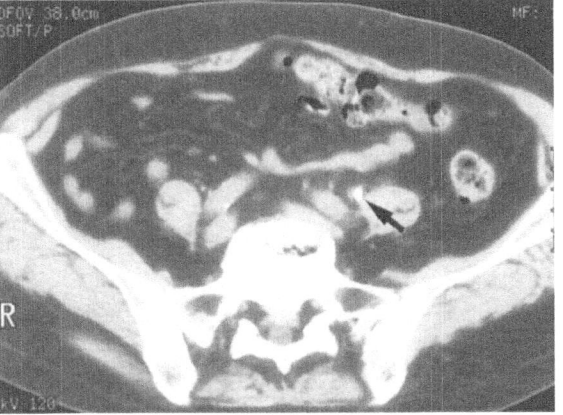

Fig. 7.22a–c. Wegener's granulomatosis of the ureter. **a** EU shows right ureterohydronephrosis secondary to a stenosis of the iliac portion of the ureter. **b** Retrograde pyelogram shows a localized narrowing with abrupt margin of the ureter. Segmental ureterectomy allows the diagnosis of Wegener's angiitis. **c** CT scan at the level of the stenosis: thickening of the left ureter wall (2-J catheter in place, *arrow*)

Similar to these observations, some exceptional cases of exclusive ureteral wall fibrosis in the settings of a systemic inflammatory disease, sensitive to corticosteroids, were reported that can be identical to idiopathic systemic fibrosis (NAMIKI et al. 1987).

The possibility of a ureteral localization must be considered in the evolution of a collagenosis. The finding of renal insufficiency must lead to the performance of renal ultrasonography in these patients to eliminate the possibility of an obstruction. If one is suspected, the hypothesis of a ureteral localization must be taken into account in the differential diagnosis.

References

Abdel-Halim RE, Al-Mashad S, Al-Dabbagh A (1985) Fluoroscopic assessment of bilharzial ureteropathy. Clin Radiol 31:89–94

Adelson GL, Saypol DC, Walker AN (1982) Ureteral stenosis secondary to retroperitoneal rhumatoid nodules. J Urol 127:124

Al-Ghorab MM (1968) Radiological manifestations of genitourinary bilharziosis. Clin Radiol 19:200–211

Arap S, Denes FT, Silva J, et al (1986) Malakoplakia of the urinary tract. Eur Urol 12:113–116

Avni EE, van Gansbeke D, Thoua Y, et al (1988) US Demonstration of pyelitis and ureteritis in children. Pediatr Radiol 18:134–139

Baskin L, Mee S, Matthay M, et al (1989) Ureteral obstruction caused by vasculitis. J Urol 141:933–935

Baumgartner BR, Alagappian R (1990) Malakoplakia of the ureter and Bladder. Urol Radiol 12:157–159

Birnbaum BA, Friedman JP, Lubat E, et al (1990) Extra-renal genito-urinary tuberculosis: CT appearance of calcified pipe-stem ureter and seminal vesicle abscess. J Comput Assist Tomogr 14:653–655

Bosniak MA, Megibow AJ, Ambos MA, et al (1982) Computed tomography of ureteral obstruction. AJR Am J Roentgenol 139:1107

Bothe AE, Christol DS (1942) Cystic disease of the upper urinary tract: pyelitis cystica and ureteritis cystica. AJR Am J Roentgenol 48:787–793

Boyarski S, Labay P, Teague N (1978) A peristaltic ureter in upper urinary tract infection – cause or effect? Urology 12:134–138

Burki A, Tanner M, Burnier E, et al (1986) Comparison of ultrasonography, intravenous pyelography and cystoscopy in detection of urinary tract lesions due to schistosomia hematobium. Acta Trop 43:139

Caine M (1967) Diseases of the ureter. In: Bergman H (ed) In the ureter. Hoeber Medical Division, New York, pp 123–157

Capdeville R, Fortier-Beaulieu M, Gauthier N, et al (1973) Les images striées du haut appareil urinaire. J Radiol Electrol 54:509

Casserly LF, Reddy SM, Rennke HG, et al (1999) Reversible bilateral hydronephrosis without obstruction in hepatitis-B associated polyarteritis nodosa. Am J Kidney Dis 43:11–14

Cheever AW, Kamel IA, Elwi AM, et al (1978) Schistosoma mansoni and S. hematobium infections in Egypt. III. Extrahepatic pathology. Am J Trop Med Hyg 27:55

Claridge M (1970) Ureteric obstruction in tuberculosis. Br J Urol 42:693–698

Cochran ST, Kanter SA (1979) Ureteric changes in polyarteritis nodosa. Br J Radiol 52:504–506

Cory DA, Tarver RD, Baker MK, et al (1987) Subepithelial pyelo-ureteric lesions in patients with nephrostomy. Br J Radiol 60:449–453

Curet P, Bousquet JC, Guillevin L, et al (1980) Manifestations urétérales des connectivites. J Radiol 61:397–403

Cutajar CL (1983) Urinary schistosomiasis. Saudi Arabia Med J 4:67–76

Dana A, Iraqj El Hussein S, Imani F, et al (1981) La bilharziose urinaire. Encycl Med Chir Paris, Radiodiagnostic V 34280 AIO – 5

Daughtridge T (1969) Mucosal folds in the upper urinary tract. AJR Am J Roentgenol 107:743–745

Dufour B (1973) Les obstructions de l'uretère lombo-iliaque à l'exclusion des tumeurs urétérales. Association Française d'Urologie Editeur, Paris

Elkin M (1990) Urogenital tuberculosis. In: Pollack HM (ed) Clinical urography, an atlas and textbook of uroradiological imaging. Saunders, Philadelphia, pp 1021–1052

Elliott GB, Moloney PJ, Clement JG (1972) Malakoplakia of the urinary tract. AJR Am J Roentgenol 116:830–837

Fein AB, McClennan BL (1986) Solitary filling defects of the ureter. Semin Roentgenol 21:201–205

Fischer R, Howard H (1948) Unusual ureterogram in a case of periarteritis nodosa. J Urol 61:393–404

Friedenberg RM (1971) Tuberculosis of the genito-urinary system. Semin Roentgenol 6:310

Friedenberg RM, Ney C, Stachenfeld RA (1968) Roentgenographic manifestations of tuberculosis of ureter. J Urol 99:25–29

Friedland GW, Forsberg L (1972) Striation of the renal pelvis in children. Clin Radiol 23:58–60

Frimmann-Dahl J (1958) Radiological investigation of urogenital tuberculosis. Urol Int 80:218–228

Galakhoff C, Hospitel S, Dana A, et al (1986) La pyélo-urétérite kystique. A propos de 40 cas. J Radiol 67:463–468

Glanz I, Grunebaum M (1976) Ureteral changes in polyarteritis nodosa seen during excretory urography. J Urol 116:731–733

Goldman SM, Fishman EK, Hartman DS, et al (1985) Computed tomography of renal tuberculosis and its pathologic correlates. J Comput Assist Tomogr 9:771–776

Gow JG (1986) Genitourinary tuberculosis. In: Walsh PC, Gittes RF, Perlmutter AD, Stamey TA (eds)Campbell's urology, vol 1, 5th edn. Saunders, Philadelphia, pp 1037–1069

Gwinn JL, Barnes GR (1964) Striated ureter and renal pelvis. Preliminary report. AJR Am J Roentgenol 91:666

Hanash KA (1971) Genito-urinary bilharziosis (schistosomiasis). In: Emmett JL, Witten DM (eds) Clinical urography, vol 2, 3th edn. Saunders, Philadelphia, pp 837–854

Hanafy HM, Youssef TH, Saad SM (1975) Radiological aspects of bilharzial (schistosomial) ureter. Urology 6:118–124

Harrow PY, McPherson DR, de Wardener HE (1963) Ureteritis emphysematosa: spontaneous ureteral pneumogram; renal and perirenal emphysema. J Urol 89:43–48

Hartman GW, Segura JW, Hattery RR (1977) Tuberculosis of urinary tract. In: Witten DM, Myers GH, Utz DC (eds) Emmett's clinical urography, vol 11, 4th edn. Saunders, Philadelphia, pp 898-921

Hill GS (1971) Experimental production of pyeloureteritis cystica and glandularis. Invest Urol 9:1-9

Hodson CJ, Edwards D (1960) Chronic pyélonephritis and vesico-ureteris reflux. Clin Radiol 11:219-231

Hollingworth P, Denman AM, Gumpel JM (1980) Retroperitoneal fibrosis and polyarteritis nodosa successfully treated by intensive immunosuppression. J R Soc Med 73:61

Hugosson C (1987) Striations of the renal pelvis and ureter in bilharziosis. Clin Radiol 38:407-409

Hugosson DO, Olsen P (1986) Early ureteric changes in schistosomia haematobium infection. Clin Radiol 37:501-503

Hyde I, Wastie ML (1971) Striations (longitudinal mucosa folds) in the upper urinary tract. I. Striated renal pelvis and ureter. Br J Radiol 44:445-456

Imray TJ, Huberty LH (1980) Isolated ureteritis emphysematosa simulating pneumatosis intestinalis. AJR Am J Roentgenol 135:1082-1083

Jacoby M (1929) Hydronephroider Krebs der Niere kombiniert mit Nierenbeckenstein, papillarer Krebs der Nierenbecken und Harnleiter, ureteritis cystica. Z Urol 23:718-728

Jorulf H, Lindjtedt E (1985) Urogenital schistosomiasis: CT evaluation. Radiology 157:745-749

Kardorff R, Traore M, Doehring-Schwerdtfeger E (1994) Ultrasonographic of ureteric abnormalities induced by schistosoma hematobium infection before and after praziquantel treatment. Br J Urol 74:7003

Kass EJ, Silver TM, Konnack JW, et al (1976) The urographic findings in acute pyelonephritis. Nonobstructive hydronephrosis. J Urol 116:544-546

Kim SH, Yoon HI, Park JH, et al (1993) Tuberculosis stricture of the urinary tract: antegrade balloon dilatation and ureteral stenting. Abdom Imaging 18:186-190

Kollins SA, Hartman GN, Carr DT, et al (1974) Roentgenographic finding in urinary tract tuberculosis. AJR Am J Roentgenol 121:487-499

Lavasse JP (1969) Les ureterites tuberculeuses chez l'homme et leur traitement en milieu sanatorial. Thèse, Marseille

Le Thi HD, De Gennes C, Wechsler B, et al (1988) Anurie par sténose urétérale bilatérale au cours d'une granulomatose de Wegener. Presse Med 17:870

Lemaitre G, Remy J, Maillard JP (1966) Les manifestations radiologiques de la bilharziose uro-génitale. J Belg Radiol 49:321-325

Levine RS, Pollack HM, Banner MP (1982) Transient ureteral obstruction after ureteral stenting. AJR Am J Roentgenol 138:325-327

Little PY, McPherson DR, de Wardener HE (1965) The appearance of the intravenous pyelogram during and after acute pyélonephritis. Lancet 1:1186-1188

Maged A (1971) Bilharzial strictures of the ureter and their treatment. J Egypt Surg Soc 6:35-54

Mariano RT, Sussman SK (1998) Sarcoidosis of the ureter. AJR Am J Roentgenol 171:1431

Metselaar HJ, ten Kate FJW, Weimar W (1985) Ureter obstruction as a complication of Wegener's granulomatosis. Eur Urol 11:63-64

Michaeli J, Mogle P, Perlberg S (1984) Emphysematous pyelonephritis. J Urol 131:203-208

Michaelis L, Guttmann C (1902) Ueber Einschlusse in Blasentumoren. Z Klin Med 47:209-221

Mougenot B, Mitranoff P, Bouissou F, et al (1978) Urétérite sténosante au cours du purpura rhumatoïde de Schonlein-Henoch. Ann Radiol 21:215-221

Namiki M, Koh F, Oka T, et al (1987) Bilateral ureteral stricture due to ureteral fibrosis. Case report. Urol Int 42:231-233

Narayana AS (1982) Overview of renal tuberculosis. Urology 19:231-237

Ney C, Friedenberg RM (1981) Diseases of the ureter. In: Ney C, Friedenberg RM (eds) Radiographic atlas of the genitourinary system, 2nd edn. Lippincott, Philadelphia

Nicolet V, Carignan L, Dubuc G, et al (1988) Thickening of the renal collecting system: a nonspecific finding at US. Radiology 168:411-413

O'Reilly PH (1986) Ureteric obstruction. In: O'Reilly PH (ed) Obstructive uropathy. Springer, Berlin Heidelberg New York, pp 138-139

Padovani J, Faure F (1977) Tuberculose renale et ureterale. Encl Med Clin Radiodiagnostic Tome V 34320-1-12, Paris

Parker MD, Clark RL (1996) Urothelial striations revisited. Radiology 198:89-91

Poole CA, Ferris AJ, Haukohl RS (1970) Radiolucent folds in the upper urinary tract. AJR Am J Roentgenol 110:529-539

Premkumar A, Lattimer J, Newhouse JH (1986) CT and sonography of advanced urinary tuberculosis. AJR Am J Roentgenol 148:65-69

Puigvert A (1974) Algo acerca de los ureteritis quistica. Arc Esp Urol 27:639-656

Rees RW, Hollands FG (1970) The ureter in renal tuberculosis. Br J Urol 42:693

Sano K, Kitajima N (1993) A case of ureteritis: a course of rapidly progressing stricture. Acta Urol Jpn 39:467

Schneiderman C, Gutmann C (1968) Malakoplakia of the urinary tract. J Urol 100:694-698

Sexton CC, Lowman RM, Nyongo AO, et al (1982) Malakoplakia presenting as complete unilateral ureteral obstruction. J Urol 128:139

Shopfner CE (1970) Urinary tract pathology with sepsis. AJR 108:632-640

Silber I, McAlister WH (1970) Longitudinal folds as an indirect sign of vesicoureteral reflux. J Urol 103:89

Smith BH (1965) Malakoplakia of the urinary tract. A study of twenty-four cases. Am J Clin Pathol 43:409-417

Spark RP, Gleason DM, de Benedetti CD, et al (1991) Is eosinophilic ureteritis an entity? 2 case reports and review. J Urol 145:1256

Spataro RF (1990) Inflammatory conditions of the renal pelvis and ureter. In: Pollack HM (ed) Clinical urography, an atlas and text book of uroradiological imaging, vol 2. Saunders, Philadelphia, pp 884-901

Stanton JJ, Maxted W (1981) Malakoplakia: a study of the literature and current concepts of pathogenesis diagnosis and treatment. J Urol 125:146-151

Tencate HW (1971) Tuberculosis of the genitourinary tract. In: Emmett JL, Witten DM (eds) Clinical urography, vol 2, 3rd edn. Saunders, Philadelphia, pp 855-930

Theander G, Wehlin L (1976) Mucosal folding in upper urinary pathways following ureterolithiasis. Acta Radiol Diagn 17:609-616

Thomas E, Hillman BJ, Stanilic T (1980) Urinary tract infection with atypical mycobacteria. J Urol 124:748-750

Umerah BC (1977a) The less familiar manifestations of schistosomiasis of the urinary tract. Br J Radiol 50:105–109

Umerah BC (1977b) Evaluation of the physiological function of the ureter by fluoroscopy in bilharziasis. Radiology 124: 645–647

Vezina JA, Leger LP, Raymond O, et al (1963) Les replis muqueux de l'arbre urinaire supérieur. J Can Assoc Radiol 14:10–19

Von Hanseman D (1983) Über Malakoplakie der Harnblase. Arch Pathol Anat 173:302–308

Wadsworth DE, McClennan BL (1983) Benign causes of acquired uretero-pelvic junction obstruction: a uroradiologic spectrum. Urol Radiol 5:77

Wang LJ, Wong YC, Chen CJ, Lim KE (1997) CT features of genitourinary tuberculosis. J Comput Assist Tomogr 21:254–258

Wasserman NF (1996) Inflammatory diseases of the ureter. Radiol Clin North Am 31:1131–1156

Williamson B, Harman GW, Hattery RR (1987) Multiple and diffuse ureteral filling defects. Semin Roentgenol 38: 407–409

Wright FM (1969) Mucosal edema of ureter and renal pelvis. Radiology 93:1309–1312

Young SW, Khalid KH, Farid Z, et al (1974) Urinary tract lesions of Schistosoma hematobium with detailed radiographic consideration of the ureter. Radiology 111: 81–84

Zagora RJ, Assimos DG, Yap MA, et al (1993) Obliteration pyelo-ureteris: a complication of stone disease in patients with urinary conduit diversion. J Urol 150:961

8 Ureters in Pregnancy

N. Grenier, H. Trillaud, and J. L. Pariente

CONTENTS

Dilatation of the collecting system is a classical phenomenon during pregnancy and is due to hormonal and extrinsic compressive factors. It may occur during the first 10 weeks of gestation but increases in frequency as pregnancy advances, predominating during the second and third trimesters (Brown 1990). Abdominal or flank pain is also a very frequent clinical problem, and is considered the most common nonobstetric cause of hospitalization during pregnancy (Maikranz and Coe 1994). In such cases, it is difficult to know whether the pain is related to acute renal obstruction, generally because of urolithiasis, or to other nonurinary causes. In this setting, imaging tests play a major role, since irradiation of the fetus has to be avoided and contrast media are generally not recommended or are contraindicated. However, since the urinary tract of a pregnant woman is often dilated after the first trimester, the radiologist faces two main dilemmas: first, differentiating the so-called physiological dilatation from a possible pathological obstruction; second, deciding between conservative and more invasive therapy.

The purpose of this review is to discuss the potential of the different imaging techniques for differentiating between physiological dilatation and pathological obstruction, and to consider their impact on treatment.

N. Grenier, MD; H. Trillaud, MD; J. L. Pariente, MD
Service de Radiologie, B.G.H. Pellegrin Tripode, Place Amélie Raba Léon, F-33076 Bordeaux Cedex, France

8.1 Physiological Dilatation of the Collecting System

Physiological dilatation can be observed in up to 90% of pregnant women during the third trimester. It may occur at the end of the first trimester and generally increases in severity as pregnancy advances. This frequency is not related to the number of pregnancies, and its regression is usual during the first 8 weeks after delivery. Dilatation is located on the upper cavities and on the lumbar ureters. Their pelvic portion is always normal. The dilatation predominates on the right side in 80%–90% of cases (Swanson et al. 1995).

Today, it is well accepted that dilatation of the collecting system is related to a mechanical compression of the ureters by the gravid uterus. This dilatation is favored by high levels of progesterone and gonadotropin, which are responsible for smooth muscle cell relaxation (Marshall et al. 1966). Several factors are in favor of this compressive mechanism: Dilatation increases with the volume of the uterus; it is predominant on the upper cavities, without dilatation of the pelvic ureter; its right-sided predominance can be explained by the different relationships between the ureters and arteries; no dilatation is observed in pregnant women with a pelvic kidney or a urinary diversion.

8.2 Acute Ureteral Obstruction During Pregnancy

Compression of the ureter by the gravid uterus can be responsible for mild or severe flank pain (Jones et al. 1979). In this context, an additional factor of obstruction, such as a stone, must be sought because it may require specific treatment and, more importantly, will rule out other abdominal or obstetrical causes.

The true incidence of urolithiasis during pregnancy is unknown because only symptomatic cases are actually identified (MAIKRANZ and COE 1994). It seems to be low, between 0.03% and 0.6% (GOLFARB et al. 1989). The incidence of symptomatic stones increases with the number of pregnancies. Although the only known predisposing factor is dilatation of the collecting system, symptomatic stones are equally frequent on both sides (KROOVAND RL 1992).

Pregnant women with urolithiasis can present with symptoms similar to those of nonpregnant patients. Renal colic is the most frequent and may initiate premature labor. Erroneous clinical diagnosis of appendicitis, diverticulitis, placental abruption, or primary premature labor may be made in around 28% of patients (GOLDFARB et al. 1989). Microscopic hematuria is present in 75%–100% of stone-bearing patients and is macroscopic in around 20% (JONES et al. 1979).

Associated renal infection or pyelonephritis is also more frequent in patients with stones. If symptoms of irritation such as frequency, urgency, or irritative voiding symptoms are common in pregnancy, pyelonephritis occurring especially after the fourth month rules out renal obstruction by urolithiasis (SWANSON et al. 1995).

8.2.1
Radiological Techniques

Until recently, excretory urography (EU) was considered the method of choice for imaging pregnant patients with suspected acute obstruction. Today, sonography plays a major role in limiting the indications of this technique, thus avoiding irradiation of the fetus and injection of contrast medium. SWARTZ and REICHLING noted that only the first trimester was a significant risk period for limited ionizing radiation exposure during pregnancy; after that time, birth defects and spontaneous abortions are unlikely (SWARTZ and REICHLING 1978).

8.2.1.1
KUB

The limitations of KUB in this context are the proportion of nonopaque urinary stones and, particularly during the third trimester, the obscuring of stones by the enlarged uterus and by the fetal skeleton. Therefore, it should not be performed before sonography, which is now the prime imaging technique in this context.

8.2.1.2
Sonography

Dilatation of the collecting system, which is almost always present, can easily be shown by sonography (FRIED et al. 1983; PEAKE et al. 1983). However, detection of a possible stone and separation of physiological dilatation from pathological obstruction of the pelvis has proven somewhat disappointing. Measurements are not used in clinical practice because the size of the cavities can be modified by the degree of bladder filling and with the patient's position, and owing to physiological variation between patients (GRENIER et al. 2000; MCNEILLY et al. 1991).

Therefore, qualitative changes are considered the most important. For the reasons mentioned above, it may be speculated that: (a) if sonography demonstrates absent or only slight dilatation on the symptomatic side, pathological obstruction can be excluded (FRIED et al. 1983); (b) a predominant left dilatation, especially with left flank pain, is highly suggestive of left pathological obstruction (Fig. 8.1). However, to enhance the value of sonography, the evaluation of the dilatation of the collecting system must include the entire ureter. MCNEILLY et al. (1991) were the first to report their experience with studying lumbar ureters in pregnancy: Since the gravid uterus, with placenta and amniotic fluid, provided a perfect acoustic window, the lumbar ureters could be visualized in 77% of hydronephrotic kidneys in asymptomatic pregnant women (88% on the right side and 52% on the left). The most important point to be examined is the level where the lower lumbar ureter crosses the common iliac artery, because this is the site of the so-called physiological compression (GRENIER et al. 2000). To do so, the patient has to lie in a contralateral oblique position and the transducer has to be positioned longitudinally in the iliac fossa. In all cases of physiological dilatation, the ureter is tapered at this site and is not dilated below (Fig. 8.2). Color Doppler is very helpful in this setting because it helps in differentiating the ureter from the iliac vessels and from the enlarged ovarian veins running close to it (Figs. 8.3, 8.4): These veins run more lateral than the ureter at the level of the pelvic brim but surround the ureter above. Identification of the ureteral stone is made easier with this approach, mostly at the lumbar level (Fig. 8.5). Color flow sonography helps here in demonstrating the dilated lumbar ureter crossing the iliac vessels (Fig. 8.6). Visualization of such a ureter crossing over the iliac vessels always means that a pathological ureteral obstruction is present below (Fig. 8.7). Stones located in the lower pelvic and

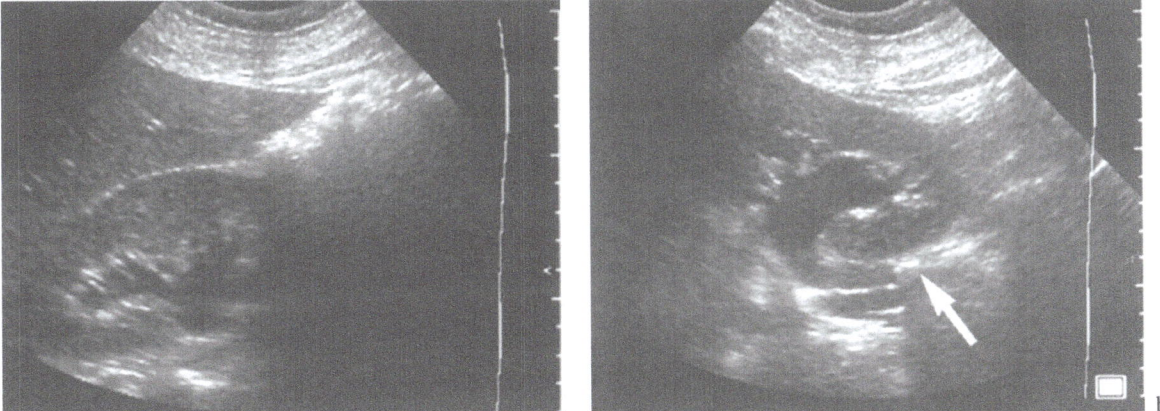

Fig. 8.1a, b. Pregnant woman with left lumbar pain during the third trimester, related to a left ureteral stone. Longitudinal sonographic images of the right (**a**) and left (**b**) kidneys show a dilatation of right (**a**) and left (**b**) collecting systems. This dilatation predominates on the left side. The stone located at the level of the left pelviureteral junction (*arrow*) is shown by this coronal transrenal approach

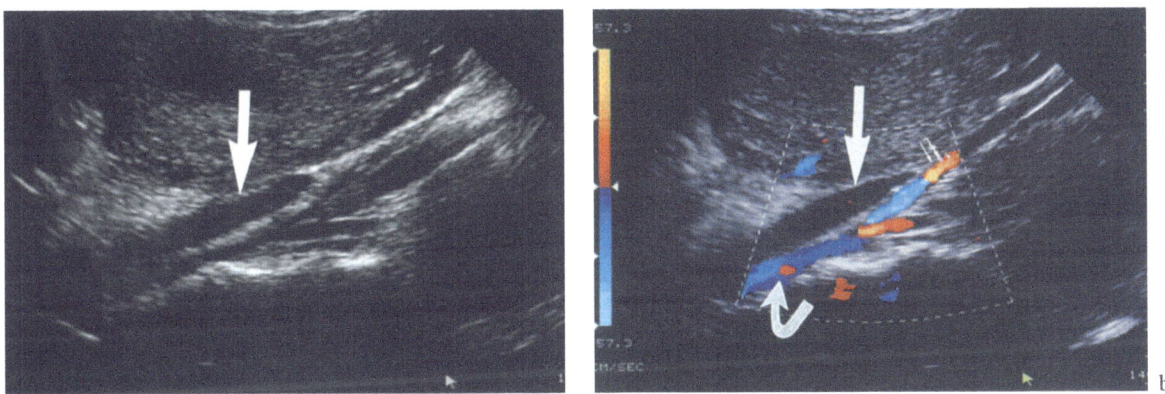

Fig. 8.2a, b. Asymptomatic pregnant woman with a physiological dilatation on the right side. The right lumbar ureter (*arrow*) is well shown on the B-mode image (**a**) and on the color flow sonogram (**b**) tapered at the level of the right common iliac artery (*double arrow*). The inferior vena cava (IVC) (*curved arrow*) is situated behind the ureter. On the left side, the aorta is visible in depth instead of the IVC (not shown)

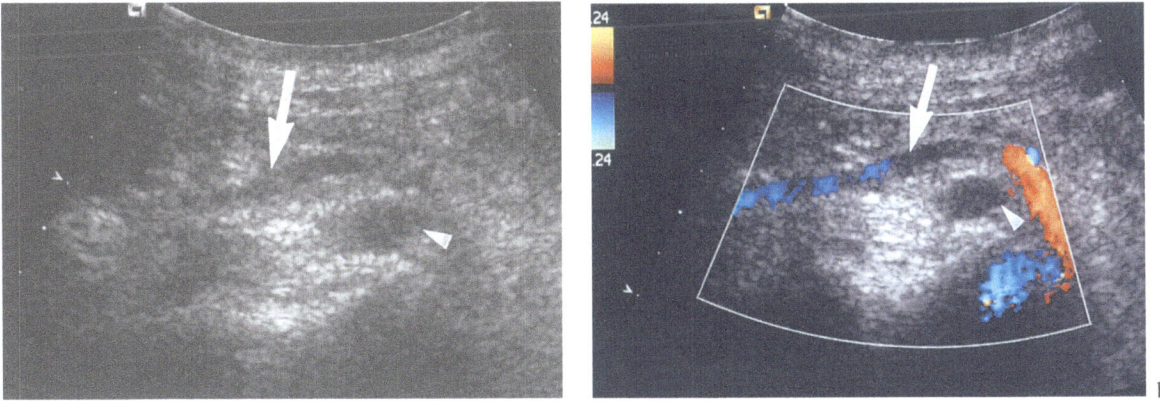

Fig. 8.3a, b. Slightly enlarged left ovarian vein. On the B-mode image (**a**), there is a tubular structure (*arrow*) crossing the iliac vessels (*arrowhead*) which could be confused with a lumbar ureter. The color flow sonographic image (**b**) shows that it is a flowing ovarian vein positioned more laterally than the ureter (not shown). No flow is detected in the iliac artery because the image was acquired during diastole

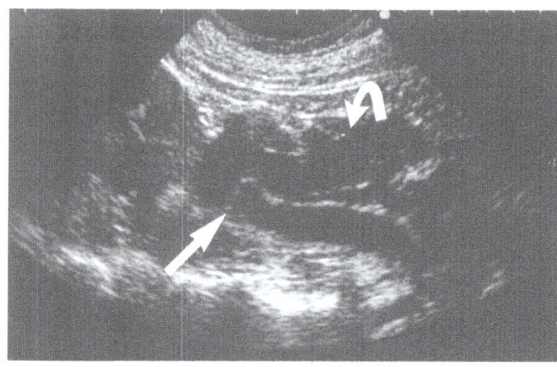
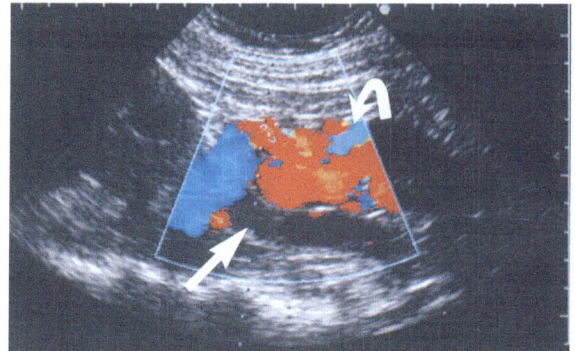

Fig. 8.4a, b. Enlarged right ovarian veins (*curved arrow*) at the lumbar level, surrounding the right ureter (*arrow*). On the B-mode image (**a**), separation of the ureter and veins is almost impossible, whereas it becomes obvious on color flow sonography (**b**)

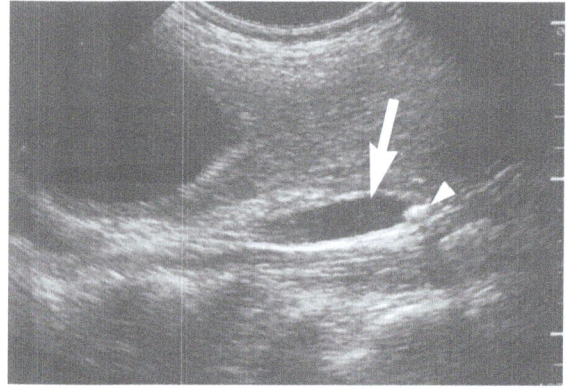
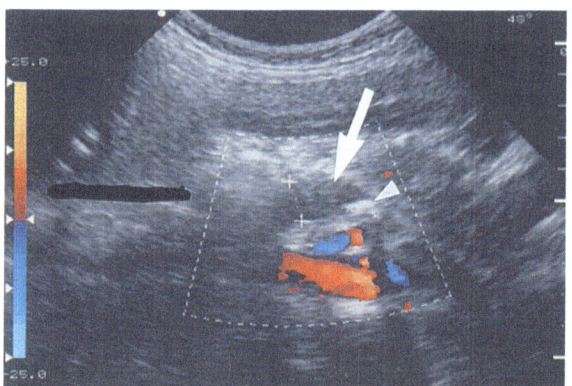

Fig. 8.5a, b. Pregnant woman with right lumbar pain during the second trimester, related to a right lumbar ureteral stone. On the B-mode image (**a**) and on the color flow sonogram (**b**), the right lumbar ureter (*arrow*) is dilated above a stone (*arrowhead*) which is blocked at the level of the right iliac artery

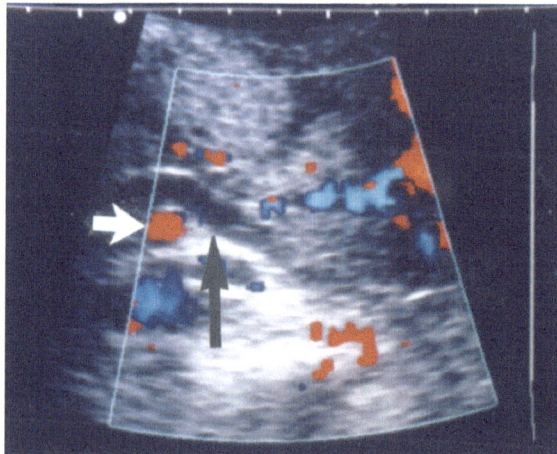

Fig. 8.6. Pregnant woman with right lumbar pain during the third trimester, related to a right pelvic ureteral stone. On the sagittal color flow sonogram the right lumbar ureter (*black arrow*) is crossing the right iliac artery (*white arrow*) and remains dilated below. No stone is detected on the upper pelvic portion of the ureter because the stone was located at the ureterovesical junction (not shown)

terminal portions of the ureter are more difficult to identify with this approach and require anterior trans-abdominal or endovaginal approaches. The endovaginal approach increases the sensitivity of detection of small calculi, as shown by LAING et al. (1994).

Color Doppler also helps in detecting small pelvic urinary stones by the twinkling artifact (Fig. 8.8). This color artifact is related to complex interactions between the US beam and the stone surface and is unchanged by the emission frequency, pulse repetition frequency, or filtering (RAHMOUNI et al. 1996). When the artifact is present, even in the absence of visible acoustic shadowing, the presence of a stone is highly probable (CHELFOUH et al. 1998). This color marker appears very helpful with small stones in difficult locations, such as the pelvic portion of the ureter, and when the ureter is not well dilated.

Color Doppler can also help by measuring the intrarenal resistivity index (RI). Platt showed that an acute and complete ureteral obstruction may induce an elevation of intrarenal RI (PLATT et al. 1993). This

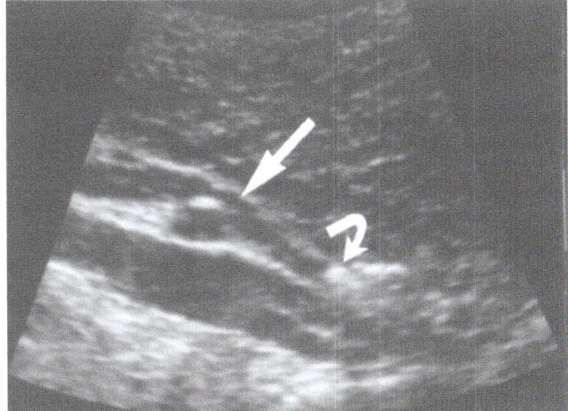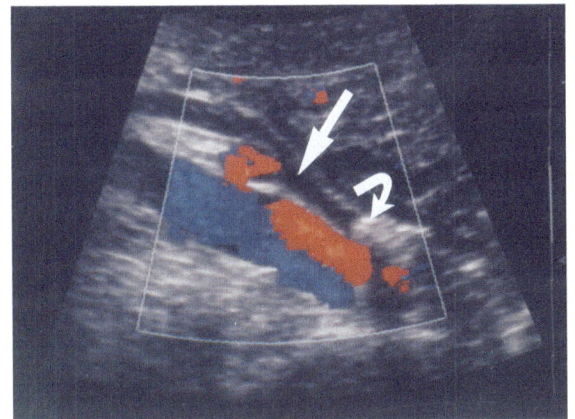

a
b

Fig. 8.7a, b. Pregnant woman with right lumbar pain during the third trimester, related to a right pelvic ureteral stone. On the sagittal B-mode image (**a**) and on the sagittal color flow sonogram (**b**), the right lumbar ureter (*white arrow*) is crossing the right iliac artery and remains dilated below. A stone is detected in the upper pelvic portion of the ureter (*curved arrow*)

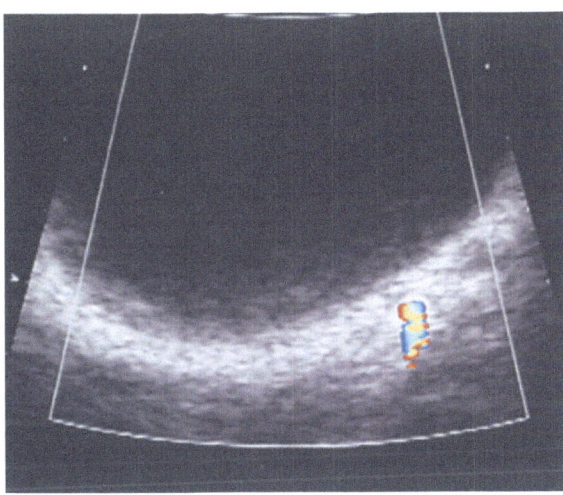

Fig. 8.8. Color twinkling artifact behind a pelvic ureteral stone with a transabdominal approach. The stone was difficult to detect on the B-mode image because it was small and without acoustic shadowing

test has a diagnostic value only when positive: If this index appears unilaterally elevated on the side of the symptoms (>0.7), then an acute and significant pathological obstruction must be present (Fig. 8.9). The ureteral jets can also be altered in such cases of obstruction, as in nonpregnant women (BURGE et al. 1991). However, the jets are not always present at the time of examination because this depends on urine density. In asymptomatic pregnant women, the absence of urinary jet may be observed unilaterally in 13% of cases (WACHSBERG 1998) when the examination is carried out in the decubitus position. In all these cases, and in the absence of any significant

obstruction, the jet reappears after the patient turns to the contralateral decubitus position. Therefore, if urinary jets are present on a symptomatic side and are symmetrical with the contralateral side, significant obstruction is unlikely. However, if urinary jets are unilaterally altered, even in the contralateral oblique decubitus position, obstruction is probable. Sometimes, when infection occurs, an echogenic sediment may be identified within the dilated collecting system (Fig. 8.10).

8.2.1.3
Excretory Urography

EU is now to be performed only if sonography is equivocal. Everything should be done to reduce the radiation dose, such as limiting the number of films and using tight collimation, low kilovoltages (60–70 kV), short exposure times and high-speed screens (BORIDY et al. 1996). During the third trimester, wide dilatation is responsible for delayed opacification of the cavities. Therefore, in these cases, a "limited urography" is recommended.

When no ureteral calculus is present, excretory urography shows a bilateral dilatation of the collecting system, predominating on the right side, with both ureters being tapered at the level of the pelvic brim (Fig. 8.11). One drawback of EU compared with sonography is that the distinction between this physiological tapering and a stone at the same level may be unclear. As for sonography, if the dilated ureter tapers to a normal caliber above that level, or below it, a stone is highly probable. Therefore, excretory urography is no longer considered to be more contributive to diagnosis than sonography.

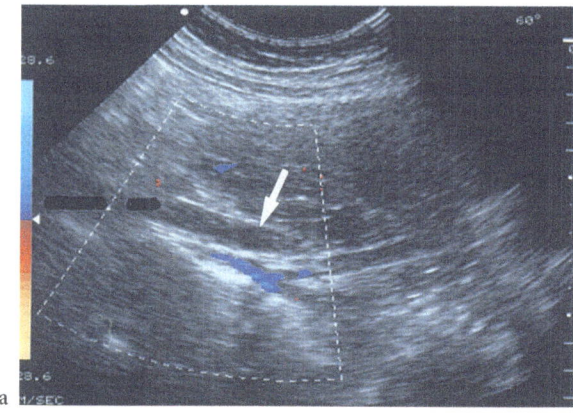

Fig. 8.9a–c. Pathological right compression of the lumbar ureter by the uterus in a 28-week pregnant woman presenting with right lumbar pain. The right lumbar ureter (*arrow*) is dilated and tapered at the level of the pelvic brim (**a**). Intrarenal spectral waveforms show an increased RI (0.83) on the right side (**b**) compared with the left side, which is normal (RI=0.65). (**c**). Stenting of the ureter provided relief of symptoms

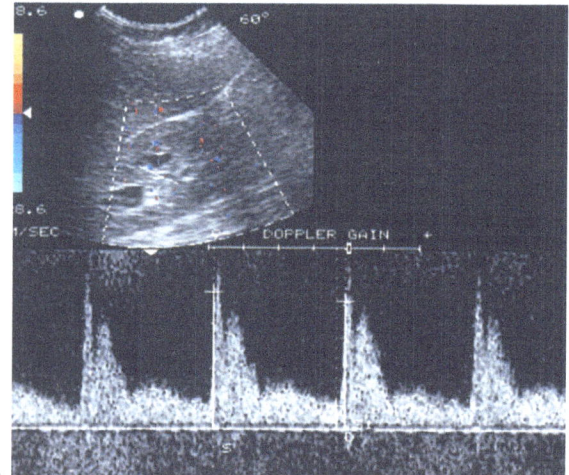

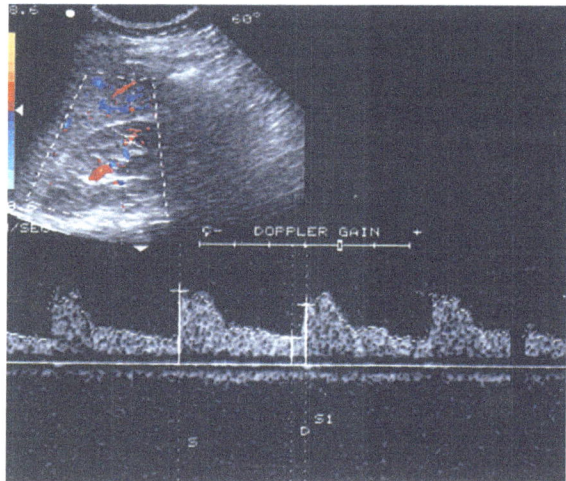

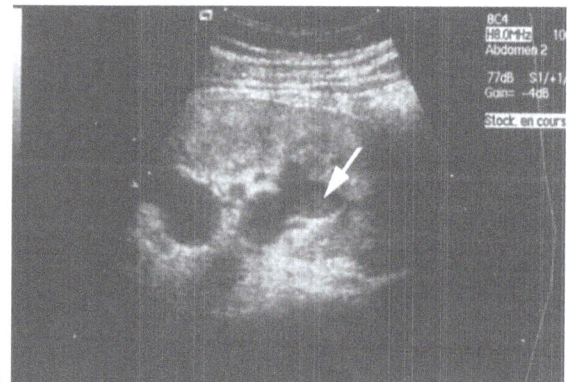

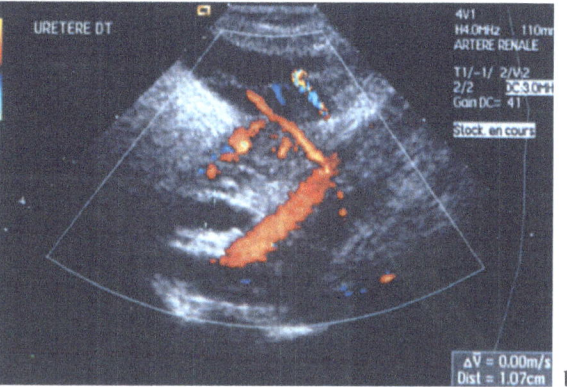

Fig. 8.10a, b. Right lumbar pain and fever in a 31-week pregnant woman. On the B-mode image (**a**), an echogenic sediment is present within the dilated cavities (*arrow*), which are "physiologically" obstructed at the pelvic brim (*b*)

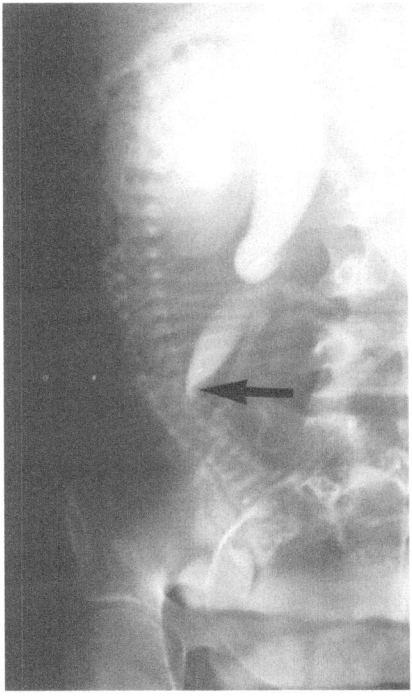

Fig. 8.11. Excretory urography in a pregnant woman with right lumbar pain during the third trimester, showing the tapered ureter at the level of the pelvic brim

8.2.1.4
Computed Tomography

The use of unenhanced CT is now growing in many institutions for the purpose of detecting ureteral stones in patients with renal colic. However, in pregnant patients, helical CT is considered too irradiating. Therefore, its use should be limited strictly to cases where renal infection must be identified.

8.2.1.5
MR Imaging

The so-called MR urography sequences are static and nonfunctional images allowing visualization of the water content of the cavities (ROTHPEARL et al. 1995). The indication for obtaining such images is the need to visualize the degree, level, and cause (if possible) of an obstruction of the upper excretory system in patients with a contraindication to contrast agents or in those with a nonfunctioning kidney. During pregnancy, this technique makes it possible to avoid irradiation and contrast agent injection because the cavities are dilated. If the ureter is tapered at the level of the pelvic brim, a "physiological" compression is highly probable (Fig. 8.12); if tapered higher or lower,

a stone is likely (Fig. 8.13) (ROY et al. 1996). ROY et al. showed that the cause of obstruction could be identified on images based on morphological criteria: physiological extrinsic compression appeared as regular tapering of the lumen, whereas stones appeared as complete filling defects with a signal void at the level of obstruction (ROY et al. 1996). Based on this preliminary experience, it seems that MR urography is now becoming the second step after sonography in the noninvasive evaluation of the excretory system in pregnancy.

8.3
Management

Clinical findings and the results of imaging remain the major criteria for targeting appropriate treatment. Medical treatment of stone obstruction is the method of choice, because 50%–80% of stones will pass spontaneously. (HENDRICKS et al. 1991). Other cases require decompression of the obstructed upper urinary tract.

Ureteral stent placement has been the modality most commonly used (LOUGHLIN 1994). Unfortunately, it requires general anesthesia and X-ray control.

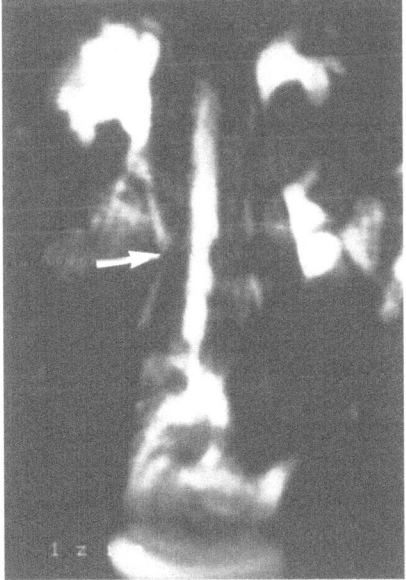

Fig. 8.12. MR urography of an asymptomatic pregnant woman. The right ureter is seen to be tapered at the level of the pelvic brim (*arrow*). (Courtesy of Dr. Haleem Kahn, Department of Radiology, Hôpital Cantonal Universitaire de Genève, Switzerland)

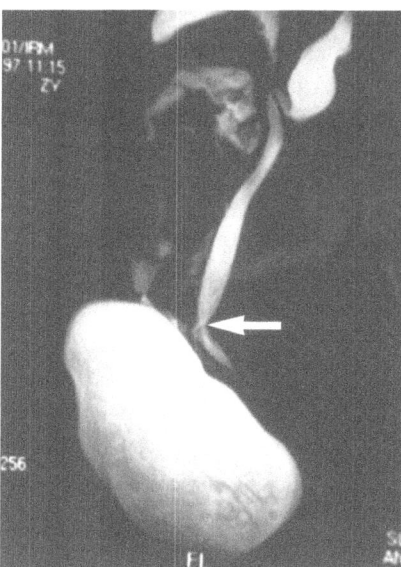

Fig. 8.13. MR urography of a pregnant woman with right lumbar pain. The MR urographic image shows a large dilatation of the right pelvocaliceal system. The proximal portion of the lumbar ureter is dilated up to a ureteral stone (*arrow*), above the pelvic brim. (Courtesy of Prof. Catherine Roy, Service de Radiologie, Hospices Civil de Strasbourg, France)

Nephrostomy under ultrasound guidance may be performed without difficulty. The disadvantages are discomfort and risk of infection.

Ureteroscopy can be performed successfully for ureteral calculus in pregnant women (RITTENBERG and BAGLEY 1988). Obstetrical monitoring is absolutely necessary during the procedure.

References

Boridy IC, Maklad N, Sandler CM (1996) Suspected urolithiasis in pregnant women: imaging algorithm and literature review. AJR Am J Roentgenol 167:869–875

Brown MA (1990) Urinary tract dilatation in pregnancy. Am J Obstet Gynecol 164:641–643

Burge HJ, Middleton WD, McClennan BL, et al (1991) Ureteral jets in healthy subjects and in patients with unilateral ureteral calculi: comparison with color Doppler US. Radiology 186:685–688

Chelfouh N, Grenier N, Higueret D, et al (1998) Characterization of urinary calculi: in vitro study of "twinkling artifact" revealed by color flow sonography. AJR Am J Roentgenol 171:1055–1060

Fried AM, Woodring JH, Thompson DJ (1983) Hydronephrosis of pregnancy: a prospective sequential study of the course of dilatation. J Ultrasound Med 2:255–259

Goldfarb RA, Neerhut GJ, Lederer E (1989) Management of acute hydronephrosis in pregnancy by ureteral stenting: risk of stone formation. J Urol 141:921

Grenier N, Pariente JL, Trillaud H, et al (2000) Dilatation of the collecting system during pregnancy: physiologic VS obstructive dilatation. Eur Radiol 10:271–279

Hendricks SK, Ross SO, Krieger JN (1991) An algorithm for diagnosis and therapy of management and complications of urolithiasis during pregnancy. Surg Gynecol Obstet 172:49

Jones WA, Correa RJ, Ansell JS (1979) Urolithiasis associated with pregnancy. J Urol 122:333–335

Kroovand RL (1992) Stones in pregnancy and children. J Urol 148:1076–1078

Laing FC, Benson CB, Disalvo DN (1994) Distal ureteral calculi: detection with vaginal US. Radiology 192:545–548

Loughlin KR (1994) Management of urologic problems during pregnancy. Urology 44:159–169

Maikranz P, Coe FL (1994) Nephrolithiasis in pregnancy. Clin Obstet Gynecol 8:375–386

Marshall S, Lyon RP, Minkler D (1966) Ureter dilatation following use of oral contraceptives. JAMA 198:782

McNeily AE, Goldenberg SL, Allen G, et al (1991) Sonographic visualization of the ureter in pregnancy. J Urol 146:298–301

Peake SL, Roxburgh HB, Langlois SLP (1983) Ultrasonic assessment of hydronephrosis of pregnancy. Radiology 146:167–170

Platt JF, Rubin JM, Ellis JH (1993) Acute renal obstruction: evaluation with intrarenal duplex Doppler and conventional US. Radiology 186:685–688

Rahmouni A, Bargion R, Herment A (1996) Color Doppler twinkling artifact in hyperechoic regions. Radiology 199:269–271

Rittenberg MH, Bagley DH (1988) Ureteroscopic diagnosis and treatment of urinary calculi during pregnancy. Urology 32:427

Rothpearl A, Frager D, Subramanian A (1995) MR urography: technique and application. Radiology 194:125–130

Roy C, Saussine C, Jahn C, et al (1996) Assessment of painful ureterohydronephrosis during pregnancy by MR urography. Eur Radiol 6:334–338

Stothers L, Lee LM (1992) Renal colic in pregnancy. J Urol 148:1383–1387

Swanson SK, Heilman RL, Eversman WG (1995) Urinary stones in pregnancy. Surg Clin North Am 75:123–143

Swartz HM, Reichling BA (1978) Hazards of radiation exposure for pregnant women. JAMA 239:1907

Wachsberg RH (1998) Unilateral absence of ureteral jets in the third trimester of pregnancy: pitfall in color Doppler US diagnosis of urinary obstruction. Radiology 209:279–281

9 Ureteral Diseases of Extrinsic Origin

V. Chabbert, B. Janne D'Othee, Ph. Otal, F. Joffre, A. Gozlan, P. Chemla

CONTENTS

The ureter is the central structure of the retroperitoneal space and the pelvic cavity. Any expansive or infiltrative pathological process in these regions may have an impact on the ureter. Most extrinsic disorders, whether tumoral or not, compress without direct extension and frequently displace the ureter. However, the mechanism of ureteral involvement by extrinsic malignancies can be different (Marincek et al. 1993; Talner 1990):

- Direct tumoral involvement of the ureteral wall (serosal, intramural, mucosal, or a combination of all of them)
- Metastatic extension to periureteral lymph nodes or periureteral fatty tissue with frequent desmoplastic reaction, so-called malignant retroperitoneal fibrosis (RPF)
- Mucosal or intramural metastases may be isolated or associated with retroperitoneal metastases. Their patterns are described in Chap. 6.

V. Chabbert; B. Janne D'Othee; Ph. Otal; F. Joffre;
A. Gozlan; P. Chemla
Service de Radiologie, Hôpital de Rangueil, 1 avenue Jean
Poulhes, 31403 Toulouse Cedex 4, France

These disorders all have in common a varying impact at a higher level, creating an obstructive syndrome of the urinary tract. Any available imaging modality must be used to assess whether or not the ureters are affected before attempting treatment of a retroperitoneal and/or pelvic disorder, in particular an expansive disorder.

Diagnosis of ureteral disorders of extrinsic origin is based on detection and identification of a peri-ureteral pathological process and evaluation of its effect on the urinary tract prior to treatment. Cross-sectional imaging techniques have spectacularly improved the diagnostic evaluation of these patients by identifying the cause of the obstruction. The new 3-D reconstruction techniques provided by helical CT scan and/or MRI both depict the morphology of the obstructed urinary tract and demonstrate the causal lesion and, if necessary, its nature.

Following an overview of the semiology, four main groups will be discussed:
- Retroperitoneal and/or pelvic tumors
- Retroperitoneal and pelvic fibrosis
- Ureteral disorders of vascular origin
- Miscellaneous disorders

9.1
General Semiology of Extrinsic Ureteral Disorders

Extrinsic ureteral disorders have a number of common radiological features which are observed in the majority of cases and can be grouped together as the "extrinsic ureter syndrome". However, this radio-logical syndrome shows variations depending on location, above all, on the type of extrinsic disorder, tumoral or infiltrative, and the presence or absence of invasion of the ureteral wall.

All these abnormalities can be observed using (a) conventional opacification techniques of the urinary tract, such as EU and/or retrograde and/or antegrade pyelography; and (b) cross-sectional imaging techniques, in particular, helical CT with reconstruction.

9.1.1
EU and Direct Opacification Techniques

KUB affords little information. It may reveal signs of an abdominal and/or pelvic water attenuation mass, displacing the intestinal loops and obliterating the psoas margin. There may be abnormal opacities, calcifications, or an area of fatty density within this mass.

EU is informative if opacification is sufficient. Changes usually affect a single ureter but may affect both, depending on the causal lesion. If tomographic images of the kidney are obtained, a retroperitoneal mass can certainly be visualized, the opacification of which depends on its soft tissue or fluid nature. However, the purpose of EU is currently not to visualize this type of lesion but to opacify the urinary tract sufficiently so as to identify the abnormalities of morphology and location which are secondary to the paraureteral lesion (Fig. 9.1). Urographic opacification of the urinary tract can be obtained immediately after CT.

A peri- or paraureteral retroperitoneal or pelvic lesion may modify morphology and function of the urinary tract above the obstruction. These abnormalities are highly variable and depend on the lumbar or pelvic location and on the duration of compression. Above the obstruction, the urinary tract may not be dilated if the impact is moderate. Dilatation is often marked, but it also varies according to the shape of the renal pelvis and its location within or outside the sinus. The whole range of functional abnormalities due to an obstructive syndrome may be observed, ranging from the deceptive picture without dilatation or delayed excretion to the silent kidney. These abnormalities may be accompanied by various degrees of destruction of the renal parenchyma. If opacification is insufficient or if the kidney is urographically silent, retrograde or antegrade opacification techniques can be used, especially if there is an obstruction requiring decompression.

Whatever the method of opacification, the abnormalities observed are identical, although they are better visualized by direct opacification techniques (PFISTER and NEWHOUSE 1978). In the future, reconstructional urography will be used increasingly to observe these abnormalities, and so it is indispensable to describe them. They are of two types, often found in association:
- *Ureteral narrowing* depends on the type and volume of the lesion and whether it is infiltrative, circumferential, or otherwise. In most cases, stenosis is eccentric, regular, progressive, more or less localized and marked. An infiltrative, circumferential pathological process causes smooth, concentric stenosis, but irregularities in the ureteral wall indicate that infiltration may extend to the wall (KUNIN and GOODWIN 1990).
- *Anomalous locations* depend essentially on the site of the causal lesion. They rarely provide any

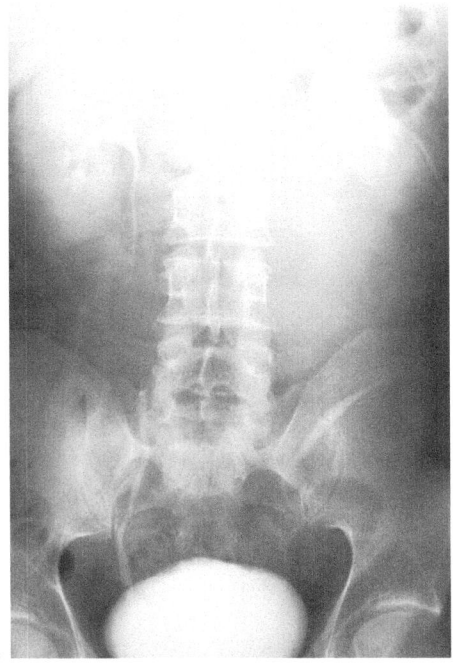

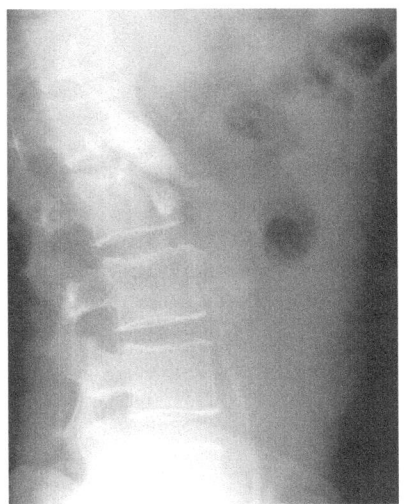

Fig 9.1a, b. Topographic abnormality of ureter related to a retroperitoneal mass. Supine (**a**) and profile (**b**) views from IVP performed in a patient with a huge right retroperitoneal mass. The upper urinary tract is slightly dilated. The lumbar ureter is compressed and forced back laterally and anteriorly by a dense retroperitoneal mass (retroperitoneal hemangiopericytoma at surgery)

indication as to etiology. At the lumbar level, one or both ureters may be laterally displaced. Maximal displacement beyond the contralateral ureter can be observed with huge tumors. They may be displaced medially or drawn to one or both sides. In the sagittal plane, displacement is usually anterior. At the pelvic level, displacement is usually posterior and one or both ureters may be deviated laterally or medially. All these anomalous locations of the ureter must be differentiated from physiological abnormalities in its position (renal ptosis, psoas muscle hypertrophy, etc.) and from surgical sequelae (CUNAT and GOLDMAN 1986).

9.1.2
Cross-sectional Imaging

The signs observed relate mainly to helical CT but can be extrapolated to MRI. The ureter is visualized during delayed acquisition after injection of contrast medium. The protocol of opacification is similar to that for EU of an obstructive syndrome. The contrast medium progresses more slowly and reaches the sloping areas. Acquisition with the patient prone helps the contrast medium descend to the level of the obstruction. CT scanning nevertheless has the advantage of following the dilated ureter without opacification, and so of identifying and analyzing the region of obstruction (MEGIBOW et al. 1982). Helical acquisition provides frontal reconstructions

similar to EU pictures and visualization by multiplanar reconstruction (MPR), maximum-intensity projection (MIP), or shaded-surface display (SSD) of the urinary tract.

Hydroureteronephrosis at an upstream level can thus be identified, as well as the anomalous locations of the ureter depending on the peri- or paraureteral pathology. The various pathological processes which affect the ureter may be detected, identified, and characterized.

The CT technique used must be adapted to the type of lesion and its presumed site (JOFFRE and PORTALEZ 1984). For certain lesions which are very localized and without great impact, sometimes discovered incidentally during EU, helical CT is guided by ureteral opacification. After making an overall scan of the abdominal and pelvic cavity, the operator must focus on the region of interest and take advantage of all the technical possibilities of helical acquisition to obtain optimal information on the suspect area (thin sections, dynamic arterial and venous opacification, 3-D reconstruction and visualization techniques). Primarily, the region of stricture should be analyzed to exclude a parietal or intraluminal pathology for which focused sections will detect only ureteral abnormalities (BOSNIAK et al. 1982). There is generally little or no change in the fatty environment around the ureter. However, a urothelial tumor with marked periureteral extension may be difficult to distinguish from a retroperitoneal or pelvic tumor invading the ureter (BECHTOLD et al. 1998). The abnormalities seen on EU or direct pyelography often make it possible to settle the question. In addition, CT cannot determine with certainty in all situations whether the ureter is invaded by an adjacent tumor or whether there is simply extrinsic compression without invasion of the wall. Finally, CT has the advantage of guiding needle biopsy, allowing the diagnosis (BARBARIC and wMcINTOSH 1981) (Fig. 9.2).

MRI techniques seem very promising in this field. Conventional sequences, associated with low-flow MR urography, provide the same type of information as helical CT regarding the ureteral obstruction, its effect at a higher level, and the extrinsic causal lesion.

9.2
Retroperitoneal and Pelvic Tumors

9.2.1
Primary Retroperitoneal Tumors
(ACKERMAN 1954)

These rare entities comprise tumors which impinge on the retroperitoneal space, independently of the various retroperitoneal organs, great vessels and lymphatics, and which are not related to any systemic disease (PATEL 1990). They develop in patients in the fifth decade, and most are malignant (BRAASCH and MON 1967). Mesodermal tumors are the most frequent and the majority are liposarcomas (20% of retroperitoneal tumors), but all soft tissue components of the retroperitoneal space may be involved. Retroperitoneal tumors can rarely be diagnosed at a early stage. The presenting signs are very vague and appear late: abdominal pain, increasing abdominal volume with a palpable mass, deterioration of the general condition. There may also be signs of compression of adjacent organs: vomiting, functional bowel complaints, problems of micturition, kidney failure, lower limb edema. The lesion may be discovered incidentally by ultrasonography or CT scan carried out for other reasons.

Conventional plain abdominal film or the scout view obtained before CT scan may provide useful information: altered location of adjacent structures (gaseous lucency) by a mass syndrome which may orient the search for the tumor site; the presence of abnormal opacities, or of "tooth-like" calcifications or fatty hyperlucency.

Ultrasonography is often the initial investigation. It shows the distension of the urinary tract and makes it possible to detect the tumoral mass. In favorable cases, it can help to locate the tumor site

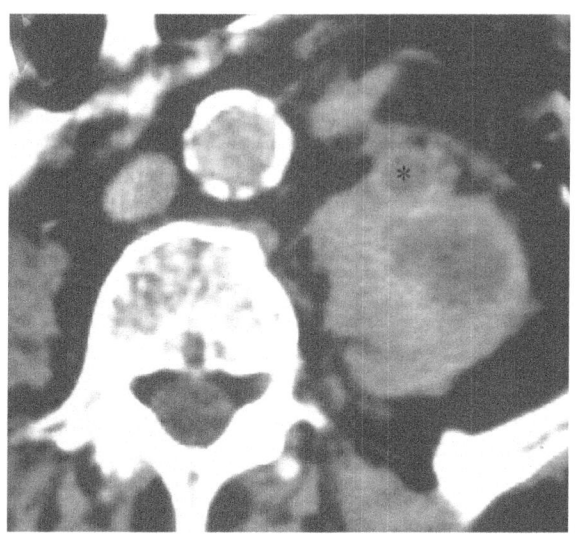

a

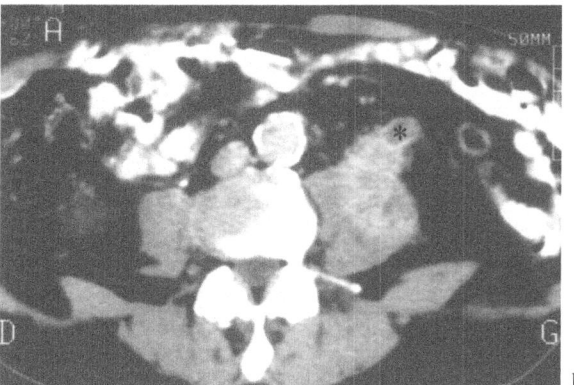

b

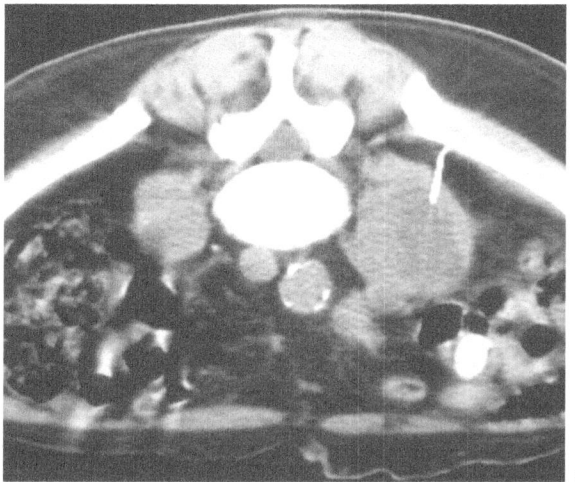

c

Fig 9.2a–c. Ureteral obstruction secondary to a tuberculous psoas abscess. **a, b** CT of the lumbar left ureter showing adhesion between a dilated ureter (*asterisk*) and a soft tissue mass that has developed into the psoas muscle. This mass is characterized by the presence of areas of enhancement and hypervascularization and areas of necrosis. The ureteral wall is thickened. **c** CT-guided needle puncture of the mass, which allowed the diagnosis of tuberculous abscess

by demonstrating the relationship of the tumor to adjacent structures, but most often the retroperitoneal site is difficult to confirm, especially if the tumor is very large. Ultrasonography gives an idea of the type of tumor by analyzing echogenicity, which may be solid (hyper- or hypoechoic), fluid, or mixed. It is also useful for guiding a biopsy.

Conventional EU is rarely carried out today. It evaluates the effect on the kidney and the displacement of the ureter, which is generally only compressed, without invasion of the wall. The spatial orientation of the displacement helps to indicate where the lesion arises. Ureteral displacement may be marked and extend beyond the midline. Direct opacification of the ureter is rarely useful.

The investigation of choice is the CT scan, which provides almost all the necessary information: conclusive diagnosis, tumor location and extent, effect on ureter and adjacent structures (LANE et al. 1989). CT diagnoses a retroperitoneal site in nearly 90% of cases (PISTOLESI et al. 1984). The most difficult problems are related to very voluminous masses, especially those originating in the anterior pararenal space (LAURENT et al. 1988). Multiplanar reconstructions are the most useful to precisely locate the tumor in the retroperitoneum and to differentiate it from a huge renal tumor. CT scan, in particular 3-D reconstruction, precisely evaluates tumor shape and the surgical possibilities: size, borders, vascular supply, relationship to and impact on adjacent structures (blood vessels, kidneys, ureter) (LEMAITRE et al. 2000) (Fig. 9.3). By assessing certain components of the tumor (calcifications, fat, single or multiple cysts, hypervascularization, necrosis), CT can provide an indication as to whether the tumor is benign or malignant and as to its histological type, but histopathological assessment is necessary for a conclusive diagnosis (COHAN et al. 1988). In primary retroperitoneal tumors, guided biopsy is generally used only if surgery is contraindicated for local or general reasons or if a retroperitoneal lymph node tumor is a differential consideration.

MRI is very promising and, like CT, provides 3-D visualization of the tumor and its effect on the urinary tract and vascular axes, but without the need for contrast medium. It also gives a better indication of tissue type even though it does not allow a sufficiently precise diagnosis.

The histological diagnosis may be suspected but can rarely be confirmed. Lipomas are generally easy to diagnose: a hypodense fat attenuation tumor, homogeneous, well circumscribed, rarely crossed by bands of opaque tissue (Fig. 9.4). These tumors exhibit a homo-

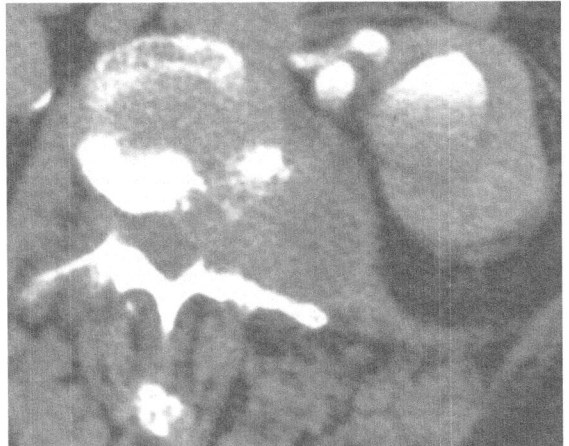

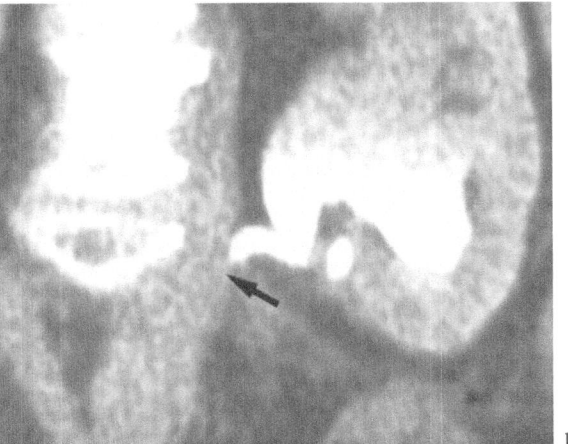

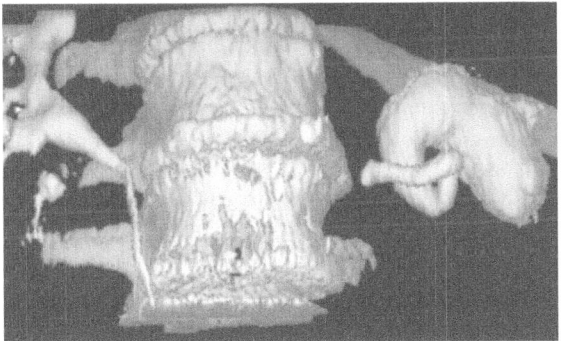

Fig 9.3a–c. Left ureteral obstruction secondary to a retroperitoneal extension of a vertebral metastasis. **a** CT axial slice shows hydronephrotic left kidney and a soft tissue retroperitoneal mass invading the psoas muscle and the retro-aortic area. Osteolytic lesion of the vertebra. **b** Frontal reconstruction shows the dilated left upper ureter with a stenosis at the level of the tumor (*arrow*). **c** SSD 3-D reconstruction demonstrating the sinuous pathway of the proximal ureter up to the stenotic area

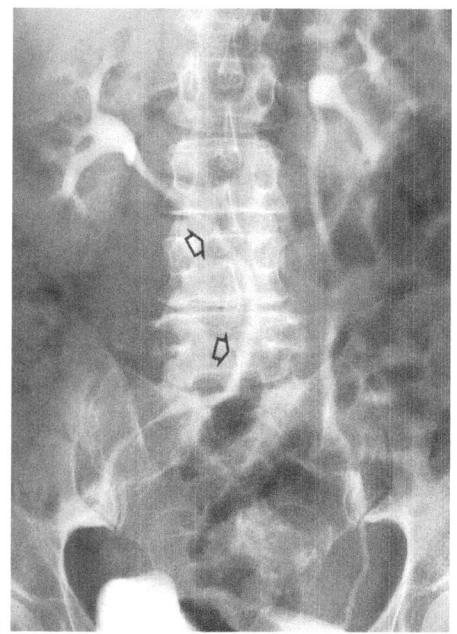

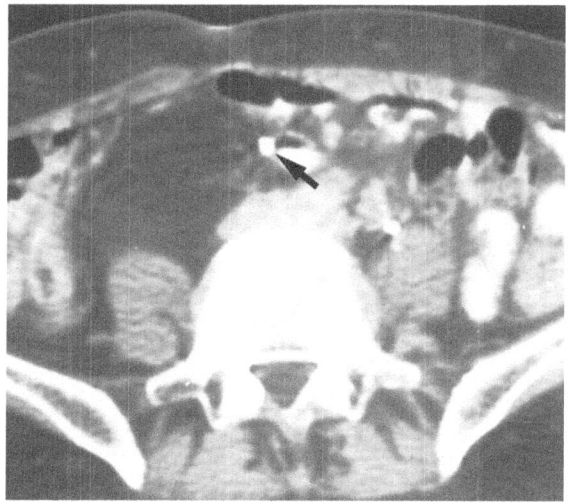

Fig 9.4a, b. Ureteral deviation secondary to a retroperitoneal lipoma. **a** EU shows medial deviation of the right ureter (*arrows*). **b** CT slice showing the retroperitoneal tumor with fatty attenuation and medial deviation of the right ureter (*arrow*)

geneous increased signal on T_1-weighted sequences. Abdominal lipomatosis is rare but may resemble a tumor. It is benign and tends to occur in obese men, in Cushing's syndrome, or after corticosteroid treatment. The diagnosis can be established by CT, obviating unnecessary surgery (LEWIS et al. 1982). The diagnosis of liposarcoma may be suggested in only 20% of cases, when fatty areas are observed in the tumor. Fat is particularly present in well-differentiated tumors, where the fatty areas are separated by dense radial linear septa of varying thickness, moderately enhanced by contrast medium. Liposarcoma may be difficult to differentiate from huge extrarenal angiomyolipoma. In the other histological forms (myxoid, pleomorphic), the diagnosis is not often suspected as the appearance is extremely varied and fatty elements are rarely found. MRI does not seem to provide any more diagnostic information than CT.

Retroperitoneal cysts are exceptional. They are easily diagnosed and must merely be differentiated from voluminous renal cysts with retroperitoneal development. Cystic lymphangiomas are rare, but a single or multilocular cystic mass separated by soft-tissue attenuation septa of varying thickness is suggestive of this diagnosis (MUNECHIKA et al. 1987). Attenuation is sometimes slightly less than with water because of the fatty lymphatic content. However, only aspiration biopsy can establish the diagnosis by identifying it. Teratoma is a possible diagnosis in case of a cystic formation with calcification. In all other cases, CT investigation shows a nonspecific soft tissue mass with highly variable

necrotic tissue and fluid and hypervascular components.

MRI identifies certain tissue types with greater precision but is rarely sufficient to indicate the histological type (SUNDARAM et al. 1987). Only the fatty component characterized by increased signal intensity on T_1- and T_2-weighted sequences can be identified. Tumors with a fluid content are also easy to identify. Well-differentiated, highly vascularized tumors (leiomyosarcoma, fibrosarcoma) are characterized by a low signal on T_1- and high signal on T_2-weighted sequences and marked enhancement after gadolinium injection. Neurogenic tumors may present increased signal intensity on T_2-weighted sequences, which is suggestive of the diagnosis. MRI is, in fact, more useful to assess the extent of these lesions and the possibilities of excision.

Tumors of the psoas compartment are individualized by their origin and their specific appearance due to their location. They are rare and often of muscular origin. They laterally displace and compress the ureter but do not usually invade it. Psoas muscle hypertrophy is easily demonstrated by a CT scan (Fig. 9.5).

9.2.2
Lymph Node Tumors

Involvement of the lymph nodes occurs mainly in hematological or metastatic disease. Both ureters are frequently affected as the lymph node chains are in a medial position, and they may be laterally displaced

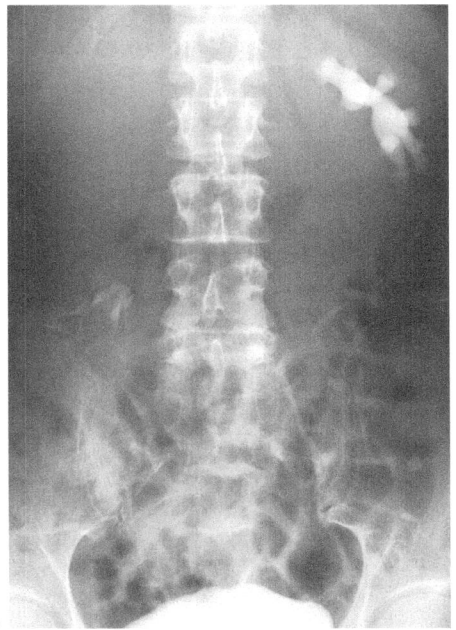

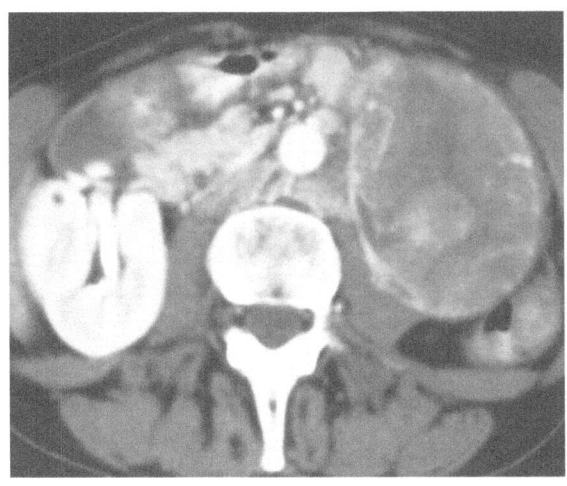

Fig 9.5a, b. Left ureteral obstruction related to a rhabdomyosarcoma of the psoas muscle. a EU: slight dilatation of the left upper urinary tract; lateral deviation of the left lumbar ureter with compression. Absence of visualization of the outer limit of the psoas muscle. b CT shows a soft tissue hypervascular and heterogeneous mass developed from the psoas muscle

either totally or in part. Urinary function may or may not be affected.

The CT scan has simplified the diagnostic approach, as in most cases lymphography is no longer necessary. Nodal areas which are not shown on lymphography can also be investigated. The limits are represented by identification of the lymph nodes in thin patients and determination of the precise criteria of lymph node involvement if hypertrophy is moderate. Diagnosis is debatable when nodes reach between 10 and 20 mm in diameter, depending on the anatomic level.

MRI is considered to be more effective in identifying lymph node chains and in spontaneously differentiating them from the vascular axes, without the need for contrast medium (LEE et al. 1984).

9.2.2.1
Lymph Node Involvement in Malignant Blood Disorders (MARGLIN and CASTELLINO 1986)

Hodgkin's disease and non-Hodgkin's lymphoma are the most frequent causes. Retroperitoneal lymph node involvement often leads to their discovery, especially in non-Hodgkin's lymphoma. Abdominal ultrasonography performed because of abdominal pain, vomiting, functional bowel complaints, or urinary symptoms may detect distension of the urinary tract associated with multiple hypoechoic masses lying between the retroperitoneal great vessels. Kidney failure due to obstruction of both ureters may be revealing, but it is usually the CT investigation which demonstrates lymph node involvement and

determines the extent and stage of progression. Retroperitoneal adenopathies usually have soft-tissue attenuation; they are homogeneous and moderately enhanced after injection of contrast medium. In Hodgkin's disease they are generally small (about 20 mm) and nonconfluent, whereas in lymphoma they are larger, confluent and compressive, sometimes necrotic, and often more diffuse and associated with mesenteric adenopathies (Fig. 9.6).

Perirenal and periureteral involvement is rare but characteristic: the ureter is surrounded by tissue which may or may not be associated with nodular or sheet-like infiltration (CHEN et al. 1988) (Figs. 9.7, 9.8). Tissue infiltration within the renal sinus may be seen and prevents the development of obstructive dilatation of the urinary tract. This may account for some observations of acute obstructive renal failure without a dilated urinary tract.

Confluent lymph nodes may cause some difficulties in diagnosis. There is rarely any debate concerning a primary medial retroperitoneal tumor which is globular, hypervascularized on CT scan, and often necrotic. On the other hand, certain cases of benign retroperitoneal fibrosis may simulate lymph node involvement if they have a polylobular contour. Inversely, a retroperitoneal lymphoma may present as a homogeneous, soft tissue perivascular mass with a regular border. Some other features are in favor of a lymphoma: ureteral displacement rather than stenotic attraction, extension beyond the renal pedicle and the iliac axes, involvement of other lymph node regions (mesentery), and, above all, anterior displacement of the great vessels,

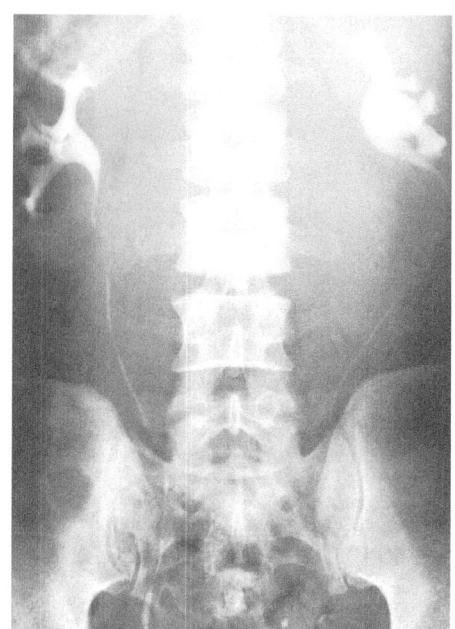

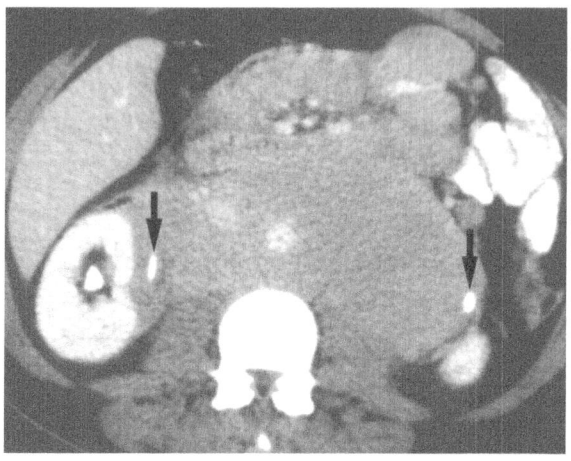

Fig 9.6a, b. Involvement of both ureters in a retroperitoneal lymphoma. a EU shows bilateral lateral displacement of lumbar ureter with compression, narrowing, and slight dilatation of the left upper urinary tract. b CT demonstrates diffuse retroperitoneal infiltration of the lymph nodes with periureteral extension (*arrows*) and multiple adenopathies of the mesentery. The infiltration displaces the aorta forward

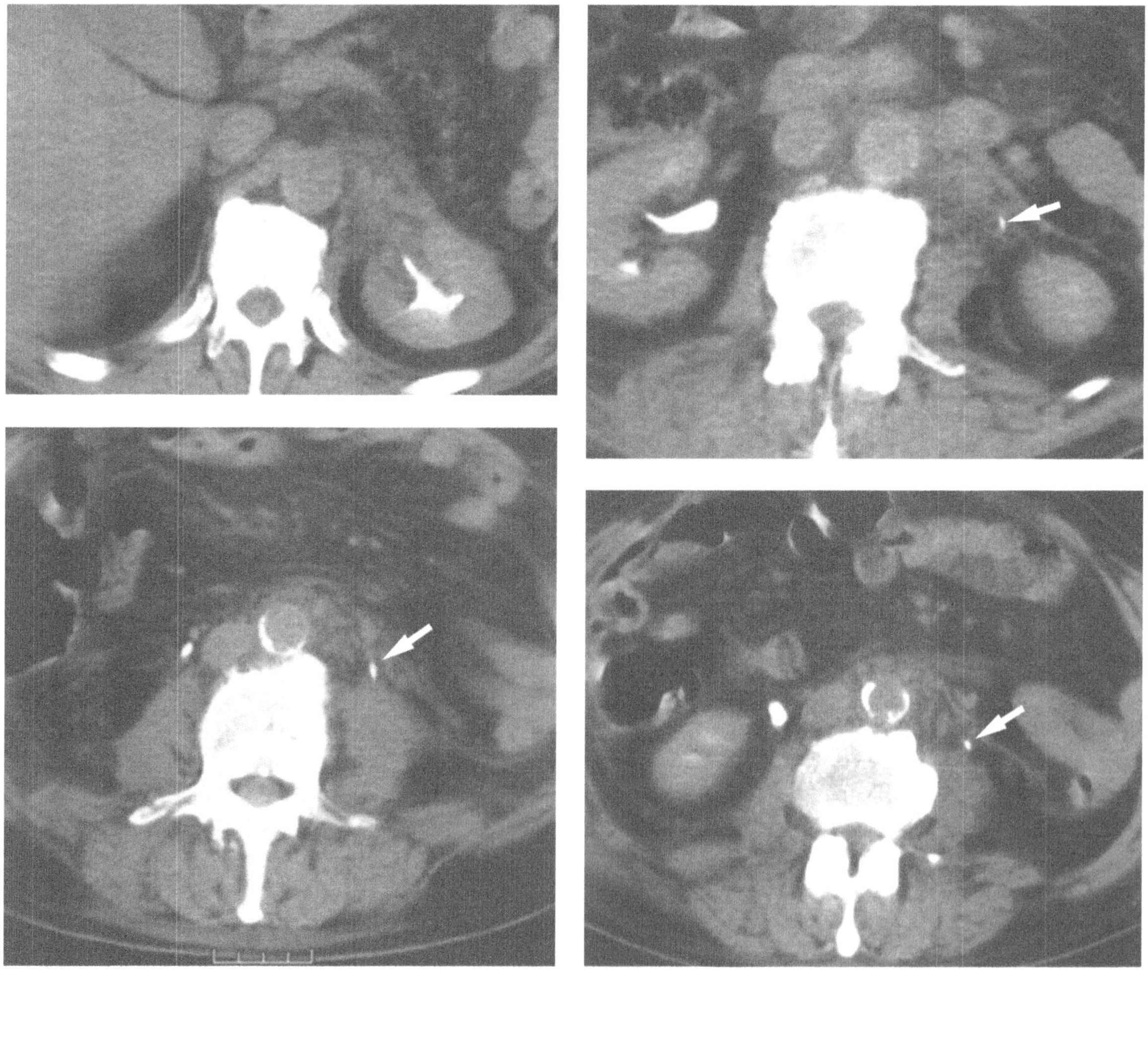

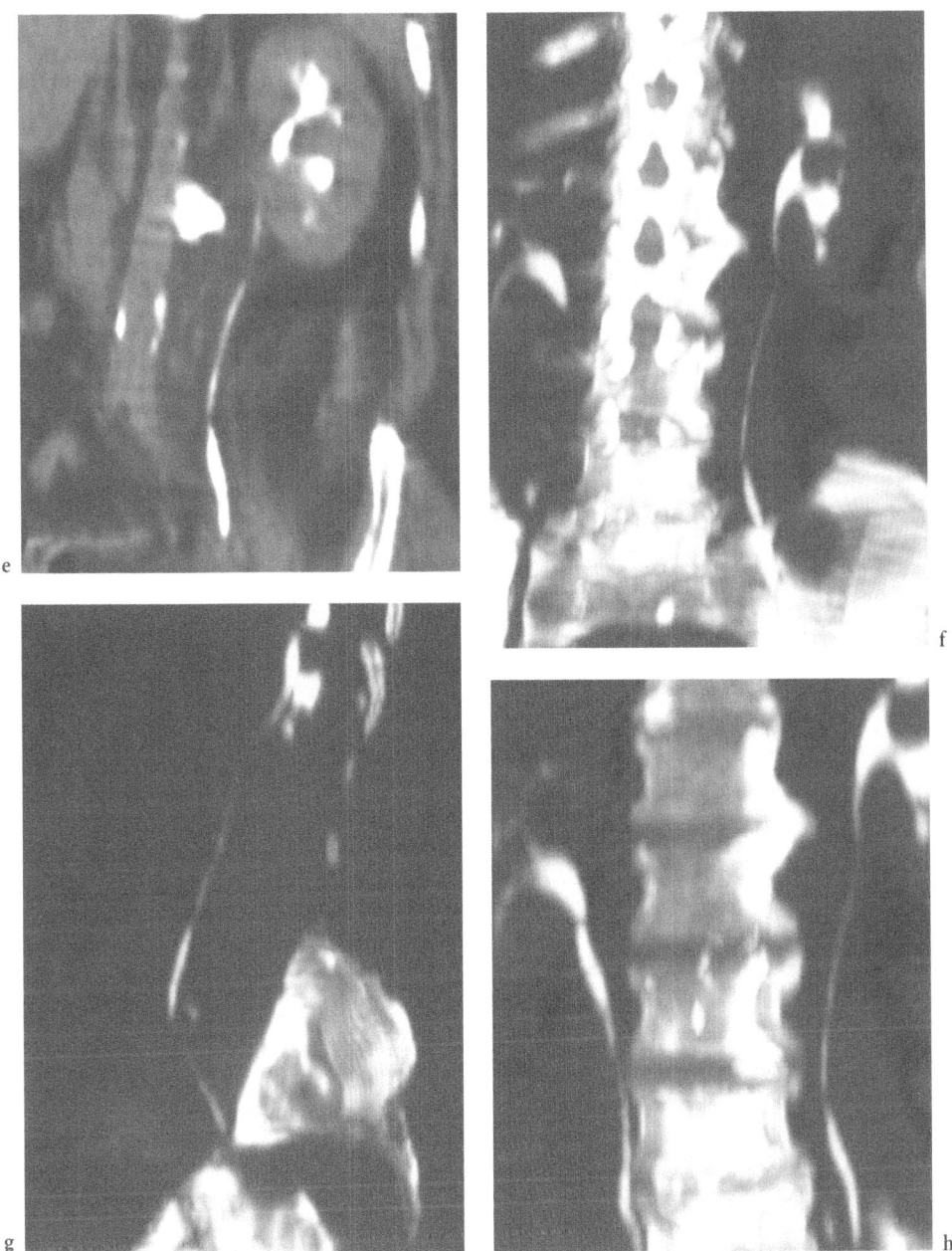

◁ **Fig 9.7a–h.** Periureteral lymphoma. **a–d** Diffuse infiltration of the left periureteral and periaortic areas by multiple soft-tissue nodules with hazy limits and thickening of the left anterior pararenal fascia. The left ureter is surrounded by streaky diffuse densities (*arrows*). **e–h** Several views of the left ureter after MIP reconstructions: tubular and moderately irregular narrowing of the lumbar part of the ureter

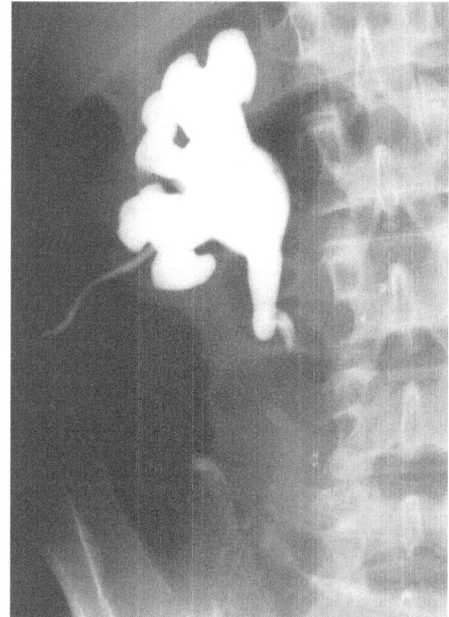

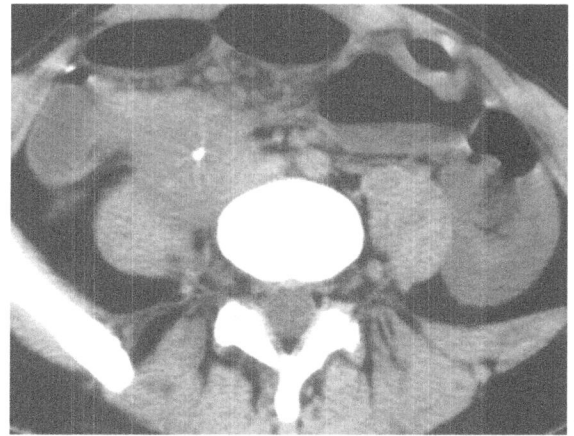

Fig 9.8a, b. Periureteral lymphoma. a Right antegrade pyelography after percutaneous nephrostomy. Ureterohydronephrosis of the upper urinary tract with total obstruction of the middle part of the lumbar ureter without topographic changes. b CT shows a soft-tissue homogeneous and well-limited mass surrounding the ureter, identified by a 2-J catheter. The diagnosis was provided by CT-guided needle biopsy

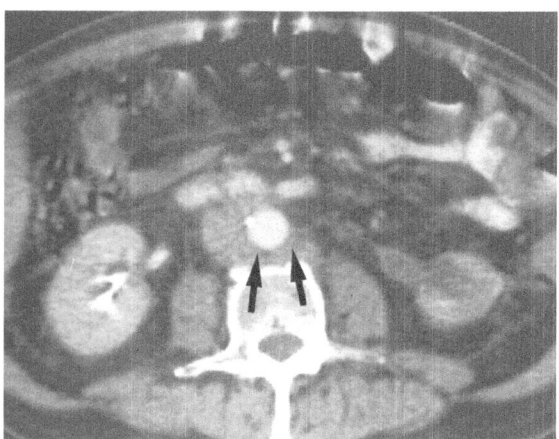

Fig 9.9. Retroperitoneal lymphoma: CT shows a periaortic soft-tissue mass with a pattern similar to that described for benign retroperitoneal fibrosis. Anterior displacement of the aorta (*arrows*) is characteristic of malignant disease and exceptional in benign RPF

which is exceptional in benign retroperitoneal fibrosis (CHISHOLM et al. 1986; DEGESYS et al. 1986) (Fig. 9.9).

Guided biopsy of the retroperitoneal adenopathies may be the only means of reaching a diagnosis if there are no other accessible sites (BARBARIC and McINTOSH 1981). Adequate sample size is necessary for diagnosing and typing a lymphoma, and a large needle (18 G) must be used. A lateovertebral, posterior retroperitoneal approach is the only possibility.

9.2.2.2
Metastatic Adenopathies

Metastatic involvement of the pelvic and retroperitoneal lymph node chains is frequent and is observed in the course of many cancers of the pelvic cavity (uterus, bladder, ovaries, prostate, testicles, rectosigmoid) and also many cancers of the lower limbs (bony or soft-tissue sarcomas, melanomas) or, more rarely, after a bronchopulmonary cancer or cancer of the breast, pancreas, stomach, or colon.

Metastatic lymph node involvement is reflected in nodal hypertrophy associated with architectural changes secondary to the presence of intranodal metastatic islets. There is some controversy concerning the size above which abdominal lymph nodes should be considered definitely abnormal. Difficulty in diagnosis arises if there is lymph node hypertrophy of hyperplastic origin, especially at the pelvic level, secondary to regional infection. Inversely, the lymph nodes may be involved even if hypertrophy is not evident. Lymphography is the only investigation which differentiates between the two types of anomaly: hypertrophy and intranodal defect. However, it is difficult to perform and to interpret and does not investigate all the retroperitoneal lymph node regions. A CT scan merely detects hypertrophy and cannot confirm its metastatic origin.

Node size can be difficult to assess at the retroperitoneal level, related to the longitudinal axis of the nodes which are parallel to the axes of the great vessels. Diagnosis is easier if hypertrophy is marked and involves several nodes which become confluent or clustered (JING et al. 1982). Adenopathies related to testicular cancer may be suggested depending on the site (Fig. 9.10): they displace the renal pelvis and proximal ureter laterally and lie at the level of the para-aortic or paracaval regions in front of the renal hilum. Retroperitoneal and/or pelvic adenopathies have soft-tissue attenuation on CT scan and enhance moderately after injection. In some cases, hypodense, more or less necrotic adenopathies may be observed, in particular after chemotherapy.

Guided transabdominal fine-needle biopsy confirms lymph node invasion with 85% reliability. Its indications depend on the type of primary tumor, the clinical context, or the therapeutic strategy adopted.

9.2.3
Pelvic Tumors

All pelvic tumors may directly affect the ureters, whether they are tumors of the lower urinary apparatus, mainly the bladder and prostate, or tumors of adjacent organs (uterus, ovaries, rectum). They are most often malignant, but benign tumors such as fibromas or ovarian cysts may compress the ureters by displacing them and lead to obstruction. In malignant tumors, ureteral involvement may be only compressive, but more frequently there is extension via the periureteral lymphatics (MARINCEK et al. 1993) or directly by the tumor itself. It is important to identify the ureteral involvement, as it modifies the therapeutic strategy (ROBERT et al. 1997).

Often both ureters are obstructed, and this is reflected by bilateral, often asymmetrical hydro-ureteronephrosis. It may be revealed by the signs of urinary obstruction (low back pain, acute renal failure). In other cases, the tumor is primary and already known, and the urinary tract must routinely be evaluated when assessing the extent of disease.

Ultrasonography is at present the essential modality to evaluate the ureteral impact. It locates the obstruction and, in emergency, percutaneous nephrostomy can be carried out under ultrasonographic guidance. It can detect an expansive process within the pelvis. EU is no longer used to assess the spread of pelvic tumors (GOLDMAN et al. 1984).

CT investigation evaluates the tumor and its impact on the ureter and gives a frontal view of this impact in urographic pictures following CT examination, if renal function is adequate, or provides reconstructed urographic representation of the dilated urinary

tract (Fig. 9.11). CT can sometimes help to indicate the mechanism of obstruction: While extrinsic compression cannot be differentiated from extension to the ureteral wall, it is possible to detect periureteral extension, especially in the context of prostate tumor. In such cases, there is tissue infiltration of the periureteral pelvic fat. If the ureter is opacified it can be identified within this infiltration. MRI is more efficient, in particular for this urographic representation, because it does not rely on urinary excretion of contrast medium. It is more informative than

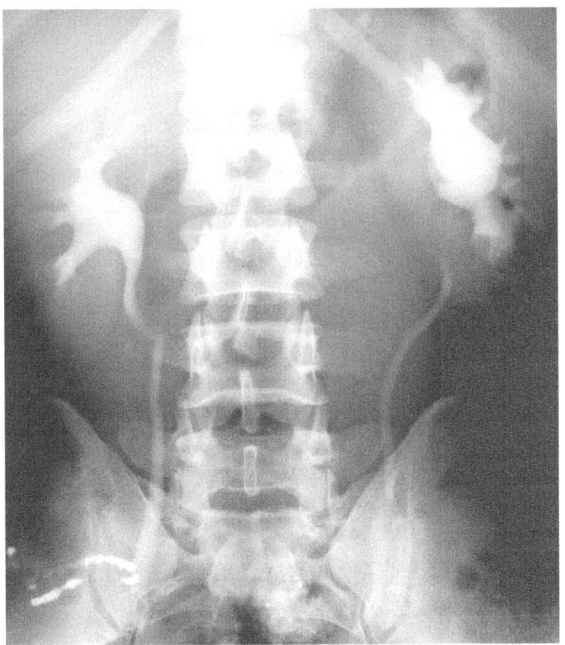
a

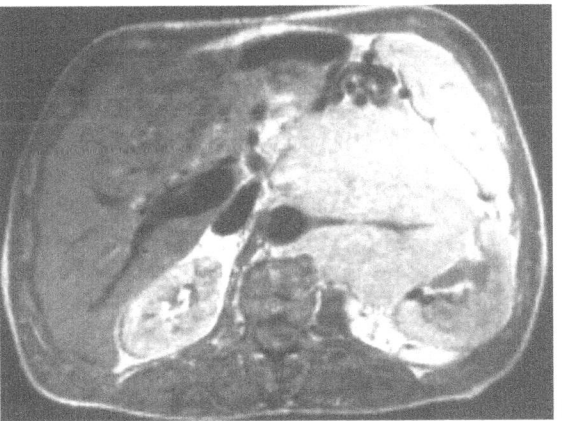
b

Fig 9.10a, b. Retroperitoneal adenopathies related to a testicular seminoma. a EU: lateral displacement of the left kidney with curvilinear deviation of the proximal ureter and moderate ureterohydronephrosis. b Axial MRI slice: SE T_2-weighted sequence shows displacement of the kidney by a lobulated mass with hypersignal developed around the renal pedicle, which is stretched

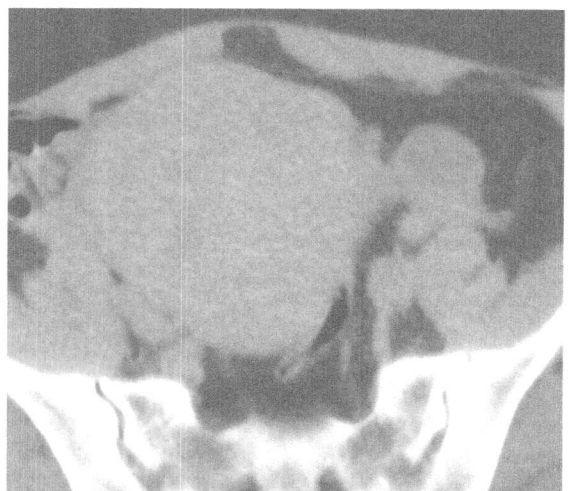

Fig 9.11a–c. Ureteral compression by a uterine fibroma. a CT axial slice shows a large soft-tissue homogeneous and well-limited uterine mass. b, c Urographic pictures after MIP and SSD reconstruction demonstrate right ureterohydronephrosis with compression of the lower part of the right ureter by the uterine mass

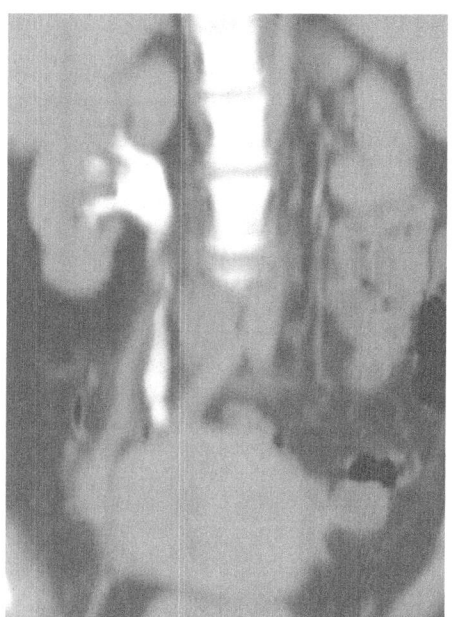

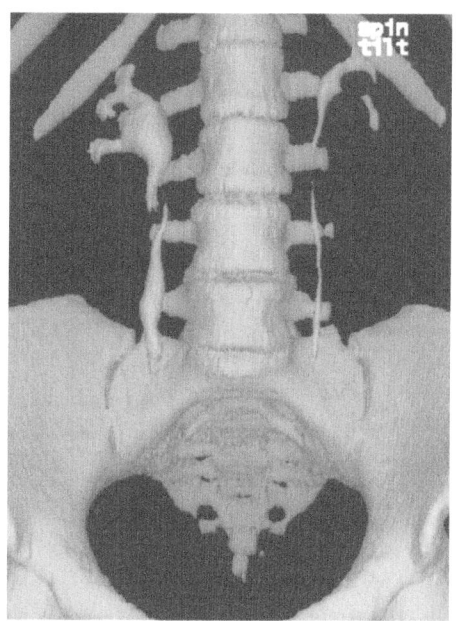

CT concerning regional and lymph node extension (Hricak 1986; Mezrich 1994). Tumor extension can be seen around the dilated ureter, which appears as a rounded structure with decreased signal intensity on T_1-weighted sequences and increased intensity on T_2.

Opacification of the ureter (on urograms following CT examination) makes it possible to analyze ureteral stenosis. The ureter is visualized on urographic images after CT scan, on MR urography or, above all, by direct opacification techniques used routinely before any attempt is made at drainage by ureteral intubation (Fig. 9.12). This stenosis involves the pelvic ureter at a variable height and is more or less bilateral (Fig. 9.13). The ureter is often displaced, either laterally or medially. Medial displacement of one of the two ureters can be seen with some gyne-cological tumors (ovarian tumor or uterine tumor within the broad ligament). Medial displacement may be observed in neoplastic pelvic fibrosis. It must not be mistaken for the medial ureteral displacement observed after therapeutic excision of the perineum and rectum. If there is any doubt, CT scan will exclude a recurrence. Stenosis is not always characteristic. Usually, blockage is total and sudden. Less commonly, the stricture is opacified, extends for several centimeters, is regular and nonspecific, more rarely irregular and suggestive of the diagnosis. Direct opacification techniques are generally the first stage of ureteral intubation using a double-J pigtail stent for urinary drainage while awaiting specific treatment of the tumoral lesion. Some of these tumors may recur after surgery and cause ureteral obstruction which

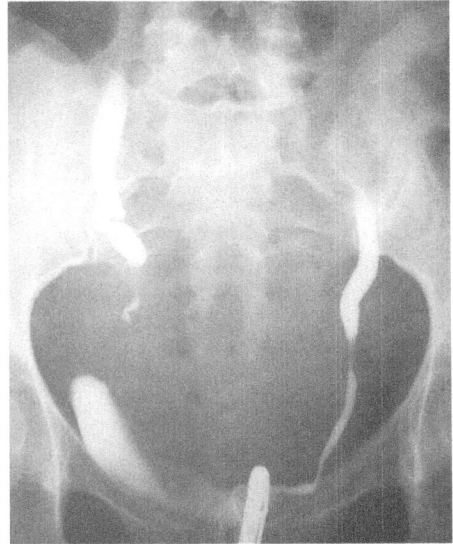
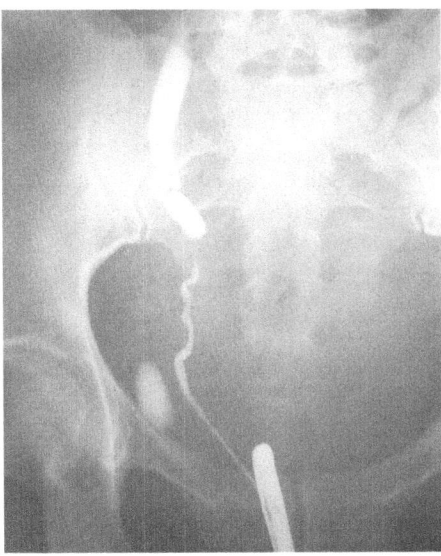

Fig 9.12a, b. Ureteral stenosis secondary to a cervical carcinoma. a, b Retrograde pyelography performed before retrograde 2-J placement for bilateral obstruction of the lower part of both ureters: smooth ureteral encasement on the left side, irregular stenosis on the right side, with possible tumoral infiltration of the ureteral wall

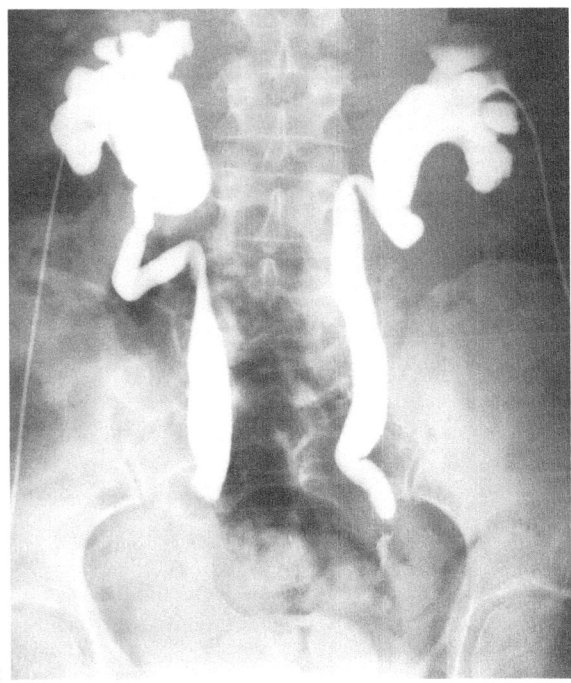

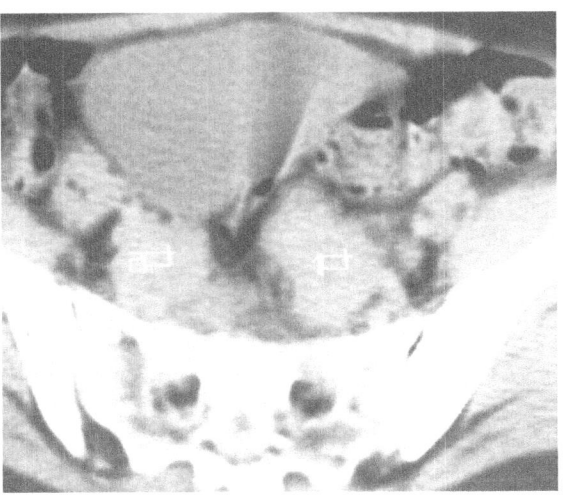

Fig 9.13a, b. Bilateral ureteral obstruction by a recurrent cervical carcinoma. a Bilateral antegrade pyelography performed after percutaneous nephrostomy for subacute renal failure. Bilateral and total obstruction of the pelvic part of the ureter. b CT slice at the level of obstruction shows bilateral soft-tissue masses with irregular outlines (p) corresponding to periureteral recurrence

can be detected by ultrasonography. MR urography may allow morphological evaluation of the effect of obstruction and differentiate a recurrent tumor from fibrosis after radiation or surgery: Recurrence is suggested by the appearance of a mass when compared with a reference CT or MR image and by a high T_2 signal with enhancement after gadolinium injection.

9.3
Retroperitoneal and Pelvic Fibrosis

Retroperitoneal fibrosis (RPF) is characterized by a localized region of reactive fibrosis, encasing the organs that traverse the retroperitoneum and principally the ureters and great vessels (AMIS 1991).

Since the descriptions by ALBARRAN and ORMOND, a variety of benign and malignant conditions have been reported as being at the origin of this entity, but the majority of cases are considered idiopathic (ALBARRAN 1905; ORMOND 1960). The diagnostic approach to RPF has been modified by advances in imaging techniques which now directly visualize the fibrotic plaque and its impact on the urinary tract, and so can follow the response to treatment (JOFFRE et al. 1989). The main difficulty is still differentiation between benign and malignant RPF, and in certain cases only histology can provide the answer.

9.3.1
Histology

The histological lesions of benign RPF are identical in appearance, whatever the etiology (CHOMETTE et al. 1986; LEPOR and WALSH 1979; MITCHINSON 1970). Gross examination shows a whitish, hard plaque with a well-defined margin, which rarely extends beyond the lateral border of the psoas and is often centered on the aortic bifurcation. Involvement is most common over the sacral promontory, from L-4 to S-1. The plaque may extend upward and reach the renal pedicle and sometimes even further toward the mediastinum, or extend downward along the iliac vessels. More rarely, it is located at the pelvic level along the iliac vessels and reaches the pelvic organs (COPLAND et al. 1981; DALLA-PALMA et al. 1981). It may also continue anteriorly along the mesenteric root. The ureters and great vessels are encased and compressed by the plaque. Cases of benign RPF extending to the ureteral wall have been described, however, as have others which spare the ureters (FRENS et al. 1982).

Microscopic examination shows a chronic inflammatory reaction of sclerosing fibrous and fatty tissue. Inflammatory foci consist of collagen clumps separated by lymphocytes, fibroblasts, and macrophages. Initially, inflammation is marked, with proliferation and vasculitis. Cellular activity decreases from the center toward the periphery of the plaque. Advanced lesions are characterized by avascular, acellular fibrous tissue (MITCHINSON 1970).

Malignant RPF is secondary to dissemination of small foci of metastatic neoplastic cells in the retroperitoneum, leading to a predominant local desmoplastic reaction (MIEZA et al. 1982). Diagnosis is difficult, as fibrosis can mask the neoplastic cells, especially if the primary cancer is unrecognized.

9.3.2
Etiology

Where there is no evident etiology, the first diagnosis is idiopathic retroperitoneal fibrosis (LEPOR and WALSH 1979). This accounts for about two thirds of RPF cases. As idiopathic RPF may be associated with other systemic disorders that have a fibrotic component, it has been included among the multifocal systemic disorders which arise from a disturbed immunological mechanism, as yet unknown. Benign RPF may be associated with fibrotic manifestations outside the retroperitoneum: mediastinal fibrosis, Riedel fibrosing thyroiditis, sclerosing cholangitis, retractile mesenteritis (LITTLEJOHN and KEYSTONE 1981). In about 15% of cases it may be associated with collagen disorders (AMIS 1991; KOEP and ZUIDEMA 1977). A vascular origin has been suggested, since the inflammatory manifestations predominate around the aorta: There is a frequent association with atheromatosis, and some authors consider the fibrosis a reaction to the presence of insoluble lipids (MITCHINSON 1986). However, this does not explain the cases of benign RPF in children.

Excessive use of certain medications is the most common etiology (12%). Methysergide, an ergot derivative, is most often incriminated (STECKER et al. 1974). Prolonged, uninterrupted use for several years is required for the development of benign RPF. However, its administration is currently decreasing. Other medications incriminated are bromocriptine, used in the treatment of certain forms of Parkinson's disease, certain analgesics and antibiotics, beta-blockers, methyldopa and hydralazine.

Benign RPF can more rarely be found after retroperitoneal "aggression". This may be sequelae of an old injury with urohematoma, or long-term complications of aortoiliac or spinal surgery or of retroperitoneal radiotherapy. Fibrosis can also be a reaction to adjacent inflammatory or infectious disorders (appendicitis, retroperitoneal abscess, spondylodiscitis, sigmoiditis, pancreatitis). Accidental leakage of barium sulfate in the retroperitoneum after barium enema frequently leads to a fibrotic reaction with obstruction of both ureters (WALTHER et al. 1987).

Perianeurysmal fibrosis, also called inflammatory aneurysm, is a relatively frequent complication of aortic aneurysms (5%–10%). Its pathological features are similar to those described for aortic atheroma (CULLENWARD et al. 1986; MITCHINSON 1984) and are dealt with elsewhere in this chapter.

Malignant RPF represents about 10% of retroperitoneal fibrosis (USHER et al. 1977). It is secondary to dissemination in the retroperitoneal fat of small

Table 9.1. Causes of retroperitoneal fibrosis (RPF)

Type of RPF	Cause
Primitive (or idiopathic) benign	
Secondary benign	Prolonged use of drugs: Methysergide Bromocriptine Beta-blockers Perianeurysmal and perivascular fibrosis Local pathology: Urohematoma Irradiation Gastrointestinal inflammation Barium extravasation Systemic fibrosing disease
Malignant	

metastatic foci, generally hematogenous, more rarely carried by the lymphatic system or the vessels around the ureter (MARINCEK et al. 1993). These metastatic foci give rise to a desmoplastic reaction within which it is always difficult to find neoplastic cells. The primary tumors most often incriminated are tumors of the breast, lung, uterus, prostate, stomach, colon, and pancreas, as well as melanoma.

9.3.3
Clinical Presentation

Retroperitoneal fibrosis is rare, occurring in about one per 200,000 population. It develops in the fifth decade, and men appear to predominate, except for drug-related benign RPF, where the sex ratio is reversed.

The clinical signs are due to the compression of retroperitoneal structures, principally the ureters. Ureteral obstruction is the main manifestation, reflected by low back pain, progressive renal failure, and sometimes renal colic or acute renal failure (ARGER et al. 1973; LEPOR and WALSH 1979). More rarely, signs of vascular compression may be observed: edema of the lower limbs, thrombophlebitis, hydrocele. Lower limb ischemia or, less commonly, gastrointestinal or renal ischemia have been described. Benign RPF may also be manifested by general signs: acute or chronic low back pain, deterioration of the general condition, weight loss, gastrointestinal problems. Elevated ESR and an inflammatory syndrome are nearly always observed.

9.3.4
Radiological Findings

New imaging techniques such as ultrasonography, CT scanning and MRI have profoundly modified

the investigation of RPF, providing more precise information on diagnosis, extent and, above all, the evolution (WITTEN 1990).

9.3.4.1
EU

EU has been a modality of choice for investigation and surveillance of RPF (JOFFRE et al. 1993). However, its status has now changed, as most of the presenting signs tend to require ultrasonography and/or CT scan for the initial evaluation. On the other hand, acquisition of urograms after CT scan must be the rule. Classically, EU demonstrates chronic obstruction of the upper urinary tract associated with ureteral abnormalities (Fig. 9.14). In 70% of cases, obstruction affects both ureters but is asymmetrical. It may, however, involve only a single ureter and is sometimes accompanied by a silent kidney (ARGER et al. 1973; JOFFRE et al. 1989).

Ureteral abnormalities are seen as ureteral stenosis at L4–5, with the stenotic part drawn toward the midline (AMIS 1991). Stenosis is regular, concentric, and progressive. However, this is seen in many ureteral disorders. In addition, some appearances are difficult to diagnose (PERSKY and HUUS 1974):
- Unilateral stenosis
- Advanced obstruction with very weak opacification of the urinary tract
- Absence of ureteral displacement

Moreover, medial deviation is nonspecific and may be encountered in normal subjects (SALDINO and PALUBINSKAS 1972). This sign is thus of value only when associated with an obstruction (ARGER et al. 1973).

EU is suggestive in half the cases but is no longer adequate for diagnosis and is rarely helpful in differentiating between benign and malignant RPF. It remains useful for assessing response to medical therapy.

9.3.4.2
Antegrade or Retrograde Pyelography

Classically, these investigations are necessary if the ureters are not sufficiently opacified on EU (MICHEL et al. 1986). Their main role is to allow percutaneous nephrostomy drainage and, if necessary, ureteral intubation with a double-J pigtail stent. Ureteral opacification shows the same abnormalities as urographic study, however, with little apparent narrowing, which would be in favor of a disorder of ureteral

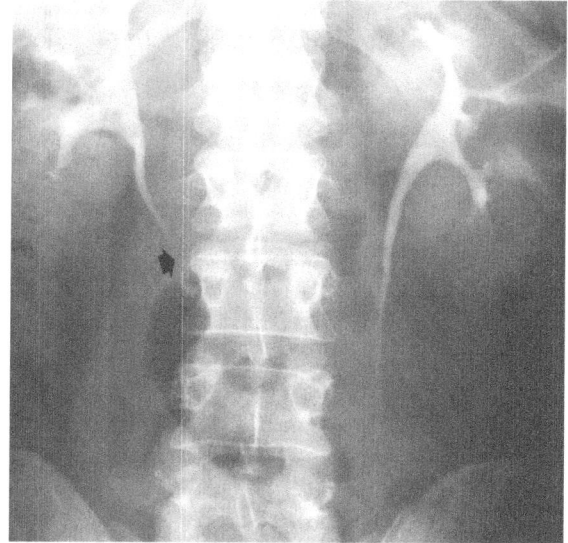

a

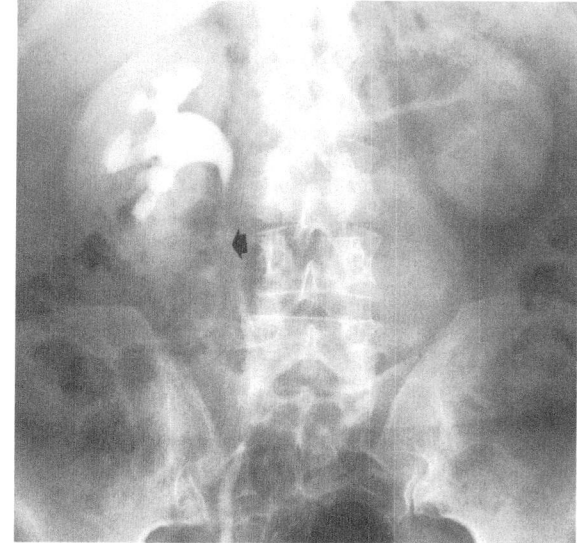

b

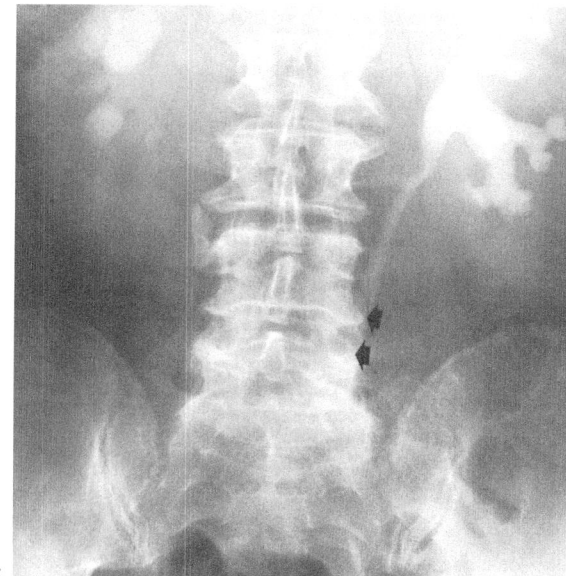

c

Fig 9.14. Different urographic patterns of a benign RPF. **a** Discrete stenosis of the right lumbar ureter (*arrow*) without obstruction and with medial displacement. Absence of abnormalities on the left side. **b** Mute left kidney with moderate bulging of left psoas muscle. Moderate obstruction of the right kidney related to a stenosis of the right lumbar ureter without medial displacement (*arrow*). **c** Asymmetrical bilateral obstruction with faint opacification on the right dilated side and moderate dilatation on the left side. The left lumbar ureter is attracted toward the midline (*arrows*)

peristalsis secondary to benign RPF (Fig. 9.15). This is confirmed by the ease of ureteral intubation, apparently without hindrance (LALLI 1977). Irregular stenosis suggests malignant RPF, but most commonly the appearance is identical to that of benign stenosis. Sometimes obstruction is total with no further opacification, whether fibrosis is malignant or benign in nature (Fig. 9.16).

9.3.4.3
Angiographic Investigations

Angiography is indicated only exceptionally today. Iliocavography can be used to guide insertion of a caval stent if the patient presents with venous complications

such as thromboembolic symptoms. Aortography is useful only if there are signs of lower limb ischemia.

9.3.4.4
Ultrasonography
(CORNUD et al. 1983; SANDERS et al. 1977)

Ultrasonography is often the initial evaluation in abdominal pain or urinary complaints. It detects urinary tract obstruction with various degrees of hydroureteronephrosis, unilateral or more often bilateral and asymmetrical, associated with more or less marked thinning of the parenchyma. The fibrous plaque is often difficult to visualize because of intervening gastrointestinal structures. It presents

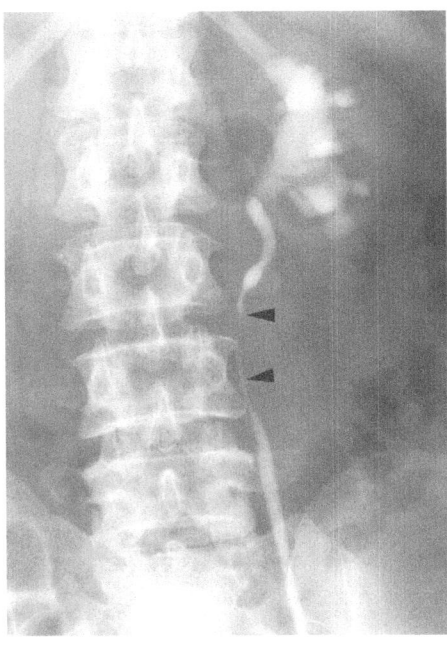

Fig 9.15. Benign RPF aspect on retrograde pyelography: Opacification of the left ureter shows smooth and moderate stenosis (*arrowheads*) with medial displacement and dilatation of the upper urinary tract

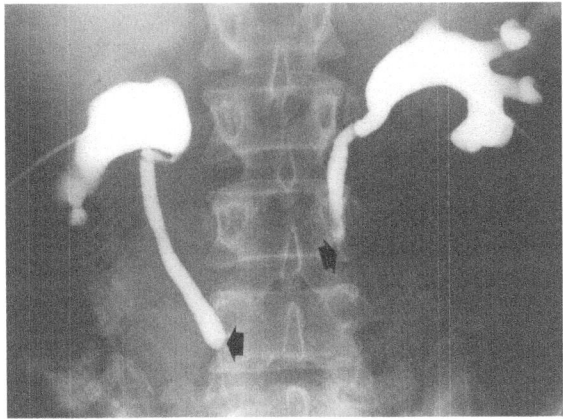

Fig 9.16. Benign RPF aspect on antegrade pyelography: Bilateral percutaneous nephrostomy for ureteral obstruction related to post-irradiation RPF. Total obstruction with medial deviation of the lumbar ureters (*arrows*)

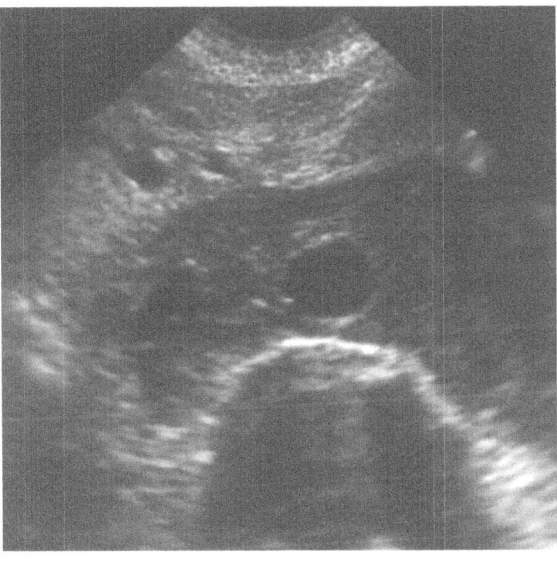

Fig 9.17. Ultrasonography aspect of a benign RPF: Perivascular hypoechoic and well-limited mass surrounding the IVC and aorta

as a hypoechoic mass, usually with a regular outline, extending anterior to the great vessels at the level of the bifurcation (Fig. 9.17).

9.3.4.5
CT Scan

CT scanning is the technique of choice, visualizing the fibrous plaque and its effect on the urinary tract (LEMAITRE et al. 1984). Contrast media are required to identify the great vessels within the fibrous plaques and to assess the effect of ureteral obstruction on renal function. Opacification of the urinary tract can be demonstrated either by multiplanar reconstruction or, more simply, by radiographs taken following CT examination (LEMAITRE et al. 2000).

The classic appearance of RPF is that of a tissue mass lying anterior to the great vessels, in particular the aorta. The anterior border is clearly outlined and usually convex. The plaque extends laterally and abuts on the psoas muscles, infiltrating the fatty space around the ureters, which are drawn toward it (FEINSTEIN et al. 1981) (Fig. 9.18). The plaque lies anterior to the sacral promontory, centered over L4–5 and S-1, and often has a linear extension with thick-

ening of the anterior pararenal fascia (BRUN et al. 1981). It has the same attenuation as the psoas muscle on unenhanced images. On post-contrast CT images, enhancement varies depending upon the maturity and the degree of inflammation of the fibrous tissue (KOTTRA and DUNNICK 1986). Uptake of contrast medium is sometimes uneven and often increased at the periphery of the plaque, whereas the central part is weakly enhanced (Fig. 9.19). Inflammation, in fact, develops from the center toward the periphery of the plaque, the center being the oldest and most

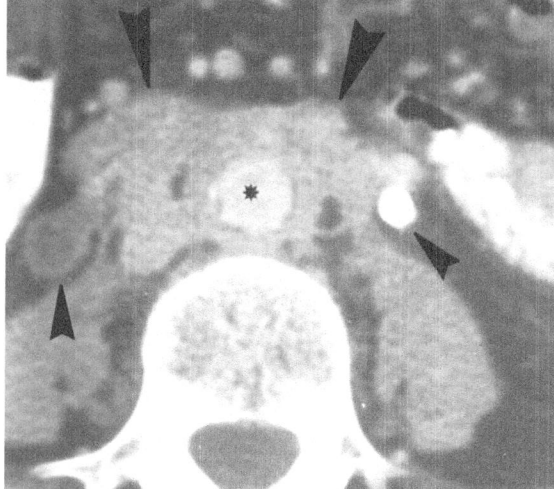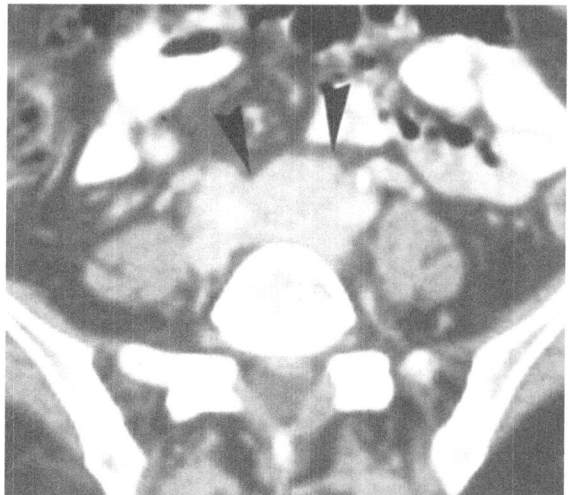

Fig 9.18a, b. Computed tomography of benign RPF. **a** Soft-tissue mass developed around the aorta (*asterisk*) with an anterior border clearly outlined (*arrowheads*). The plaque extends laterally infiltrating the fascias and the fatty space around the ureters (*arrowheads*). The left ureter is opacified, the right ureter is not. The IVC is not identified. **b** Extension of the plaque around the iliac vessels and anterior to the sacral promontory (*arrowheads*)

fibrotic part (DALLA-PALMA et al. 1981). Injection of contrast medium visualizes the great vessels. The aorta is well opacified and in benign forms is only exceptionally displaced anteriorly; its wall is often thickened, atheromatous and calcified (BROOKS et al. 1989). The vena cava is often poorly visualized and is sometimes thrombotic above the plaque (CHISHOLM et al. 1986). Sections at the level of the kidneys reveal hydroureteronephrosis, unilateral or more often bilateral, immediately above the plaque. If the plaque extends to the kidneys, dilatation is slight due to nondistensibility of the renal pelvis. Multiplanar

reconstructions give a urographic representation of obstruction above the plaque.

A number of unusual appearances may be encountered and make diagnosis difficult. The plaque may extend upward around the kidneys and/or along the renal pedicles in the sinus (ROTHSCHILD et al. 1986), sometimes above the kidneys toward the hepatic pedicle or the mesentery, sometimes with stenosis of the gastrointestinal tract and more rarely the mediastinum (DEGESYS et al. 1986; HULNICK et al. 1988). Exclusively pelvic forms exist, as well as forms located only around both kidneys (COPLAND et al.

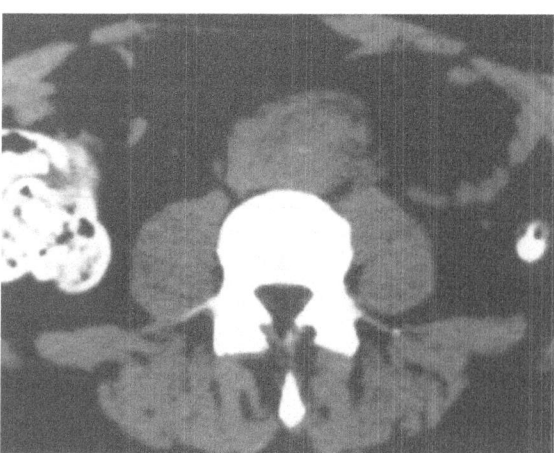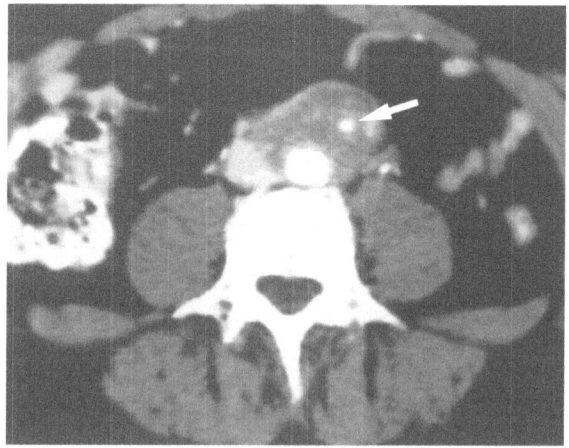

Fig 9.19a, b. Computed tomography of a benign RPF. **a** Slice before injection shows the plaque with an attenuation similar to the psoas muscle. **b** Following injection of CM, enhancement of the peripheral part of the plaque more than of the central part. Inferior mesenteric artery is surrounded by the plaque (*arrow*)

1981; AYUSO et al. 1999) (Fig. 9.20). These perirenal forms reach the sinus and infiltrate the renal pelvis and the calices without involving the ureter (YANCEY and KAUDE 1988). The morphology of the plaque may vary: pseudonodular appearance mimicking retroperitoneal adenopathies, pseudotumoral or pseudocystic areas, or a limited, scarcely visible form generally located at the crossing of the ureter and the iliac vessels (FELDBERG and VAN WAES 1987). The ureters may be spared.

CT scan may reveal the primary cause: Besides the perianeurysmal forms discussed below, uro-hematoma, gastrointestinal abscess, and barium granuloma may be found. Malignant RPF may have exactly the same appearance (CHISHOLM et al. 1986), although certain signs may be suggestive: more extensive areas of fibrosis, often a lower location, anterior displacement of the great vessels (Figs. 9.21, 9.22). The neoplastic context is not always evident, and trial treatment with corticosteroids can be given before biopsy is considered. These particular forms mainly raise the possibility of retroperitoneal neoplastic extension and above all of retroperitoneal lymphomas. Infiltrative retroperitoneal lymphomas are usually easy to diagnose. Confluent adenopathies may simulate a fibrous plaque but usually present as a much more extensive polylobular, multinodular mass. The ureters tend to be displaced laterally and the great vessels may be displaced anteriorly, but these changes are not always specific (DEGESYS et al. 1986). Retroperitoneal amyloidosis is difficult to differentiate from retroperitoneal fibrosis but remains exceptional (GLYNN et al. 1989).

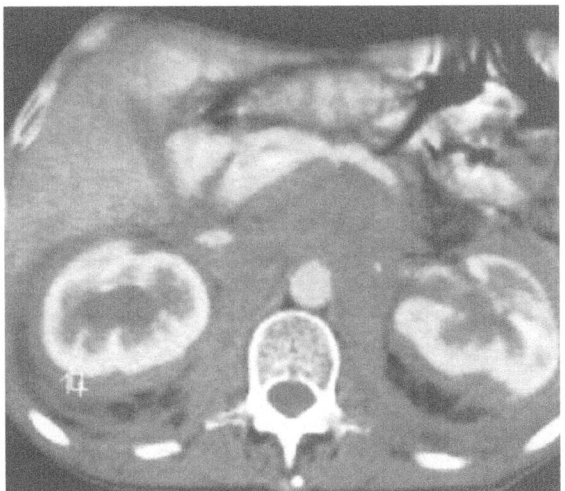

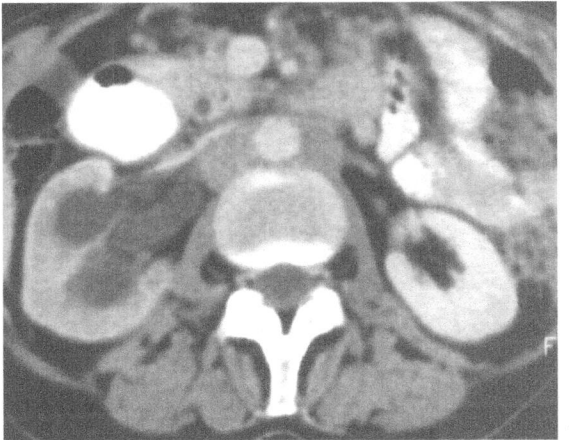

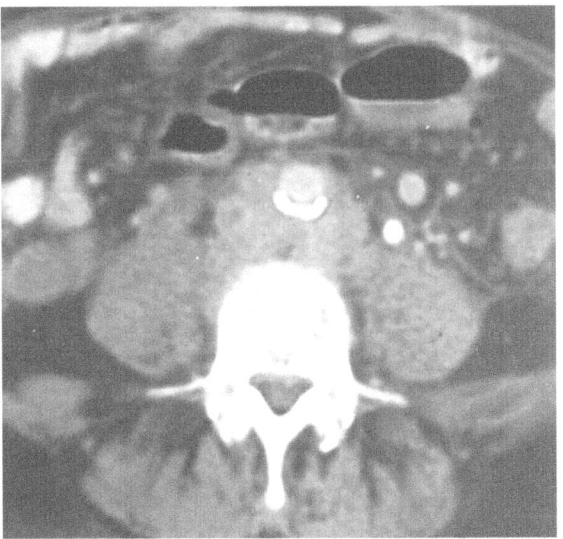

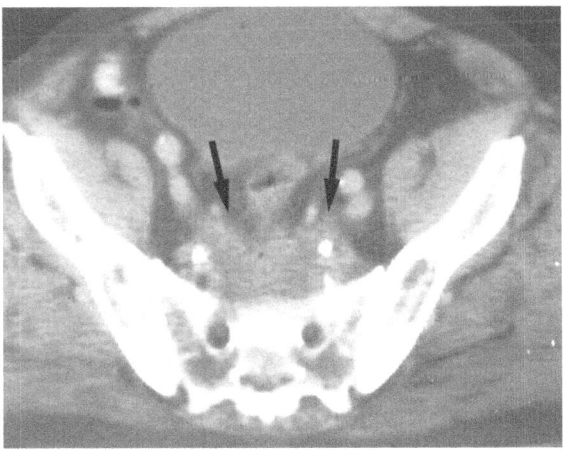

Fig 9.20. Computed tomography of a benign pelvic RPF: Development of the plaque anterior to the sacrum with encasement of both pelvic ureters (*arrows*)

Fig 9.21a–c. Some aspects of malignant RPF. **a** Extensive soft-tissue mass developed around the aorta with perirenal bilateral infiltration. **b** Localized periaortic plaque similar to a benign RPF. **c** Anterior displacement of calcified aorta, which is characteristic but not specific of malignant RPF

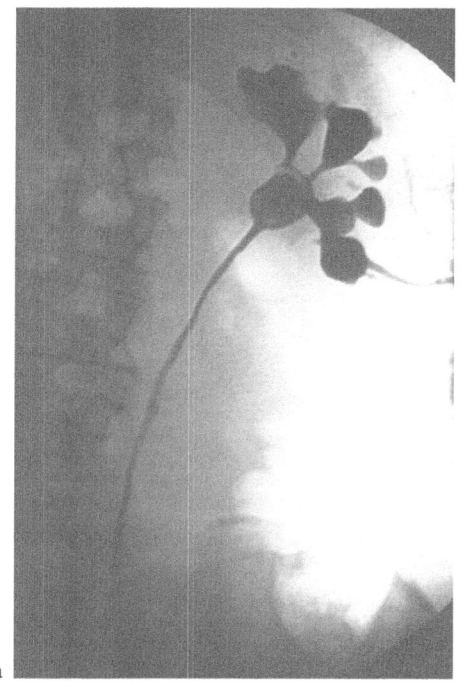

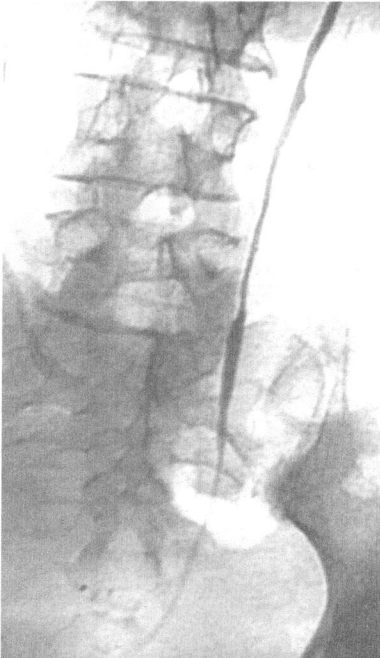

Fig 9.22a–d. Malignant RPF. a, b Antegrade left pyelography shows multiple irregular narrowing of the whole ureter. c, d Computed tomography shows diffuse soft-tissue mass infiltrating the retroperitoneal space with extension to the pelvic cavity

a

b

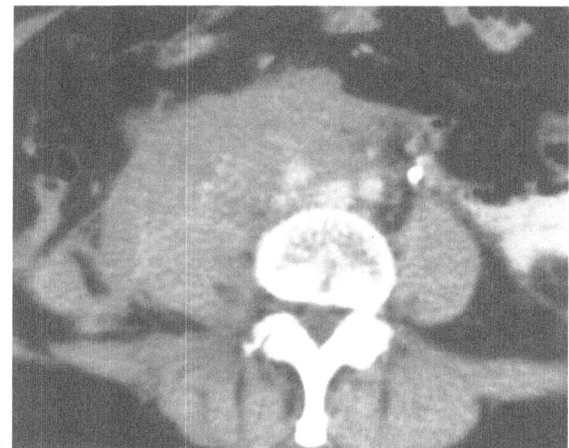

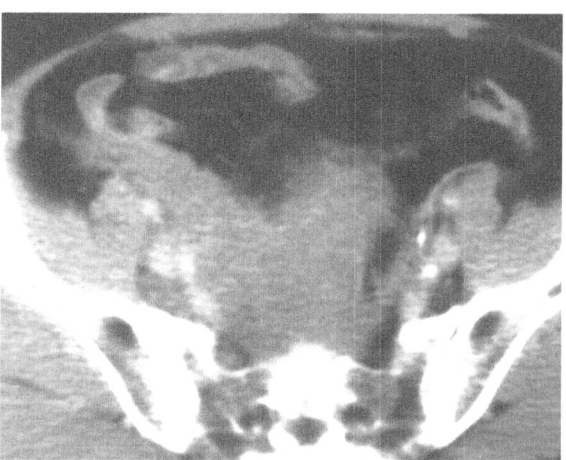

c

d

9.3.4.6
MRI

MRI has definite advantages over the CT scan: three-dimensional evaluation of the plaque, urographic and vascular visualization, better tolerance by patients with renal failure, and characterization of the plaque. MRI effectively distinguishes between active inflammatory tissue and mature, organized fibrous tissue. Recent benign RPF has decreased signal intensity on T_1- and increased signal on T_2-weighted sequences when there is a considerable inflammatory component (Fig. 9.23). Advanced forms or those which have been treated by corticosteroids have decreased

signal intensity on T_2-weighted sequences (BROOKS et al. 1990). Use of gadolinium chelates provides further information related to differences in vascularization: MRI differentiates mature benign RPF from malignant RPF, which has increased signal intensity on T_2-weighted sequences (HRICAK et al. 1983). However, differentiation is not possible with early forms in the inflammatory stage (ARRIVE et al. 1989). Both malignant and benign RPF enhance after gadolinium injection (MULLIGAN et al. 1989; YANCEY and KAUDE 1988).

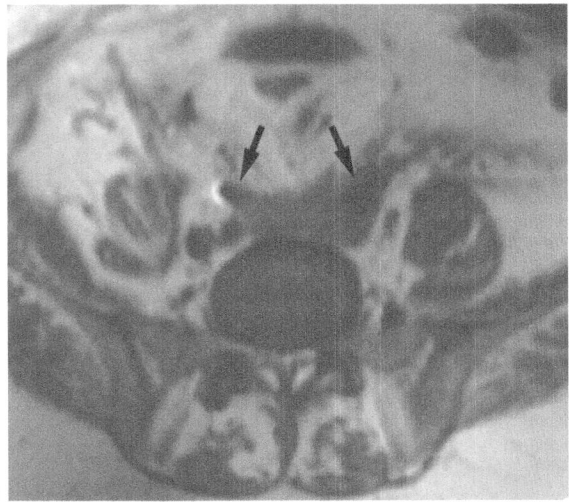
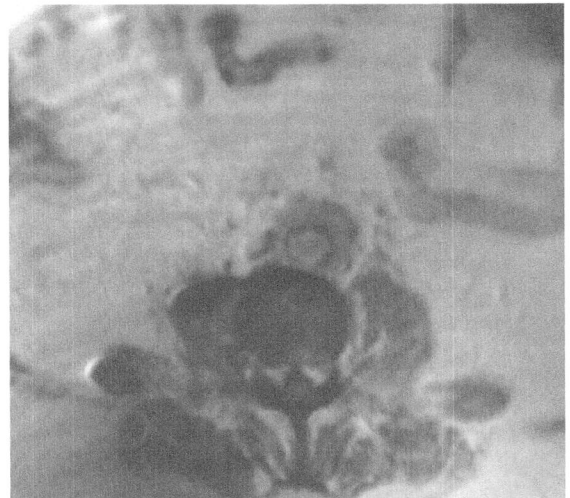
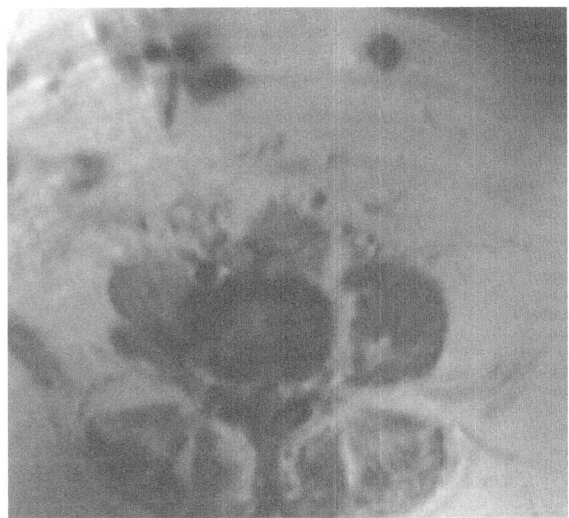

Fig 9.23a–c. MRI of benign RPF. **a** T$_1$-weighted slice at the level of the promontory shows the plaque with a low signal intensity. The plaque includes the ureters (*arrows*). **b, c** T$_2$-weighted slices showing an increased signal corresponding to a moderate inflammatory component

9.3.4.7
Periureteral Malignant Fibrosis

The abundance of lymphatics and blood vessels around the ureter explain the frequency of metastatic spread only in this area (MARINCEK et al. 1993),

The primary tumors most often concerned are tumors of the bladder, prostate and cervix, but distant primary tumors can produce periureteral metastases (pancreas, stomach, breast, colon). Similarly with more diffuse malignant RPF, such metastases tend to give a desmoplastic reaction, which explains the radiological findings (see Chap. 6).

Antegrade or retrograde pyelography shows multiple narrowing of the lumen with a filiform and irregular stenosis and sometimes a corkscrew pattern. Absence of ureteral displacement is characteristic (Figs. 9.24, 9.25).

CT slices demonstrate ureteral wall thickening with streaky densities of the periureteral space. The perirenal fascias can be thickened, and in some cases the ureter is surrounded by multiple small, nodular soft-tissue densities corresponding to periureteral hypertrophied lymph nodes (Fig. 9.25). In some cases it is difficult to differentiate thickening of the ureteral wall by metastatic disease from periureteral neoplastic infiltration (Fig. 9.26). Periureteral histological needle biopsy is needed in these cases, particularly if the primary tumor is unknown (USHER et al. 1977).

9.3.4.8
Interventional Radiology

Interventional radiology plays an important role in RPF. It provides further diagnostic information for guided biopsy, although this is of limited value as

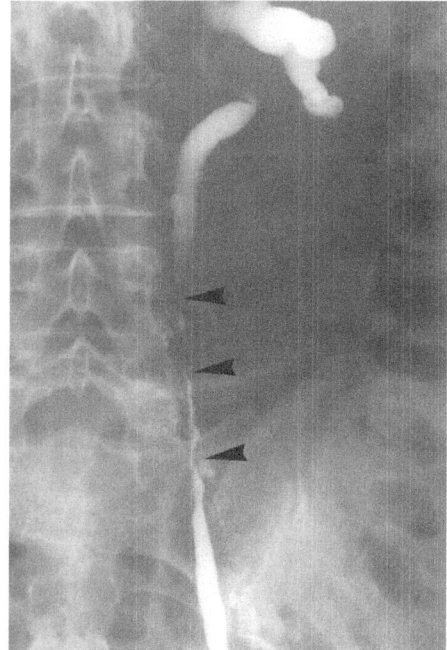

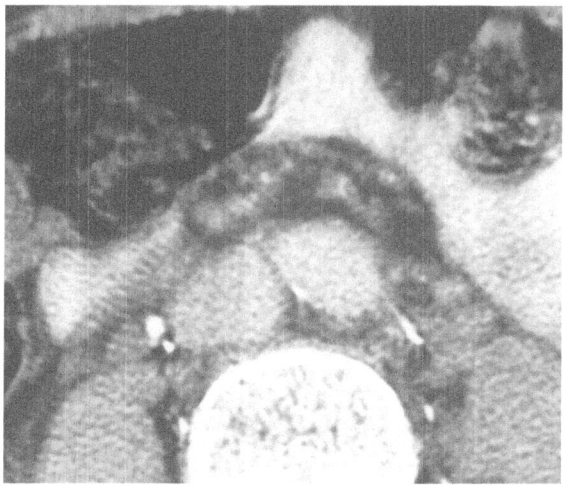

Fig 9.24a, b. Periureteral malignant RPF after cervical cancer. a Retrograde pyelography shows irregular stenosis of the left lumbar ureter without deviation and with multiple irregular imprints, probably related to adenopathies poorly opacified after a previous lymphography (*arrowheads*). (From JOFFRE et al. 1993) b CT shows multiple nodular periureteral soft-tissue densities with tissular heterogeneous infiltration of the periureteral fat

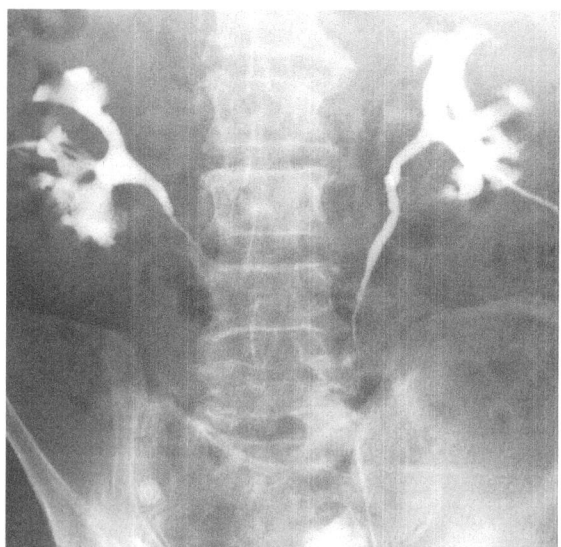

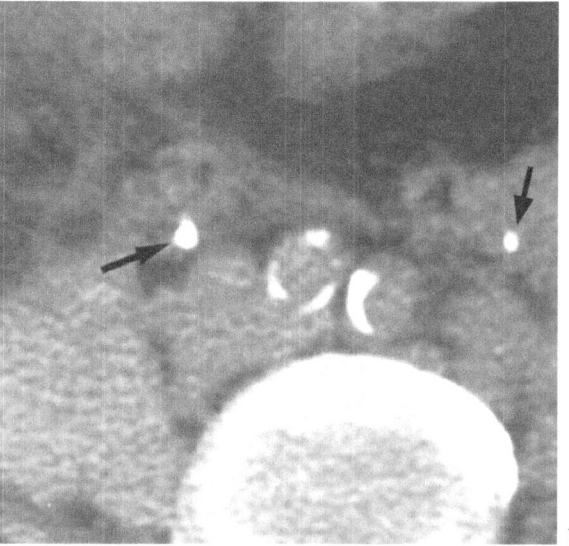

Fig 9.25a, b. Periureteral malignant RPF after bladder cancer. a Bilateral antegrade pyelography after percutaneous nephrostomy shows irregular and extensive stenosis of both ureters. b CT shows irregular infiltration of the periureteral fat of both ureters with mass effect on the left side (*arrows*)

it rarely retrieves neoplastic cells, which are often difficult to identify within the fibrotic desmoplastic reaction. It is of interest, however, for detecting a lymphoma mimicking benign RPF.

Percutaneous nephrostomy can be performed for emergency decompression of the distended urinary tract above an obstruction causing an episode of severe kidney failure. A temporary diversion can be created above the obstruction while waiting for

medical therapy to take effect and for internal derivation with insertion of a double-J pigtail stent. Some authors have suggested completing this temporary palliative treatment with antegrade or retrograde dilatation of the stenosis by balloon catheter, similar to that used for vascular dilatation (DOWNEY et al. 1987). The results are only moderately satisfactory, and there is no guarantee that this type of treatment permanently relieves the occlusion.

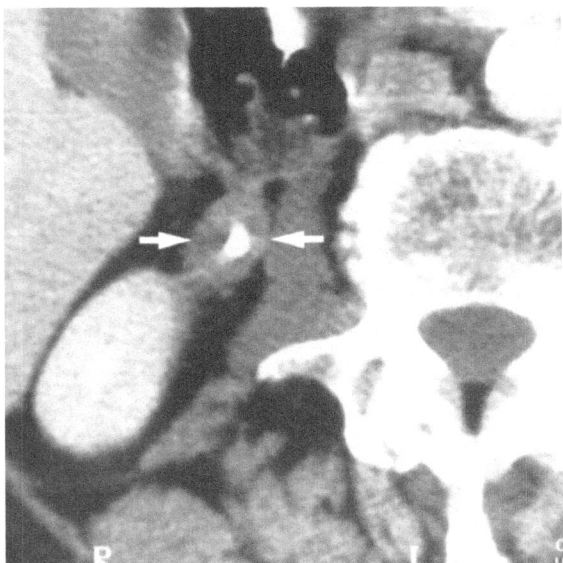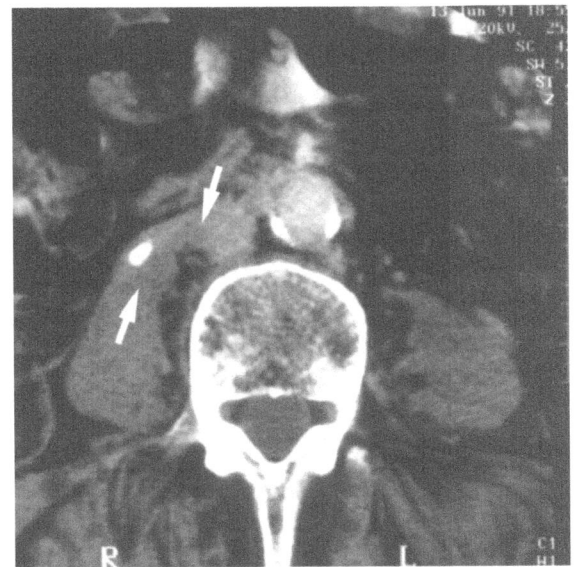

Fig 9.26. Periureteral malignant RPF after a prostatic cancer. **a** CT slice shows a periureteral thickening with clear outlining of the outer border (*arrows*): ureteral metastasis or periureteral malignant extension? **b** CT slice at a lower level shows extension of the soft tissue densities to the psoas muscle and the great vessels, indicating a periureteral infiltration (*arrows*)

9.3.4.9
Strategy for Diagnosis, Treatment, and Surveillance

EU has long been the reference investigation, because the majority of patients present with abdominal symptoms which draw attention to the urinary tract. However, ultrasonography is being performed more and more frequently as the initial investigation, especially if renal function is impaired. If ultrasonography is normal or equivocal, EU can then be performed. In the remaining cases, if one or both ureters are obstructed, whether the plaque is visualized or not, EU is generally not done. Depending on the clinical presentation, direct opacification with antegrade or retrograde drainage is performed. Observation of an extrinsic ureteral obstruction is the indication for a CT scan, which must always be followed by urographic images or pseudourographic reconstructions. CT is the reference investigation for assessing the extent of the plaque and monitoring the efficacy of treatment (Brooks et al. 1987). The role of MRI has still to be defined. It probably provides the most valuable information, though cost and accessibility may limit its use in certain countries. It may be proposed instead of CT if the patient has severe renal failure or major iodine allergy, or in pregnancy (Yuh et al. 1989).

Treatment of retroperitoneal fibrosis has a dual aim: to treat the causative disorder and to palliate its effect on the urinary tract by preserving as much as possible the function of the renal parenchyma. If the RPF is drug related, it is imperative to discontinue the medication. In practice, if the obstruction is not severe and renal function is preserved, medical treatment with corticosteroids can be initiated along with temporary drainage using a double-J pigtail stent. Fast improvement of the clinical symptoms and radiological patterns frequently occurs (Smith et al. 1986).

Ultrasound and above all CT enable surveillance of the fibrotic plaque, whose regression depends on its age, and of a decrease in obstruction (Figs. 9.27–9.29). However, in this field EU seems more adequate to assess functional recovery, in particular after withdrawal of the double-J pigtail stent at about 3 months (Fig. 9.28). Some authors advocate surgical treatment when obstruction persists despite medical therapy and renal function is still acceptable. Other teams turn systematically to surgery. Two types of procedure are proposed: (a) ureteral release by ureterolysis and separation from the fibrotic plaque by intraperitonealization (Fig. 9.30), and (b) ureteral replacement, in general by ileoplasty when ureterolysis is not possible (Fig. 9.31). In both cases, EU is the most suitable technique for assessing the efficacy of the result (Brooks et al. 1987). The radiological appearance after these procedures is characteristic: lateral, arc-shaped ureteral deviation after intra-

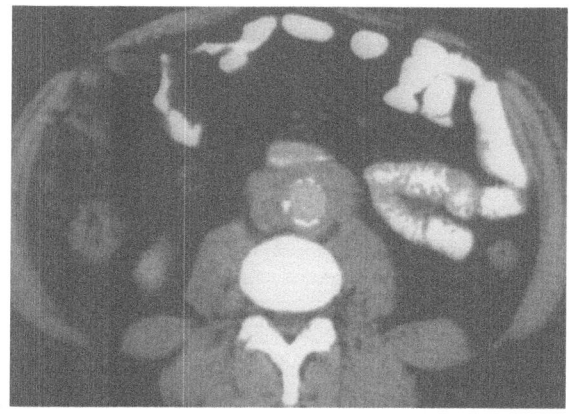

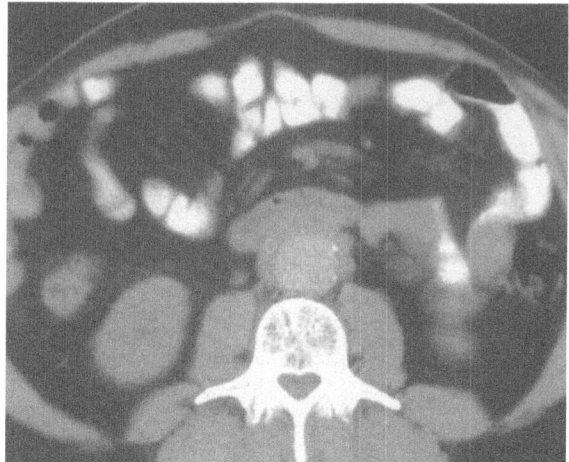

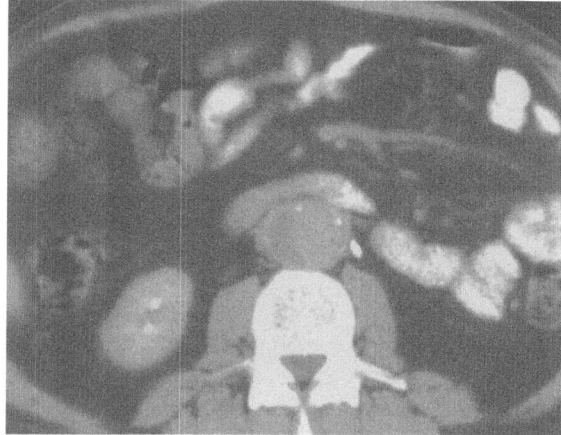

Fig 9.27a–c. CT surveillance of a benign RPF. a Typical aspects of periaortic RPF (Oct. 9, 1995). b Decrease of plaque after corticosteroid treatment (Nov. 18, 1996). The diameter of the aorta is increased. c Plaque has almost disappeared but the aorta is aneurysmal (Jan. 22, 1997)

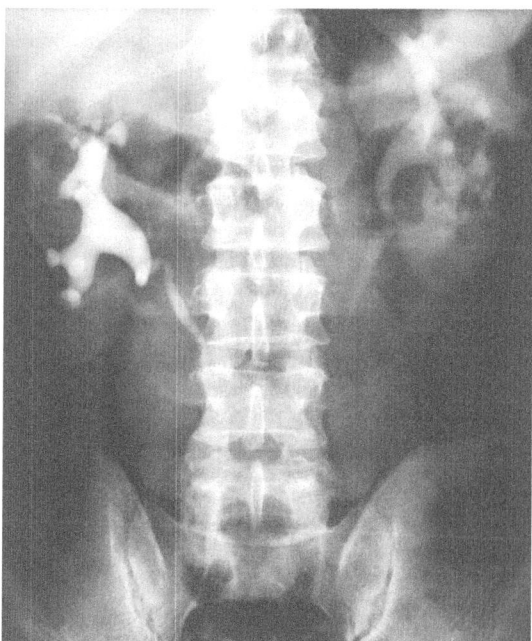

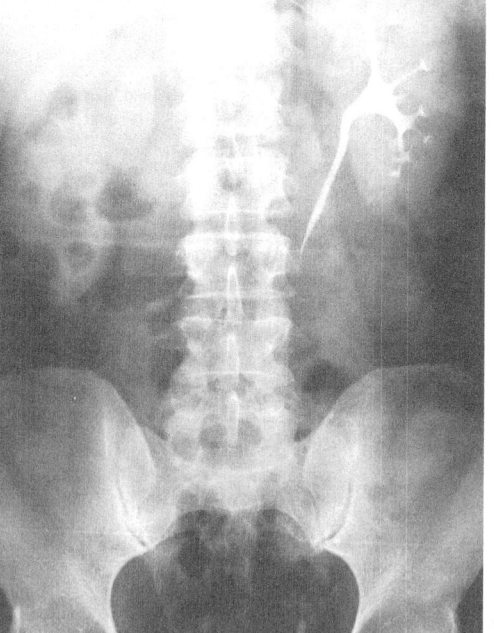

Fig 9.28a, b. EU surveillance of a benign RPF. a EU shows a typical aspect of RPF with moderate and asymmetrical bilateral obstruction of the upper urinary tract. Medial deviation of both lumbar ureters. b EU performed after 1 year of treatment with corticosteroids shows improvement on the left side and mute obstructed kidney on the right side after withdrawal of the 2-J catheter

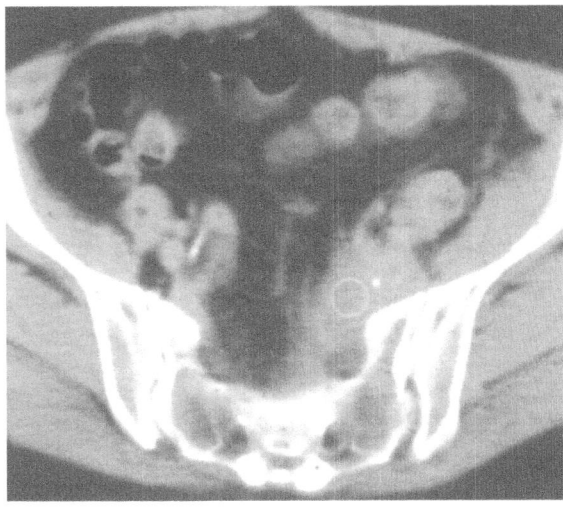

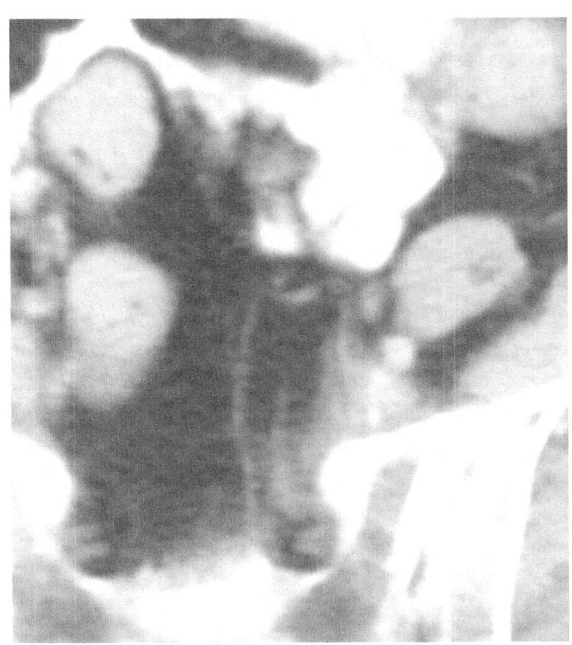

Fig 9.29a, b. CT surveillance of a benign RPF. a CT shows a pelvic benign fibrous plaque developed in the left lateral border of the pelvic brim (Dec. 18, 1995). b Decrease of plaque after corticosteroid treatment (Oct. 14, 1996)

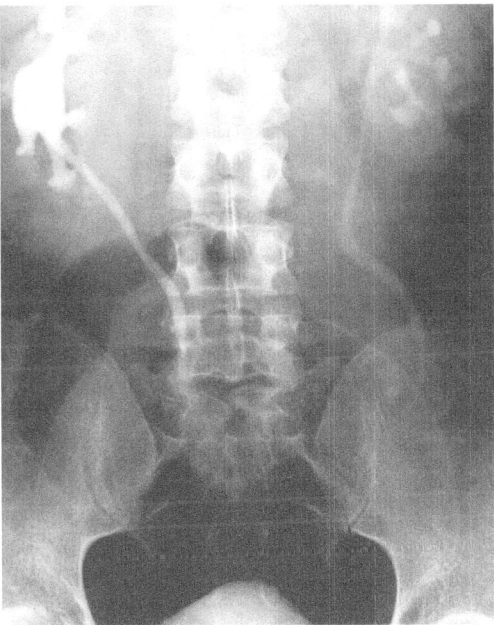

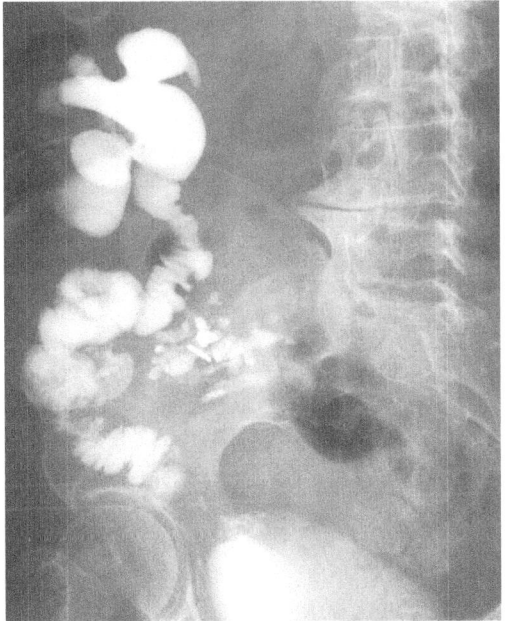

Fig 9.30. Ureterolysis for a benign RPF: EU shows typical lateral deviation of the left ureter related to the intraperitonealization

Fig 9.31. Ureteroileoplasty for benign RPF

peritonealization, appearance of the small intestine intervening between the renal pelvis and the bladder after ileoplasty.

The long-term prognosis of benign RPF depends on renal impairment. If this is not severe, if corticotherapy is started early, and if the surgical repair functions adequately, long-term results are excellent in 90% of cases (HIGGINS et al. 1988). In malignant RPF, corticosteroids are usually ineffective and this suggests the diagnosis if it has not already been established. Prognosis is bleak and treatment is simply palliative by ureteral intubation, except in cases where treatment of the primary tumor may be effective (USHER et al. 1977).

9.4
Extrinsic Ureteral Disorders of Vascular Origin

There are different relationships between the ureters and the vascular system: (a) The vascularization of the ureter may be compromised and result in ureteral ischemia, the consequences of which are multiple. (b) Periureteral vascular structures, either arterial or venous, may produce ureteral obstruction by compression because of their abnormal topography, their caliber and/or their number. (c) Periureteral vessels may be responsible for parietal impressions.

The interest in their identification is twofold: (a) to detect a vascular disease responsible for the abnormality, and (b) to exclude nonvascular causes of ureteral filling defects.

9.4.1
Ureteral Ischemia

The vascularization of the ureter is very fragile and poor (Winfield and Mazer 1990). Many pathological conditions may be causally involved in ureteral ischemic phenomena, and most of them will be discussed in other chapters. The main etiologies of ureteral ischemia are as follows:
- Diffuse arterial disease (periarteritis nodosa, inflammatory arteritis)
- Trauma by bullet (shock wave)
- Iatrogenic trauma (retroperitoneal surgery, renal transplantation, ureterointestinal anastomosis)
- Post-radiation ureteritis
- Inflammatory aortoiliac aneurysm
- Retroperitoneal tumors that alter ureteral vascularization

Their general consequences are of variable severity: ureteral hypotonia with dilation and evacuation delay, progressive centered and regular ureteral stricture with upstream consequences of varying significance, necrosis with ureteral perforation and contrast medium extravasation.

An exceptional case of ureteral fibrotic obstruction with multiple smooth filling defects secondary to a thromboembolic infarct of the ureteral wall related to atrial fibrillation was recently reported (Davia et al. 1995).

9.4.2
Ureteral Obstruction of Arterial Origin

Ureteral obstructions of arterial origin are rare and related to causes of varying incidence, mostly acquired. They can be schematically separated into three distinct groups:
- Ureteral obstruction secondary to an aortoiliac aneurysm
- Ureteral complications of aortoiliac vascular surgery
- Ureteral obstruction due to aberrant artery

9.4.2.1
Ureteral Obstructions Secondary to an Aortoiliac Aneurysm and Aortoiliac Atheroma

9.4.2.1.1
Aortoiliac Aneurysms

Ureteral relationships with Aortoiliac aneurysms (AIAs) are very close and some topographic changes of the ureter are often demonstrated by EU, such as bilateral external deviation or unilateral external deviation associated with medial traction (Peck et al. 1973) (Fig. 9.32).

AIAs are also a potential cause of uni- or bilateral ureteral obstruction. This may be due to direct compression by the aneurysmal sac. In rare cases, a uni- or bilateral ureteral obstruction may also be related to collection of blood secondary to aneurysmal fissure (Datta et al. 1979). In most cases, however, stricture is secondary to a perianeurysmal inflammatory fibrosis (PIF) of variable extension (Drake et al. 1977). This entity has been well identified since the first descriptions were made (James 1935). PIF, the mechanism of which is still debated, involves mostly the abdominal aorta and less frequently the common and internal iliac arteries. The English literature insists on the inflammatory mechanism and calls this entity "inflammatory aneurysm" or "periaortitis". The incidence of this entity varies among reported series; 5%–23% of AIAs are discovered during surgery (Cullenward et al. 1986). Most authors report a rate of approximately 10% (Culp and Bernatz 1981). On the other hand, the frequency of reported ureteral obstructions is lower by far: Fewer than 100 cases were reported by several authors (Boissieras et al. 1984; Loughlin and Kearney 1984). Available etiopathogenic hypotheses based on clinical and histological evidence are multiple and varied, but all authors agree that the obstruction is not related to

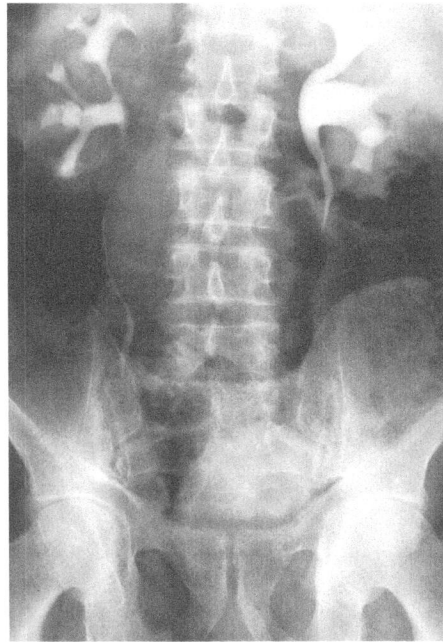
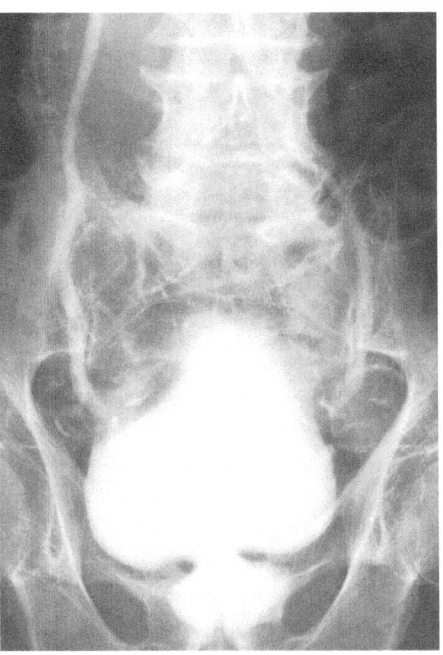

a   b

Fig 9.32a, b. Extrinsic compression of ureters by AIA. **a** EU shows external deviation of the right lumbar ureter and medial attraction of the left ureter. **b** EU shows deviation of both lumbar and pelvic ureters by calcified AIA and external compression of the bladder (postoperative enlargement of the prostatic urethra)

the AIA itself, but rather to the surrounding fibrous plaque (Savarese et al. 1986). The plaque first results in disturbances of ureteral peristalsis, which may explain the occurrence of moderate obstruction. Then it surrounds the ureter without invading it (Vint et al. 1980). The PIF is extensive and may involve adjacent viscera (duodenum and duodenoje-junal angle, inferior vena cava, sigmoid mesocolon). The histopathological structure of the fibrous plaque is similar to that of benign idiopathic RPF. Its topography is identical, involving only the anterior and lateral sides of the aorta. The fibrous process encompasses the adventitia. A lymphoplasmocytic infiltrate is invariably found. The presence of the fibrous plaque seems to protect the aneurysm from fissure, the rate of which (15%) is clearly lower than that of simple aneurysms (40%) (Walker et al. 1972).

Macroscopic and microscopic appearance of AIAs is strictly identical to that of aneurysms without PIF (Kittredge and Gordon 1987). These two entities are clearly related, and the perianeurysmal inflammatory reaction is obviously secondary to the aneurysm. This is confirmed by the topography of PIF (which is located predominantly at the level of the greatest diameter of the aneurysmal sac) and by its regression after the aneurysm has been treated (Cullenward et al. 1986). The observation of Kittredge, whereby a PIF developed over several months between two con-

secutive CT examinations, is demonstrative of this close relationship (Kittredge and Gordon 1987). However, the mechanism of this event is not precisely known. The first hypothesis proposed involved the presence of microperforations in the aneurysm with minimal blood extravasation and development of a periaortic fibrous reaction. Histological observations did not support this hypothesis: No blood pigment or hemosiderin-carrying macrophages were found. An autoimmune hypothesis has also been presented, as well as an increase of the inflammatory reaction commonly seen in the AIA wall in front of the endoluminal thrombus (Mitchinson 1984). The favorable influence of corticotherapy in some recent cases, as well as the histological appearance, argue for this last hypothesis (Clyne and Abercrombie 1977). No infectious factor has ever been demonstrated. A recent observation of spontaneous resolution of the fibrous plaque raises additional doubts regarding the exact nature of this lesion (Robbe and Dixon 1984).

PIFs are more commonly found in men (90%), and their associated aneurysms are exactly identical to those seen in classic atherosclerotic AIAs (Savarese et al. 1986). They often consist of aortic or aortoiliac aneurysms, more rarely of isolated iliac aneurysms or hypogastric aneurysms (Villani et al. 1985; Leflot et al. 1978).

Ureteral involvement is bilateral in most cases

(about 60%) (LOUGHLIN and KEARNEY 1984). This may be responsible for an obstructive acute renal failure in up to 18% of cases (BOISSIERAS et al. 1984). The left ureter is more frequently involved. Clinical presentation is usually nonspecific. Pain is invariably present and occasionally acute. In 35% of cases, symptoms (abdominal pain or mass) indicate the possibility of an aortic aneurysm. Lower limb edema may point to compression of the inferior vena cava. The urological clinical presentation (10%) may include loin pain, hematuria, and urinary tract infection (CULP and BERNATZ 1981). Biological examinations are poorly characteristic, but renal failure may exist in 20% of cases and an increased sedimentation rate in 50% of cases. Given the lack of specificity of these signs and symptoms, a systematic search for renal consequences seems compulsory in the preoperative workup of AIAs. This may be done either with renal ultrasonography, with computed tomography, or with post-angiography urographic pictures.

9.4.2.1.2
Imaging

Imaging methods are of varying importance. Abdominal plain X-rays provide nonspecific information that could point to the presence of an AIA: arciform calcifications of the aneurysmal wall, soft-tissue opacity of the aneurysmal mass.

Ultrasonography (CULLENWARD et al. 1986) provides essential data. When perfect technical conditions are met during completion of the examination, it may be sufficient by itself to confirm the diagnosis of AIA. Ultrasonography demonstrates the AIA, its caliber, its extension toward the iliac and renal arteries, and the existence of an endoluminal thrombus and parietal calcifications. The intra-aneurysmal flow is evaluated by color Doppler ultrasonography. Examination of renal areas shows the presence of a pyelocaliceal dilatation and the morphological status of the parenchyma. The PIF plaque usually appears as a periaortic hypoechoic ring, the thickness of which is uniform and ranges between 10 and 20 mm. (Fig. 9.33).

Today, EU is seldom performed as such, but more often as post-CT or post-angiography complementary urographic pictures. It demonstrates a uni- or bilateral pyelocaliceal and ureteral dilation, which is of varying severity and seldom symmetric. It is related to an extended regular filiform stenosis of extrinsic origin and associated to topographic abnormalities of the ureters. Most of the time, these are forced laterally, contrary to simple benign RPF

(SAVARESE et al. 1986). A unilateral attraction may also coexist (PECK et al. 1973). The association of vascular arciform aortoiliac calcifications to an adjacent ureteral stricture should call to mind this diagnosis (ALLIBONE and SAXTON 1980).

Helical CT provides the most complete information on the full spectrum of morphological data that are necessary for the therapeutic approach (Fig. 9.34). The diagnosis of the aneurysm, its precise morphological evaluation, the renal consequences, the demonstration of the fibrous plaque and its anatomic relation with the ureters constitute the main information provided by this examination in nearly all cases (DIXON et al. 1984). Multiplanar reconstructions allow adequate visualization of the relationships between the ureters and the fibrous plaque (Fig. 9.35). Depending much less on patient morphotype, its efficiency is far superior to that of ultrasonography. The fibrous plaque is found on the anterolateral aspect of the aorta as a dense homogeneous area with regular or irregular limits, of variable thickness, resulting in obliteration of perivascular fatty spaces (MEGIBOW et al. 1980).

After intravenous injection of an iodinated contrast medium, plaque enhancement may vary from intense or moderate and delayed to nearly absent in relation to the inflammatory status of the plaque (VINT et al. 1980; CULLENWARD et al. 1986). Three-dimensional reconstructions enable precise determination of the craniocaudal extension of the plaque.

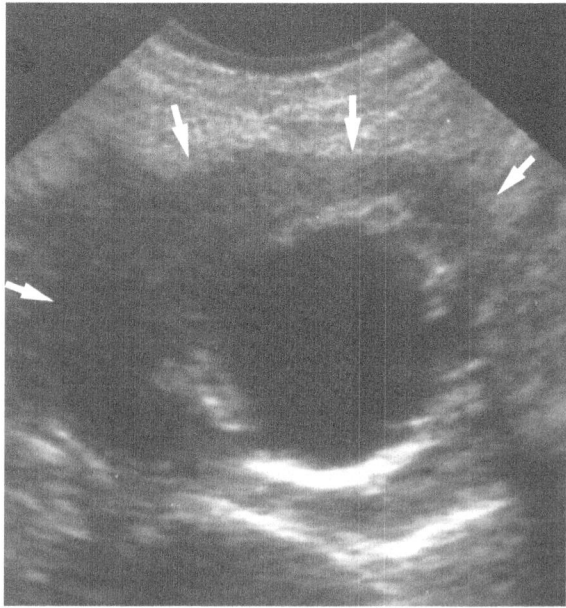

Fig 9.33. Perianeurysmal fibrosis: Ultrasonography shows a hypoechoic zone (*arrows*) surrounding a dilated aorta with hyperechoic and partially calcified wall

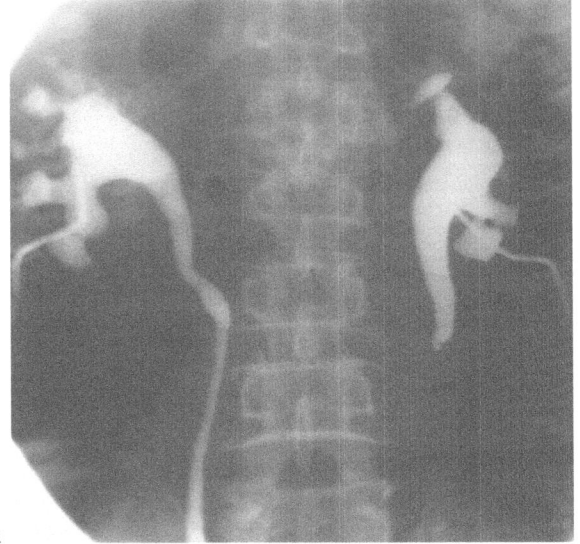

a

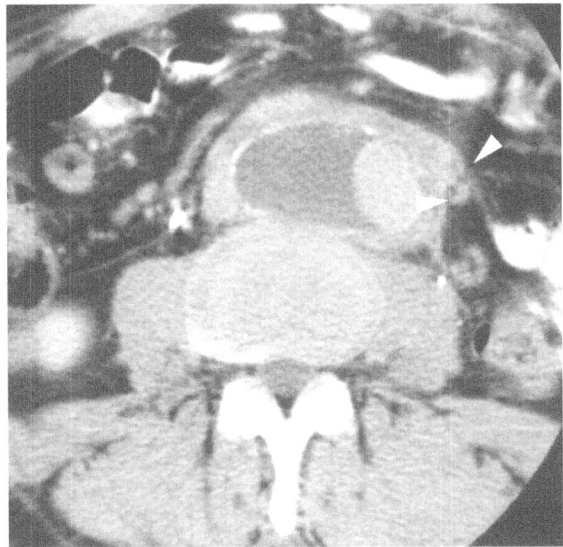

b

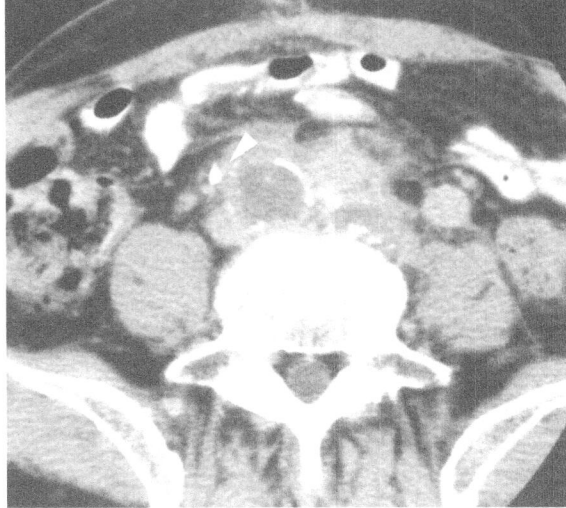

c

Fig 9.34a–c. Perianeurysmal fibrosis. a Bilateral antegrade pyelography in a 58-year-old patient with bilateral obstructive renal insufficiency. Total occlusion of the left lumbar ureter. External deviation of the right lumbar and iliac ureter with dilatation of the upper urinary tract. b, c CT slices show partially thrombosed AIA with tissular plaque around the anterior and lateral borders of the aneurysm. The left ureter is against the plaque in b (*arrowhead*), the right in c (*arrowhead*)

Retroperitoneal lymphomas, metastatic retroperitoneal adenopathies, and benign and malignant retroperitoneal fibroses may produce CT appearances similar to those of the fibrous plaque of PIF (DEGESYS et al. 1986). However, the association between an AIA and a fibrous plaque is so suggestive that there is usually little doubt. The hypothesis of a perianeurysmal hematoma due to fissure may be discussed but the latter spontaneously appears hyperdense in most cases and does not enhance after contrast medium injection.

MRI combines the interests of a three-dimensional view of the aneurysm and information concerning the plaque and the intra-aneurysmal flow (CULLENWARD et al. 1986). Its capabilities in density resolution make it easy to detect the fibrous plaque as a hypointense perianeurysmal area on both T_1- and T_2-weighted images (Fig. 9.36), with more or less enhancement after intravenous gadolinium injection. Uro-MRI sequences enable exact definition of the relations between the ureter and the plaque and also show the ureteral obstructive syndrome. Currently, angiography has no precise role to play in the diagnosis of the AIA. Direct opacification of the ureter may be performed as the first step of a ureteral intubation.

The documented evidence of a PIF leads to surgical treatment, given the association between vascular and ureteral lesions. Although the risk of fissure is reduced by the presence of the plaque, the problem of ureteral obstruction must be solved. On the other hand, ablation of the aortic lesion results in regression of fibrous lesions (BASKERVILLE and BROWSE 1987).

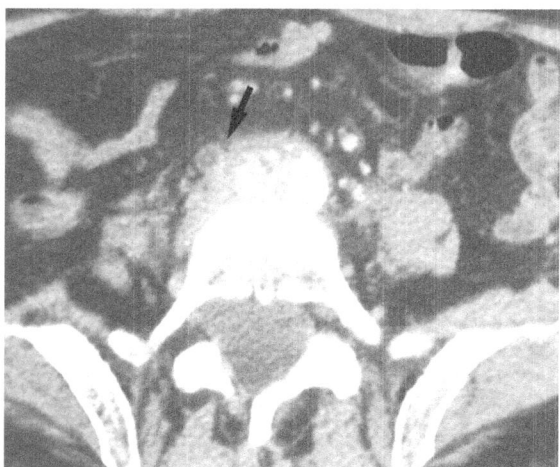

Fig 9.35a–c. Perianeurysmal fibrosis. a Axial CT slice at the level of the aortoiliac bifurcation demonstrates dilated and calcified iliac arteries surrounded by a soft-tissue density plaque. Nonopacified right ureter is adherent to the plaque (*arrow*). b, c Coronal MPR reconstructions showing the zones of obstruction with adhesion of the ureters to the plaque (*arrows*)

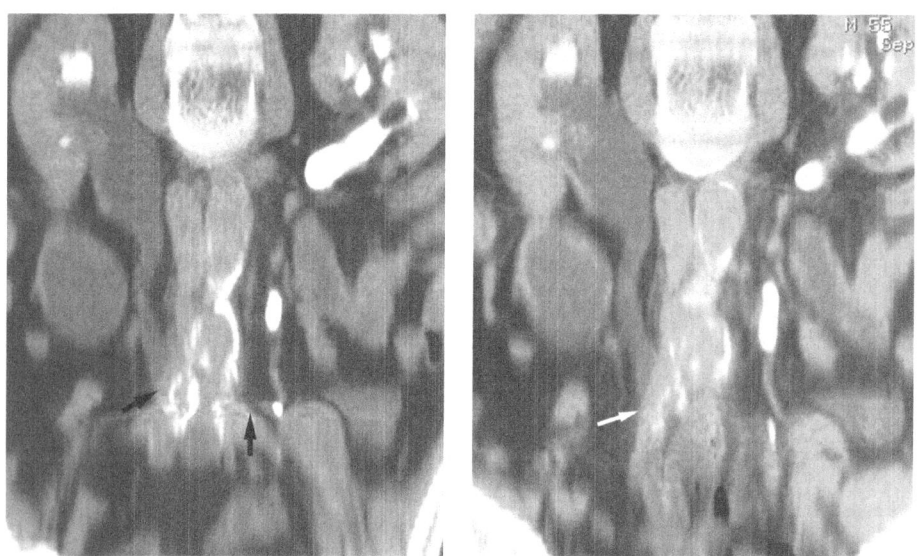

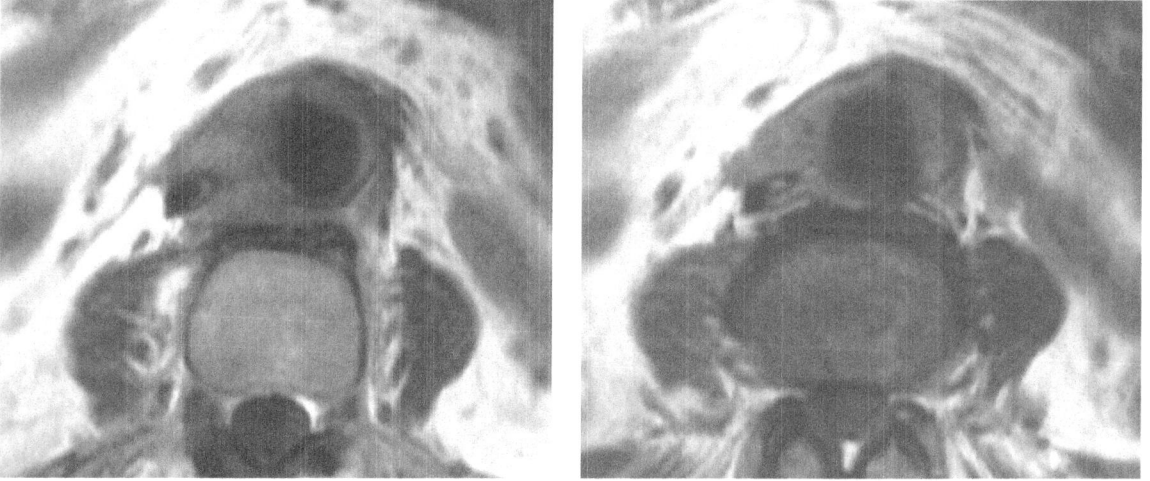

Fig 9.36a, b. Perianeurysmal fibrosis. a, b Axial TSE T_1-weighted sequences show an intermediate signal plaque around an ectatic and partially thrombosed aorta

Surgical treatment thus consists of curing the aneurysm by grafting, along with release of the ureters (ureterolysis) and occasionally intraperitonealization of the ureters. Some authors advocate the systematic preoperative use of corticosteroids, in order to reduce the inflammatory component, to facilitate surgical dissection, and to reduce postoperative morbidity and mortality (CLYNE and ABERCROMBIE 1977).

A recent survey of the postoperative course demonstrated that PIF persists longer than previously thought (77% of patients). Progression of the disease was even observed in some cases with ureteral involvement, suggesting the need for long-term surveillance of these patients (VON FRITSCHEN et al. 1999).

9.4.2.1.3
Special Cases of Periarterial Aortoiliac Fibrosis

Several cases of periarterial fibrosis related to atheroma have been reported in the literature (MITCHINSON 1984, 1986). CT made it possible to identify this specific entity. CT shows a plaque similar to most cases of perianeurysmal RPF, except that in this condition the aorta is not dilated. The plaque is often limited and localized. The ureter is obstructed when it crosses the iliac artery (Figs. 9.37, 9.38). The most common characteristic of these patients is the presence of important atheromatous and nonaneurysmal aortoiliac lesions with diffuse and large calcifications of the arterial wall at the level of the plaque.

The role of hypersensitivity to antigens from the atheromatous plaque was previously emphasized (MITCHISON 1984).

The management of these patients is identical to that for benign RPF and requires either medical treatment by corticosteroids and/or urological treatment, according to the importance of ureteral obstruction.

9.4.2.2
Ureteral Complications
of Vascular Aortoiliac Surgery

These complications are rare in comparison to other possible complications of aortoiliac prostheses: periprosthetic infection, false aneurysm, thrombosis, aortodigestive fistula. HIGGINS nevertheless considers that half of all surgical ureteral lesions are due to vascular surgery. Three groups of complications may be defined (HIGGINS 1967).

9.4.2.2.1
Ureteral Injuries and Necroses

Ureteral injuries are exceptional and are revealed in the early postoperative period. Injuries related to a surgical wound of the ureter lead to the formation of a postoperative urinoma, which is an extremely serious condition, as the urinoma is in contact with a prosthetic material. Ureteral necroses may result from wounding of ureteral vessels during dissection and lead to a devitalization of the ureter wall.

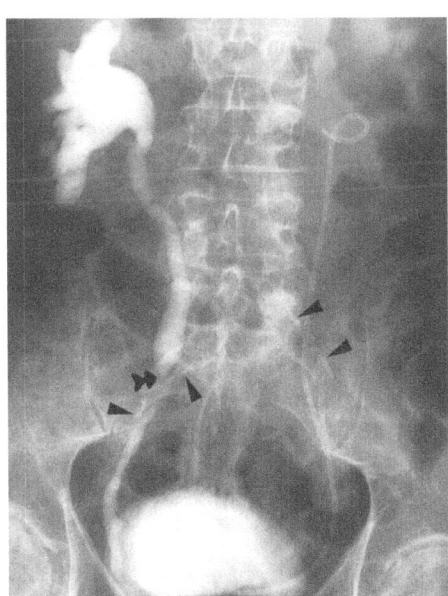
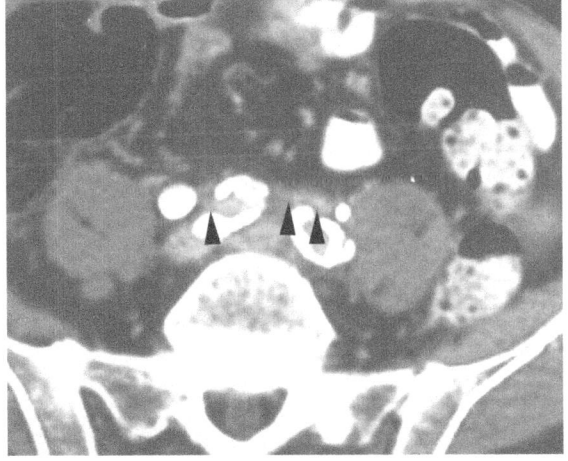

Fig 9.37. Periarterial RPF. **a** EU shows absence of opacification of the left urinary tract despite the presence of 2-J catheter. The right upper urinary tract is obstructed, and opacification demonstrates a narrowing at the crossing of right iliac artery (*arrow*). The iliac arteries are heavily calcified (*arrowheads*). **b** CT slice at the level of pelvic brim shows both iliac arteries with important calcifications of the arterial wall. The anterior part of the vessel is surrounded by a thin plaque of soft-tissue density (*arrowheads*). Both ureters are adherent to the plaque

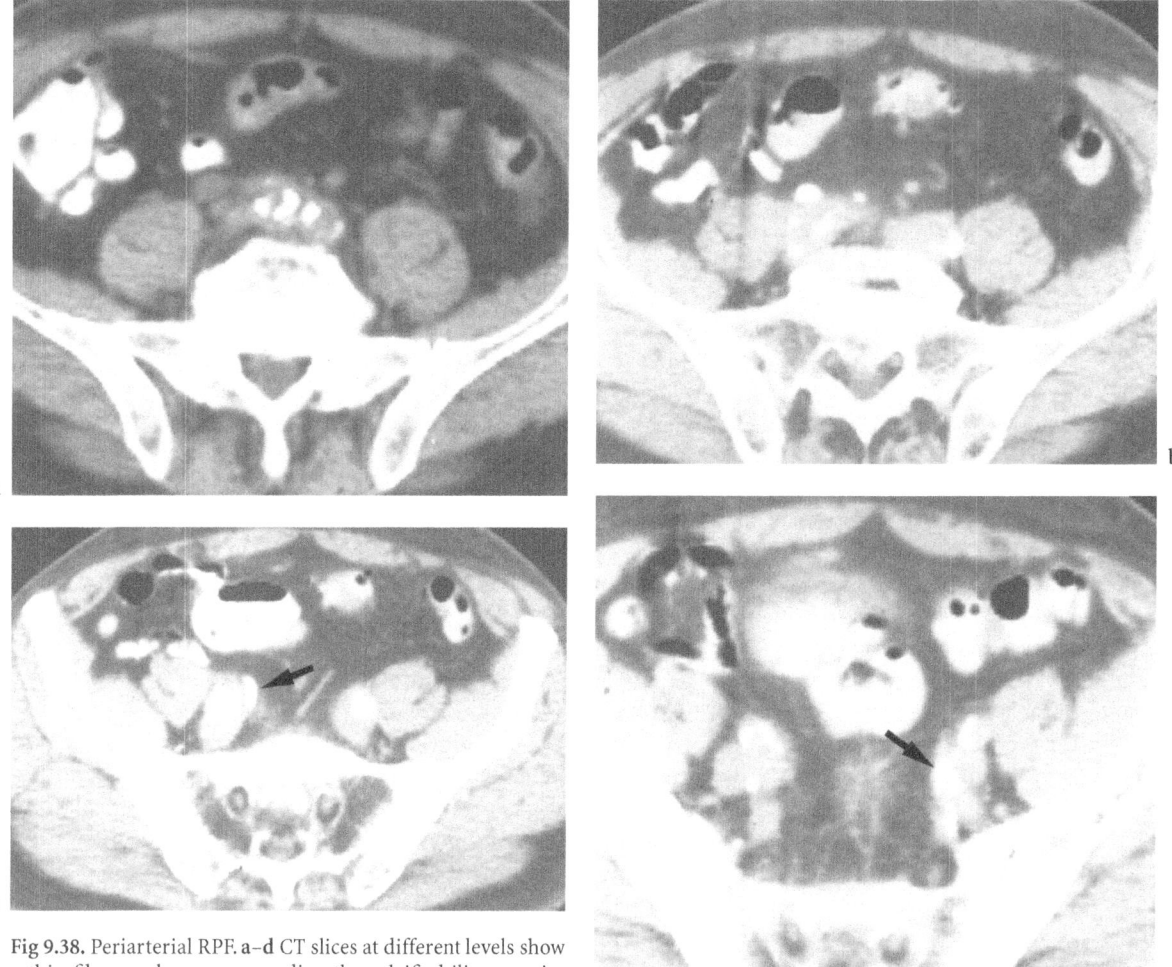

Fig 9.38. Periarterial RPF. **a–d** CT slices at different levels show a thin fibrous plaque surrounding the calcified iliac arteries and obstructing both ureters (*arrows*)

9.4.2.2.2
Ureteroarterial Fistulas

The occurrence of ureteroarterial fistulas is discussed in Chap. 11.

9.4.2.2.3
Ureteral Obstructions

Ureteral obstruction also is a rare clinical situation: Since the first case report by Lytton appeared in 1966, Tracy found 17 cases in the literature in 1979 and reported four supplementary cases (Lytton 1966; Tracy et al. 1979). In most cases, they consisted of aortoiliac or aortofemoral bypasses related to obstructive or aneurysmal disease. One case of obstruction after a portocaval shunt has been reported. (Manco et al. 1982).

According to Frusha, an obstruction occurs in 10% of cases (Frusha et al. 1982). In Heard's experience, obstructions are more frequent: In 30% of cases, an obstruction of variable severity is noted during the first postoperative year (Heard and Hinde 1975). In one half of cases this obstruction is transitory and regresses after 1 year (Goldenberg et al. 1988). It can also be asymptomatic and discovered by chance (Schubart et al. 1985).

There are several different causes of ureteral obstruction.

Technical Causes. Accidental ligation of the ureter is rare, and the related obstruction might regress spontaneously or after dilatation if resorbable thread has been used (Harshman et al. 1982). According to Tracy, the most frequent causative factor (73% of cases) is an iliac vascular prosthesis placed in front of the ureter and compressing it on the posterior osseous plane (Fig. 9.39) (Tracy et al. 1979). As it is normally attached to the reclined posterior parietal

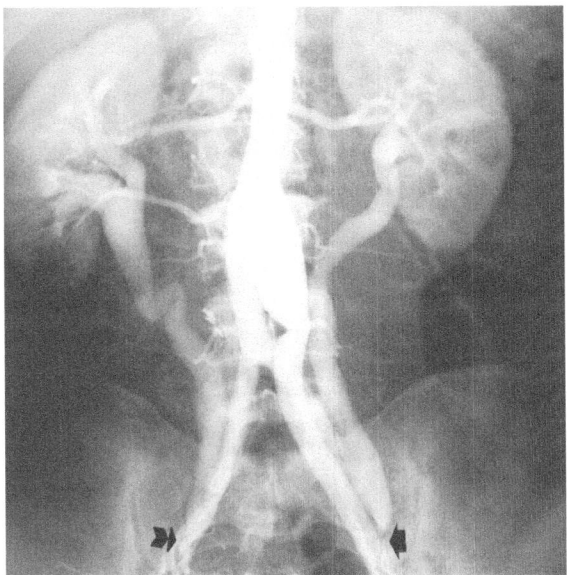

Fig 9.39. Ureteral bilateral obstruction secondary to vascular aortoiliac surgery: Aortography shows an aorto-bi-iliac bypass. Opacification of both ureters shows bilateral obstruction at the level of crossing with the iliac parts of the bypass (*arrows*). The vascular prostheses compresses the ureters on the posterior osseous plane

peritoneum, the ureter is not always isolated during surgical intervention. Opinions are nevertheless not unanimous on this topic. According to Thomas, given the number of completed operative bypasses, the absence of ureter separation at surgery is not the origin of the obstruction (Thomas et al. 1983). Prosthetic pulsations have been incriminated: Lytton thinks that a fibrosis of the ureteral wall would occur secondary to the compression of the ureter between a pulsating prosthesis and an atheromatous artery (Lytton 1966).

Inflammatory Mechanism. Inflammatory stenosis could be secondary to the development of a more or less extensive periprosthetic fibrotic reaction (Rhind and Bradford 1977). This fibrosis could be due to surgical tissular damage by ischemia or prolonged clamping, to the existence of a residual hematoma, or to the development of a periprosthetic inflammatory reaction (Petrone et al. 1974). This periprosthetic fibrosis might combine with the aforementioned compressive mechanical factor to result in ureteral obstruction. Finally, a ureteral obstruction may be observed in cases of periprosthetic abscesses.

Whatever the incriminated mechanism, there seems to be a significant connection between the existence of an obstruction and the presence of a prosthetic complication (infection, anastomotic

ectasia, thrombosis) (Schubart et al. 1985). The urological complication may reveal a purely vascular problem. Clinical symptoms depend on the mechanism and associated lumbar pain, occasional renal colic, fever in case of urinary tract infection, and renal insufficiency in bilateral cases. The occurrence of these signs is either early (i.e., within the first few weeks) – rather related to a mechanical or septic cause – or delayed (i.e., beyond 1 year) – rather related to a perivascular fibrosis reaction. A delay in appearance of more than 5 years has been observed. Ultrasonography performed in this condition detects a dilatation of the excretory tract. Helical CT provides nearly all required information. Thanks to the different kinds of spatial reconstruction, it allows visualization of both the urinary tract and the prosthetic bypass (Fig. 9.40). The anatomic relations are defined and the periprosthetic atmosphere may be analyzed. Opacification of the urinary tract by EU or directly is still often requested by the urologist, although it is seldom necessary. The evolution varies depending on the authors. Given the evolution and frequency of this kind of complications, it is difficult to propose a strategy for the postoperative follow-up of these patients. Systematic pre- and postoperative EU as proposed by Tracy does not appear necessary anymore (Tracy et al. 1979; Thomas et al. 1983). Surveillance may rely on sequential ultrasonographic examinations during the first year.

The treatment is based on reintervention on the surgical bypass associated with ureterolysis. Intraperitonealization of the ureter may be added in some cases. Preservation of normal anatomic relations between the ureter and the vascular compartment (the ureter should always remain anterior to the prosthesis) should prevent the occurrence of such complications.

9.4.2.3
Ureteral Obstruction Due to Aberrant Arteries

The existence of multiple renal arteries may be responsible for ureteral obstruction (Lee et al. 1997). The presence of such a lower polar renal artery is classically responsible for a UPJ obstruction. More rarely, this anomaly can concern the proximal ureter. EU shows a short segment of lumbar ureter upstream from the vascular imprints which has the main characteristics of arterial origin: a band-like linear print with sharp edges. Helical CT angiography precisely demonstrates the relationships between the artery and the ureter (Lee et al. 1997) (Figs. 9.41, 9.42).

Other exceptional arterial causes of ureteral

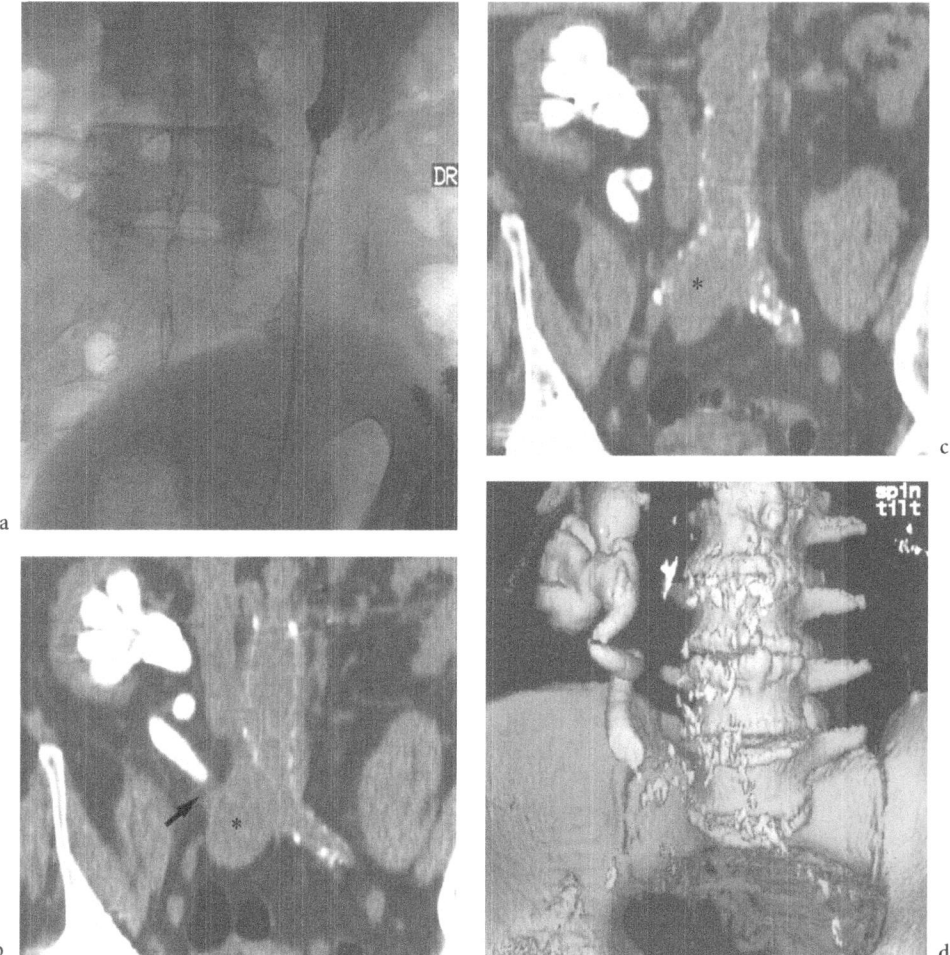

Fig 9.40a–d. Right ureteral obstruction secondary to anastomotic false aneurysm. **a** Antegrade pyelography in prone position shows obstruction of the terminal part of the lumbar ureter. **b, c** CT MPR reconstructions demonstrate the false aneurysm (*asterisks*) and the right ureterohydronephrosis with the obstruction area (*arrow*). **d** CT SSD reconstruction does not provide any additional information

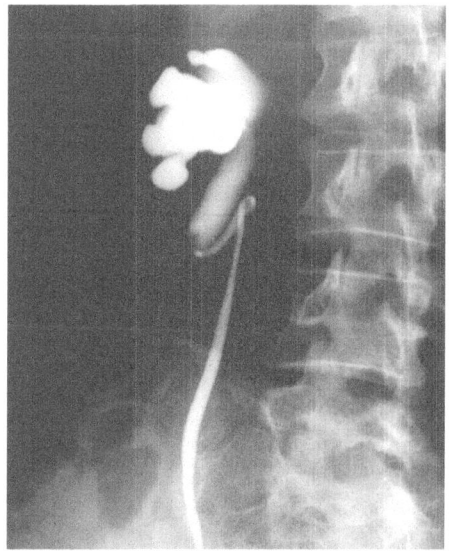

Fig 9.41. Ureteral obstruction due to aberrant artery: Retrograde pyelography shows right upper urinary tract obstruction related to a plication of the proximal lumbar ureter secondary to a crossing with right renal polar artery confirmed by surgery

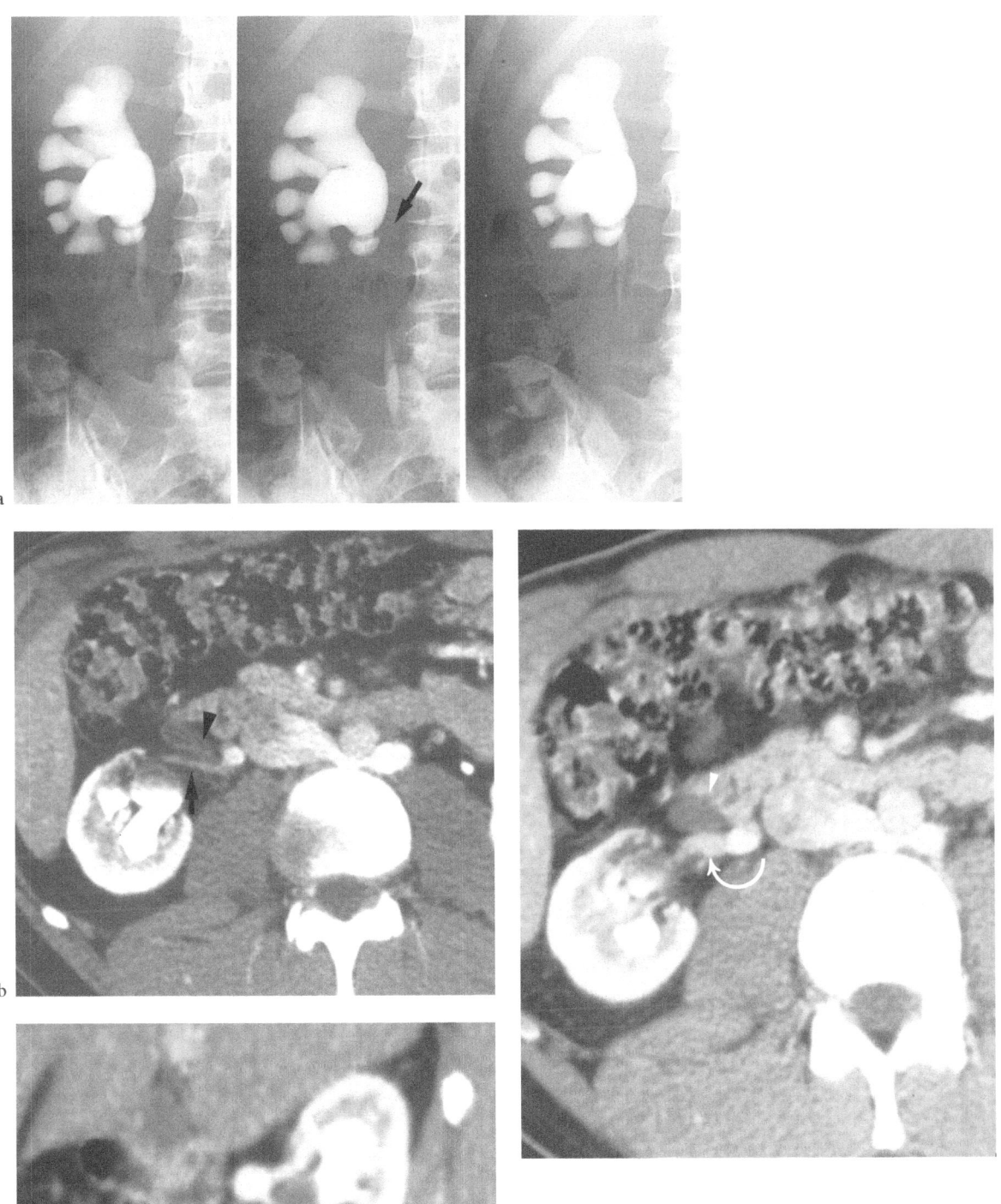

Fig 9.42a–d. Ureteral obstruction due to aberrant artery. a Several urographic views in different positions show ureterohydronephrosis with dilatation of the initial segment of the ureter upward to a ureteral plication (*arrow*). b, c Axial CT slices show the crossing between the right ureter (*arrowhead*) and the polar inferior renal artery (*arrow*) and vein (*curved arrow*). d Profile MPR reconstruction shows the crossing of the ureter with polar inferior renal vessels (*arrow*)

obstruction have been reported: the ureter crossing the iliac artery from behind (Hanna 1972), obstruction secondary to thrombosed aberrant umbilical artery in children (Read and Devine 1975). The diagnosis of these rare anomalies is generally peroperative (Quattlebaum and Anderson 1985).

9.4.3
Ureteral Obstructions of Venous Origin

Ureteral obstructions of venous origin encompass mainly two major pathological conditions: the retrocaval ureter, i.e., an embryogenic abnormality of the inferior vena cava (IVC), and the ovarian vein syndrome, the existence of which remains the subject of discussion.

9.4.3.1
Retrocaval Ureter

Retrocaval ureter is a congenital abnormality corresponding to the retrocaval or – more appropriately – circumcaval route of the lumbar ureter. It consists of an abnormality in the embryological development of the IVC, and the term "preureteral IVC" would actually be more suitable. This is a rare condition: Since the first description, approximately 150 cases were reported in 1971 and 200 in 1979 (Hochstetter 1893; Shown and Moore 1971; Carrion et al. 1979).

The origin of ureteral obstruction relates to embryological development of the IVC (Mayo et al. 1983). In the embryo, the ureter is located between the right posterior cardinal vein (ventral) and the supracardinal vein (dorsal), which forms the origin of the infrarenal segment of the IVC. In case of abnormal persistence of the right posterior cardinal vein, the ureter comes to surround the IVC from behind and medially and is then pushed against the rachidian plane (O'Reilly 1986). Fibrous changes in the retrocaval portion of the ureter also contribute to the obstruction (Dufour 1973). Other types of retrocaval ureter have been described: ureteral obstruction by a periureteral venous ring secondary to a longitudinal duplication of the IVC (Hattori et al. 1986; Sasai et al. 1986; Dillon and Camputaro 1991), bilateral retrocaval ureter secondary to a double vena cava, left retrocaval ureter in the case of a situs inversus (Gladstone 1929; Brooks 1962).

As symptoms are not at all specific, the diagnosis is a difficult one clinically and therefore is usually made radiologically. The retrocaval ureter may be asymptomatic or may manifest as signs related to the ureteral

obstruction (pain, urinary tract infection). Although congenital, it has rarely been reported in children and most often appears in the adult from the fifth decade on. It is more frequent in men than in women.

EU is often not sufficient to indicate the diagnosis (McElhinney and Dorsey 1948). It allows a schematic distinction between two appearances (Bateson and Atkinson 1969): Type I is typical with an suggestive ureteral course associated with an upstream ureterohydronephrosis. Type II is more difficult to diagnose, as its more external course is less characteristic; its effects on the evacuation of the upstream urine flow are moderate. In both cases, the level of crossing may vary from L-I to L-4. In the first case, the deviation of the right ureteral course is extremely characteristic and corresponds to the "Randall sign". In front of the L3-4 level, the pelvic ureter presents a "bayonet" route, with medial deviation immediately below the dilated zone (Figs. 9.43, 9.44). The ureter follows a horizontal or slightly ascending segment with a J or an L appearance of the prestenotic segment. Visualization of the circumcaval segment depends on peristalsis, on the dose and type of contrast medium injected, on the importance of ureteral contractions, and on the radiological projection. The underlying portion of the ureter is vertical and more or less medial and cannot be seen in some cases.

Ultrasonography enables detection of obstruction and tends to replace EU as a first-line examination (Murphy et al. 1987). The relationship between the dilated ureter and the IVC can be demonstrated by color Doppler ultrasonography.

CT is currently the most appropriate method for visualizing simultaneously the IVC and the ureter and precisely determining their relation in the three space planes, providing all the required information for future treatment (Gefter et al. 1978; Lautin et al. 1988). CT should make it possible to avoid the completion of an RUP and/or cavography and provide a precise description of the relation between both ureters and the IVC (Hattori et al. 1986). Post-injection scans clearly demonstrate that the opacified ureter surrounds the IVC from behind (Fig. 9.44). The latter most often has a relatively lateral position in relation to the embryological abnormality. In some rare cases, the retrocaval position of the ureter is not visualized: Only the posterior orientation of the ureter and a smooth, tapered narrowing may then be detected (Lautin et al. 1988). 3-D reconstructions provide easier recognition of the different kinds of anomalies of IVC and the close relationships with the ureter (Dillon and Camputaro 1991; Pienkny et al. 1999).

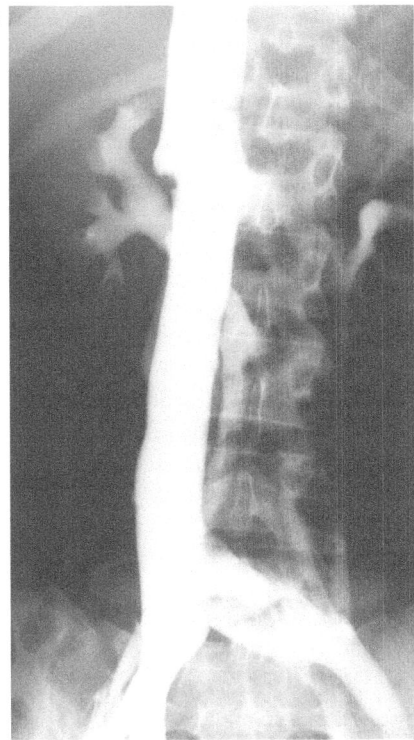

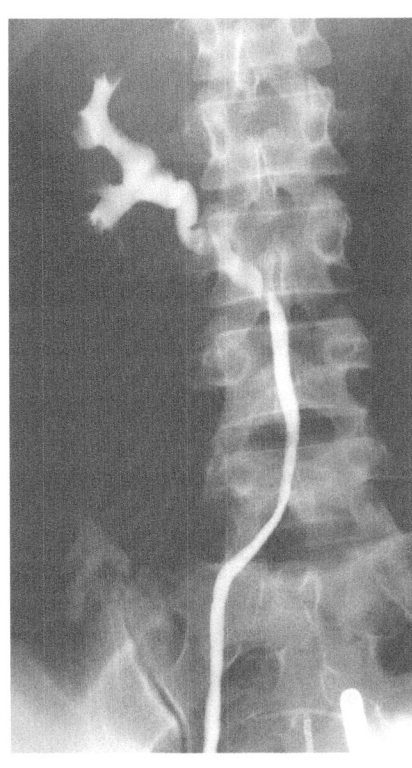

Fig 9.43a, b. Retrocaval ureter.
a Simultaneous opacification
of right upper urinary tract
by intravenous injection of
CM and IVC by cavography.
Course of right ureter is
clearly seen behind the IVC.
There is a slight dilatation of
the upper urinary tract. **b** Retrograde pyelography shows
medial deviation of the right
lumbar ureter

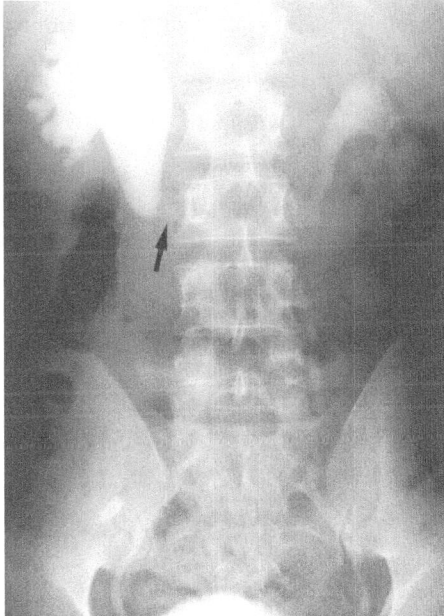

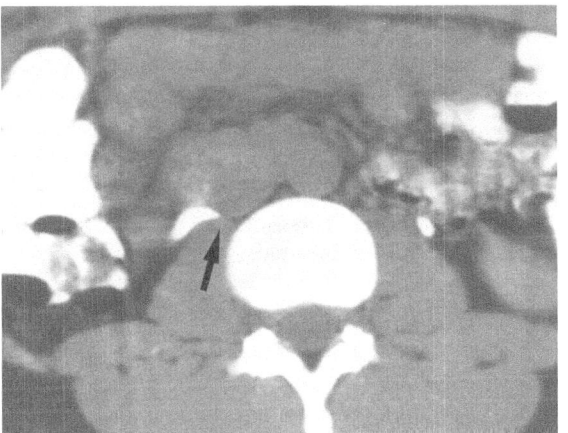

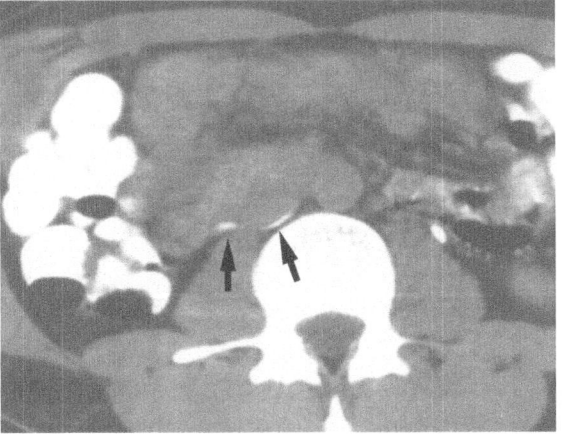

Fig 9.44a–c. Retrocaval ureter. **a** EU shows right ureterohydronephrosis with a "bayonet" route of the right lumbar ureter
(*arrow*). **b, c** CT slices demonstrate the retrocaval course of
the lumbar ureter (*arrows*)

The diagnosis of retrocaval ureter is usually an easy one: Other causes of medial deviation of the ureter (hypertrophy of the psoas muscle, retroperitoneal fibrosis) are most often bilateral and thus easy to exclude. Similarly, ureteral hypotonia with vascular compression (ovarian vein) will be easily eliminated. Ureteral obstructions by aberrant veins are more difficult to exclude (PSIHRAMIS 1987).

In the rare cases of periureteral venous rings, CT diagnosis is more difficult, as ureteral compression is moderate and topographic abnormalities are less evident.

MRI is able to provide the same information as CT. Use of diuretic renography can be proposed to exclude clinically non significant obstruction (PIENKNY et al. 1999).

The treatment of retrocaval ureter is based on surgical uncrossing, with sectioning of the excretory tract if ureteral alterations exist, and restoration of the continuity. Late results are usually good and depend on the extent of consequences on the upper urinary tract.

9.4.3.2
The Ovarian Vein Syndrome

Compression of the ureter by an abnormal ovarian vein may result in two distinct clinical entities that must be considered separately: (a) syndromes of the ovarian vein strictly speaking, which correspond to an anatomoclinical entity, and (b) thrombophlebitis of the ovarian vein.

The ovarian vein syndrome was first described by Clark (CLARK 1964). It remains a controversial entity. It is defined by a moderate ureteral obstruction secondary to an extrinsic compression of the lumboiliac ureter by an ovarian vein of abnormal volume and situation (HUBMER 1978). This syndrome most often concerns the young, multiparous woman. Clinical presentation includes lumbar pain, recurrent urinary tract infections, and even acute pyelonephritis. Symptoms begin either during the second half of pregnancy or postpartum, or during the premenstrual period, occasionally reinforced by estrogen-progesterone treatment. Occurrence of this syndrome in a nulliparous patient is exceptional.

Risk factors and etiopathogenic hypotheses are numerous, so that there remains some doubt as to the existence itself of this syndrome.

9.4.3.2.1
Anatomic Factors

The particular relation between the right ovarian vein and the ureter accounts for the nearly exclusively right-sided location. Following an oblique course from lateral to medial, the right ovarian vein crosses indeed the anterior aspect of the ureter in front of L5–S1, at the level of the pelvic inlet. The craniocaudal level of this crossing may vary and, whatever the level, the ureter is flattened against the psoas muscle or the iliac vessels (Fig. 9.45). The ovarian vein is poorly valved, which explains its dilation during pregnancy. The left ovarian vein crosses the corresponding ureter much higher and compressive problems are more scarce on this side, as the left ureter does not rest on any hard posterior plane at that level (LASSNIG and FRICK 1978). Some observations of this syndrome on the left side were described, as well as bilaterally in exceptional cases (MELNICK and BRAMWITT 1971).

9.4.3.2.2
Mechanical Factors

The increase in caliber of the ovarian vein during pregnancy, up to threefold, is extremely important. After delivery the ovarian vein may involute over a few weeks, but after several births it may remain dilated, in particular owing to loss of valvular competence. Thrombophlebitis of the ovarian vein may maintain the increase in caliber and the compressive phenomena. Ptosis of the right kidney could also play a role.

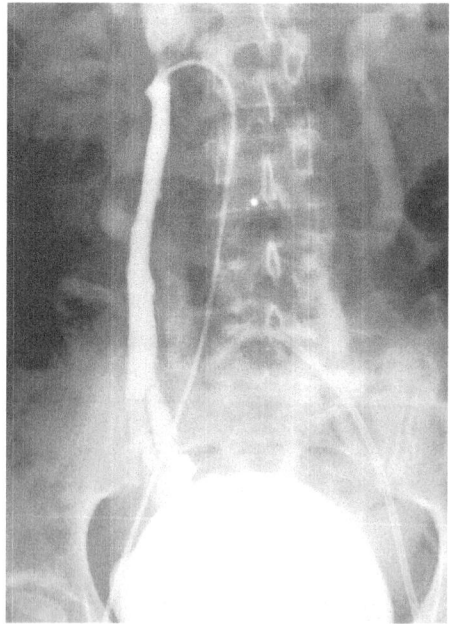

Fig 9.45. Ovarian vein syndrome? Retrograde opacification of the right ovarian vein shows crossing of the vein with the lumbar ureter, which is moderately dilated

9.4.3.2.3
Hormonal Factors

Hormonal factors may account for the ureteral hypotonia. The diagnosis is suspected on the basis of urographic findings. The typical image is represented by a medial incurvation of the right ureter at the level of L-5. Compressed segments appear as an extrinsic gutter-like lacuna with bluffed edges, oblique downward and laterally. Distension is usually moderate. RUP is necessary in exceptional cases to confirm the diagnosis. The same applies for ovarian vein phlebography: Even if it allows causal confirmation of the vein in the compressive phenomena, its clinical relevance is poor (PEREIRA et al. 1969).

Multiple arguments raise questions regarding the existence of this syndrome (DURE-SMITH 1979). The multiplicity of risk factors, the absence of an unequivocal and precise etiology, and above all the lack of a reproducible experimental model make the proper identification of this syndrome difficult. Similarly, moderate and ill-defined clinical symptoms and the low importance of radiological modifications lead us to think that in many cases this diagnosis should not be asserted with certainty, and that another cause of obstruction should always be searched for (vesicoureteral reflux, lithiasis). In some exceptional cases, this diagnosis may be retained because of the importance of clinical signs and of the upstream consequences seen at EU.

Symptomatic treatment is sufficient in most cases. Surgical intervention, including ureterolysis and resection of the ovarian vein, may sometimes be necessary and produces excellent results (DUFOUR 1973).

9.4.3.3
Thrombophlebitis of the Ovarian Vein

Thrombophlebitis is an anatomoclinical entity described by AUSTIN that has to be distinguished from the ovarian vein syndrome (AUSTIN 1956). Its place in this chapter results from its ureteral effects, which are frequent but inconstant and for years constituted the basis of radiological diagnosis. Most cases happen during the postpartum period, sometimes in the context of septicemia after gynecological surgery. Lumbar and pelvic pain and fever are the hallmarks of the clinical picture. Its frequency is about 0.18% after delivery. Venous stasis, hypercoagulability, and obstetrical maneuvers are all risk factors.

Although the disease typically concerns women, one similar case was described in the left testicular vein (KRETKOWSKI and SHAH 1977).

The diagnosis should be suggested by a clinical history of acute postpartum pyelonephritis with sterile urine, lumbar and pelvic pain, or fever that appears early between the first and fourth days after delivery.

The vital prognosis is relation to the extension of the thrombus to the IVC and to the embolic risk (RAJA-RAO et al. 1980). The right side is more frequently concerned, but some thromboses may be bilateral. Clinical diagnosis is often difficult and most frequently oriented towards a pelvic, adnexal, or appendicular infectious disease; in the past, it was sometimes discovered at surgical intervention only. Classical methods (EU, cavography) are often imprecise and tend to be replaced by color-Doppler ultrasonography, by CT and/or MRI examination, the first two being more frequently used in case of an abdominal emergency (DARNEY and WILSON 1977; SCHAPIRA and MITTY 1974). Ultrasonography may indicate ureteral obstruction and demonstrate the thrombosed vein as a hypoechoic rounded structure with hyperechoic center located to the right of the IVC (SAVADER et al. 1988).

Ureterohydronephrosis may be found as a sequela of an ovarian vein thrombophlebitis, due to a perivenous fibrous scarred proliferation encompassing the lumbar ureter. CT can show an infrarenal retroperitoneal tubular mass and, after contrast injection, a central lacuna that corresponds to the thrombus (ANGEL and KNUPPEL 1984; SAVADER et al. 1988). Some recent observations illustrated the interest of using MRI for this diagnosis: T_2-weighted sequences show a target appearance of the vein, consisting of a hypointense center, an intermediate hyperintense area, and a peripheral hypointense area (MARTIN et al. 1988; SAVADER et al. 1988). These new imaging techniques, in particular MRI, may show the extension to the IVC. Ultrasonography may be used for the follow-up after medical treatment (anticoagulation and antibiotic therapy).

9.4.3.4
Other Venous Compressions

There have been some other rare reported cases of venous compressions. Some are exceptional cases of retroiliac ureters: The ureter passes between the artery and the vein or behind these two vessels. This abnormality may be found on both sides, separately or simultaneously (HOCK et al. 1972; HANNA 1972).

Other cases are embryological abnormalities of the IVC due to abnormal persistence of horizontal branches that join the cardinal veins together. These persisting veins form rings that surround and obstruct the ureter. Similarly, ureteral obstructions due to anastomotic veins between gonadal veins and the IVC or between lumbar veins and the IVC were described (PSIRHAMIS 1987). These exceptional observations have a urographic appearance similar to that of the retrocaval ureter. CT scan with 3-D reconstructions is the only modality that indicates the diagnosis by showing the aberrant venous course and the absence of a normal course of the ureter behind the IVC (DILLON and CAMPUTARO 1991).

A ureteral obstruction by a gonadal vein has also been demonstrated by CT (MEYER et al. 1992), and an inferior vena cava filter and other filtering devices can cause right ureteral obstruction (Figs. 9.46, 9.47)

9.4.4
Vascular Ureteral Impressions

Vascular ureteral impressions comprise several radiological abnormalities, discovered mainly at EU and corresponding to lacunar images in relation to a narrow contact between the ureter and a normal or abnormal vascular structure, either arterial or venous. These abnormalities are usually asymptomatic and benign. Their identification may be difficult and their observation may occasionally raise diagnostic problems. Indeed, they are characterized by the fact that they are not accompanied by any effect on the evacuation of the urinary tract and do not provoke any obstructive syndrome. CHAIT demonstrated particularly well the different etiologies of these vascular impressions, by distinguishing pressure defects without clinical significance and pressure defects which represent collateral pathways in relation to a vascular obstructive pathology, either arterial or venous (CHAIT et al. 1971).

9.4.4.1
Diagnostic Problems

Vascular impressions may be isolated or multiple, and either localized or involving a more or less extensive segment of the ureteral course. The urographic identification of these pressure defects relies on several common observations, the sum of which suggests the diagnosis. They may be seen on all pictures showing the ureter, whatever the opacification mode (WINFIELD and MAZER 1990). They consist of extrinsic compression images: pelviureteral notch "scalloping" attached by obtuse angles to the wall, persisting filling defect, corkscrew appearance of the ureter. A particular appearance is a serpentine band-like print

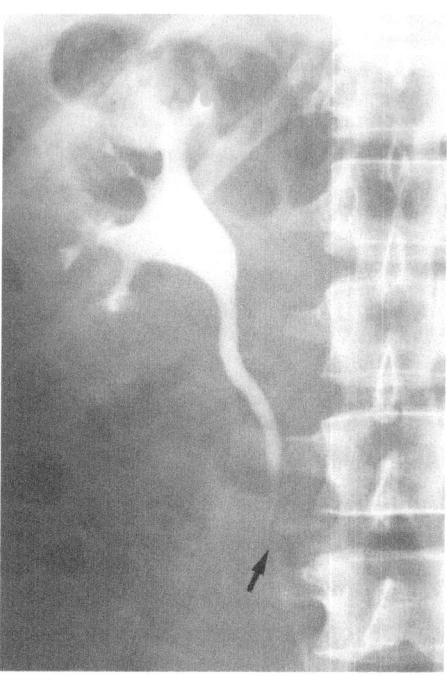

Fig 9.46. Right ureteral deviation by an Adams de Wiese device (*arrow*)

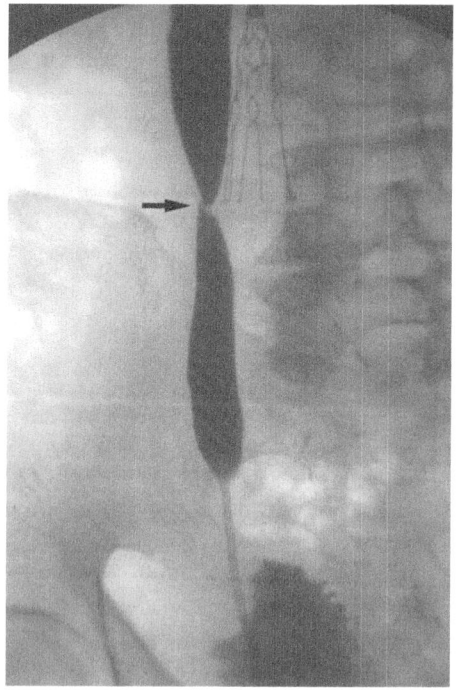

Fig 9.47. Ureteral stenosis related to a Greenfield IVC filter (*arrow*)

along the ureteral course that must be differentiated from ureteral peristaltic waves and that points toward a print due to dilated ureteral vessels. Sharp edges are suggestive of an arterial nature, fuzzy and shading off aspects rather of a venous origin. These prints may be seen on every picture and are invariably located at the same level. Their topography depends on the etiology or on the arterial or venous origin. They are more easily seen on filling films immediately after compression release than on an empty, contracted, or evacuating ureter. Some marks, however (in particular venous prints), tend to disappear more easily in case of endoureteral hyperpressure (prolonged compression, filling under pressure at RUP). These images of venous impressions also vary depending on position changes (increase in orthostatism and in prone position).

Angiography, either arterial (aortography, selective renal arteriography) or venous (inferior cavography by bifemoral approach, selective renal or gonadal phlebography), classically confirms the diagnosis. The examination is motivated by the urographic appearance. Ultrasonography (KAUZLARIC and BARMEIR 1984) and especially helical CT currently provide diagnostic details on the vascular nature and the origin of such lesions (RADIN et al. 1986; BJORGUINSSON and FRIEDMAN 1984).

Thus, the combination of these radiological signs may call to mind the vascular nature of these ureteral impressions. The differential diagnosis includes ureteral compressions of extrinsic origin and some parietal lesions of the ureter. Indicative elements are the semiologic characteristics of vascular prints, their topography, their morphology, which varies according the degree of emptying of the urinary tract and the degree of hyperpressure, and finally their usually asymptomatic character. In doubtful cases, an angiographic and mainly CT study will determine their nature precisely. It seems acceptable for the majority of authors to replace angiography by helical CT for assessment of relationships between vessels and the ureter (ROUVIERE et al. 1999).

9.4.4.2
Etiologies

The relationship between lacunar ureteral images and vascular origin is most often made at EU. However, the diagnosis relies primarily on angiographic examination and more recently on CT, which makes it possible to determine the arterial or venous nature as well as the cause of these vascular prints:

- Vascular impressions of arterial origin:
  - Compression of the lumbar ureter by an aberrant renal artery
  - Periureteral collateral arteries secondary to a renal artery stenosis
  - Periureteral collateral arteries secondary to an aortoiliac occlusion
  - Ureteral print by aortoiliac or hypogastric aneurysm
  - Thrombosed umbilical artery
  - Retroiliac ureter
- Vascular impressions of venous origin:
  - Periureteral varices
  - Collateral veins secondary to an occlusion of the IVC
  - Collateral veins secondary to an occlusion of the superior vena cava and azygos vein
  - Collateral veins secondary to portal hypertension
  - Collateral veins secondary to pancreatic cancer and segmental portal hypertension
  - Ovarian vein syndrome

Identification of these anomalies allows in some cases the demonstration of underlying and previously unknown diseases.

9.4.4.2.1
Vascular Ureteral Impressions of Arterial Origin

Depending on the artery concerned, different types of ureteral prints of arterial origin may be encountered. Some are found with high frequency in the normal subject and do not have any pathological significance. They need only to be recognized at film reading and interpretation. Others are seen in certain specific arterial pathologies, involving particular aspects depending on their etiologies.

Ureteral Vascular Imprints in Relation with Normal Arteries. As previously seen, some accessory renal arteries may be responsible for ureteral compression. They consist mainly of supernumerary inferior polar renal arteries that originate on the lower abdominal aorta or sometimes on the common iliac artery. The marks are either a crossing image of the incriminated vessel with the ureter, or a lateral or medial scalloping on the ureteral edge.

Ureteral prints due to the iliac axes represent one of the classic images of physiological narrowing of the ureter, located in front of the sacroiliac joints or sacral wings. At that level, the ureter crosses the iliac axes, and a minimal fusiform dilation of the upstream ureter is often present. This physiological narrowing may occasionally favor the blocking of lithiasis at that level.

Arterial Impression in Relation to an Obstructive Arterial Pathology. Urographic appearances correspond to prints secondary to the existence of collateral pathways. They may occasionally be the revealing factor. Ureteral prints observed in these cases are related to hypertrophy of the ureteral arteries. The images of vascular origin extend along the whole lumbar portion of the ureter, with a serpentine appearance (Fig. 9.48). Hypertrophy of these vessels is most often due to the existence of a renal artery stenosis, either atheromatous or dysplastic (CHAIT et al. 1971; KIRSCHNER and TWIGG 1967). Such images may also be observed with an increase of the arterial renal flow, for example, in highly vascularized renal adenocarcinoma. Occlusion of the infrarenal abdominal aorta and iliac arteries may also be responsible for periureteral collateral ways. Contrary to the previous situation, the blood flow of the ureteral artery will be directed to the pelvis and the lower limbs.

Much rarer are ureteral prints in relation to col-

lateral pathways secondary to obstructive lesions of the digestive arteries. NORFRAY relates one case of arterial marks on the right ureter secondary to the development of a hypertrophied duodenopancreatic artery after occlusion of the celiac trunk at its origin, and opacification of the hepatic artery and the splenic artery from the superior mesenteric artery. Similarly, localized marks on the left lumbar ureter secondary to hypertrophy of the arch of Riolan may be found (NORFRAY and NUDELMAN 1974).

Ureteral Prints in Relation to an Aneurysmal Pathology. Aneurysms of the abdominal aorta and its branches may promote anterior and lateral displacement of one or even both ureters in some cases. Sometimes, lateral displacement of one ureter may be observed along with attraction of the contralateral ureter (PECK et al. 1973). These modifications often are parallel and lateral to the arciform calcifications of the aneurysmal wall. The importance of lateral displacement and the length of ureter involved is a function of the size and the topography of the aneurysm. The ureter may also be laminated, but the existence of signs of obstruction should

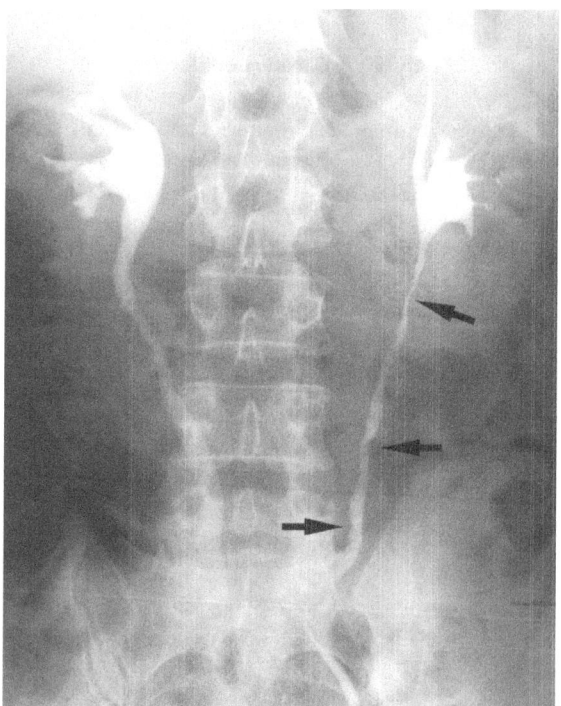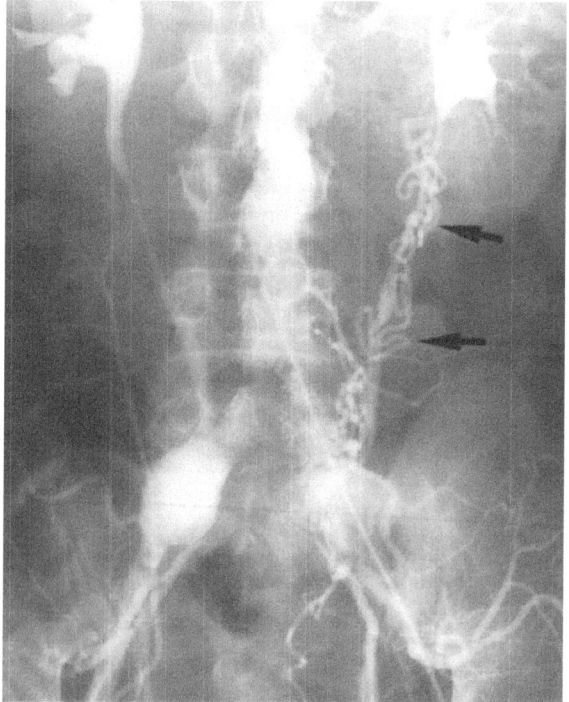

a   b

Fig 9.48a, b. Vascular ureteral impression of arterial origin. **a** EU shows multiple ureteral notches of the left lumbar ureter (*arrows*). **b** Late view of aortography shows arterial collateral circulation originating from the left iliac artery and visualizing the dilated left ureteral arteries (*arrows*). These collateral vessels allow opacification of intrarenal arterial branches, and the diagnosis of left renal artery stenosis is suspected

raise suspicion of an associated PIF. The presence of similar abnormalities on the pelvic ureter points to the diagnosis of an iliac artery aneurysm.

On abdominal plain roentgenograms, the identification of arciform calcifications of the arterial wall in front of the ureter may suggest the diagnosis, which is based on angiography and/or new imaging techniques (ultrasonography and CT)

9.4.4.2.2
Ureteral Impressions of Venous Origin

Ureteral impressions of venous origin may also be of multiple origin. In some cases, their etiopathology is straightforward (such as thrombosis of the infrarenal IVC). Their presence often is not related to a precise physiopathological mechanism (ureteral varices). In some rare cases, they may be symptomatic (hematuria from ureteral varices, ureteral obstruction from ovarian vein thrombophlebitis).

Gonadal Veins. Gonadal veins may produce a physiological vascular stamp by crossing with the right ureter at the L3–4 level, or even lower in some cases (up to the sacroiliac joint). The gonadal vein crosses the ureter following a very oblique axis coursing laterally and downward. On the left side, this crossing is located higher, just after the pelviureteral junction. The role played by gonadal veins in the right ovarian vein syndrome has been discussed above in this chapter (CLARK 1964).

Idiopathic Periureteral Varices. Idiopathic periureteral varices correspond to venous ectasias that predominate at the lumbar level and involve the gonadal or periureteral veins. These two venous networks often are anastomosed together. The varices are usually found in the male adult patient and are extremely rare in children (BRAEDEL and SCHINDLER 1981; KAUFMAN and MAXWELL 1984; PADOVANI et al. 1984). In some cases, they may be associated with varicoceles or varices of the broad ligament (BERGMAN and COPELAND 1983). They are usually isolated. Often latent and found at EU, they nevertheless merit recognition because of their occasional symptomatic character, being the origin of recurrent painless macroscopic hematuria. Their identification is important when one is deciding on a potential surgical (or endovascular) treatment. They may be bilateral, although they are more often reported on the left side. They are often associated with renal pelvic localizations. Their diagnosis, suggested by EU and less frequently by

ultrasonography, classically relies on angiographic examination (BRAEDEL et al. 1977; KAUSLARIC and BARMEIR 1984).

These periureteral varices may be identified on CT as multiple nodular or curvilinear densities, enhanced after contrast medium injection. Their diameter is about 5–6 mm. Diagnosis is improved by helical CT acquisition and 3-D reconstruction.

Their etiopathology remains a matter of discussion; they might be caused by the same mechanisms invoked for the ovarian vein syndrome, the formation of varicoceles in men and of varices of the broad ligament in women. There are nevertheless particular anatomic factors that may account for the left-sided predominance:

- Length of the course of gonadal veins on the left side
- Penetration at 90° of the left gonadal vein into the renal vein
- Venous valvular incompetence
- Compression of the left gonadal vein by the descending colon
- The aortomesenteric angle ("nutcracker phenomenon") (BEINART et al. 1982; NISHIMURA et al. 1986) (Fig. 9.49)

These idiopathic periureteral varices must be differentiated from secondary ureteral varices.

Collateral Venous Pathways. Collateral venous pathways correspond to the development and hypertrophy of a venous collateral network. They are met in various conditions, most often in thromboses affecting the inferior caval system or its branches.

Thrombosis of the infrarenal IVC, whatever its origin (retroperitoneal fibrosis, cruoric thrombosis, agenesis or malformation of the IVC, neoplastic invasion of the IVC, therapeutic caval interruption), may promote the development of a periureteral venous network of pelvic origin (Fig. 9.50). Similarly, neoplastic or cruoric thrombosis of the renal vein (particularly on the left side) leads to the creation of pathways draining blood away from the kidney, in particular periureteral collaterals (Fig. 9.50). Much more rarely, periureteral collaterals veins may be found at the level of the reno-azygo-lumbar arch, in case of occlusion of the azygos vein or thrombosis of the superior vena cava. The presence of a cancer of the pancreatic tail may produce splenic or even renal vein obstruction, which results in dilation of periureteral veins. Ureteral imprints secondary to portosystemic derivation pathways have also been reported (KESHMIN and JOFFRE 1956). In case of

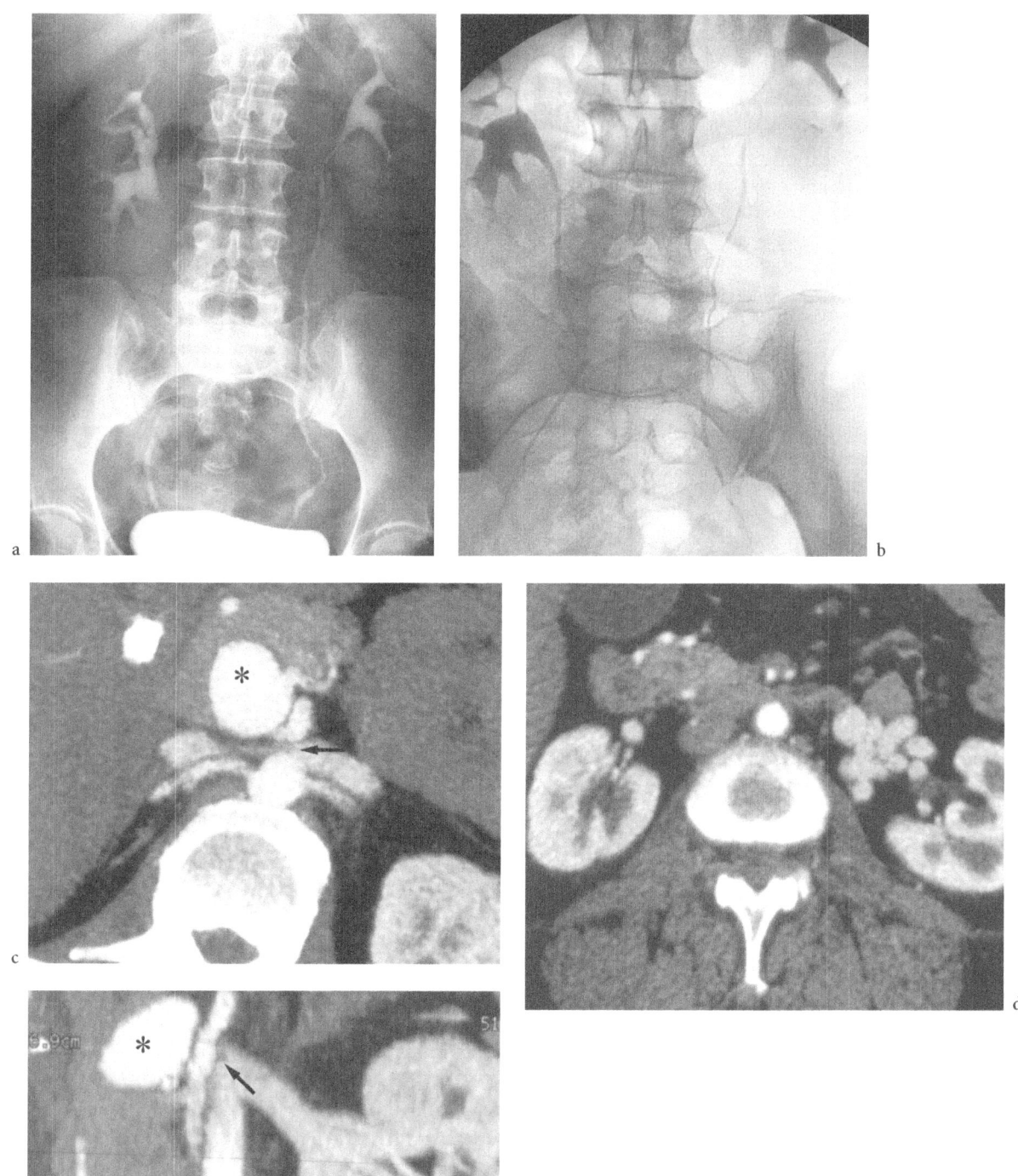

Fig 9.49a–e. Venous ureteral impressions by "nutcracker" phenomenon. **a, b** EU views of left ureter with multiple imprints of extrinsic origin. **c** CT axial slice demonstrates narrowing of the left renal vein between the aorta and the mesenteric artery (*arrow*). The left renal vein is also compressed by an aneurysm of a branch of the mesenteric artery (*asterisk*). **d** CT axial slice shows opacification of periureteral varices. **e** MIP reconstruction shows the aneurysm (*asterisk*), the nutcracker syndrome (*arrow*), and the periureteral varices

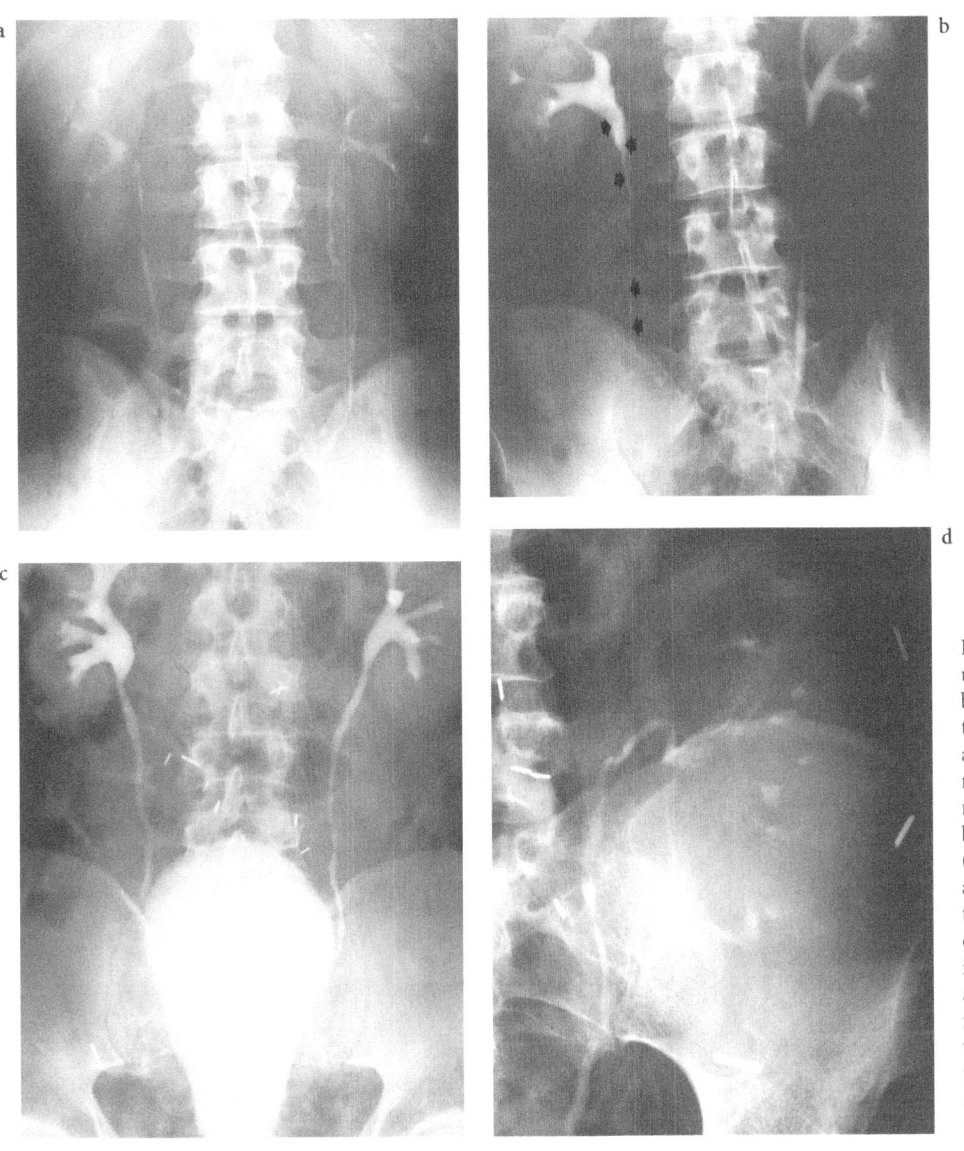

Fig 9.50a–d. Venous ureteral impressions by IVC or renal vein thrombosis. **a, b** EU in a patient with bilateral renal vein thrombosis: multiple imprints of both lumbar ureters (*arrows*). **c** EU in a patient with IVC thrombosis: bilateral venous ureteral impressions and "pear-shaped" bladder. **d** EU in a patient with renal vein thrombosis on a transplanted kidney shows multiple pelvic and ureteral notches

huge adenocarcinomas of the right kidney, communications between perirenal veins and the superior mesenteric system may also exist. Ureteral imprints have also been described in high-flow arteriovenous renal fistulas or in severe congestive cardiac insufficiency (Radin et al. 1986).

Vascular opacifications of the caval system help to determine the level and the type of obliteration, but helical CT examination is of great value in determining the etiology and, in particular, in distinguishing cruoric from neoplastic thromboses (Glazer et al. 1984). These modalities also provide a pseudoangiographic view. MRI should certainly provide interesting information in this kind of disease.

9.5
Other Extrinsic Ureteral Disorders

9.5.1
Retroperitoneal and Pelvic Lipomatosis

Diffuse fatty infiltrative lesions of the pelvic cavity and less commonly of the retroperitoneum are rare conditions (Lewis et al. 1982). Their etiology is unclear; they are encountered mainly in black males and are often associated with obesity. Cushing's disease and corticotherapy have also been incriminated. The lesions are composed of hypertrophic, normal but unencapsulated fat, differing in this from lipomas. They develop preferentially in the regions around the rectum and bladder. They generally present as urinary symptoms related to ureteral and bladder compression (low back pain, frequency, dysuria) or rectal compression (tenesmus). The patient frequently complains of pelvic congestion and heaviness. Clinical examination rarely shows a suprapubic mass, and no localized mass is found on digital pelvic examination.

Diagnosis relies on radiography. Plain abdominal film may show opacities of fatty density and displacement of gas-filled structures. EU shows bilateral hydroureteronephrosis if the location is pelvic. The ureters are symmetrically displaced, either laterally or more often toward the midline (Moss et al. 1972). The bladder shows a "reverse pear" shape, and its floor is raised (Fig. 9.51). The appearance of bladder deformity is nonspecific, and several diagnoses should be considered (Saxton 1990):

- Diffuse pelvic adenopathy, giving an appearance of arc-shaped deviation or ureteral compression at many sites
- Inferior vena cava obstruction, leading to pelvic edema and often accompanied by ureteral notching
- Pelvic hematoma in certain contexts (injury, anticoagulant treatment)
- Bilateral iliac aneurysms, resulting in localized ureteral compression

If lipomatosis is retroperitoneal, the kidneys and ureters are displaced laterally and upward, and the urinary tract and pyelocaliceal cavities are stretched, as there is often an extension to the renal sinuses (Fig. 9.52). This lipomatosis raises the possibility of a median retroperitoneal tumor, in particular a nodal tumor. These various diagnoses are generally differentiated by ultrasonography and above all by CT. Pelvic ultrasonography may be hyperechoic; CT scan is the most useful technique, as it establishes the diagnosis (Werboff et al. 1979). It detects diffuse infiltration of the pelvic and/or retroperitoneal cavity by fat-density tissue (Lewis et al. 1982) (Fig. 9.53). It reveals any impact on the adjacent organs and in particular on the urinary apparatus. CT shows cephalad displacement and "pear-shaped" bladder narrowing, straightening of the rectum, elevation of the sigmoid, and medial displacement and dilatation of the ureters. It thus excludes the other causes of diffuse pelvic infiltration and also psoas muscle hypertrophy, which is the most frequent differential diagnosis (Bree et al. 1976). MRI visualizes the extent of lipomatosis in the various spatial planes (Demas et al. 1988). Association with cystitis glandularis or cystica has frequently been noted (Fig. 9.54). Long-term prognosis is mediocre as there is no effective treatment apart from attempting to preserve renal function by ureteral intubation.

9.5.2
Extrinsic Ureteral Pathology of Gastrointestinal Origin

The urinary and gastrointestinal tracts are in close proximity in multiple regions (Balfe and Bova 1990). The right ureter is in close relationship with the distal ileum, cecum, and appendix particularly if retrocecal. The left ureter is behind the jejunal loops. The terminal right and left ureters are close to the anterolateral wall of the rectum and separated from it by fat.

The ureters are affected by diseases of the gastrointestinal tract via two main mechanisms, sometimes associated (Banner 1987):
- Direct extension of active inflammatory or tumoral diseases
- Extrinsic compression secondary to abscess or tumor

Whatever the mechanism, the radiological appearance is summarized by obstructive uropathy, generally unilateral, with or without ureteral displacement, with smooth, tapered stenoses of the ureter at differ-

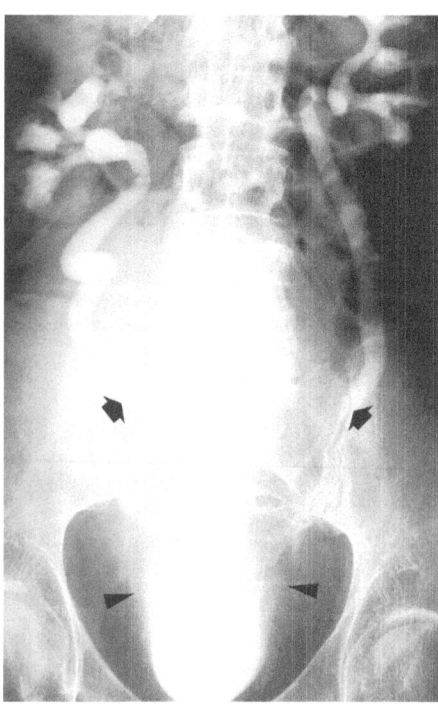

Fig 9.51. Pelvic lipomatosis: EU shows bilateral ureterohydronephrosis; lumbar ureters are laterally deviated and obstructed (*arrows*). Pear-shape change of the bladder (*arrowheads*)

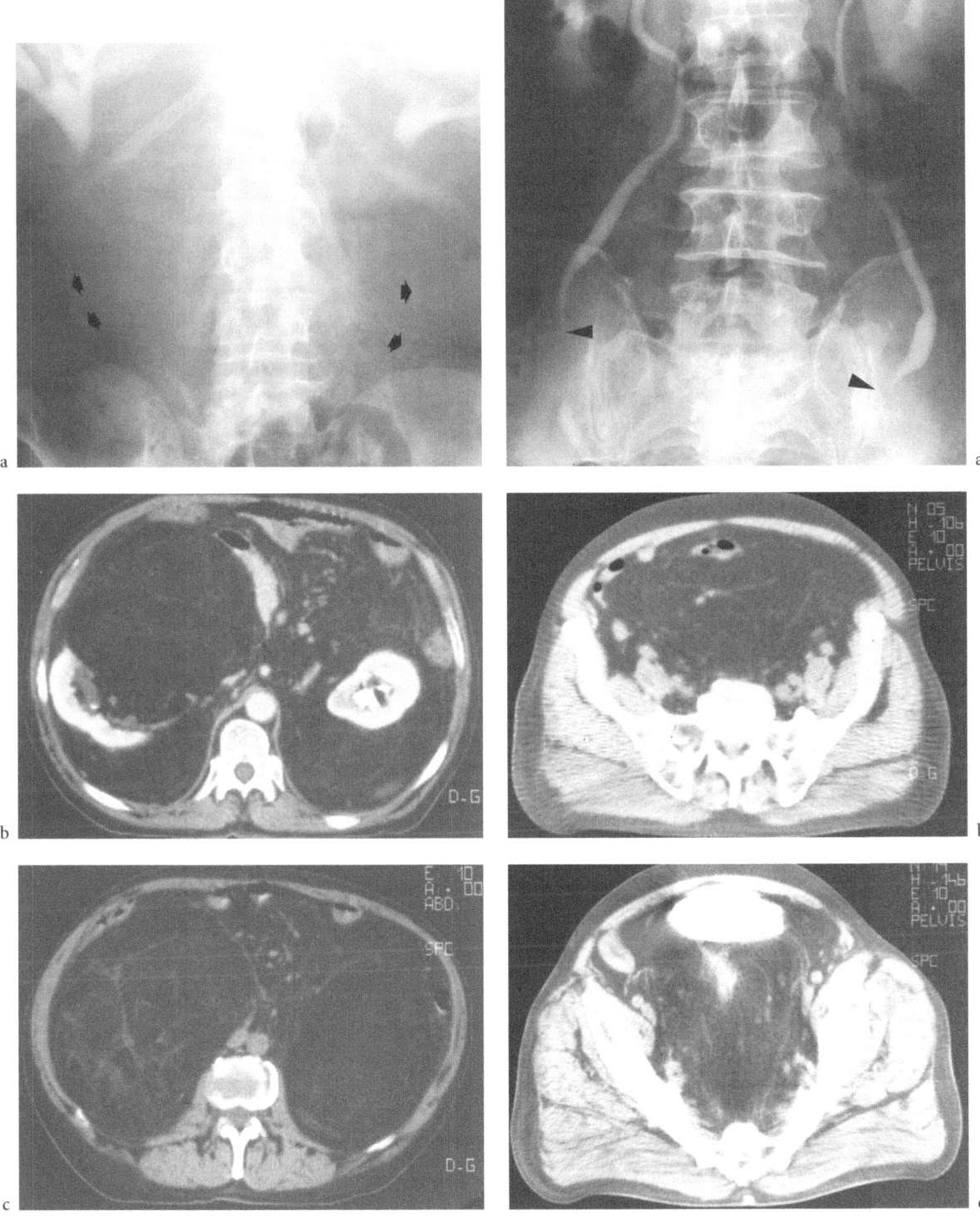

Fig 9.52a–c. Retroperitoneal lipomatosis. a EU shows bilateral deviation of both lumbar ureters and kidneys (*arrows*). Multiple fat densities in the retroperitoneum. b, c CT shows huge lipomatous retroperitoneal masses with mass effect on kidneys and intestinal tract

Fig 9.53a–c. Pelvic lipomatosis. a EU shows moderate dilatation of ureters, which are deviated laterally (*arrowheads*) by a pelvic mass. b, c CT shows diffuse infiltration of the pelvic cavity by fatty tissue with displacement of the bladder and rectum

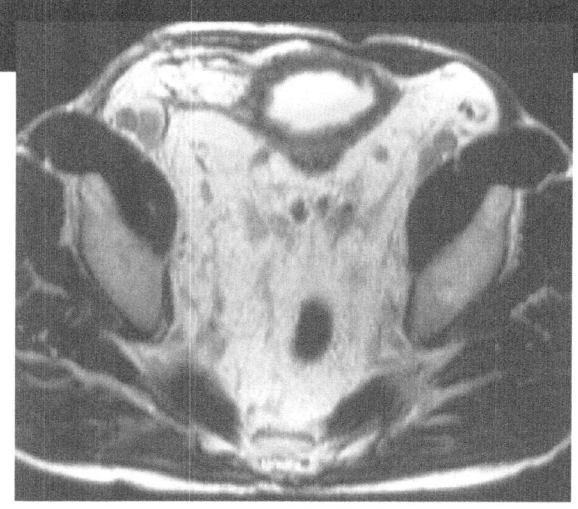
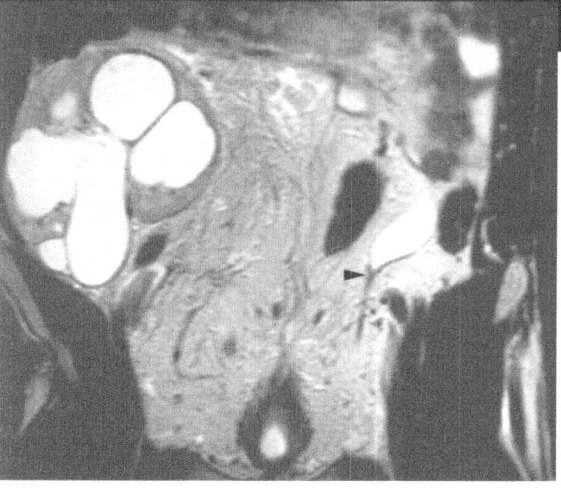

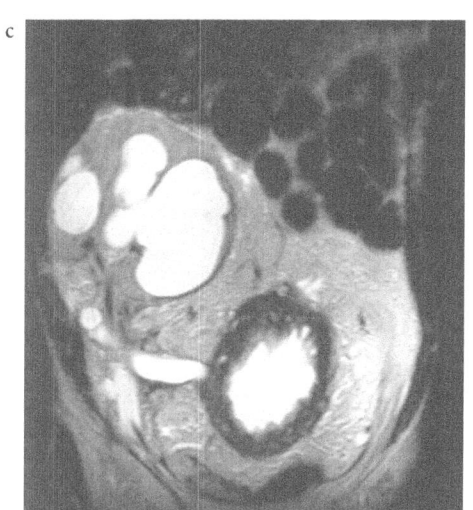
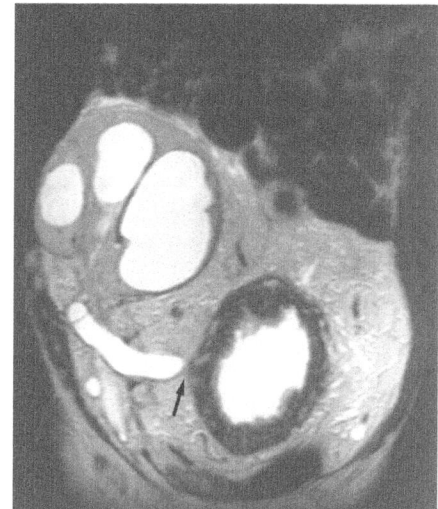

Fig 9.54a–d. Pelvic lipomatosis. **a–d** Axial and coronal MRI slices with T_2-weighted sequences show diffuse fatty infiltration of the pelvic cavity. Left native dilated ureter is visible in **b** with narrowing related to the lipomatosis (*arrowhead*). Slices **c** and **d** show ureterohydronephrosis of a transplanted kidney related to thickening of the bladder wall secondary to cystitis glandularis (*arrow*)

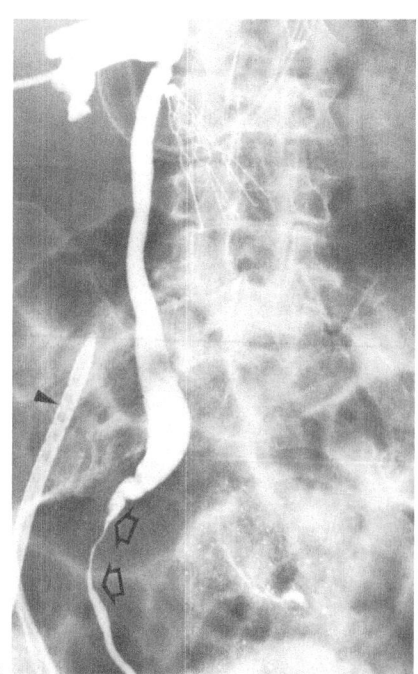
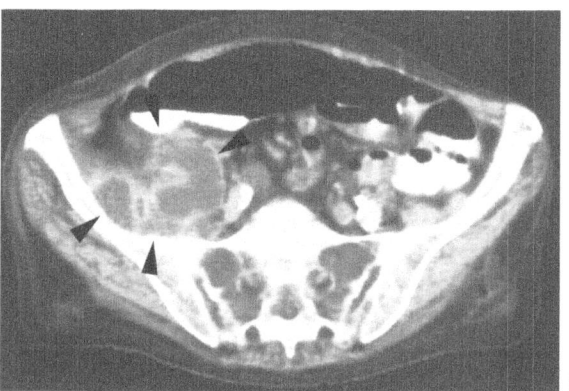

Fig 9.55a, b. Ureteral obstruction secondary to Crohn's disease. **a** antegrade pyelography via a percutaneous nephrostomy catheter shows right ureterohydronephrosis related to narrowing of the ureter, which is deviated and compressed (*arrows*). Note a drainage catheter in place in a retroperitoneal abscess (*arrowhead*). **b** CT shows pelvic abscess of the ilio-psoas compartment (*arrowheads*)

ent levels, mainly at the pelvis brim. CT scan at the level of stenosis provides information regarding gastrointestinal inflammatory or tumoral diseases.

9.5.2.1
Inflammatory Diseases

Ureteral involvement occurs in 15%–23% of patients with Crohn's disease (SHIELD et al. 1976; FLECKEN-STEIN et al. 1977). The main cause of obstruction is retroperitoneal abscess, generally in the right psoas compartment, related to ileitis (Fig. 9.55). Stenosis

may rarely be caused by chronic retroperitoneal inflammation with fibrotic reaction (retroperitoneal fibrosis). Bilateral obstruction and ureteral fistulas are exceptional (McMANAMON et al. 1985). Treatment must be conservative by ureteral intubation with a double-J pigtail stent. Surgery is technically difficult and obstruction often stationary.

The left ureter is the most likely to be affected by diverticulitis. The frequency is less than 0.5% (NEY et al. 1986). The most common type of involvement is ureteral stenosis by extrinsic compression and displacement secondary to pelvic abscess (Fig. 9.56).

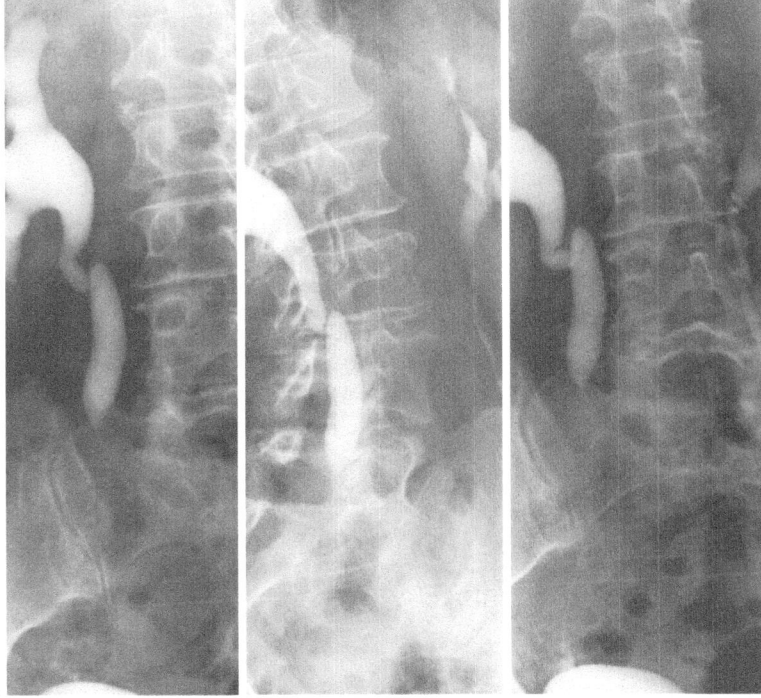

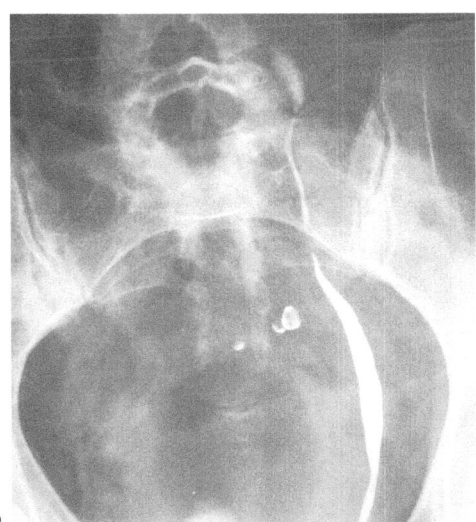
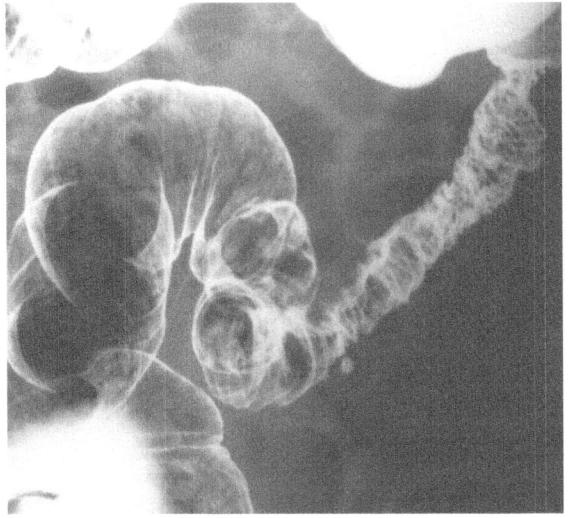

a

b

c

Fig 9.56a–c. Ureteral obstruction secondary to diverticulitis. **a** EU views in prone position show left ureterohydronephrosis with obstruction of the left iliac ureter. **b** Retrograde pyelogram shows tubular stenosis of the left ureter at the pelvic brim level. **c** Barium enema shows spiculated sigmoid with diverticula and signs of diverticulitis

Obstructive uropathy is less frequent than bladder involvement.

The proximity of retrocecal appendices and the right ureter can explain ureteral stenosis secondary to inflammation, and retrocecal perforated appendicitis with retroperitoneal abscess may cause right hydronephrosis by compression (JONES and BARIE 1988) (Fig. 9.57). Urinary symptoms occur in 17% of cases of appendiceal abscesses and EU shows hydroureteronephrosis in 50% of cases.

Due to fascial boundaries between the pancreas and retroperitoneal spaces, a pancreatic pseudocyst may extend to the ureters, mainly the left, and obstruct them (Fig. 9.58). Right ureteral obstruction can also be secondary to thickening of renal fascia secondary to pancreatitis (MOREHOUSE et al. 1983).

9.5.2.2
Tumoral Diseases

Carcinomas of the gastrointestinal tract and pancreas may infiltrate the retroperitoneum either directly or, more often, by metastatic extension. Such spread can lead to urinary obstruction, generally due to malignant retroperitoneal fibrosis or more rarely to ureteral metastasis (PUECH et al. 1987). Both ureters can be obstructed, mainly at the pelvic brim, secondary to cancer of the colon, stomach, or duodenum. Medial ureteral deviation must be differentiated from the normal appearance secondary to proctosigmoidostomy (SPILLANE et al. 1951) (Fig. 9.59). Pancreatic carcinoma can cause ureteral obstruction by encasement and also ureteral notching by occlusion of the left renal vein (WARDEN et al. 1981).

9.5.2.3
Fecal Impaction

A huge fecal mass in the rectum or sigmoid in patients with long-standing constipation may cause ureteral obstruction, frequently associated with bladder outlet obstruction (HALLER et al. 1976). The precise mechanism has not been definitively demonstrated (SHOPFNER 1968).

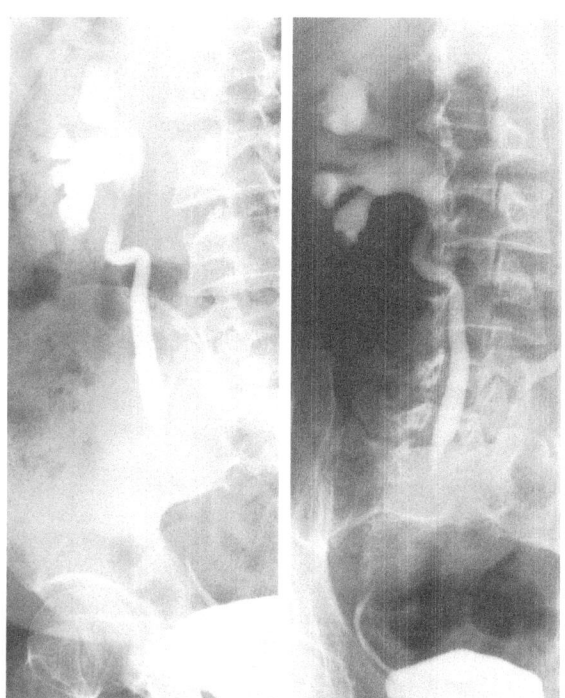

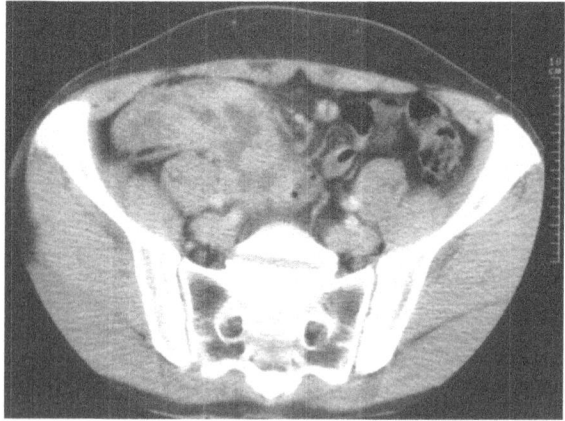

Fig 9.57a–c. Ureteral obstruction related to an appendicular abscess: **a** EU views show obstruction of the right pelvic ureter with dilatation of the upper urinary tract. **b, c** CT shows inflammatory mass of the right pelvic area with signs of abscess

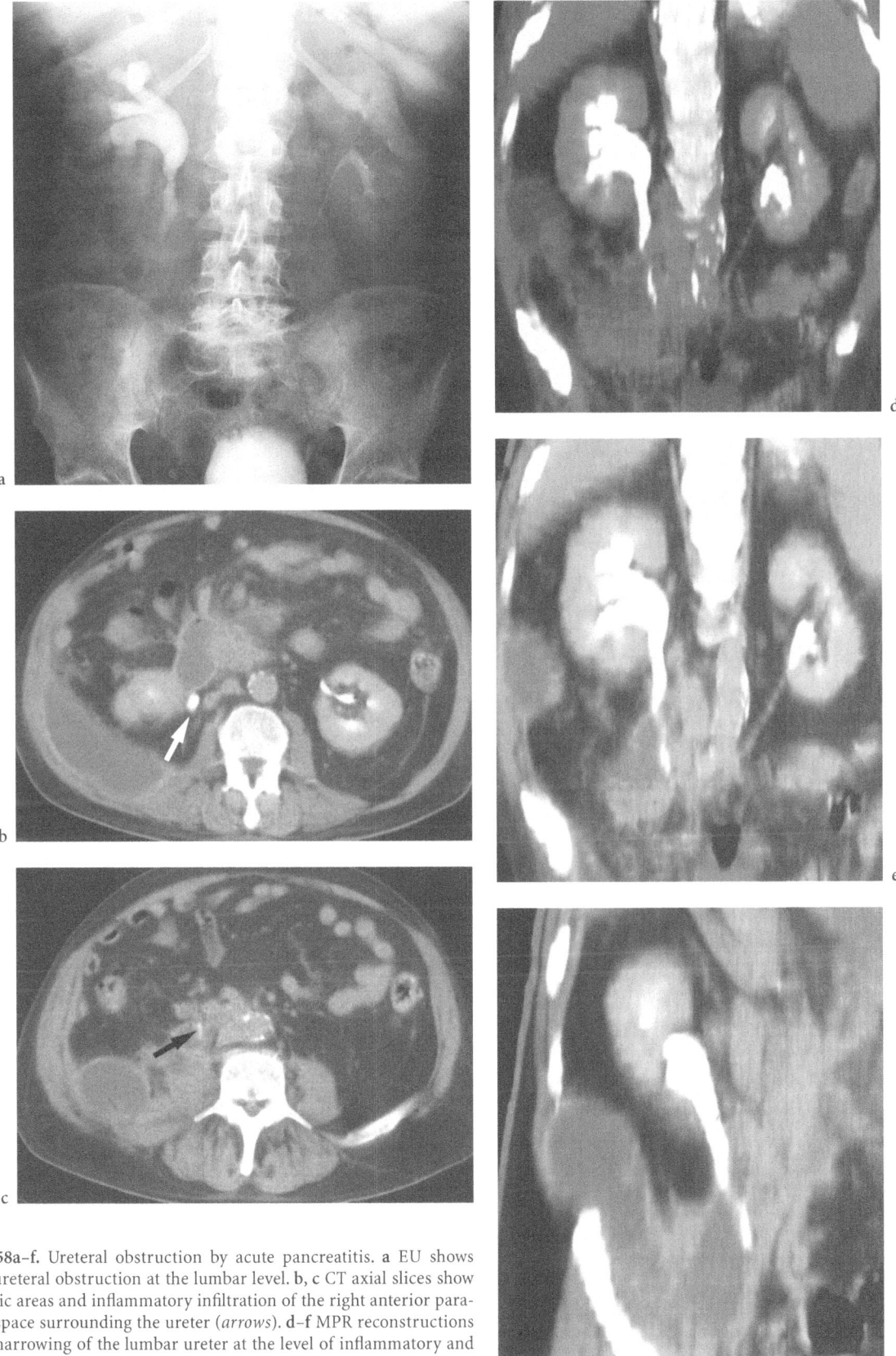

Fig 9.58a–f. Ureteral obstruction by acute pancreatitis. **a** EU shows right ureteral obstruction at the lumbar level. **b, c** CT axial slices show necrotic areas and inflammatory infiltration of the right anterior pararenal space surrounding the ureter (*arrows*). **d–f** MPR reconstructions show narrowing of the lumbar ureter at the level of inflammatory and cystic changes related to pancreatitis

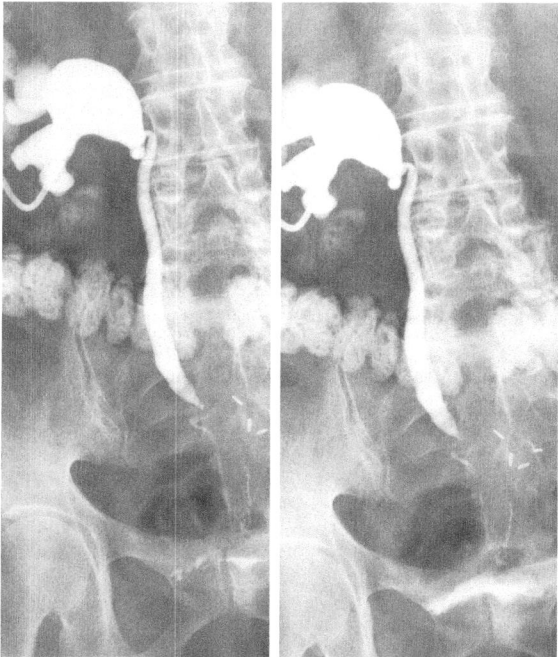

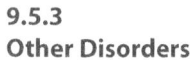

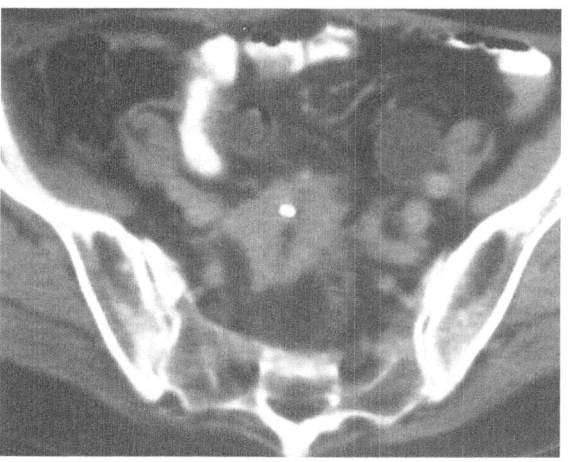

Fig 9.59a, b. Ureteral obstruction secondary to a recurrent rectal carcinoma: **a** Antegrade pyelography in prone position via a percutaneous nephrostomy catheter shows left uretero-hydronephrosis related to an obstruction of the left pelvic ureter, which is medially deviated. **b** CT shows a tumoral mass in the pelvic area corresponding to a recurrence after proctosigmoidostomy

9.5.3
Other Disorders

9.5.3.1
Uterine Prolapse

Uterine prolapse, secondary to multiple pregnancies with difficult delivery, can be responsible for cystocele and ureteral abnormalities (ELKIN et al. 1972). Ureteral obstruction has been reported in 30%–90% of women with severe prolapse (GREGOIR et al. 1976). Obstruction is related to several factors (KONTO-GEORGOS et al. 1985): inferior displacement of the trigone, compression between the uterus and levator muscles. Ultrasonography should be proposed for screening elderly women with prolapse. EU is warranted only if there is obstruction. Bilateral, usually symmetrical hydroureteronephrosis is associated with cystocele and bilateral medial displacement, stretching, narrowing and sometimes kinking of the ureters (Fig. 9.60). These changes are easily shown on erect EU and can decrease or disappear with decubitus and manual suppression of the cystocele (ELKIN et al. 1972).

9.5.3.2
Retroperitoneal and Pelvic Collections

The mass effect of retroperitoneal and pelvic collections can cause ureteral compression with deviation and obstruction at a higher level. Such collections

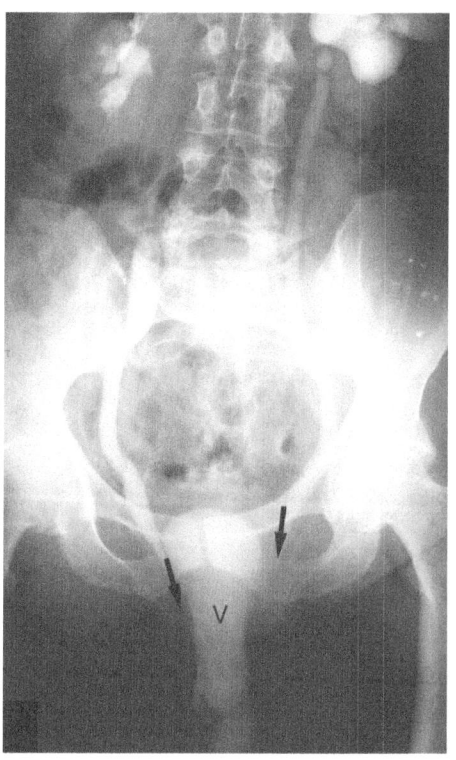

Fig 9.60. Ureteral obstruction related to uterine prolapse: EU shows moderate bilateral ureterohydronephrosis with displacement and stretching of the ureters (*arrows*) following the cystocele (*V*)

may be spontaneous, post-traumatic, or postoperative. A urinoma, hematoma, abscess, or lymphocele may be encountered. Collections within the psoas compartment may have an identical effect on the ureter. Ultrasonography and especially CT scan are the modalities of choice for detecting a collection and assessing the effect on the ureter. Diagnosis of the type of collection depends on its radiographic appearance and the clinical context.

- Retroperitoneal hematoma is the most frequent cause of retroperitoneal or pelvic collections. Helical CT is the technique of choice. Unenhanced acquisition shows characteristic high density. Early acquisition with contrast injection is very useful to detect some specific causes: hemorrhagic tumor, spontaneous or post-traumatic vascular lesions.
- A retroperitoneal or pelvic abscess is often secondary to obstructive or postoperative uropathy. It is characterized by fluid collection with thick, hypervascularized, sometimes septated walls and slightly elevated water attenuation, around 20 HU.
- A urinoma is in general paraureteral and well circumscribed and has water attenuation. A delayed CT scan may sometimes show opacification of the sac by the iodinated contrast medium because of persisting communication with the urinary tract.

If diagnosis is doubtful, guided fine-needle aspiration with bacteriological and biochemical analysis of the fluid sample determines its nature. Percutaneous drainage of the collection may be necessary, thus resolving the collection and relieving ureteral compression. If drainage fails, is difficult, or is not an option, it may be advisable to drain the urinary tract above the obstruction, either by nephrostomy or by insertion of a double-J pigtail stent.

9.5.3.3
Others

Miscellaneous disorders that have been reported (TALNER 1990) include:
- Extrinsic ureteral obstruction secondary to inflammatory retroperitoneal adenopathy: tuberculosis, brucellosis, actinomycosis, sarcoidosis
- Granulomas secondary to foreign substances
- External or medial deviation by bladder diverticula (Fig. 9.61)

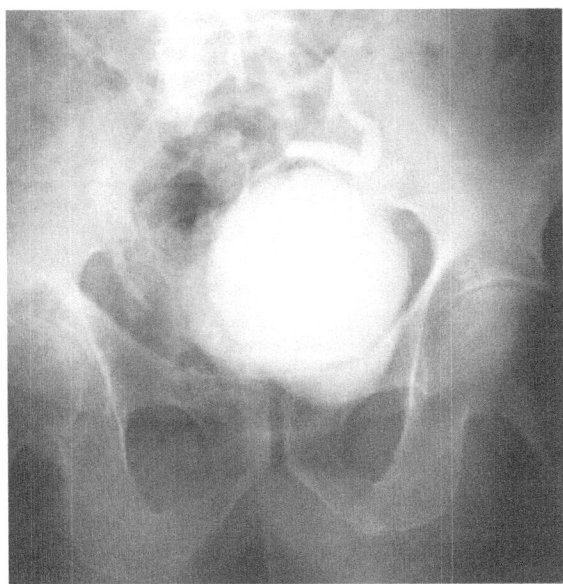

Fig 9.61. Medial deviation and moderate obstruction of the left ureter related to bladder diverticulum

References

Ackerman LV (1954) Atlas of tumor pathology. Section VI, fascicles 23–24: Tumors of the retroperitoneum, mesentery and peritoneum. Armed Forces Institute of Pathology, Washington DC, pp 12–13

Albarran J (1905) Rétention rénale par péri-urétérite: libération externe de l'uretère. Assoc Fr Urol 9:511–517

Allibone GW, Saxton HM (1980) The association of aorto-iliac aneurysms with ureteral obstruction. Urol Radiol 1: 205–210

Amis ES (1991) Retroperitoneal fibrosis. AJR Am J Roentgenol 157:321–329

Angel JL, Knuppel RA (1984) Computed tomography in diagnosis of puerperal ovarian vein thrombosis. Obstet Gynecol 63:61–64

Arger PH, Stolz J, Miller WT (1973) Retroperitoneal fibrosis: an analysis of the clinical spectrum and roentgenographic signs. AJR Am J Roentgenol 119:812–821

Arrive L, Hricak H, Tavares NJ, et al (1989) Malignant versus nonmalignant retroperitoneal fibrosis: differentiation with MR imaging. Radiology 172:139–143

Austin OG (1956) Massive thrombophlebitis of the ovarian vein. Am J Obstet Gynecol 72:428–429

Ayuso JR, Garcia-Criado A, Caralt TM, et al (1999) Atypical retroperitoneal fibrosis: MRI finding. Eur Radiol 9:937–939

Balfe DM, Bova JG (1990) Genito-urinary manifestations of gastrointestinal diseases. In: Pollack HM (ed) In clinical urography: an atlas and text book of uroradiological imaging, vol 1. Saunders, Philadelphia, pp 961–979

Banner MP (1987) Genitourinary complications of inflammatory bowel diseases. Radiol Clin North Am 25:199–209

Barbaric ZL, MacIntosh PK (1981) Periureteral thin needle aspiration biopsy. Urol Radiol 2:181–185

Baskerville PA, Browse NL (1987) Periaortic fibrosis: progression and regression. J Cardiovasc Surg 28:30–31

Bateson EM, Atkinson D (1969) Circumcaval ureter: a new classification. Clin Radiol 20:173

Bechtold RB, Chen MYM, Dyer RB, Zagoria RJ (1998) CT of the ureteral wall. AJR Am J Roentgenol 170:1283–1289

Beinart C, Sniderman KW, Saddekni S (1982) Left renal vein hypertension: a cause of occult hematuria. Radiology 145:647–650

Bergman MH, Copeland M (1983) Filling defect of ureterogram caused by varicose ureteral vein. J Urol 70:17

Bjorguinsson E, Friedman AC (1984) Notching of the ureter: CT demonstration of periureteral collaterals. J Comput Assist Tomogr 8:1213–1216

Boissieras P, Serise JM, Medina M, et al (1984) Anevrysmes aortiques abdominaux compliqués de sténoses urétérales. Chirurgie 110:571–578

Bosniak MA, Megibow AJ, Ambos MA, et al (1982) Computed tomography of ureteral obstruction. AJR Am J Roentgenol 138:1107–1113

Braasch JN, Mon AB (1967) Primary retroperitoneal tumors. Surg Clin North Am 47:663–671

Braedel HU, Schindler E (1981) Demonstration, importance and origin of renal varices. Urol Radiol 2:241–244

Braedel HU, Schindler E, Sheldon-Polsky M (1977) Selective renal phlebography in the diagnosis of renal pelvic and ureteric varices. Br J Urol 49:365–370

Bree RL, Green B, Keiller DL, et al (1976) Medial deviation of the ureter secondary to psoas muscle hypertrophy. Radiology 118:691–695

Brooks AP, Reznek RH, Webb JA, et al (1987) Computed tomography in the follow-up of retroperitoneal fibrosis. Clin Radiol 38:597–601

Brooks AP, Reznek RH, Webb JA (1989) Aortic displacement on computed tomography of idiopathic retroperitoneal fibrosis. Clin Radiol 40:51–52

Brooks AP, Reznek RH, Webb JA (1990) Magnetic resonance imaging in idiopathic retroperitoneal fibrosis: measurement of T1 relaxation time. Br J Radiol 63:842–844

Brooks RJ (1962) Left retrocaval ureter associated with situs inversus. J Urol 88:484–486

Brun B, Laursen K, Sorensen IN, et al (1981) CT in retroperitoneal fibrosis. AJR 137:535–538

Carrion H, Gatewood J, Politano U, et al (1979) Retrocaval ureter: report of 8 cases and the surgical management. J Urol 121:514

Chait A, Matasar KW, Fabian CE (1971) Vascular impressions of the ureters. AJR Am J Roentgenol 111:729–749

Chen HH, Panella JS, Rochester D, et al (1988) Non-Hodgkin lymphoma of ureteral wall: CT findings. J Comput Assist Tomogr 12:157–158

Chisholm RA, Coltart RS, Cooper P, et al (1986) Circumferential para-aortic masses: computed tomographic observations. Clin Radiol 37:531–535

Chomette G, Tranbaloc P, Delcourt A, et al (1986) Anatomie pathologique de la fibrose rétropéritonéale idiopathique. Chirurgie 112:343–348

Clark JC (1964) The right ovarian vein syndrome. In: Emmett JL (ed) Clinical urography: an atlas and textbook of roentgenologic diagnosis, 2nd edn. Saunders, Philadelphia, pp 1227–1236

Clyne CA, Abercrombie GF (1977) Perianeurysmal retroperitoneal fibrosis: two cases responding to steroids. Br J Urol 49:463–468

Cohan RH, Baker ME, Cooper C, et al (1988) Computed tomog-

raphy of primary retroperitoneal malignancy. J Comput Assist Tomogr 12:804

Copland RFB, Wilson S, Snell ME (1981) Idiopathic pelvic fibrosis: a variant of retroperitoneal fibrosis? Urology 18:567–571

Cornud F, Blangy S, Sibert A, et al (1983) Echographie abdominale dans le diagnostic et la surveillance des fibroses rétro-péritonéales. J Radiol 64:111–115

Cullenward MJ, Scanlan KA, Pozniak MA, et al (1986) Inflammatory aortic aneurysm (periaortic fibrosis): radiologic imaging. Radiology 159:75–82

Culp O, Bernatz PF (1981) Urological aspects of lesions in abdominal aorta. J Urol 86:150

Cunat JS, Goldman SM (1986) Extrinsic displacement of the ureter. Semin Roentgenol 21:188–200

Dalla-Palma L, Rocca-Rossetti S, Pozzimucelli RS, et al (1981) Computed tomography in the diagnosis of retroperitoneal fibrosis. Urol Radiol 3:77–83

Darney PD, Wilson EA (1977) Intravenous pyelography in the diagnosis and management of post-partum ovarian vein. Thrombophlebitis: a case report. Am J Obstet Gynecol 127:439–440

Datta NC, Henson GF, Vauchan ED (1979) Leaking left hypogastric aneurysm causing bilateral ureteric obstruction. Urology 13:646–649

Davia M, Borczuk A, Bennett B, et al (1995) Ureteral obstruction caused by a thromboembolic infarct. J Urol 153:402–403

Degesys GE, Dunnick NR, Silverman PM, et al (1986) Retroperitoneal fibrosis: use of CT in distinguishing among possible causes. AJR Am J Roentgenol 146:57–60

Demas BE, Avallone A, Hricak H (1988) Pelvic lipomatosis: diagnosis and characterization by magnetic resonance imaging. Urol Radiol 10:198

Dillon EH, Camputaro C (1991) Nonobstructing periureteric venous ring: diagnosis with conventional and three-dimensional reconstruction CT. AJR 157:997–998

Dixon AK, Mitchinson MJ, Sherwood T (1984) Computed tomographic observations in periaortitis: an hypothesis. Clin Radiol 35:39–42

Downey DB, O'Connell D, Donohow J (1987) Percutaneous balloon dilatation of a midureteric obstruction caused by retroperitoneal fibrosis. Br J Urol 60:84–85

Drake SG, Glass RE, Eadie DG (1977) Abdominal aortic aneurysms, peiraneurysmal fibrosis and ureteric obstruction and deviation. Br J Surg 64:649–653

Dufour B (1973) Les obstructions de l'uretère lombo-iliaque à l'exclusion des tumeurs urétérales. Association Française d'Urologie, Paris

Dure-Smith P (1979) Ovarian syndrome: is it a myth? Urology 13:355–364

Elkin M, Goldman SM, Meng CH (1972) Ureteral obstruction in patients with uterine prolapse. Radiology 115:411–419

Feinstein RS, Gatewood OM, Goldman SM, et al (1981) Computerized tomography in the diagnosis of retroperitoneal fibrosis. J Urol 126:255–259

Feldberg MA, Van Waes FG (1987) Computed tomography of pseudocysts in retroperitoneal fibrosis. J Comput Assist Tomogr 11:485–487

Fleckenstein P, Knudsen L, Pedersen F, et al (1977) Obstructive uropathy in chronic digestive inflammatory diseases. Scand J Gastroenterol 12:519–523

Frens PH, Dardenne AN, Van Cangh PJ (1982) Retroperitoneal fibrosis infiltrating ureter. Urology 19:300–301

Frusha JD, Porter JA, Batson RC (1982) Hydronephrosis following aorto-femoral bypass grafts. J Cardiovasc Surg 23:5

Gefter WB, Arger PH, Hulherm CB (1978) Computed tomography of circumcaval ureter. AJR Am J Roentgenol 131:1086–1087

Gladstone RJ (1929) Development of the inferior vena cava in the light of recent research with special reference to certain abnormalities and current description of the ascending lumbar and azygos vein. J Anat 64:70–93

Glazer GM, Francis IR, Gross BH (1984) Computed tomography of renal vein thrombosis. J Comput Assist Tomogr 8:288–293

Glynn TP Jr, Kreipke DL, Irons JM (1989) Amyloidosis: diffuse involvement of retroperitoneum. Radiology 170:726

Goldenberg SL, Gordon PB, Cooperberg PL, et al (1988) Early hydronephrosis following aortic bifurcation graft surgery: a prospective study. J Urol 140:1367

Goldman SM, Fishman EK, Rosenshein NB, et al (1984) Excretory urography and computed tomography in the initial evaluation of patients with cervical cancer: are both examinations necessary? AJR Am J Roentgenol 143:991–996

Gregoir W, Shulman CC, Chantrie M (1976) Ureteric obstruction associated with uterine prolapse. Eur Urol 2:29

Haller JO, Berdon WE, Slovis TL, et al (1976) Excretory urographic demonstration of ureteral displacement by sigmoid fecal impaction simulating retroperitoneal tumors. J Urol 113:302–303

Hanna MK (1972) Bilateral retro-iliac artery ureters. Br J Urol 44:339–343

Harshman MW, Pollack H, Banner MP, et al (1982) Conservative management of ureteral obstruction secondary to suture entrapment. J Urol 127:121

Hattori N, Fujikawa J, Kubo K et al (1986) CT diagnosis of peri-ureteric venous ring. J Comput Assist Tomogr 10:1078–1079

Heard G, Hinde G (1975) Hydronephrosis complicating aortic reconstruction. Br J Surg 62:334–347

Higgins CH (1967) Ureteral injuries during surgery: a review of 87 cases. JAMA 199:82–88

Higgins PM, Bennet-Jones DN, Naish PF, et al (1988) Non-operative management of retroperitoneal fibrosis. Br J Surg 75:573–577

Hochstetter F (1893) Beiträge zur Entwicklungsgeschichte des Venensystems der amnioten Säuger. Morphol Jahrb. Leipzig 20:543

Hock E, Purkayastha (1972) Retroiliac ureter. J Urol 107:37

Hricak H (1986) MRI of the female pelvis: a review. AJR Am J Roentgenol 146:1115–1122

Hricak H, Higgins CB, Williams RD (1983) Nuclear magnetic resonance imaging in retroperitoneal fibrosis. AJR Am J Roentgenol 141:35–38

Hubmer G (1978) The ovarian vein syndrome. Eur Urol 13:355–364

Hulnick DH, Chatson GP, Megibow AJ, et al (1988) Retroperitoneal fibrosis presenting as colonic dysfunction: CT diagnosis. J Comput Assist Tomogr 12:159–161

James TGI (1935) Uremia due to aneurysms of the abdominal aorta. Br J Urol 7:157

Jing B, Wallace S, Zornoza J (1982) Metastases to retroperitoneal and pelvic nodes: computed tomography and lymphangiography. Radiol Clin North Am 20:511–530

Joffre F, Portalez D (1984) Apport de la scanographie dans l'exploration des voies urinaires supérieures. Radiol J Cepur 4:21–24

Joffre F, Lerumeur Y, Kasbarian M, et al (1989) L'imagerie actuelle des fibroses rétropéritonéales bénignes (FRPB). Feuill Radiol 29:321–376

Joffre F, Cinqualbre A, Rousseau H (1993) Imagerie des fibroses rétropéritonéales benignes. Encycl Med Chir (Paris France) Radiodiagnostic Nephrologie – Urologie 34-290-A-1013 p

Jones W, Barie P (1988) Urological manifestations of acute appendicitis. J Urol 139:1325–1328

Kaufman JJ, Maxwell MH (1984) Ureteral varices. AJR Am J Roentgenol 92:346–350

Kauzlaric D, Barmeir E (1984) Ultrasonic detection of renal varices and ureteric varices. J Clin Ultrasound 12:569–571

Keshmin JG, Joffre A (1956) Varices of the upper urinary tract and their relationship to portal hypertension. J Urol 76:350–356

Kirschner LP, Twigg HC (1967) Ureteral vascular impression. AJR Am J Roentgenol 100:426–430

Kittredge RD, Gordon R (1987) Inflammatory aneurysm of aorta: development documented by computed tomography. J Comput Tomogr 11:128–131

Koep L, Zuidema GD (1977) The clinical significance of retroperitoneal fibrosis. Surgery 81:250–257

Konto-Georgos L, Vassilopoulos P, Tentes A (1985) Bilateral severe hydroureteronephrosis due to uterine prolapse. Br J Urol 57:360

Kottra JJ, Dunnick NR (1986) Retroperitoneal fibrosis. Radiol Clin North Am 34:1259–1275

Kretkowski R, Shah N (1977) Testicular vein syndrome. Unusual cause of hydronephrosis. Urology 10:253–254

Kunin M, Goodwin WE (1990) The encased ureter: bullet and bodkin pattern, a reliable radiographic sign. Br J Urol 6:471–474

Lalli AF (1977) Rétroperitoneal fibrosis and inapparent obstructive uropathy. Radiology 122:339–342

Lane RH, Stephens DH, Reiman HM (1989) Primary retroperitoneal neoplasms: CT findings in 90 cases with clinical and pathologic correlation. AJR Am J Roentgenol 152:83–89

Lassnig H, Frick J (1978) Left spermatic vein syndrome. Eur Urol 4:141–143

Laurent F, Drouillard J, Dorcier F, et al (1988) Scanographie des tumeurs rétropéritonéales primitives. Feuill Radiol 28:349–358

Lautin EM, Haramai N, Frager D, et al (1988) CT diagnosis of circumcaval ureter. AJR Am J Roentgenol 150:591–594

Lee JKT, Heiken JP, Ling D, et al (1984) Magnetic resonance imaging of abdominal and pelvic lymphadenopathy. Radiology 153:181–188

Lee JY, Chung JW, Kim SH (1997) Proximal ureter obstruction caused by a lower polar renal artery: demonstration with spiral CT angiography. J Comput Assist Tomogr 21:641–642

Leflot A, Weiller M, Pignon L, et al (1978) Compression ureterale par anevrysme artériel hypogastrique. A propos de deux observations. J Radiol Electrol 59:571–574

Lemaitre G, Renouard O, Kasbarian M (1984) Usefulness of computed tomography in the diagnosis and follow-up of retroperitoneal fibrosis. J Belge Radiol 67:13–19

Lemaitre L, Ala Edine C, Dubrulle F, et al (2000) Retroperitoneum and ureters. In: Terrier F, Grossholz M, Becker CD (eds) Spiral CT of the abdomen. Springer, Berlin Heidelberg New York, pp 277–317

Lepor H, Walsh P (1979) Idiopathic retroperitoneal fibrosis. J Urol 122:1–6

Lewis VL, Shaffer HA jr, Williamson BRJ (1982) Pseudo-tumoral lipomatosis of the abdomen. J Comput Assist Tomogr 6: 79–82

Littlejohn GO, Keystone EC (1981) The association of retroperitoneal fibrosis with systemic vasculitis and HLA-B27: a case report and review of the literature. J Rheumatol 8:665–669

Loughlin K, Kearney G (1984) Ureteral obstruction secondary to perianeurysmal fibrosis. Urology 24:332–336

Lytton B (1966) Ureteral obstruction following aortofemoral bypass grafts. Surgery 59:918–922

Manco LG, Kuchtas S, Evans JA (1982) Ureteral obstruction following vascular graft surgery. Urol Radiol 4:47–48

Marglin SI, Castellino RA (1986) Selection of imaging studies for newly presenting patients with non-Hodgkin lymphomas. Semin US CT MR 7:2–8

Marincek B, Scheidegger JR, Studer UE, et al (1993) Metastatic diseases of the ureter: patterns of tumoral spread and radiologic findings. Abdom Imaging 18:88–94

Martin B, Tubiana JM, Habra A (1988) IRM et thrombose post-partum de la veine ovarienne: à propos d'un cas. Ann Radiol 31:251–254

Mayo J, Gray R, St Louis E, et al (1983) Anomalies of the inferior vena cava. AJR Am J Roentgenol 140:339–345

McElhinney PP, Dorsey JW (1948) Retrocaval ureter: case report. J Urol 59:497

McManamon P, Reddy R, MacLaughlin E (1985) Urological complications in Crohn's disease. J Assoc Can Radiol 36:230–233

Megibow AJ, Ambos HA, Bosniak MA (1980) Computed tomographic diagnosis of ureteral obstruction secondary to aneurysmal disease. Urol Radiol 1:211–215

Megibow AJ, Mitnick JS, Bosniak MN (1982) The contribution of computed tomography to the evaluation of obstructed ureter. Urol Radiol 4:95–104

Melnick GS, Bramwitt DN (1971) Bilateral vein ovarian syndrome. AJR Am J Roentgenol 113:509

Meyer JI, Wilbur AC, Lichtenberg R (1992) Ureteric obstruction by the right testicular vein: CT diagnosis. Urol Radiol 13:233–236

Mezrich R (1994) Magnetic resonance imaging applications in uterine cervical cancer. MRI Clin North Am 2:211–243

Michel JR, Dufour B, Grunfeld JP (1986) Fibrose rétropéritonéale: diagnostic radiologique. Chirurgie 112:360–363

Mieza M, Rotstein JM, Geffen A (1982) CT demonstration of periureteral fibrosis of malignant etiology. J Comput Assist Tomogr 6:290–293

Mitchinson MJ (1970) The pathology of idiopathic retroperitoneal fibrosis. J Clin Pathol 23:681–689

Mitchinson MJ (1984) Chronic periaortitis and periarteritis. Histopathology 8:589–600

Mitchinson MJ (1986) Retroperitoneal fibrosis revisited. Arch Pathol Lab Med 110:784–786

Morehouse HT, Thornhill BA, Altermann DD (1983) Right ureteral obstruction associated with pancreatitis. Urol Radiol 7:150–152

Moss AA, Clark ME, Goldberg HI et al (1972) Pelvic lipomatosis: a roentgenographic diagnosis. AJR Am J Roentgenol 115:411–419

Munechika H, Honda M, Kushihashi T, et al (1987) Computed tomography of retroperitoneal cystic lymphangiomas. J Comput Assist Tomogr 11:116–119

Mulligan SA, Holley HC, Koehler RE, et al (1989) CT and MR imaging in the evaluation of retroperitoneal fibrosis. J Comput Assist Tomogr 13:277–281

Murphy RJ, Casillas J, Becerra JL (1987) Retrocaval ureter: computed tomography and ultrasound appearence. J Comput Tomogr 11:89–93

Ney C, Cruz FS, Carvajal S, et al (1986) Ureteral involvement secondary to diverticulitis of the colon. Surg Gynecol Obstet 163:215–218

Nishimura Y, Fushiki M, Yoshida M, et al (1986) Left renal vein hypertension in patients with left renal bleeding of an unknown origin. Radiology 160:663–667

Norfray JF, Nudelman EJ (1974) Visceral collateral arterial circulation: another cause of ureteral notching. J Urol 112: 172–173

O'Reilly PH (1986) Ureteral obstruction. In: O'Reilly PH (ed) Obstructive uropathy. Springer, Berlin Heidelberg New York, pp 151–152

Ormond JK (1960) Idiopathic retroperitoneal fibrosis: an established clinical entity. JAMA 174:1561–1568

Padovani J, Grangier MI, Faure F, et al (1984) Les varices urétérales essentielles chez l'enfant. A propos de quatre observations. Ann Radiol 27:482–486

Patel SK (1990) Retroperitoneal tumors and cysts. In: Pollack HW (ed) Clinical urography: an atlas and text book of urological imaging, vol 3. Saunders, Philadelphia, pp 2413–2457

Peck DR, Bhatt GM, Lowman RM (1973) Traction displacement of the ureter: a sign of aortic aneurysm. J Urol 109:983–986

Pereira RM, Ferreira AA, Lane E (1969) Diagnosis of the right ovarian vein syndrome. Am J Obstet Gynecol 103:888

Persky L, Huus JC (1974) Atypical manifestations of retroperitoneal fibrosis. J Urol 111:340–344

Petrone AF, Dudzinski J, Maniatas W (1974) Ureteral obstruction secondary to aorto-femoral by-pass. Ann Surg 179: 192–196

Pfister RC, Newhouse JH (1978) Radiology of the ureter. Urology 1:15–39

Pienkny AJ, Herts B, Streem B (1999) Contemporary diagnosis of retrocaval ureter. J Endourol 13:721–722

Pistolesi GF, Procassi C, Cavdona R, et al (1984) CT criteria of the differential diagnosis in primary retroperitoneal masses. Eur J Radiol 4:127–138

Psihramis KE (1987) Ureteral obstruction by a rare venous anomaly: a case report. J Urol 138:130–132

Puech JL, Song MY, Joffre F, et al (1987) Ureteral metastases: computed tomographic findings. Eur J Radiol 7:103–106

Quattlebaum R, Anderson A (1985) Ureteral obstruction secondary to a patent umbilical artery in a 79-year-old man: a case report. J Urol 134:347

Radin DR, Ray MJ, Harrison E, et al (1986) CT demonstration of ovarian varices. J Comput Assist Tomogr 10:361–362

Raja-Rao AK, Zucker M, Sacks D (1980) Right ovarian vein thrombosis with extension to the inferior vena cava. Br J Radiol 53:160–161

Read BP, Devine PC (1975) Vascular distal ureteral obstruction. J Urol 114:762–764

Rhind JR, Bradford R (1977) Retroperitoneal fibrosis following aortic surgery. Br J Urol 49:552

Robbe IJ, Dixon AK (1984) Spontaneous resolution of ureteric obstruction in perianeurysmal retroperitoneal fibrosis. Br J Urol 57:92–95

Robert Y, Rocourt N, Rigot JM, et al (1997) Retentissement de la grossesse et des affections génitales sur l'appareil urinaire. Encycl Med Clin (Elsevier, Paris), Radiodiagnostic Urologie Gynécologie 31–110-A-10, 8 p

Rothschild E, Ganeval D, Michel JR, et al (1986) Les fibroses rétropéritonéales, diagnostic et évolution. Chirurgie 112: 356–359

Rouviere O, Lyonnet D, Berger P (1999) Uretero-pelvic junction obstruction. Use of helical CT for pre-operative assessment: comparison with arterial angiography. Radiology 213:668–673

Saldino RM, Palubinskas AJ (1972) Medial placement of the ureter: a normal variant which may simulate retroperitoneal fibrosis. J Urol 101:582–585

Sanders RC, Duffy T, McLoughlin MG, et al (1977) Sonography in the diagnosis of retroperitoneal fibrosis. J Urol 118: 944–946

Sasai K, Sano A, Imanaka K, et al (1986) Right vein ureteric venous ring detected by computed tomography. J Comput Assist Tomogr 10:349–35

Savader SJ, Otero RR, Savader BL (1988) Puerperal ovarian vein thrombosis: evaluation with CT, US and MR imaging. Radiology 167:637–639

Savarese RP, Rosenfeld JC, de Laurentis DA (1986) Inflammatory abdominal aortic aneurysm. Surg Gynecol Obstet 162: 405–410

Saxton HM (1990) Pelvic lipomatosis. In: Pollack HM (ed) Clinical urography: an atlas and textbook of uroradiological imaging, vol 3. Saunders, Philadelphia, pp 2458–2468

Schapira HE, Mitty HA (1974) Right ovarian vein septic thrombophlebitis causing ureteral obstruction. J Urol 112: 451–453

Schubart P, Fortner G, Cummings D, et al (1985) The significance of hydronephrosis after aortofemoral reconstruction. Arch Surg 120:62

Shield DE, Lytton B, Weiss RM et al (1976) Urologic complications of inflammatory bowel diseases. J Urol 115:701–706

Shopfner CE (1968) Urinary tract pathology associated with constipation. Radiology 90:865

Shown TE, Moore CA (1971) Retrocaval ureter: 4 cases. J Urol 105:497

Smith S, Bosniak MA, Megibow AJ, et al (1986) CT demonstration of rapid improvement of retroperitoneal fibrosis in response to steroid therapy. Urol Radiol 8:104–107

Spillane RJ, Kaiser TF, Prather GC (1951) Medial deviation of ureters complicating carcinoma of rectum and sigmoid and proctosigmoidostomy. Surg Gynecol Obstet 93:273

Stecker JF, Rawls HP, Devine CJ, et al (1974) Retroperitoneal fibrosis and ergot derivatives. J Urol 112:30–32

Sundaram M, McGuire MH, Schajowicz F (1987) Soft tissue masses: histologic basis for decreased signal (short T2) on T2-weighted MR images. AJR Am J Roentgenol 148: 1247–1250

Talner LB (1990) Specific causes of obstruction. In: Pollack HM (ed) Clinical urography: an atlas and textbook of uroradiological imaging, vol 2. Saunders, Philadelphia, pp 1629–1751

Thomas JM, McMortensen NJ, Bayliss CR (1983) Ureteric obstruction after Dacron vascular replacement. Am R Coll Surg Emg 65:383–388

Tracy D, Eisenberg R, Hedgecock M (1979) Urinary obstruction resulting from vascular prosthetic graft surgery. AJR Am J Roentgenol 132:415

Usher SM, Brendler H, Ciavarra VA (1977) Retroperitoneal fibrosis secondary to metastatic neoplasia. Urology 9: 191–194

Villani U, Leoni S, Mora A (1985) Unilateral hydro-uretero-nephrosis secondary to iliac aneurysm. Urology 16:62–63

Vint VC, Usselman JA, Warmath MA, et al (1980) Aortic perianeurysmal fibrosis: CT density enhancement and ureteral obstruction. AJR 136:577–580

Von Fritschen U, Malzfelfd E, Clasen A (1999) Inflammatory abdominal aortic aneurysm: a postoperative course of retroperitoneal fibrosis. J Vasc Surg 30:1090–1098

Walker DI, Bloor K, Williams G, et al (1972) Inflammatory aneurysm of the abdominal aorta. Br J Surg 59:609

Walther JM, Romas NA, Lowe FC (1987) Barium granuloma: an unusual cause of unilateral ureteral obstruction. J Urol 138:614–616

Warden SS, Fiveash JG Jr, Tynes WV, et al (1981) Urological aspects of pancreatic adenocarcinoma. J Urol 125:265–267

Werboff LH, Korobkin M, Klein RS (1979) Pelvic lipomatosis: diagnosis using computed tomography. J Urol 122: 257–261

Winfield AC, Mazer MJ (1990) Vascular abnormalities of the lower urinary tract. In: Pollack HM (ed) Clinical urography: an atlas and textbook of uroradiological imaging, vol 3. Saunders, Philadelphia, pp 2210–2221

Witten DW (1990) Retroperitoneal fibrosis. In: Pollack HC (ed) Clinical urography: an atlas and textbook of uroradiological imaging, vol 3. Saunders, Philadelphia, pp 2469–2483

Yancey JM, Kaude JV (1988) Diagnosis of perirenal fibrosis by MR imaging. J Comput Assist Tomogr 12:335–337

Yuh WT, Barloon TJ, Sickels WJ, et al (1989) Magnetic resonance imaging in the diagnosis and follow-up of idiopathic retroperitoneal fibrosis. J Urol 141:602–605

10 Miscellaneous

L. Bouchard, P. Rischmann, T. Smayra, R. Chemali, M. Soulie,
S. Moussouni, Ph. Otal, F. Joffre

CONTENTS

L. Bouchard, MD; T. Smayra, MD; S. Moussouni, MD;
Ph. Otal, MD; F. Joffre, MD
Service de Radiologie, Hôpital de Rangueil, 1, avenue Jean
Poulhès, 31403 Toulouse Cedex 4, France
P. Rischmann, MD; M. Soulie, MD
Service d'Urologie, CHU Rangueil, 1, avenue Jean-Poulhès,
31403 Toulouse Cédex 4, France
R. Chemali, MD
Service de Radiologie, Hôpital Saint Georges, Achrafieh,
Beirut, Lebanon

10.1
Traumatic and Iatrogenic Lesions of the Ureter

This chapter covers a number of ureteral lesions which are caused by direct aggression of external origin, whether it be a real post-traumatic lesion or an iatrogenic trauma, which is by far the most frequent. The anatomic lesions are sometimes identical and consist of ruptures and stenoses. On the other hand, the clinical presentation, diagnosis, and problems of management can vary and lead to the study of these lesions as separate entities. The aim of imaging techniques is to identify the location, the importance, and the type of lesion, and the presence of leaks and of associated lesions.

10.1.1
Noniatrogenic Ureteral Trauma

The small caliber of the ureter, the fact that it is situated deeply, mobile and well protected, make ureteral traumas exceptional. The frequency is estimated to be 1% of all traumas of the urinary tract (Presti et al. 1989). The ureter may present a pure traumatic lesion or can be involved indirectly in a case of retroperitoneal trauma, in particular renal, with urohematic retroperitoneal collection, causing impact on the ureter through compression. This situation, with no direct involvement of the ureter, must be excluded from this chapter.

Penetrating lesions are the most frequent causes of traumatic noniatrogenic lesions and represent 85% of traumatic lesions of the ureter (Presti et al. 1989). They are dominated by gunshot wounds (Holden et al. 1976). They are accompanied most often by intra-abdominal lesions that may involve the retroperitoneal great vessels and the small bowel, along with the other intra-abdominal organs (Steers et al. 1985). A gunshot wound can also be responsible for an indirect trauma of the ureter, the shock wave possibly being responsible for ureteral ischemia, thus leading to a remote stenosis or a ureteral fistula (LIROTT et al. 1977). Urgent laparotomy is often warranted and radiological techniques do not play a role in the diagnosis. Direct visualization of the ureteral injury is the most accurate diagnostic modality and justifies thorough surgical exploration of the abdomen following penetrating trauma (MEDINA et al. 1998). It happens sometimes that an insufficient surgical exploration misses the diagnosis. It will be made remotely, with the appearance of clinical signs of retroperitoneal collection (lumbago, fever, tenderness) (SARRAMON and SERNY 1975). Ultrasonography and CT will then allow the diagnosis of urinoma and reveal its extent.

The lesion is generally unilateral, but a recent case of rupture of both ureters by a single bullet was reported (CECCONI et al. 1986). In these cases or in case of a single kidney, anuria may appear. Stab wounds are more uncommon but are increasing. They raise the same diagnostic problems as gunshot wounds.

Ureteral ruptures by closed trauma are less frequent (BRIGHT and PETERS 1977b). They are seen mostly in infants, because of the higher mobility of their kidneys and their greater elasticity. Three hypotheses are considered: a blow to the vertebral column, brutal stretching by hyperextension, or tear from deceleration (PALMER and DRAGO 1981). The right ureter is more frequently involved, but it is not clear why this is so. The simultaneous involvement of both ureters is exceptional (AINSWORTH et al. 1966). The tear is most frequently total and concerns the proximal ureter (BRUEZIERE et al. 1975; FRIEDEN-

BERG et al. 1963). The diagnosis is difficult, because it often involves multiple trauma and the hematuria is inconstant. It is in fact rare that clinical signs point towards a urinary lesion and lead to an EU that shows the contrast fluid leak associated with normal upper urinary tract cavities. EU must also be performed in case of abdominal gunshot wound if the path seems to involve the urinary tract, if the ureteral lesion is missed on laparotomy, or if it is hidden by other traumatic lesions.

In the majority of cases the diagnosis is delayed. Remote from the trauma site, signs of retroperitoneal collection appear: lumbago, fever, lumbar region tenderness. The collection can be suspected on KUB and EU films that show shifting of the inferior renal pole and of the ureter, normal appearing cavities, and contrast medium extravasation with single ureter opacification (BECKLEY and WATERS 1972; CARLTON 1978). These examinations may be inconclusive, however, (PRESTI et al. 1989), mainly if EU is performed too close to the trauma (McGINTY and MENDEZ 1977). The leak is seen in only 25% of cases because of ureteral spasm (LANG 1981). A urinary obstruction is rare. Direct opacification of sites remote from the trauma is often more precise for assessing the location and the presence of a leak or of a fistula, as well as its type (LANG 1981; LABERGE et al. 1979) (Figs. 10.1a, b, 10.2). In some circumstances, the diagnosis is not made until many years later, with the discovery of a mute obstructive kidney and ureteral stenosis, associated or not with a urinoma (PETERS and SAGALOWSKY 1986) (Fig. 10.3).

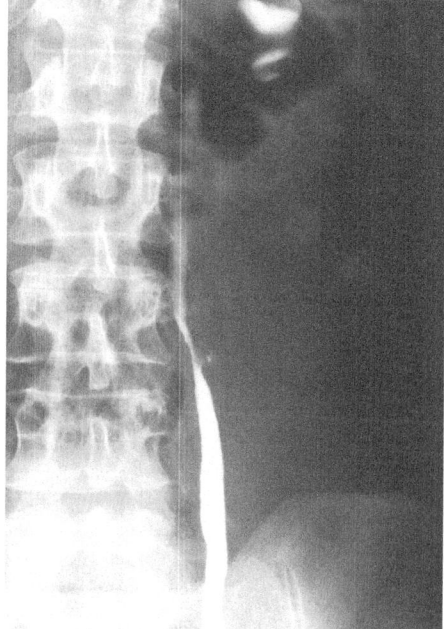

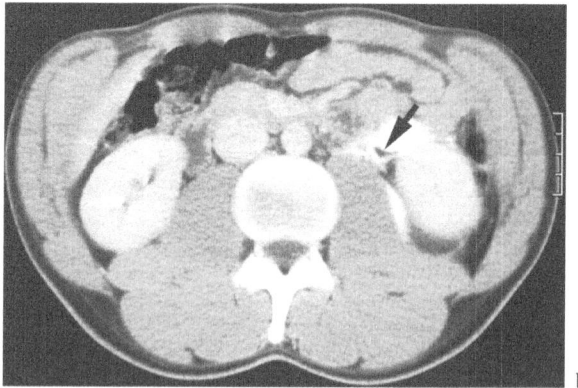

Fig. 10.1a, b. Gunshot wound of left ureter: a RUP shows a blind-ended, pseudodiverticular extravasation of contrast medium at the middle part of the left lumbar ureter. b CT: round lacunar image inside the leak, corresponding to the nonopacified ureter (*arrow*)

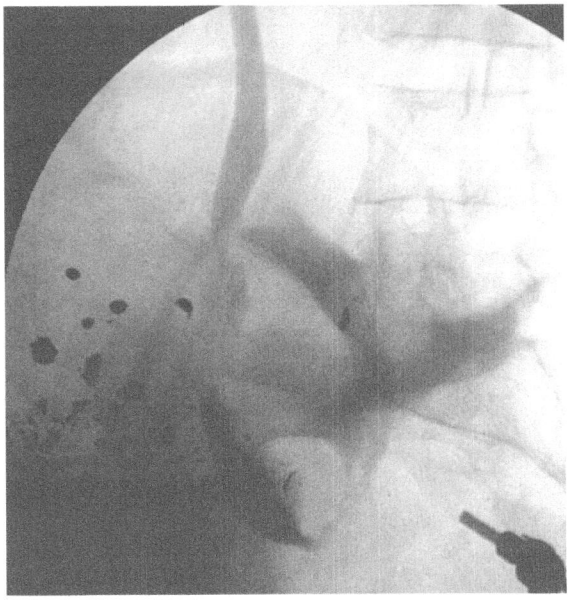

Fig. 10.2. Gunshot wound of the right ureter: Antegrade pyelography shows extravasation of contrast medium in front of multiple bullet fragments

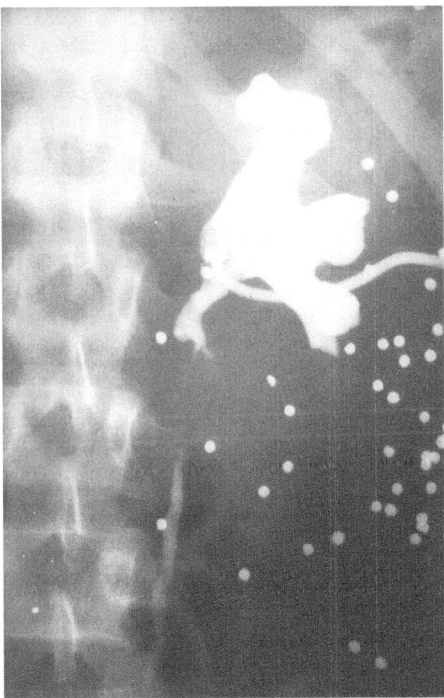

Fig. 10.3. Gunshot wound of the left ureter: Late examination with nephrostomy catheter shows narrowing of the upper part of the lumbar ureter

The broad indications for ultrasonography and CT in case of abdominal trauma permit earlier detection of a ureteral trauma even if the kidney is functioning insufficiently: the sensitivity for detecting a minor leak is excellent, and the density measurement allows the differentiation of a urine leak from one of blood (Fig. 10.1a, b). KENNEY described a group of signs particularly suggestive of a rupture of the pyelo-ureteral junction or the lumbar ureter (KENNEY et al. 1987):

1. Contrast leak in paramedial location of the perirenal region, with liquid sometimes extending beyond the perirenal space region
2. Round lacunar or linear image inside the leak, corresponding to the nonopacified ureter (Fig. 10.1a, b)
3. No opacification of the underlying ureter
4. Absent parenchymal lesions

CT also permits the evaluation of lesions to neighboring structures and the detection of air in the ureter that may suggest communication with a digestive organ.

The treatment of traumatic rupture of the ureter relies, in the case of an incomplete lesion, on antegrade or retrograde ureter intubation with 2-J catheters (STEERS et al. 1985). A uretero-ureteral anastomosis is warranted in complete ruptures when possible. It is sometimes necessary to move the kidney to overcome loss of ureteral material, but frequently, nephrectomy is the only therapeutic solution because of late diagnosis (McGINTY and MENDEZ 1977).

Traumatic lesions of the upper urinary tract can have a late impact on the ureter through the fibrotic organization of a urohematic collection (DUFOUR 1973) (Fig. 10.4a–f). The frequency of obstruction phenomena secondary to this type of lesion is difficult to determine precisely. Obstruction related to a simple retroperitoneal hematoma, without associated urinary extravasation, is exceptional. It is more frequent in case of urohematoma. Detection of a urinary extravasation associated with a retroperitoneal hematoma is then an important factor that CT must look for.

10.1.2
Iatrogenic Traumatic Lesions

The ureter, a central element of the retroperitoneum and especially of the pelvic cavity, is one the first structures to receive a traumatic lesion during abdominal and pelvic surgery. In addition, the multiplicity of urological or radiological endoureteral

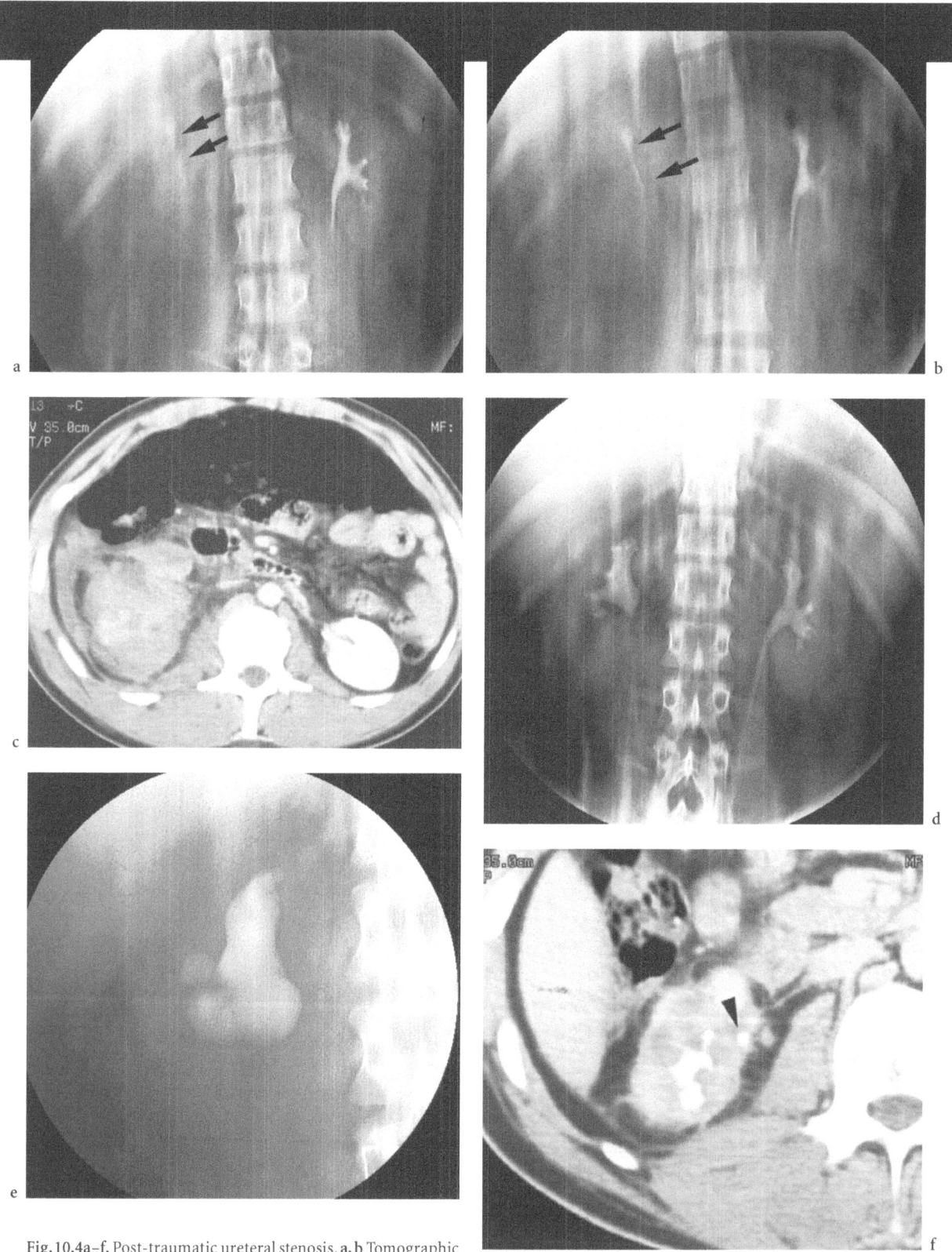

Fig. 10.4a–f. Post-traumatic ureteral stenosis. **a, b** Tomographic picture during EU performed after a right renal trauma. Faint opacification of the right upper urinary tract (*arrows*). The right kidney is not visible inside an important perirenal collection. **c** CT: presence of a large and probably urohematic collection of the perirenal space without clear identification of the kidney. **d** EU performed 1 month later shows improvement of the opacification of the right upper urinary tract with slight pelvis dilatation. **e** Six months later, EU shows clear obstruction of the upper urinary tract with pelvicaliceal dilatation and absence of visualization of the lumbar ureter. **f** After injection of contrast medium, CT shows irregular and retracted lower pole of the kidney with caliceal dilatation. The right ureter is attracted and included in a scarred retractile zone, which explains the stenosis (*arrowhead*)

procedures frequently lead to traumatic lesions of variable severity (SELZMAN and SPIRNAK 1996).

10.1.2.1
Surgical Trauma

Surgical trauma to the ureter is an important problem that surgeons encounter. Two main categories of lesions can be found: obstruction by accidental ligature during reperitonization and rupture by partial or total section of the ureter. The perioperative devascularization in case of extensive ureteral dissection can also play a role and be responsible for a ureteral fistula or a delayed stenosis due to retraction sclerosis, particularly if preoperative radiotherapy was performed (LANG 1973). Ureteral lesions appear in 1% of all abdominopelvic interventions (WEINBERG 1967), hysterectomy being the principal cause of these complications (BRIGHT and PETERS 1977a; DOWLING et al. 1986), followed by vascular and urological surgery (HIGGINS 1967). For some authors, the frequency of ureteral traumas during radical pelvic interventions reaches 30% (SOLOMONS et al. 1960; SHIGELTON et al. 1969). Other interventions that can be responsible for ureteral lesions (BENOIT et al. 1983; BORSKI and SMITH 1960) are indicated in Table 10.1. The ureteral complications of vascular surgery are detailed in Chap. 9.

The frequency of these ureteral lesions is explained by the tight anatomic relationship (<1 cm) between the ureter and the gonadal vessels at the level of the pelvic brim, the ureter, and the uterine artery at the level of the broad ligament (ZHIRI et al. 1987). The proximity of the ureter to the cervical region, its similarity to a venous structure, can explain the frequency of these traumas that occur more frequently during the ligature of the lumbo-ovarian ligament. These traumas are more frequent and severe when regional anatomy is modified by the original disease (inflammation, neoplasia) or previous treatments (MATTINGLY and BORKOWF 1978). The type of approach, vaginal or abdominal, does not influence the rate of these complications. However, the rate seems higher with laparoscopic surgery, particularly for colorectal lesions.

The systematic practice of EU preoperatively in pelvic tumoral lesions does not appear justified any longer. The preoperative screening for ureteral involvement does not seem to have an impact on the frequency of postoperative ureteral complications. In addition, the presence of ureteral obstructive involvement can be depicted by preoperative ultrasonography or CT.

The frequency of ureteral complications after pelvic surgery, particularly if an obstructive syndrome exists,

Table 10.1. Iatrogenic traumatic lesions of the ureter

1. Surgical trauma
   Gynecologic surgery
      Hysterectomy
      Subtotal or total
      Salpingectomy
      Cesarean
   Urologic surgery
      Ureterolithotomy
      Ureteral resection with end-to-end anastomosis
      Ureterolysis
      Ureteroileoplasty
      Total or partial cystectomy with bladder replacement
      Bladder diverticula removal
      Radical prostatectomy
      Colpocystopexy
   Others
      Sympathectomy
      Orthopedic surgery for pelvic trauma or hip disease
      Abdominal aorta repairs
      Lumbar disk surgery
      Retroperitoneal lymphadenectomy
      Abdomino-perineal amputation
      Retroperitoneal or pelvic tumor removal
2. Nonsurgical trauma
   RUP
   Ureteral stenting
   Retrograde stone removal
   Ureteroscopy
   Transurethral resection of prostate or bladder tumor
   Endoscopic ureterocele incision
3. Miscellaneous
   Percutaneous sympatholysis
   Translumbar aortography
   Percutaneous chemonucleolysis
   Forceps delivery
   Celioscopic tubal occlusion

justifies for some authors the prophylactic placement of a 2-J catheter (ANSONG et al. 1985).

The diagnosis of a ureteral traumatic lesion can be made during surgery, with the wound then being repaired at the same time. In fact, however, the findings are frequently more delayed. The symptoms and signs are the appearance of lumbar or pelvic pain, frequently associated with fever. More rarely there are signs of urinary fistula, cutaneous or vaginal, or a finding of hematuria. The trauma may be discovered many years later, the symptoms and signs being a function of the severity of the ureteral stenosis. In some types of intervention (colpocystopexy of the MARSCHALL-MARCHETTI type) the ureteral trauma can be bilateral during vaginal fixation and manifests as early postoperative anuria (PERSKY and GUERRIERE 1976).

The radiological diagnosis is given by EU or by US. The most frequent radiological manifestation is a ureteral obstruction, mostly pelvic (FLYNN et al. 1979). Most of the lesions are complete stenosis, abrupt, centered, and regular, the ureter having a convex blind end. In case of incomplete obstruction, there is a short diaphragm-like stenosis. In case of colpocystopexy, the obstruction is often bilateral and associated with morphological modifications of the bladder giving it a "pseudo-ureterocele" pattern (HERITIER et al. 1988).

Complications such as fistulas are rare: ureterocutaneous fistula, or more frequently ureterovaginal fistula, or simple urinoma (Fig. 10.5). Retrograde opacification can be done to show a fistula poorly visible on EU.

CT can show the extent of a urinoma (Fig. 10.6a, b). Its sensitivity is excellent and opens the way to interesting therapeutic solutions since percutaneous nephrostomy can allow the healing of a fistula (PERSKY et al. 1981; LANG 1981). It can also allow in certain good cases, to wait for the spontaneous resolution of the ureteral obstruction: the current use of resorbable can allow a spontaneous disappearance of the ligature with disappearance of the stenosis (HARSHMAN et al. 1982). Antegrade or retrograde ureteral catheterization can also be done on a temporary basis to heal a fistula or calibrate a stenosis (SIEBEN et al. 1988; STEERS et al. 1985). The use of angioplasty balloons is also possible to dilate the stenosis (BANNER et al. 1983). Reparative surgery of the ureter is based on the type of the lesion, its etiology, and possibly the results of uroradiological techniques (FLYNN et al. 1979).

10.1.2.2
Iatrogenic Endourologic Traumas

The increased frequency of endoureteral operations raises the risk of traumatic lesions of the ureter. Traumas related to endoureteral procedures represent between 75% and 80% of ureteral traumas, occurring most frequently after ureteroscopy (SELZMAN and SPIRNAK 1996). However, continual technological progress and increased experience on the part of the operators are making these techniques more and more secure.

The majority of these complications are diagnosed intraoperatively, e.g., an abnormal path of the catheter or extravasation of contrast medium during opacifi-

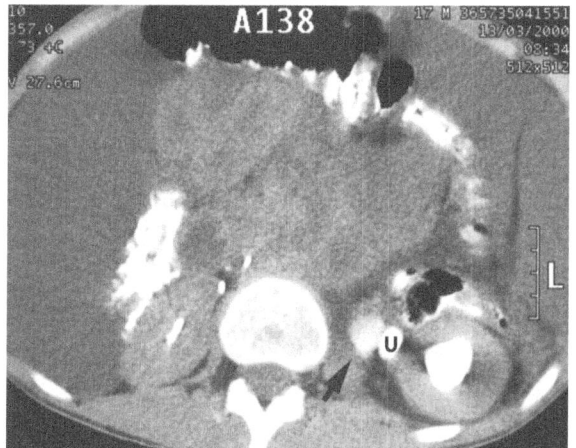

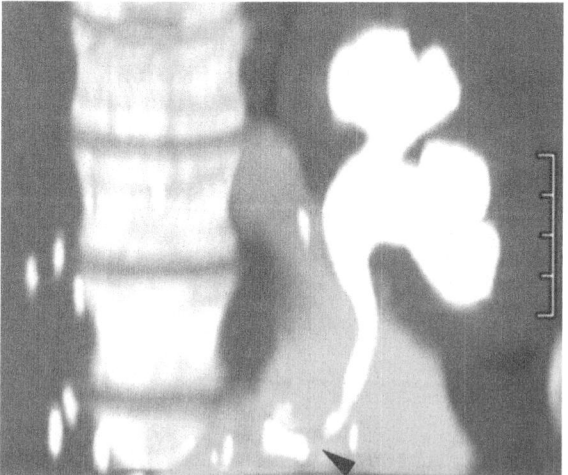

Fig. 10.6a, b. Post-surgical ureteral trauma. **a** Postoperative CT performed in a young male patient after retroperitoneal lymphadenectomy. Chylous ascites and extravasation of contrast medium (*arrow*) around the left lumbar ureter (*U*). **b** MIP reconstruction shows ureterohydronephrosis secondary to ureteral obstruction with extravasation (*arrowhead*)

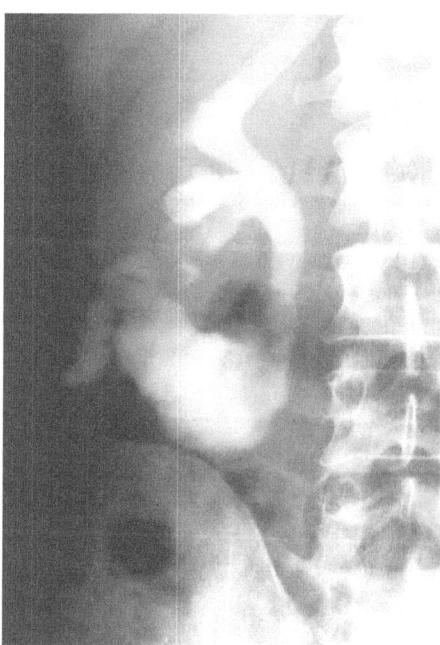

Fig. 10.5. Extravasation of contrast medium from the right lumbar ureter during EU performed after surgical ureterostomy for ureteral stone

cation (LANG 1990). However, they might be missed, hidden by spasmodic and edematous phenomena (PETERSON and SCHULZE 1987). Depending on the clinical signs, the imaging techniques (EU and/or US) may visualize either signs of extravasation or fistula, or more rarely an obstruction or evidence of retroperitoneal or pelvic collections (HUFFMAN 1989; SCHULTZ et al. 1987). The majority of these lesions, in particular extravasations, are minor and heal spontaneously, but sometimes interventional radiourologic procedures are necessary: nephrostomy, ureteral 2-J catheter, ureteral dilatation (BANNER et al. 1983; LANG 1981; MAILLET et al. 1987; PERSKY et al. 1981). Surgical repair is rarely indicated.

Special mention must be made of retrograde techniques for stone extraction under endoscopic control (Dormia catheter, Zeiss catheter) (CARLTON 1978). Previous weakening of the ureter (edema, ureteritis, dilation) and the size of calculi explain the relatively high frequency of severe complications that can lead to real ureteral stripping. The techniques of stone extraction are being abandoned, however, in favor of ureteroscopy. The latter can also be responsible for ureteral lesions. First described by PEREZ CASTRO, this technique has gained popularity in recent years for the treatment of ureteral lithiasis as well as for the diagnosis of some ureteral lesions, particularly tumors (PEREZ-CASTRO et al. 1982). The results of some series (SCHULTZ et al. 1987; WEINBERG et al. 1987) show that complications are about 5%–10% but seem to decrease to 2%–3% with an experienced operator. The frequency seems also to be related to the diameter (<10 mm) and to the rigidity of the endoscope (HUFFMAN 1989). Ureteral perforations represent the most frequent complications (Fig. 10.7). They are generally detected during peroperative radiological opacification and are treated immediately by placement of a temporary 2-J catheter (HORROW et al. 1997). Failure of retrograde techniques can lead to obstructive edema of the meatus, which requires antegrade catheterization (Figs. 10.8, 10.9). More rarely, there is residual stenosis, which can also be treated with a 2-J catheter, or a complete ureteral rupture requiring surgical treatment. Stenoses are encountered principally in previously weakened ureters (radiation lesions, for example). The endoscope can cause traumatic lesions to the mucosa and submucosa in these cases and alter the vascularization of the ureter. The use of endoureteral therapeutic methods such as electrohydraulic, ultrasonographic, or laser lithotripsy may also lead to a parietal lesion (perforation, intraparietal lithiasis inclusions). Ureteral stripping generally requires prompt reimplantation of the ureter.

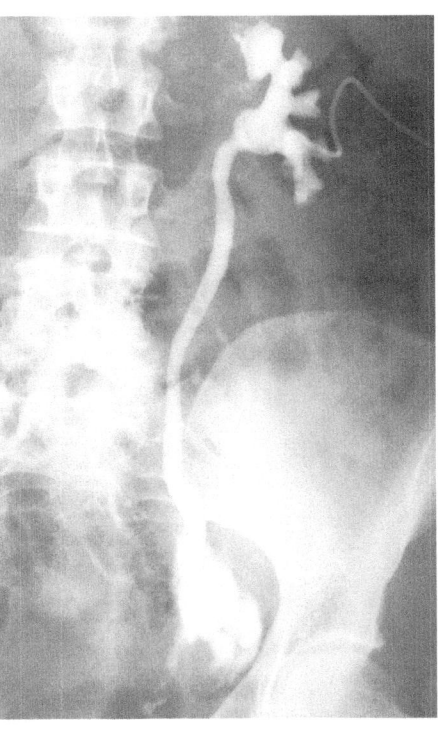

Fig. 10.7. Antegrade pyelography after retrograde extraction of a ureteral stone: extravasation of contrast medium

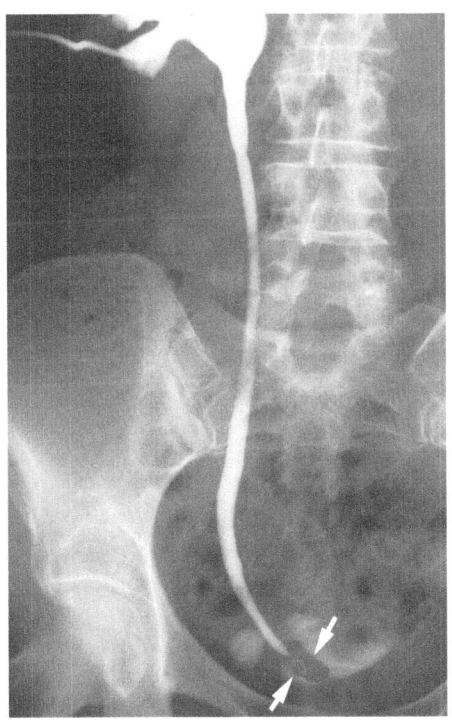

Fig. 10.8. Antegrade pyelography performed after multiple attempts at retrograde catheterization of the right ureteral meatus: presence of stenosing edema around the intramural part of the ureter (*arrow*) treated by antegrade placement of a 2-J indwelling catheter

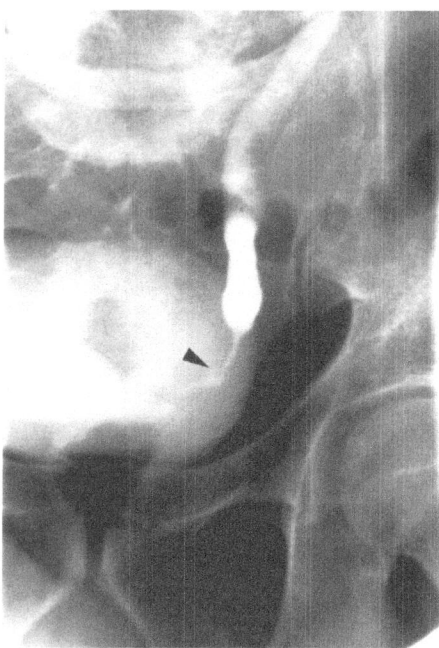

Fig. 10.9. Ureteral stenosis after retrograde extraction of a distal ureteral stone (*arrowhead*)

In addition to these endoureteral manipulation techniques, ureteral traumas by puncture or accidental lesions in the course of translumbar aortography (LOPEZ et al. 1978), or during more recently introduced techniques of interventional radiology such as chemonucleolyis or percutaneous sympatholysis (DONDELINGER and KURDZIEL 1984) must be mentioned. The proximity of the ureter to the vertebral column explains how it might be accidentally damaged by the injection of the aggressive drugs used, in case of imperfect needle positioning. This is the principal reason why the interventional radiologist performs these procedures under CT guidance, following iodinated intravenous ureteral opacification.

10.1.3
Other Iatrogenic Ureteral Lesions

Other iatrogenic lesions of the ureter are represented essentially by post-radiation stenoses. These appear mostly after treatment of uterine cervical cancer (GRAHAM and ABAD 1967). The ureter is the organ "target and symptom" of post-therapeutic complications of uterine cervical cancer (ZERBIB et al. 1983). Their frequency is evaluated at between 1% and 8%, but it may be higher if radiotherapy is associated with surgery, which increases ureteral vascular lesions (SHINGLETON et al. 1969). It seems more elevated for

ZERBIB (39%) but remains lower than that for stenoses from neoplastic recurrence (ZERBIB et al. 1983; RHAMY and STANDER 1962). Although the ureter is relatively resistant to radiation, a periureteral fibrotic reaction may be seen secondary to post-radiation tumoral necrosis (UNDERWOOD et al. 1977).

The lesion is characterized by a narrowing secondary to inflammation that creates endarteritis, ischemia, and evolution toward fibrosis that extends to the periureteral space (SHINGLETON et al. 1969). The necessity of differentiating this type of lesion from a tumoral recurrence is obvious (GRAHAM and ABAD 1967).

The radiological aspect is nonspecific. EU, or direct exploration when obstruction is severe, shows a long, uni- or bilateral, centered and regular lesion of the pelvic ureter (Figs. 10.10, 10.11). Few radiological elements make it possible to distinguish between a radiation stenosis and a neoplastic relapse. However, two points should be noted:

1 The presence of a suspended stenosis is in favor of a relapse (ZERBIB et al. 1983).
2 The stenotic topography outside the radiation area is also in favor of a neoplastic stenosis.

Only the clinical elements can aid the diagnosis: appearance many years after treatment, unilateral topography, and the lack of pelvic compressive signs or of general signs all point to a radiation origin.

CT shows the absence of pelvic mass or of signs of perivesical infiltration, but CT alone cannot differentiate between a tumoral relapse and post-radia-

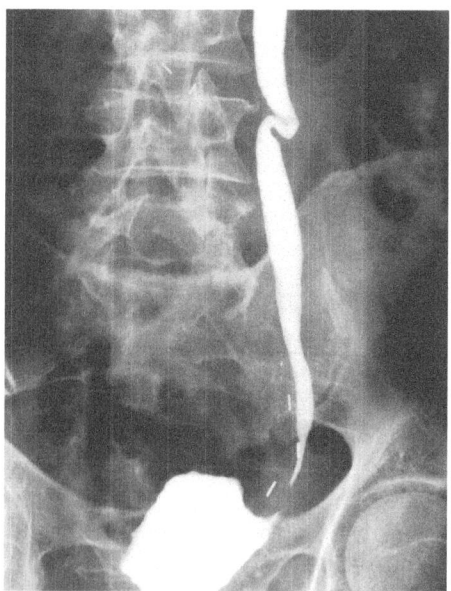

Fig. 10.10. Post-radiation ureteral stenosis: filiform, regular, centered narrowing of the lower part of the left ureter

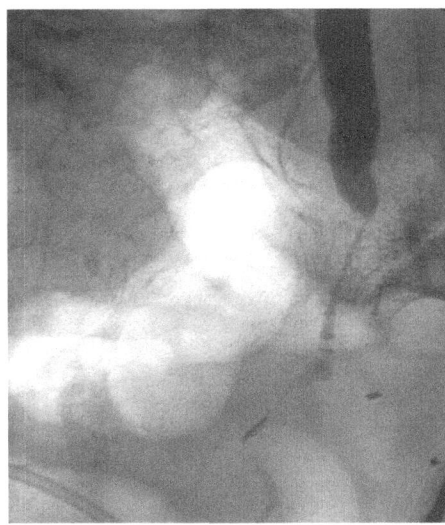

Fig. 10.11. Post-radiation ureteral stenosis: tight, regular, centered, with slight angulation narrowing of the lower part of the left ureter

tion pelvic fibrosis. MRI with gadolinium injection gives diagnostic arguments by showing enhancement in neoplastic relapse. Biopsy guided by ureteral opacification or CT allows a more precise diagnostic approach, avoiding laparotomy (FREIMAN et al. 1978). It is noncontributory when negative, however.

Other iatrogenic ureteral lesions have been described after vena cava clipping (WRENN and ASSIMOS 1988).

10.2
Spontaneous Rupture of the Ureter

Spontaneous rupture of the ureter is an exceptional event that is unrelated to iatrogenic maneuvers, recent urologic surgery, urinary trauma, and preexisting urinary disease (COULON et al. 1998). With an early diagnosis it can actually benefit from new therapeutic modalities of interventional uroradiology. A spontaneous ureteral rupture is practically always secondary to a urinary obstruction.

The diagnosis can be clinically suspected when, during an apparently simple renal colic, signs of complication appear. Pain at the level of the lumbar fossa, frequently associated with fever, should suggest performing EU. The decompressive effect of ureteral rupture makes it possible to opacify the upper excretory tract and thus to visualize ureteral leakage (Figs. 10.12; 10.13a, b). This can be located at any level. EU can identify the ureteral origin of the leakage and eliminate a retroperitoneal collection sec-

ondary to leakage by fornix rupture, which is much more frequent (DIAMOND and MARSHALL 1982).

Ultrasonography can show a retroperitoneal urinary collection, i.e., a urinoma, which is the consequence of rupture. This collection is located at the posteroinferior part of the renal fossa in rupture of the lumbar ureter. The collection is pelvic, subperitoneal, when the pelvic ureter ruptures. An intraperitoneal rupture of the pelvic ureter is possible (COULON et al. 1998). CT is particularly efficient by showing the leakage of contrast material and opacification of the collection, even in cases where EU is negative. RUP is classically performed in case of inconclusive EU. ^{99m}TC DTPA scintigraphy can also detect leakage (BARASCH et al. 1988).

The etiology is most frequently lithiasis (ORKIN 1952). However, spontaneous rupture of the ureter has been described secondary to a low-level obstruction, particularly of prostatic origin (CAMPBELL et al. 1982).

Whatever the etiology, some local factors are necessary to explain the rupture (BORKOWSKI and CANPLICZKA 1974). The stone, by itself, can tear and weaken the ureteral wall during its passage (KAPLAN et al. 1987). At the level of the blockade, ischemic necrosis may eventually occur (NEWMAN et al. 1974). The association of edematous phenomena or additional ureteritis can also explain the rupture. A case of post-lithiasis spontaneous rupture was reported in

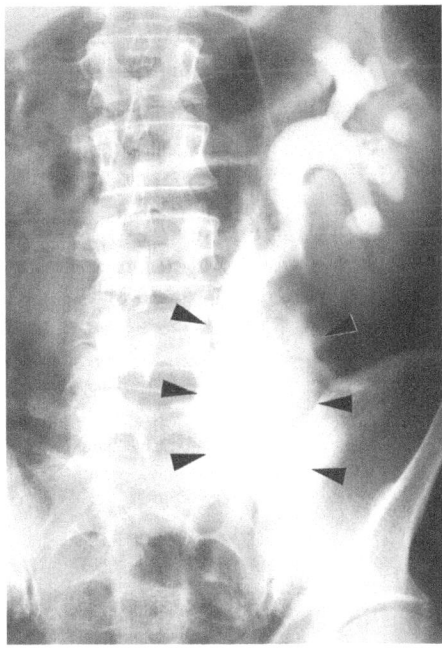

Fig. 10.12. EU during left renal colic: signs of acute obstruction with periureteral extravasation (*arrowheads*)

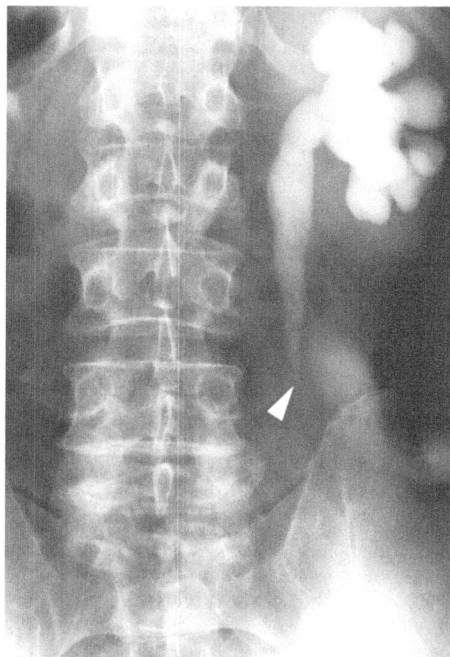
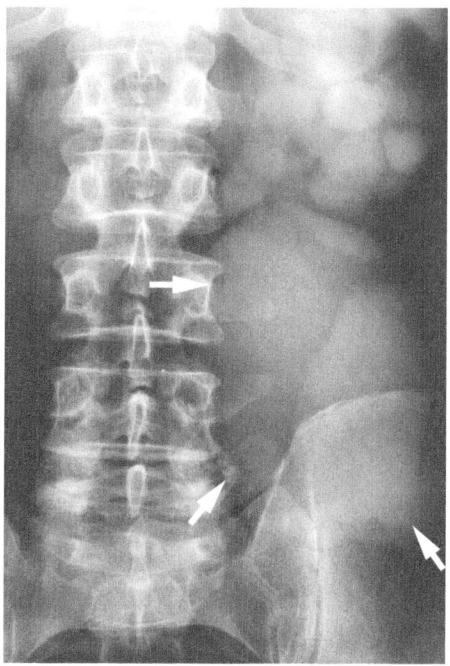

a   b

Fig. 10.13a, b. EU in a patient with previous history of left renal colic. **a** Signs of chronic obstruction with ureterohydronephrosis, lumbar ureteral stenosis, and extravasation of contrast medium (*arrowhead*). **b** Opacification of a large urinoma below the left kidney (*arrows*)

a patient with Cushing syndrome, which is known to weaken tissues (Fuse et al. 1985). The overdose of a highly osmolar contrast medium may also be implicated through inducing hyperdiuresis (Becopoulos et al. 1979; Schwartz et al. 1966).

Spontaneous rupture of the ureter requires fast treatment. Besides classical surgical drainage methods, the radiologist can propose efficient, less aggressive methods: Percutaneous nephrostomy allows external urinary drainage and thus decompresses the excretory tract, with spontaneous closure of the rupture orifice within a few days. It is sometimes necessary to complete the percutaneous nephrostomy with an ureteral catheterization (Goel et al. 1996). It is also possible to drain the urinoma percutaneously under echographic or CT guidance. These two simultaneous drainage procedures should provide a simple and definitive solution.

10.3
Ureteral Fistulas

Ureteral fistulas correspond to an abnormal communication between the ureteral lumen and a neighboring structure. The various etiologies and anatomic types have in common the therapeutic problems they raise.

Most fistulas are related to important ureteral and/or periureteral tissue lesions, secondary to the association, in variable proportions, of different factors: (a) tissue lesions from previous surgery, (b) inflammatory phenomena, (c) post-radiation lesions, (d) tumoral infiltration (Table 10.2). This explains the difficulty of surgical treatment and the frequency of surgery failure (Lang 1981): Nephrectomy is necessary in 20% of cases, with 10% mortality (Higgins 1967).

Imaging, dominated by direct opacification, is essential. It allows the diagnosis, depicts the exact anatomic type and its impact on the urinary tract, and thus leads to the best treatment (Kelais 1971). More and more, these patients can and must benefit from interventional radiology techniques (Maillet et al. 1987). Retrograde ureteral catheterization is most often impossible in the case of fistula.

Occurrence, diagnostic strategy, and therapeutic problems are dependent on the exact anatomic type of fistula and the etiology: infectious, tumoral, or iatrogenic.

10.3.1
Ureterovaginal Fistulas

Ureterovaginal fistulas are the most frequent type (Fig. 10.14). They generally occur in the same settings

Table 10.2. Etiology of ureteral fistulas

Uretero-vaginal fistulas
   Radiosurgical treatment of uterine neoplasia
   Abdominal or vaginal hysterectomy
   Obstetrical trauma
Uretero-cutaneous fistulas
   Post-surgical (renal transplantation, aorto-iliac surgery, ureteroplasty)
   Penetrating trauma of ureter (gunshot or stab wound)
Uretero-intestinal fistulas
   Penetrating injury
   Pelvic radiotherapy and/or surgery
   Inflammatory intestinal diseases (Crohn's disease, diverticulitis, appendiceal abscess)
Uretero-lymphatic fistulas
   Retroperitoneal tumors
   Retroperitoneal lymphadenectomy
   Filariasis
   Aorto-iliac surgery
Uretero-retroperitoneal fistulas
   Penetrating injury
   Ureteral lithiasis
   Ureteral surgery
   Psoas abscess
   Iatrogenic ureteral injury
Uretero-vascular fistulas
   Aortic aneurysm
   Aorto-iliac surgery
   Ureteral intubation
Miscellaneous
   Uretero-peritoneal
   Uretero-uterine
   Uretero-tubal
   Uretero-pancreatic

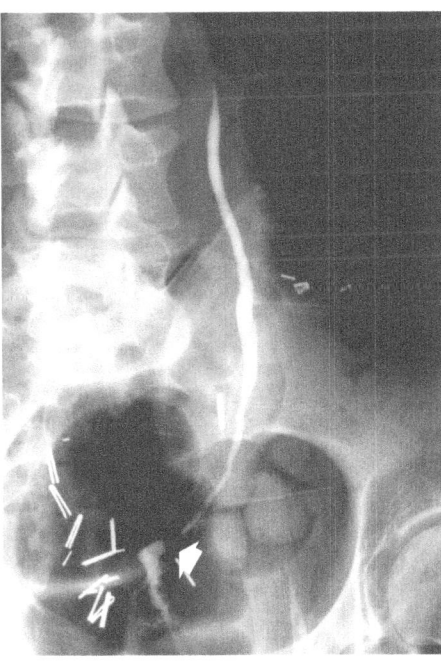

Fig. 10.14. Antegrade pyelography for ureterovaginal fistula (*arrow*) following radical hysterectomy

as vesicovaginal fistulas but are much rarer, usually occurring after radiosurgical treatment of advanced pelvic neoplasia, and particularly after treatment of uterine cervical cancer. The development of irradiation and surgical techniques has led to a clear drop in the frequency of these fistulae from 10% to about 1%. The presence of a diffuse atherosclerosis, the association of irradiation and/or chemotherapy with excessive vascular clipping at certain regions (crossing of the ureter with the uterine artery), and dissection of the ganglia chains can compromise ureteral vascularity. At this level, the vascularity of the pelvic ureter is in fact poor, insured essentially by a branch of the internal iliac artery.

The fistula appears most frequently in the weeks after surgery (BUNKIN 1967), following a painful lumbar episode. It manifests frequently as incontinence associated with normal micturition (BOLLACK and REINHARDT 1977). Intravenous injection of patent blue allows screening for vaginal fistula, but radiological urographic opacification is necessary to differentiate a ureterovaginal from a vesicovaginal fistula; the association of the two is possible (GOODWIN and SCARDINO 1980). Antegrade pyelography is often necessary.

10.3.2
Ureterocutaneous Fistulas

Ureterocutaneous fistulas are most frequently secondary to ureteral surgery, occurring mainly after ureteroileoplasty, uretero-ureteral anastomosis, or a ureteral deviation intervention (BETTMAN et al. 1983). Certain conducive factors are frequently encountered (chronic infection, radiotherapy, chemotherapy). Fistulas can be seen also after uretero-ureteral anastomosis in a renal transplantation, or after aortoiliac surgery (Fig. 10.15a, b). More rarely, ureteral fistula follows a penetrating trauma (gunshot wound or lithotomy). EU is often insufficient if an upper obstruction exists, and opacification of the fistula tract from the cutaneous orifice might be necessary (Fig. 10.16a, b).

10.3.3
Ureterointestinal Fistulas

Ureterointestinal fistulas can be of very different etiologies. Penetrating gunshot wounds are rarely incriminated. Extensive pelvic surgery, in particular for cancer, associated or not with radiation treatment, and pelvic radiotherapy alone can also be responsible.

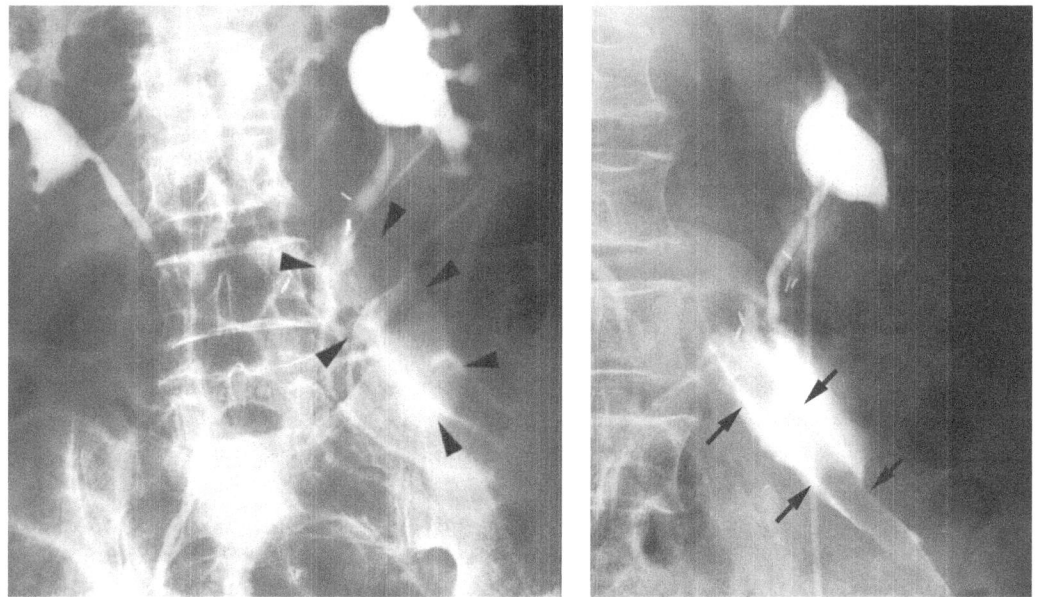

a   b

Fig. 10.15a, b. Ureterocutaneous fistula secondary to left aorto-femoral bypass. **a** EU shows left upper urinary tract obstruction with extravasation of contrast medium (*arrowheads*). **b** Antegrade pyelography confirms ureteral extravasation around the graft, which is seen as a negative image surrounded by contrast medium (*arrows*). CM follows the graft up to the groin

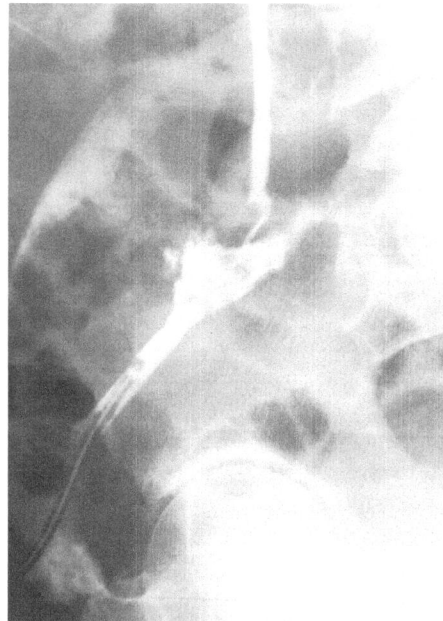

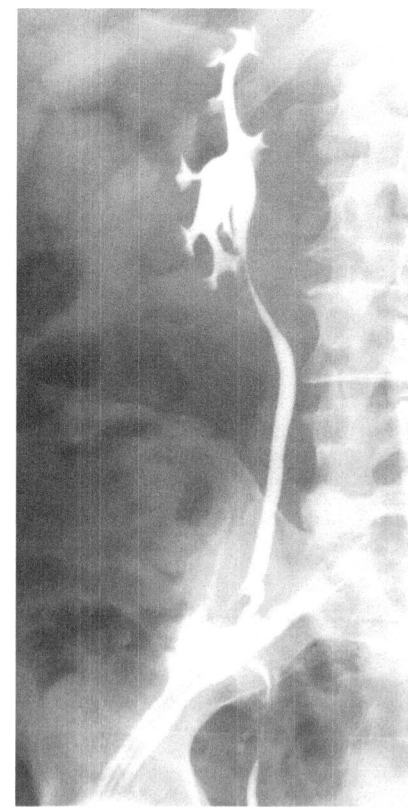

a

b

Fig. 10.16a, b. Ureterocutaneous fistula secondary to right aorto-femoral bypass. Opacification via the cutaneous orifice of the fistula: visualization of the whole urinary tract secondary to a fistula near the ureteral crossing with the bypass

Crohn's disease is currently the principal cause of ureterointestinal fistula (SMITH and WILLIAMS 1972). However, this type is clearly less frequent than ileovesical fistulas and occurs late in the course of the disease. Other chronic inflammatory diseases of the alimentary tract are also potential causes of fistulas in this anatomic region. They can happen, of course during ileocecal tuberculosis, which is rare nowadays, but are found mostly in cases of diverticular sigmoiditis or appendicular abscess (WINTER and WILLIAMS 1972). Ureterocolonic fistulas can be encountered in the settings of huge invading or necrotic colonic tumors, encasing the ureter. Exceptional cases of ureterointestinal fistula secondary to lithiasis or tumoral ureter obstruction have also been described (FERRIE 1985). The communication is made most frequently with the colon, but the ileum, and more rarely the duodenum and the jejunum can be involved.

The diagnosis can be suspected in the presence of signs of intestinal irritation, watery diarrhea, and fecaluria or pneumaturia. Hyperchloremic acidosis and hypokalemia are practically constant. Radiological diagnosis is difficult and is performed mostly with direct opacification of the urinary tract (Fig. 10.17a, b). The presence of air in the ureteral lumen is rarely seen on KUB. The digestive opacification techniques that are useful to identify possible inflammatory lesions of the alimentary tract rarely show the fistula. However, CT can demonstrate it on condition that the digestive tract is not previously opacified (Fig. 10.17c–e).

10.3.4
Ureterolymphatic Fistulas

Ureterolymphatic fistulas (LANG 1973) are exceptional. They are generally secondary to retroperitoneal lymphatic obstruction, particularly tumoral, but can occur following a retroperitoneal node dissection or after vascular aortoiliac surgery. More rarely, ureterolymphatic fistulas have been described as a complication of filariasis. The communication with lymphatic channels is difficult to prove and requires direct antegrade or retrograde pyelography, rather than lymphography.

10.3.5
Ureteroretroperitoneal Fistulas

Ureteroretroperitoneal fistulas make a persistent communication between the ureteral lumen and a newly formed retroperitoneal cavity, corresponding to a urinoma. A calculous disease is frequently responsible for these chronic urinomas. This type of urinoma can also be encountered following a penetrating wound or trauma after ureter surgery, uretero-ureteral anastomosis, replacement surgery or uretero-intestinal anastomosis. In case of gunshot wound of the abdomen, the associated shock wave causes easily missed tissue lesions that can be secondarily responsible for a uretero-retroperitoneal fistula, in relation to ureteral ischemia (ROHNER 1971). Via the same mechanism, some ureteral catheters can be responsible for ischemia by parietal compression, in particular if the vascularity of the ureter is already compromised (surgical history, radiotherapy) (TEUTON et al. 1987). A psoas abscess can exceptionally be responsible for a retroperitoneal fistula, but fistula between the ureter and a urinoma inside the psoas muscle is possible (Fig. 10.18a–e).

These fistulas are sometimes of small diameter, and the communication between the ureter and the cavity is often difficult to see on EU and/or antegrade or retrograde pyelography (Fig. 10.19a). The new imaging techniques are useful to appreciate the volume, the topography, and the extent of the urinoma. CT can also detect a small communication, by showing progressive opacification of the urinoma (Figs. 10.18a–e; 10.19b).

10.3.6
Ureterovascular Fistulas

Ureterovascular fistulas are secondary to a communication between the ureter and the aorta and/or iliac arteries, whether these arteries are normal, aneurysmal, or have been replaced with a prosthesis (REINER et al. 1975). No more than 50 observations of this type have been reported in the literature (QUILLIN et al. 1994; WHEATLEY et al. 1981). Fistulas between the ureter and a vein are less frequent (TEUTON et al. 1987). The increase in the number of endourological procedures has led to a higher frequency of these complications. They were always deadly in the past, but their prognosis is getting better thanks to improvement of diagnosis and treatment.

The etiologies are various; many conducive factors are found (JAFRI et al. 1987) and frequently mixed (DAUPLAT et al. 1985). The performance of an instrumental endoureteral procedure represents the most frequent cause, whether the involved artery is pathological or not. It might be a difficult ureteroscopy or an endoscopic ureterotomy for stenosis, but more

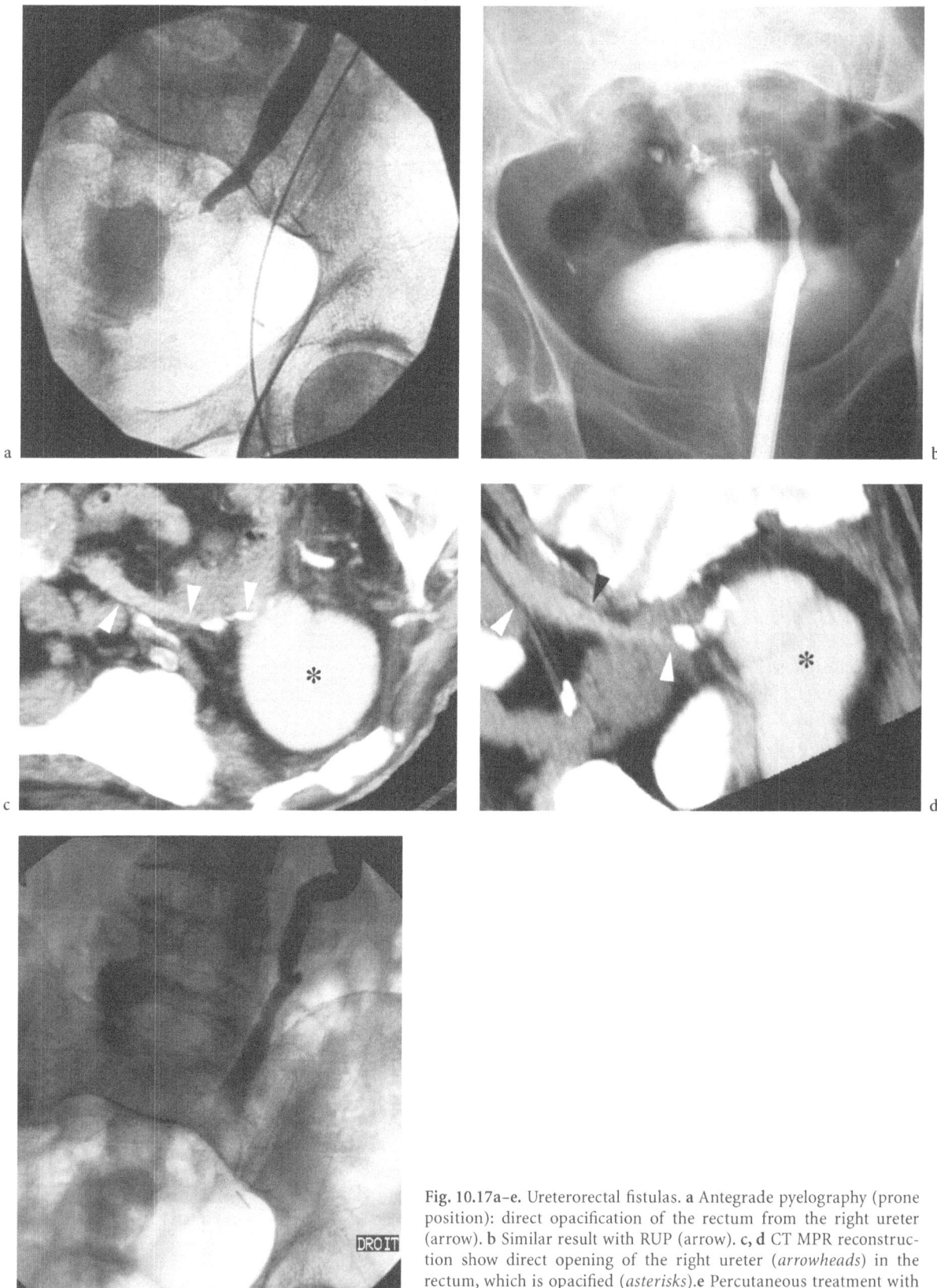

Fig. 10.17a–e. Ureterorectal fistulas. **a** Antegrade pyelography (prone position): direct opacification of the rectum from the right ureter (*arrow*). **b** Similar result with RUP (*arrow*). **c, d** CT MPR reconstruction show direct opening of the right ureter (*arrowheads*) in the rectum, which is opacified (*asterisks*).**e** Percutaneous treatment with temporary antegrade balloon occlusion: control antegrade pyelography in prone position

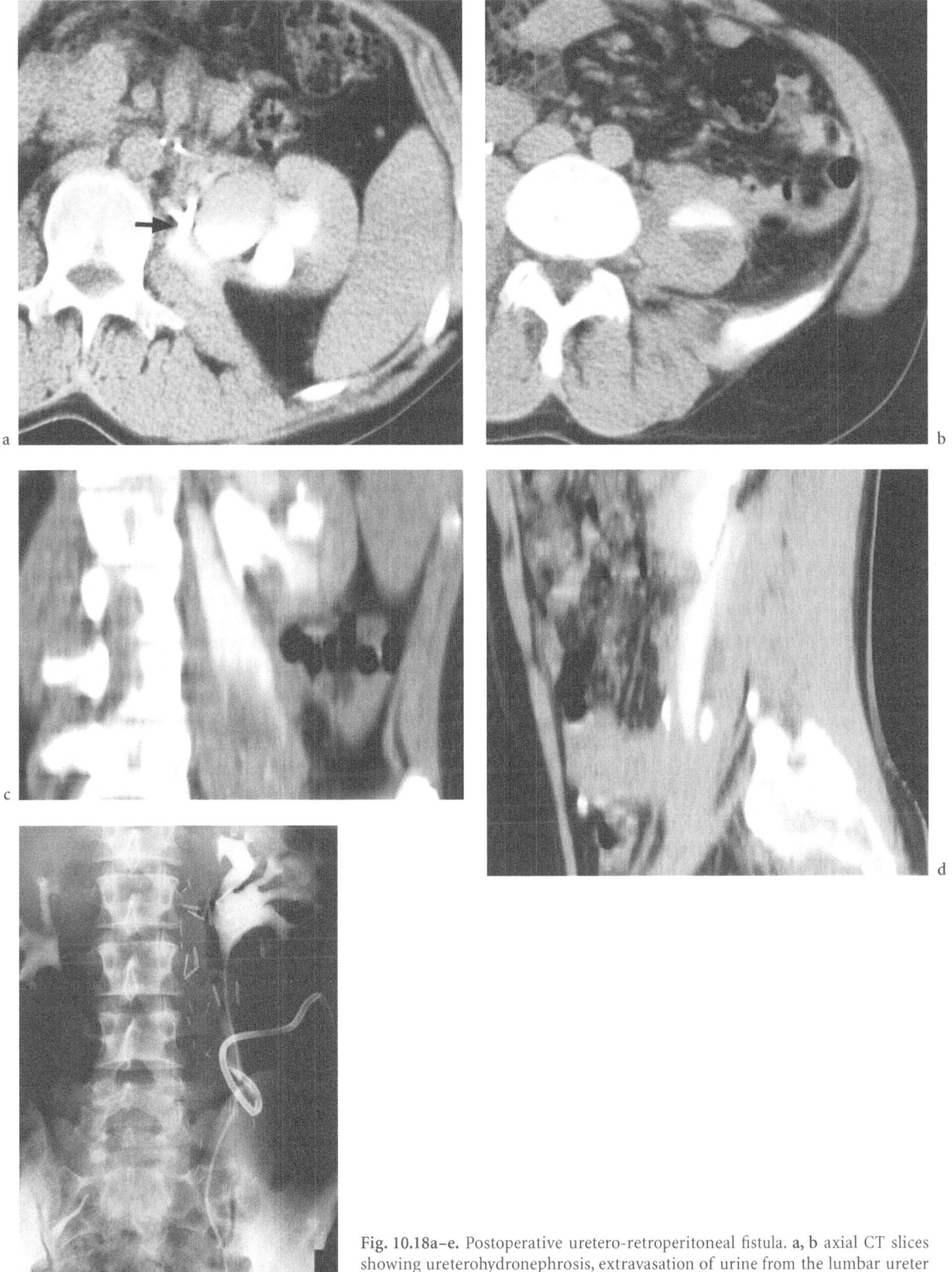

Fig. 10.18a–e. Postoperative uretero-retroperitoneal fistula. **a, b** axial CT slices showing ureterohydronephrosis, extravasation of urine from the lumbar ureter (*arrow*), urinoma inside the psoas muscle with fluid level. **c, d** Coronal and sagittal reconstructions demonstrate opacification of the urinoma. **e** Treatment with antegrade 2-J intubation and urinoma drainage

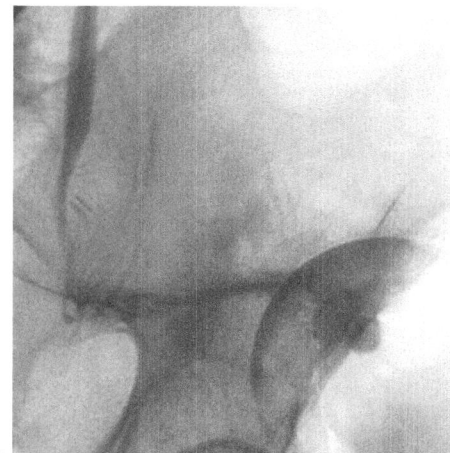

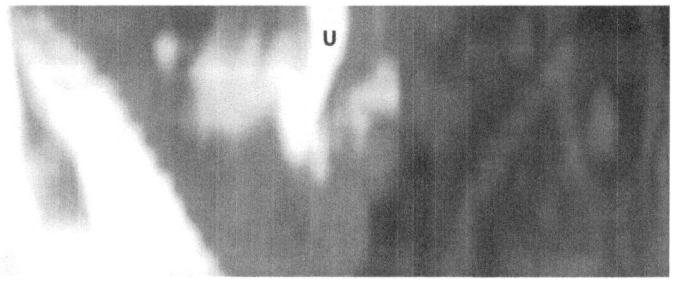

Fig. 10.19a, b. Postoperative uretero-retroperitoneal fistula. **a** Antegrade pyelography shows retroperitoneal extravasation. **b** CT reconstruction shows similar result with periureteral (*U*) opacification

frequently these fistulas appear following prolonged ureteral catheterization (SMITH 1984). The stiffness of 2-J catheters may cause erosion of the ureteral wall at the contact of the artery pulse (NELSON and FRIED 1981; ADAMS 1984). The use of new materials (silicon) has made this type of lesion exceptional.

The second cause is arterial disease: A fistula might result from an atheromatous or mycotic aneurysm opening into the ureter (JAFRI et al. 1987) or an arterioureteral fistula may form following stitch loosening of an aorto-iliac bypass (WHEATLEY et al. 1981). Arterioureteral fistulas with communication between an arterial aneurysm and a ureteral stump after nephrectomy are also seen. The presence of a ureteral obstruction secondary to the vascular anomaly frequently plays a role. Some other factors favoring ureteral ischemia are also indicated (DAUPLAT et al. 1985): pelvic cancerous excision, history of pelvic radiotherapy, periureteral or perianeurysmal fibrosis, local ureteral inflammatory fixation of the ureter against the external iliac artery. Such fistulas were reported in cases where a 2-J catheter was placed in pregnant women, with the dilated ureter pressing against the iliac artery (SMITH 1984). Arterioureteral fistulas have also been described in the setting of uretero-intestinal anastomosis (KELLER et al. 1990). On the whole, the most frequent context is that of a patient with a 2-J catheter associated with surgery and/or a history of pelvic irradiation.

In all cases, hematuria is the first sign, usually intermittent, often preceding cataclysmic hematuria (AHLBORN et al. 1986). It is important to stress the necessity of an accurate and early diagnosis: A correct diagnosis allows efficient treatment in about 90% of cases, whereas misdiagnosis leads to 52% mortality (KELLER et al. 1990). The diagnosis is dif-

ficult because the index of suspicion is low. EU most frequently shows a mute or slightly opacified kidney (NELSON and FRIED 1981). Antegrade or retrograde ureteropyelography does not always show the communication (TOOLIN et al. 1984). CT can visualize the communication, particularly in cases where an iliac aneurysm is involved (JAFRI et al. 1987; BAUM et al. 198) (Fig. 10.20a, b).

Angiography investigation is the most contributive test, providing the most precise information, because bleeding is often intermittent and difficult to detect. Selective opacification of the internal iliac artery is necessary on different views. At the same time, the 2-J catheter can be shifted to provoke bleeding, but this requires the placement of an occlusive balloon catheter in the hypogastric artery in case of massive bleeding (KELLER et al. 1990). Embolization can be proposed as an alternative to surgical bypass. The two techniques can be combined in some cases (QUILLIN et al. 1994). The use of a covered vascular endoprosthesis may be an appropriate solution if an associated iliac artery aneurysm is found. At the same time, embolization of the internal iliac artery can be done to control the bleeding along with arterial endovascular reconstruction to ensure coverage of the arterial lesion (ROUSSEAU et al. 1996).

It is possible that a rise in the frequency of this type of fistula can be expected, because of the increased use of 2-J catheter placement and the consistently high number of aortoiliac revascularization and ureteral derivation operations (CASS and ODLAND 1990). Intermittent macroscopic hematuria in a patient with these two factors should indicate the diagnosis, and early diagnosis can avoid serious developments. Interventional radiology then plays an increasingly important role in this condition.

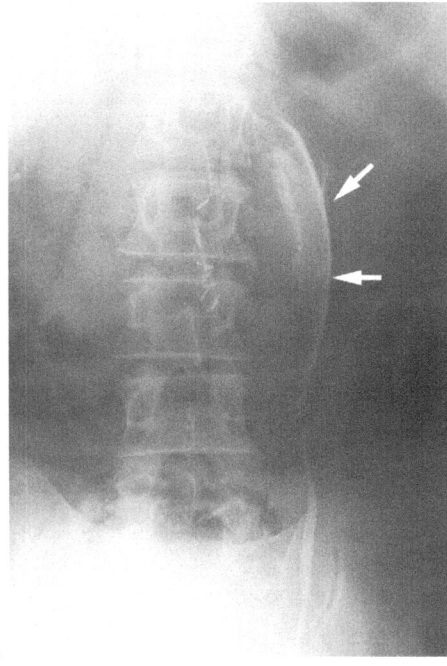

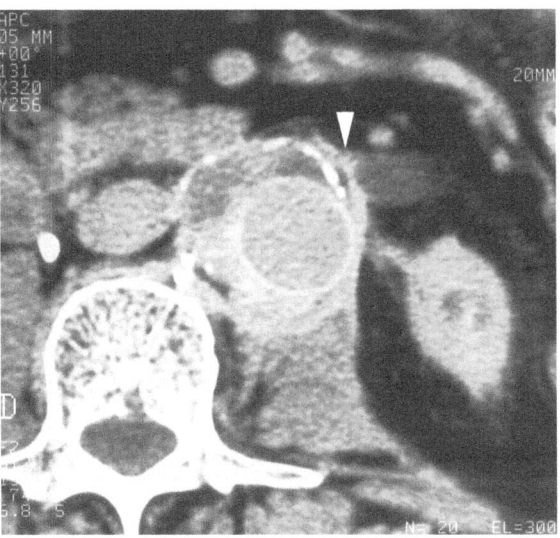

Fig. 10.20a, b. Aorto-ureteral fistula. a RUP shows opacification of the curvilinear wall of an aortic aneurysm (*arrow*). b CT slice demonstrates the aneurysm and adhesion of the left ureter to the aortic wall (*arrowheads*)

10.3.7
Miscellaneous

Other types of fistulas are reported but are less frequent:

- Ureteroperitoneal fistula, generally postoperatively after stitch loosening of a ureterointestinal anastomosis, or after ureteral trauma during intestinal surgery. Besides the use of classic direct opacification, CT can show signs of urinary ascites with enhancement after injection of contrast medium (HIRSCH 1985).
- Ureterouterine fistula secondary to uterine revision of a large necrotic tumor
- Ureterotubal fistula
- Ureteropancreatic fistula, exceptionally encountered after gunshot wounds. The shock wave caused by the projectile can be responsible for diffuse ischemic lesions, leading to avascular necrosis of the pancreas and the ureter. This phenomenon is exacerbated by the released pancreatic enzymes (ROHNER 1971).

10.3.8
Problems of Radiological Diagnosis
and of Treatment

Although ureteral fistulas differ according to their etiology and anatomic type, the problems of radiological diagnosis are frequently identical. EU is frequently unable to opacify the urinary tract sufficiently. Direct investigations are necessary and fine-needle antegrade pyelography is preferred: besides the diagnostic information it provides (level and importance of the fistula, associated obstruction) (FRITZSCHE 1986), it offers the possibility of draining the urine and at the same time treating the fistula and the obstruction. RUP is performed only if the distal ureteral segment is not opacified. CT with 3D reconstruction can delineate the fistula, its site, and the associated obstruction (Fig. 10.21a–c).

Therapeutic management via the antegrade percutaneous route is in fact justified by the difficulties of surgical treatment (FRITZSCHE 1986; LANG 1981). Nowadays, interventional radiology has proven its efficiency in treating most ureteral fistulas. Only some failures of radiological treatment and some arterioureteral fistulas require surgical treatment. The different therapeutic modalities for ureteral fistulas are developed in Chap. 12.

10.4
Ureteral Hernias

Ureteral hernias are rare; about 130 cases have been reported in the literature (CURRY 1990). Most were detected during a surgical intervention; few were diagnosed preoperatively by radiological examination (POLLACK et al. 1975; CRESPI 1980). Many cases remain

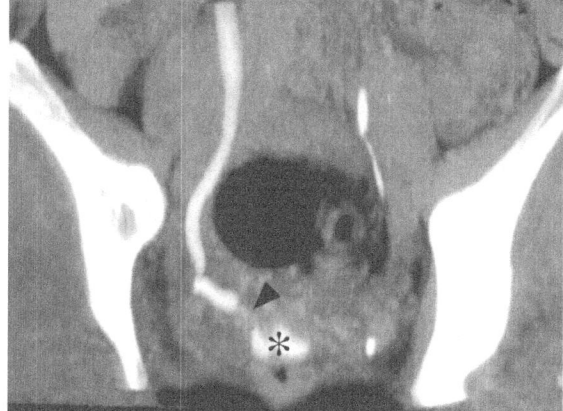

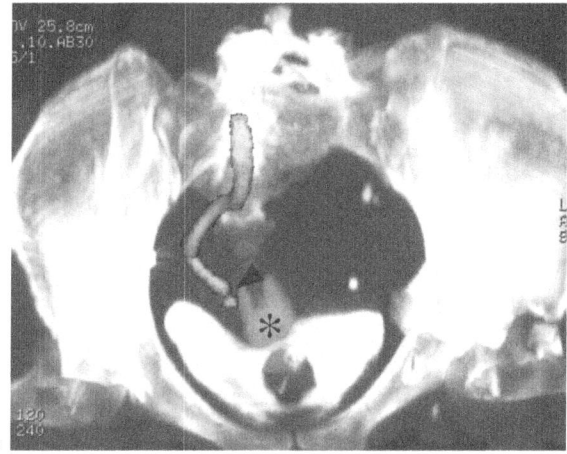

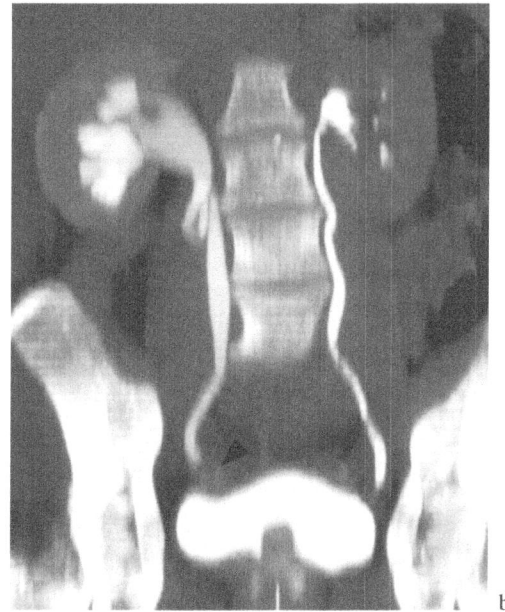

Fig. 10.21a–c. CT 3D reconstruction of a fistula (arrowheads) between right ureter and vagina (*asterisk*). a, b MIP; c SSD

asymptomatic and are misdiagnosed. The majority of ureteral hernias are inguinal (65%) and appear principally in men. In three of four cases they are on the right side, but they can be bilateral. More rare are the femoral hernias, seen particularly in women (30%). In 25% of cases a bladder hernia is associated. As for any inguinal hernia, the ureter can be intraperitoneal (the ureter being in the hernia sac) or more rarely extraperitoneal (no sac is found). Intraperitoneal hernia can be due to congenital adhesion of the ureter to the posterior parietal peritoneum, which pulls the ureter during hernia migration. Extraperitoneal hernias may be secondary to a congenital adhesion of the ureter to the genitoinguinal ligament (CURRY 1990). The ureter becomes herniated during testicular migration.

Sciatic hernias are exceptional findings (5%), because they are usually asymptomatic and accidentally discovered. Thus, in fact, they probably have a higher frequency (OYEN et al. 1987). The hernia occurs in the greater sciatic foramen. It is secondary to atrophy of the piriformis muscle, which is encountered in neuromuscular diseases, hip diseases, or other disturbances of the lower limb.

Other ureteral hernias reported are thoracic ureteral hernia through the foramen of Bochdalek (CURRY 1990), parailiac internal hernia between the psoas muscle and the iliac vessels, obturator hernia (WEINGARTEN et al. 1996; POLLACK et al. 1975), and retrocrural herniation through a diaphragmatic defect (CATALANO et al. 1998).

The performance of EU is crucial when the clinical symptoms are unclear but point towards the urinary tract, e.g., intermittent or colicky lumbar pain. In most cases, the patients are adults approximately 50 years of age; ureteral hernia in the infant is exceptional. The radiological diagnosis is easy when the ureter is in an abnormal extra-abdominal location, but the intermittent nature of the hernia phenomenon explains the frequent lack of this finding and the necessity of suspecting the diagnosis based on indirect signs (Fig. 10.22a, b). It may then be necessary to perform maneuvers that cause the hernia to occur. The most suggestive sign is the presence of a pelvic ureteral loop, single or sometimes double, with a vertical axis. This finding should prompt oblique and lateral views and sometimes erect or prone films,

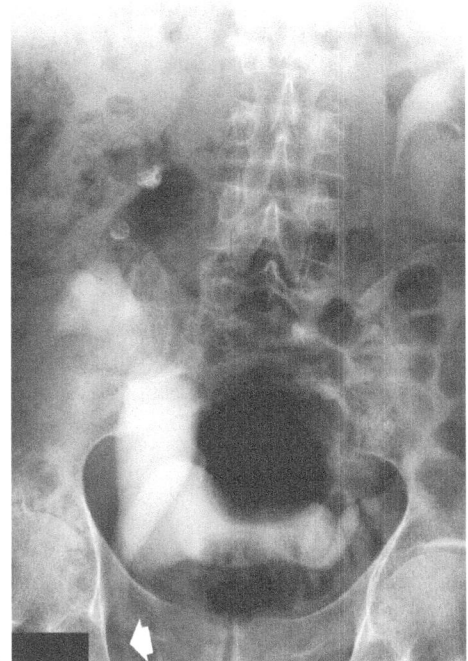
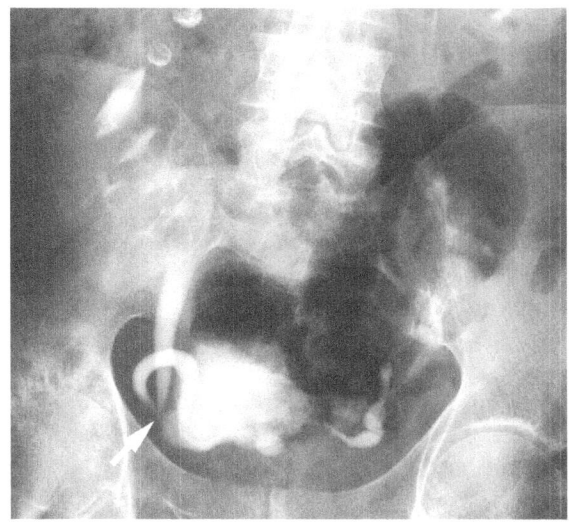

Fig. 10.22a, b. Inguinal hernia of ureter. **a** EU shows right urinary obstruction with abnormal pathway of right ureter outside the pelvis (*arrow*). **b** X-ray picture made after setting of a right inguinal hernia shows the curled aspect of the pelvic ureter (*arrow*) and a decrease in obstruction

centered on the pelvis and the scrotum to show the hernia. The existence of an inguinal hernia can be coupled with topographic modifications of the ureter, without ureteral hernia: A medial shift by attraction towards a contralateral hernia or a lateral shift, with the ureter being pushed away by herniated intestinal loops, can be found.

Sciatic hernias are characterized by the presence of a ureteral loop in front of the sciatic foramen (Fig. 10.23). The loop is known as "curlicue" ureter, and the lateral view shows the posterior orientation of the loop and the extrapelvic location of the ureter. This allows the elimination of some ureteral loops found in the sinuosity of the iliac artery, the loop having in this case an anterior orientation (OYEN et al. 1987). Renal ptosis can be associated as well as pelvic ectopy of the kidney. In some cases, the hernia is responsible for an obstruction syndrome.

CT examination has allowed the detection of some sciatic hernias (ARAT et al. 1996; SPRING et al. 1983). It may show the loop appearance and the ectopic course. This technique allows the detection of possible related abnormalities and reveals the different structures involved in the herniation and relationships with the abnormal ureter, providing for accurate presurgical mapping (CATALANO et al. 1998; OYEN et al. 1987).

Finding of a ureteral hernia is exceptional, but the possibility of such a lesion must be considered in case of surgical intervention for a large inguinal hernia,

particularly by a "sliding mechanism", in order to avoid iatrogenic ureteral trauma. Surgical treatment is reserved for symptomatic patients, but in specific cases percutaneous reduction with placement of an internal 2-J stent provides a new and minimally invasive therapeutic approach in poor surgical candidates or elderly patients (WEINTRAUB et al. 2000).

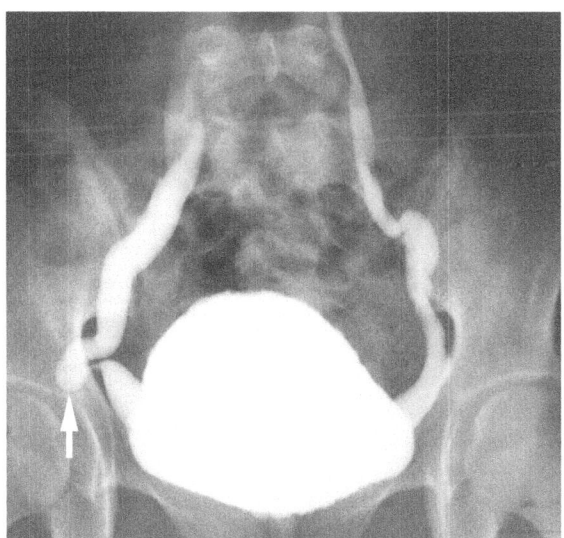

Fig. 10.23. Sciatic hernia of ureter demonstrated during voiding cystography: abnormal course of the right ureter through the sciatic foramen (*arrow*)

10.5
Ureteral Endometriosis

Endometriosis is a frequent disease (10%–20% of nonmenopausal women) that corresponds to endometrial proliferation in an abnormal topography. Two types of endometriosis are reported: internal endometriosis or adenomyosis, corresponding to small foci of endometrium in the myometrium and the uterine wall, and external endometriosis or true endometriosis, of extra-uterine topography. This disease generally affects women 30–40 years old, rarely after menopause, and its most frequent locations are ovarian, tubal and periuterine, but distant locations (thoracic) may exist (FAGAN 1974). Urinary tract involvement is rare, and then mainly the bladder is concerned (1%) (ASBESHOUSE and ASBESHOUSE 1960). Pure ureteral locations have seldom been reported since the first case was published (CULLEN 1977). LUCERO found 106 locations reported in the literature and AMAR found 157 cases (LUCERO et al. 1988; AMAR et al. 1989). These can be of two anatomic types (KERR 1966). Most frequent is the extrinsic form that results from the periureteral extension of a genital endometriosis. This form develops insidiously in the pelvis and leads to a real "frozen pelvis", similar to a neoplastic lesion (AMAR et al. 1989). If the diagnosis is suspected needless surgery can be avoided. The pure ureteral form is unusual. STIEHM says that the extrinsic form is four times more frequent than the pure ureteral one (STIEHM et al. 1972). But POLLACK criticizes this statement because the distinction cannot be made radiologically (POLLACK and WILLIS 1978). In exceptional cases, both types of lesion occur together (MOURIN-JOURET et al. 1987).

Three theories have been proposed concerning the pathogenesis of this condition (LUCERO et al. 1988). According to the embryological theory, these ectopic locations can have their origin in the remnants of the Wolff and Muller channels. The metaplastic theory suggests metaplasia of peritoneal cells following inflammatory, traumatic, or hormonal injuries. The migration theory is more attractive. It suggests that endometrial cells are transported, whether by the lymphatic or the hematologic route or tubally, to the level of the peritoneal cavity during menstruation, or also following surgical trauma (SAMPSON 1940; MOURIN-JOURET et al. 1987). Multiple ectopic locations are in favor of this last theory (BULKELEY et al. 1965), but it is possible that the origin varies. All abnormal locations of endometrial tissue are under hormonal stimulation of the endometrium. Hormone-dependent histological modifications (prolif-

eration, necrosis, desquamation) are identical. These locations do not act like neoplastic lesions but can, via a mass effect or a fibrotic reaction, have an impact on neighboring structures (OLDER 1990).

Anatomic lesions are different in the two forms. In the extrinsic form, endometrial cells reach the periureteral connective tissue but do not cross the adventitia. In contrast, in the intrinsic form the endometrial glands and connective tissue develop in the muscle layers of the ureter, leading to reduction of the lumen or polypoid intraluminal development andall. In both cases, lesions are accompanied by a more or less localized pelvic fibrosis, due to repeated bleeding; they are unresponsive to hormonal treatment and resemble a neoplastic process (BUCKSPAN et al. 1985).

The clinical symptomatology is poor. There may be lumbar or pelvic pain, dysmenorrhea, hematuria, or dysuria in a nonmenopausal woman. Sometimes there is renal failure related to bilateral ureteral involvement (MOURIN-JOURET et al. 1987). The exacerbation of signs during monthly periods, noted by some patients, is in fact rare, and the diagnosis is frequently delayed.

EU is the test classically performed first. If the location is periureteral it normally shows a unilateral stenosis – sometimes bilateral, but most frequently asymmetrical – of the pelvic ureter a few centimeters above the meatus, at the level of the insertion of the ureterosacral ligaments (POLLACK and WILLIS 1978). This stenosis is centered smooth and covers many centimeters (Fig. 10.24). More rarely, a simple lateral

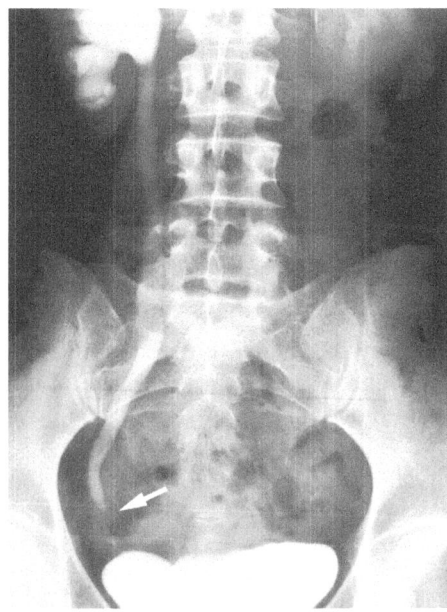

Fig. 10.24. Ureteral endometriosis. EU shows right urinary obstruction secondary to a centered smooth stenosis of the right pelvic ureter (*arrow*)

shifting with angulation or internal concavity secondary to the fibrotic phenomena is found (TALNER 1990. Sometimes the lumen is not opacified. In the majority of cases there is a ureterohydronephrosis above, sometimes with a mute kidney (TENCATE 1977; KANE and DROVIN 1985). This obstruction may long remain asymptomatic, and endometriosis manifests later at this site than elsewhere (STIEHM et al. 1972).

Retrograde opacification delineates the lesions better, but the aspect is most frequently poorly specific, suggesting conditions such as stenosing ureteral tumors, tuberculosis, and especially an extrinsic periureteral involvement (tumoral invasion or benign pelvic fibrosis). CT shows the presence of a periureteral mass of tissue density or a cystic aspect, sometimes with spontaneous hyperdensity secondary to

pelvic hemorrhage (PLOUS et al. 1985; ROY et al. 1993) (Fig. 10.25a–d). A pseudotumoral diffuse infiltration of the pelvis can also exist.

True ureteral endometriosis is rarely suggested by EU where a more or less tight stenosis is found. The image of an intraureteral lacuna with a cupula shape, seen during EU or RUP, also raises difficult problems for diagnosis, leading to discuss a budding ureteral tumor (KAPLAN and KUDISH 1974; REDDY and EVANS 1974). CT cannot differentiate because in both cases there is a zone of tissue density at the level of the stenosis with thickening of the ureteral wall (ROY et al. 1993). Ureteroscopy with biopsy appears to be very useful for this diagnosis (PURENA et al. 1985). Endoluminal ultrasonography following retrograde opacification can demonstrate the parietal location of the lesion (Fig. 10.26a–d).

Fig. 10.25a–d. Bilateral ureteral endometriosis. **a** EU shows bilateral urinary obstruction secondary to stenosis of both pelvic ureters. **b** RUP of the left ureter: tight, short, smooth stenosis with ureteral shifting of the narrowed area. **c, d** CT slices show the narrowed zone without evident mass. Some periureteral fat tissue infiltration is visible on the right side

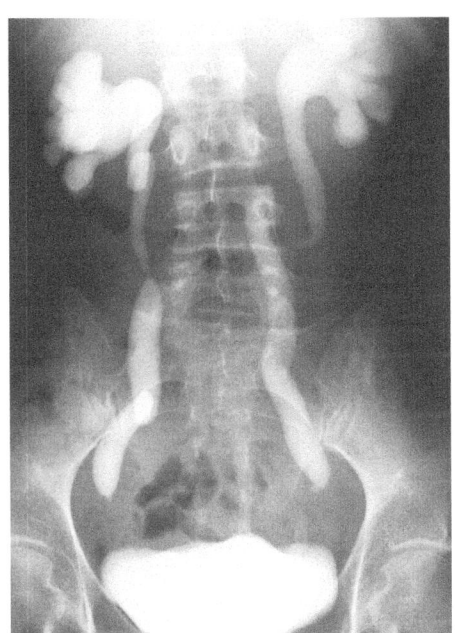

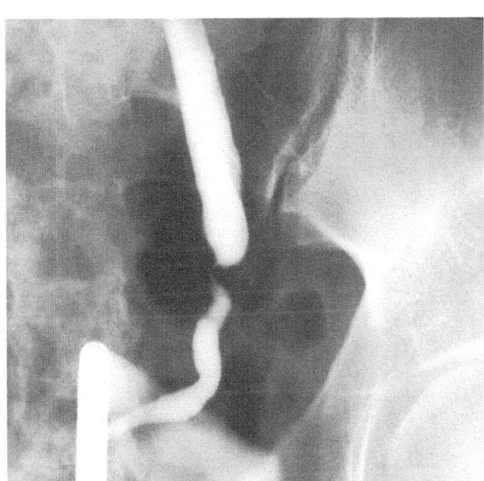

a

b

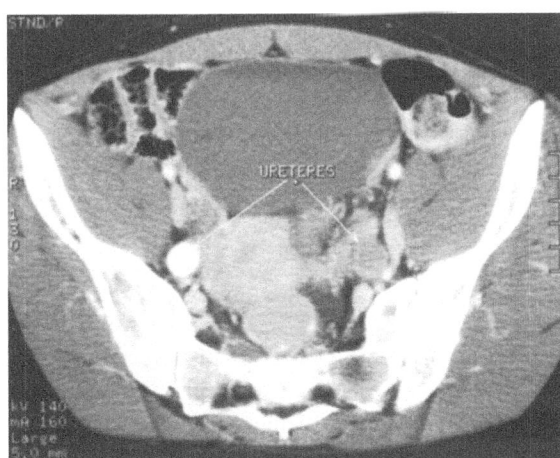

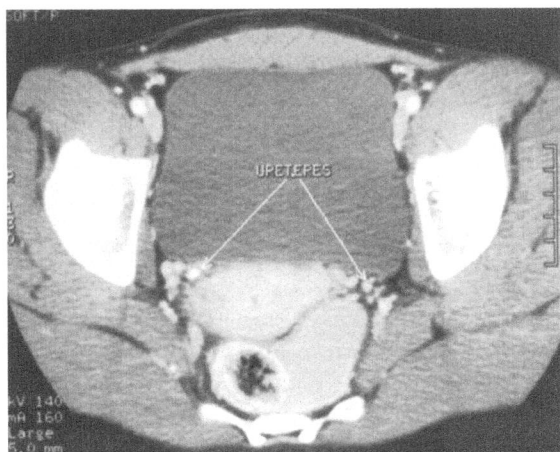

c

d

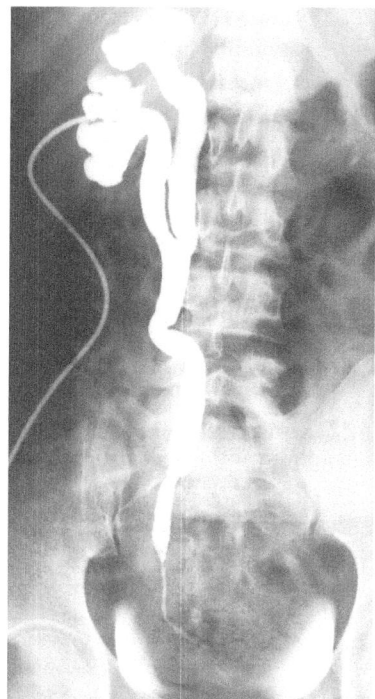

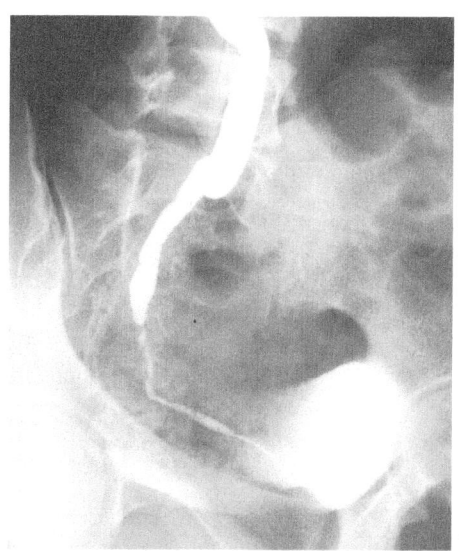

Fig. 10.26a–d. Intrinsic ureteral endometriosis. a, b Antegrade pyelographic view via a nephrostomy catheter: right urinary obstruction secondary to a long, centered, smooth stenosis of the right pelvic ureter. c, d Endoluminal ultrasonography shows diffuse homogeneous thickened wall of the right pelvic ureter up to the intramural portion (d)

a

b

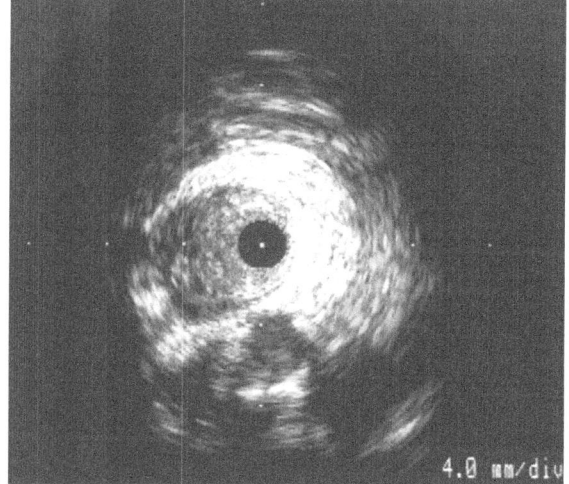

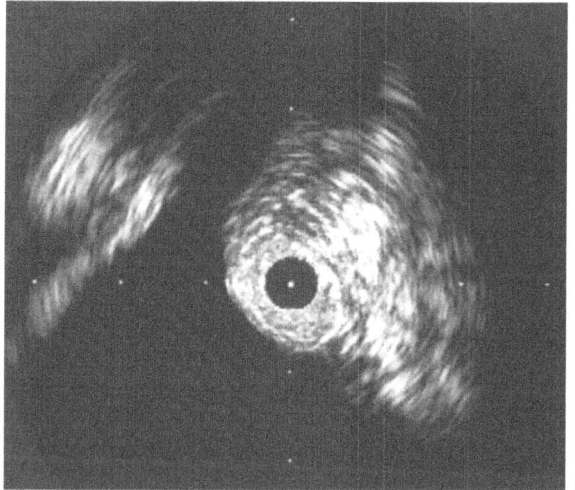

c

d

Cystoscopy is useful for diagnosis because a ureteral localization can be associated with vesical involvement.

MRI must be mentioned here; it detects endometriosis by showing a hypersignal on T_1 and T_2 weighted sequences, at the level of the periureteral region, because of the hemorrhagic character of the lesion (Roy et al. 1993). Uro-MRI sequences can complete this information, showing a uretero-hydronephrosis secondary to pelvic obstruction with the characteristic signal (Fig. 10.27a–g).

The diagnosis of ureteral endometriosis is often difficult. However, it must be suspected in case of obstruction of the pelvic ureter in a young woman,

the involvement of menopausal women being exceptional (Plous et al. 1985). Early diagnosis can prevent the evolution to irreversible and difficult-to-treat renal lesions. Celioscopic investigation of the pelvis often makes it possible to detect and biopsy associated lesions.

The treatment is based on combined surgery and hormone therapy. Although regression of some ureteral obstructions has been reported after hormone treatment with LHRH agonists in association with a 2-J catheter, particularly when the diagnosis was early, surgical treatment is usually necessary to identify ureteral endometriosis and re-establish the continuity of the ureter. According to the degree of

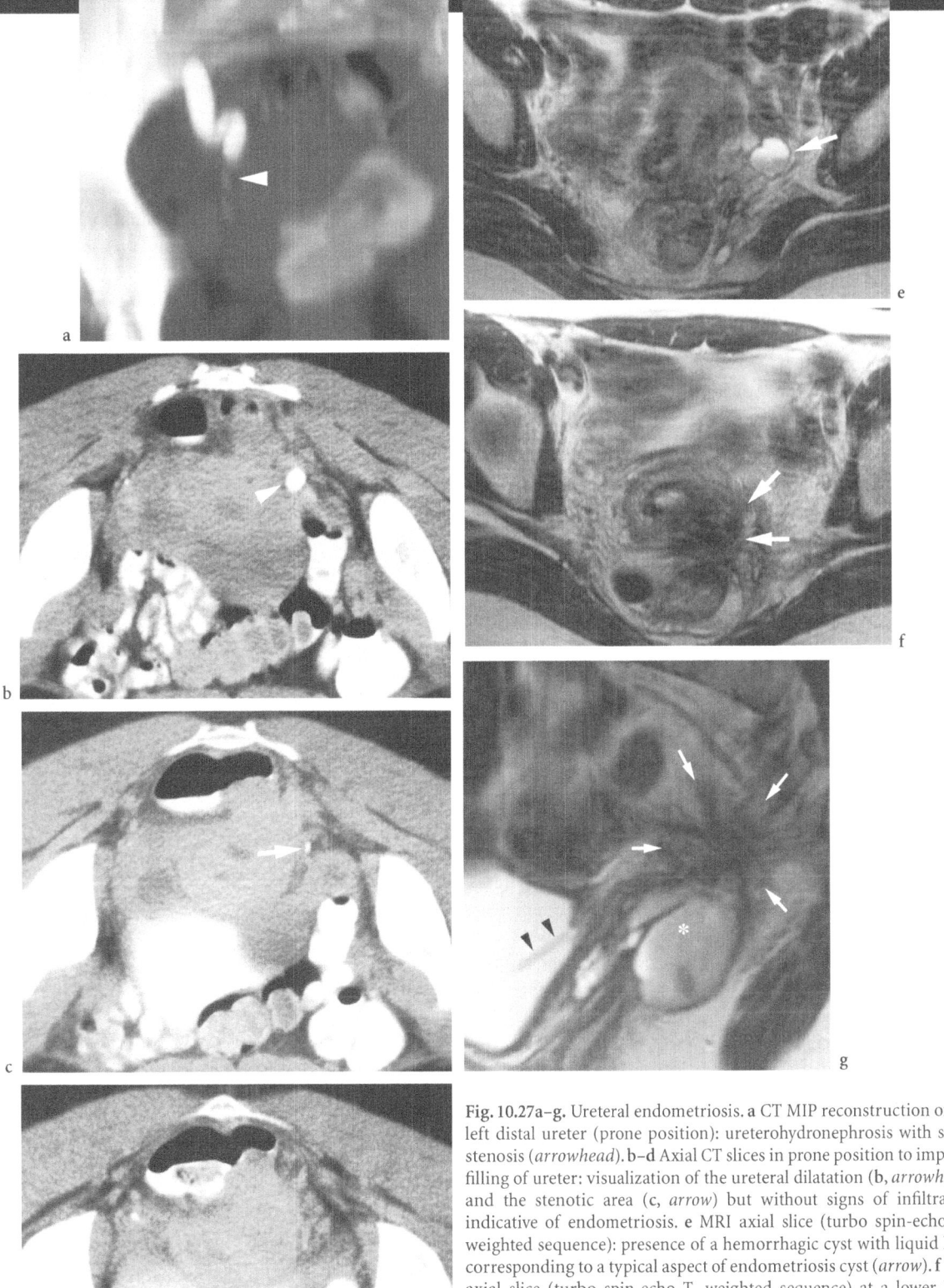

Fig. 10.27a–g. Ureteral endometriosis. **a** CT MIP reconstruction of the left distal ureter (prone position): ureterohydronephrosis with short stenosis (*arrowhead*). **b–d** Axial CT slices in prone position to improve filling of ureter: visualization of the ureteral dilatation (**b**, *arrowhead*) and the stenotic area (**c**, *arrow*) but without signs of infiltration indicative of endometriosis. **e** MRI axial slice (turbo spin-echo T_2-weighted sequence): presence of a hemorrhagic cyst with liquid level corresponding to a typical aspect of endometriosis cyst (*arrow*). **f** MRI axial slice (turbo spin-echo T_2-weighted sequence) at a lower level shows retracted stellar infiltration of the left parauterine area surrounding the distal part of the left ureter, which is not visible (*arrows*). **g** MRI left parasagittal slice (turbo spin-echo T_2-weighted sequence). Another endometriosis cyst is visible (*asterisk*) below the distal part of the left ureter, which is indicated by the 2-J catheter visible in the bladder (*arrowheads*). The cyst is surrounded by the probably fibrotic infiltration, which explains the ureteral stenosis (*arrows*)

obstruction and pelvic infiltration, nephroureterectomy, ureterolysis, a resection anastomosis, or ureteroileoplasty can be proposed.

The silent evolution of ureteral endometriosis and the difficulties of diagnosis suggest a need for regular radiological surveillance of the urinary tract (particularly using US) in women with genital endometriosis (KAPLAN and KUDISH 1974).

10.6
Other Diseases of the Ureteral Wall

10.6.1
Ureteral Pseudodiverticulosis

This rare affection of the ureter must be differentiated from other diverticular diseases of the ureter (CULP 1947). Real diverticula of the ureter are of congenital origin. They constitute a complete ureteral wall and correspond to an aborted duplication or "blind ureter". Most frequently there is a tube parallel to the ureter and ending in a bulging extremity; more rarely, a sacciform diverticulum, orthogonal to the axis of the ureter, is encountered (HOSPITEL et al. 1986).

Ureteral pseudodiverticulosis seems to be an acquired disease, the origin of which is still poorly elucidated (BENACERRAF and FABERT 1974). It differs from congenital diverticula by presenting as multiple lesions. It was described by HOLLY in 1957 and only 50 cases had been reported at that time (HOLLY and SUMCAD 1957), but the frequency is probably underestimated. It corresponds to multiple small expansions across the muscular layers of the wall (WASSERMAN et al. 1985). An increasing number of authors now consider it to be a preneoplastic lesion favoring the development of a urothelial tumor, but this is a point of controversy (PARKER et al. 1989).

The circumstances under which ureteral pseudodiverticulosis is discovered are various (GOLDMAN et al. 1977). The patients are always adult men, usually over 60 years of age. The most frequent major sign is hematuria, more rarely a UTI or signs of obstruction are seen, generally involving the lower apparatus. In some cases, these pseudodiverticular images are associated with urolithiasis or with an excretory tract tumor, particularly of the bladder. Association with transitional cell carcinoma is encountered in 30%–60% of cases (PARKER et al. 1989).

More than 50% of these anomalies are revealed by EU, particularly after ureter compression, but also on a post-voiding film that shows stasis of the diver-

ticular cavities (Fig. 10.28). Retrograde or antegrade ureteropyelography show theses anomalies better, particularly when good ureteral distension can be obtained (Figs. 10.29, 10.30). Pseudodiverticula are very small outpouchings of the lumen, less than 4 mm in diameter, implanted perpendicular to the ureteral lumen and of sacciform morphology (GOLDMAN et al. 1977; CREED et al. 1980)). These diverticula are multiple in nine of ten cases, and one of two patients has more than ten diverticula (up to 25 have been reported for one ureter). Three patients in four have bilateral involvement (Fig. 10.31). It predominates at the upper part of the lumbar ureter. The involved ureteral segment is often narrowed but not obstructed.

No evolution was noted in patients followed up over many years. There was no modification or disappearance of reported pseudodiverticula, even after suppression of associated lesions.

The exact origin of this anomaly is unclear, since few have been examined to date. By analogy to colonic diverticula, some authors, in particular Khonsari, suggested the possibility of pulsation diverticulum at the point of vascular penetration or congenitally weak zones (KHONSARI and OLIVIER 1971). This hypothesis was weakened by the histological studies of COCHRAN, which showed the existence of an epithelial proliferation of the wall and particularly the muscular layer with pseudodiverticular formation (COCHRAN et al. 1980). It may then represent reactive hyperplasia of

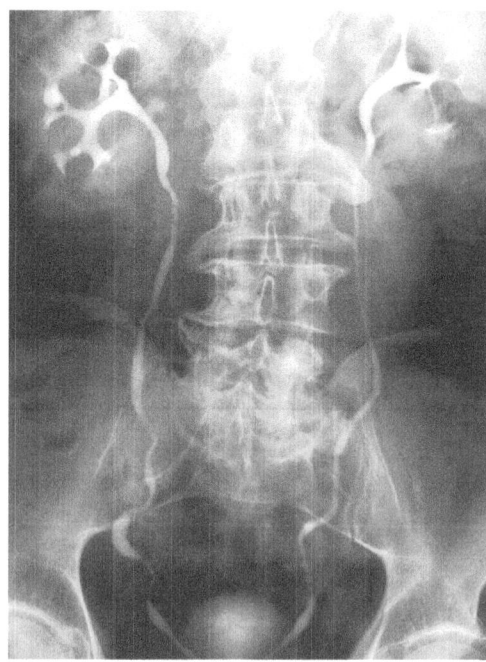

Fig. 10.28. Incidental discovery of bilateral ureteral pseudodiverticulosis on EU

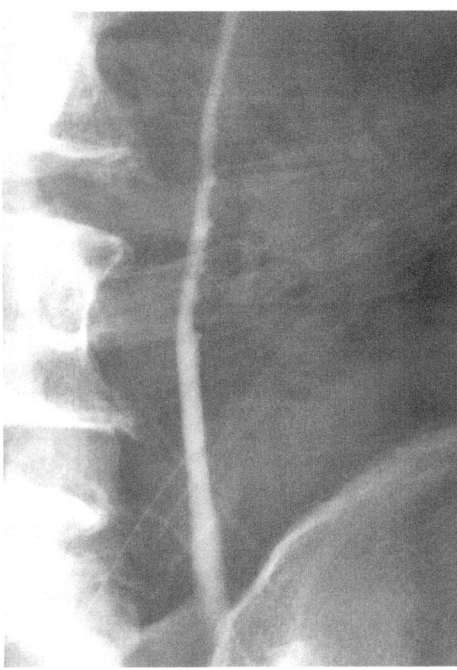

Fig. 10.29. Pseudodiverticulosis on RUP in a patient with bladder cancer. Presence of atypical cells on urine cytology study

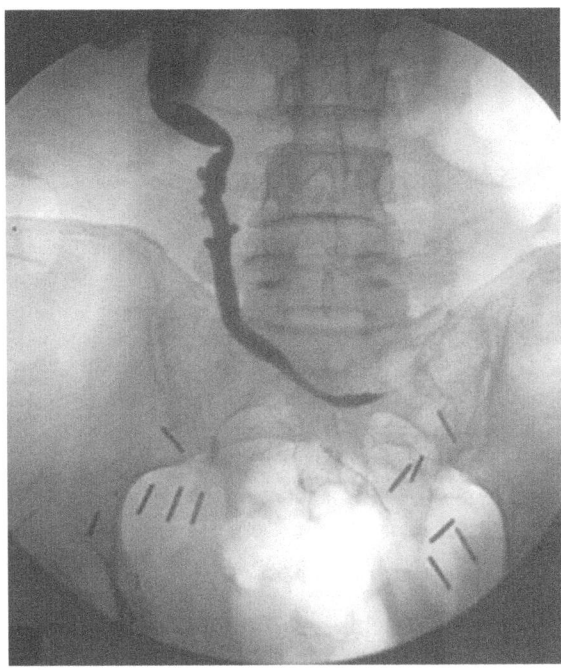

Fig. 10.30. Ureteral pseudodiverticulosis on antegrade pyelography. This patient has complete obstruction of a ureterointestinal anastomosis

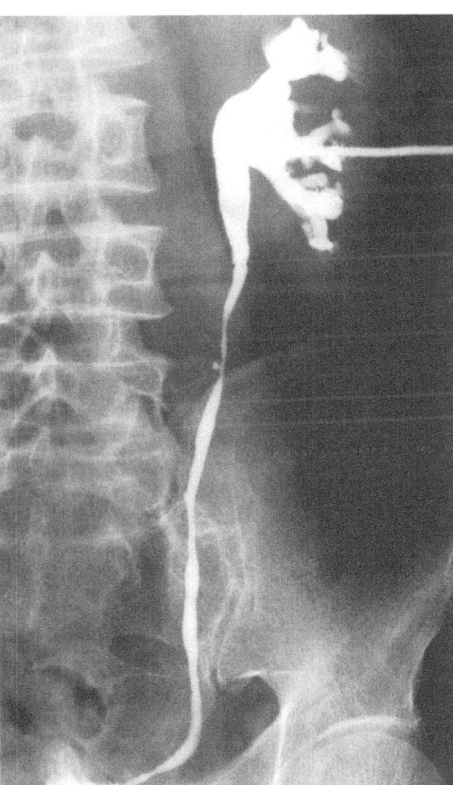

Fig. 10.31. Isolated ureteral pseudodiverticulosis associated with ureteral lithiasis, demonstrated during antegrade pyelography for left renal obstruction

the urothelium secondary to chronic inflammatory processes and/or stasis (PARKER et al. 1989; LESTER and KYAW 1973). However, this anomaly remains rare in these situations. It is possible that these factors favor the formation of pseudodiverticula only in cases where there are weak zones at the level of vascular penetration (HOLLY and SUMCAD 1957).

Wasserman found this anomaly in 11% of the ureters studied post mortem, without infections and/or obstructive context (WASSERMAN et al. 1985). The pseudodiverticula he found are smaller than those seen in vivo, which explains the difference of frequency from that in the already published series. In all cases, the zone of pseudodiverticulosis is the location of glandular and/or cystic ureteritis lesions (WASSERMAN et al. 1988).

The existence of hyperplastic anomalies and atypical cells of the mucosa, as well as the presence of associated urothelial tumors in a higher number of cases than normal, have raised the hypothesis of a preneoplastic status. These tumors are most frequently vesical, but ureteral or pelvicaliceal localizations can exist (COCHRAN et al. 1980; KENNEY and WASSERMAN 1987). ARCIOLA reported a urothelial tumor that developed inside a diverticulum (ARCIOLA et al. 1984). The cytological studies done by WASSERMAN showed, with the exclusion of four patients who were known to have urothelial cancer, atypical cells in five of 11 cases (WASSERMAN et al. 1985). In a more recent study, WASSERMAN reported urothelial malignancy in 46% of 37 patients who were found to have pseudodiverticulosis on EU or RUP (WASSERMAN et al. 1991) The majority of the tumors involved the bladder (65%). The association between pseudodiverticula and radiolucent filling defects or strictures is highly suggestive of urothelial tumor in these situations. Identification of diverticula, even a single one, strongly suggests the possibility of urothelial tumor, either synchronous or metachronous. The occurrence of a tumor 10 years after identification of pseudodiverticula has been reported by KENNEY (KENNEY and WASSERMAN 1987). Thus, close monitoring of these patients is necessary, including half-yearly cytology and annual cystoscopy (WASSERMAN et al. 1991). Evaluation of the upper collecting system is required only in patients with positive findings. WASSERMAN has reported four cases of pseudodiverticula patterns secondary to metastatic malignancy in a study of postmortem ureters (WASSERMAN 1994). This author suggests that, in the presence of pseudodiverticula in a cancer patient with no obstruction and no reversal after medical management, closer monitoring for future ureteral obstruction is needed.

10.6.2
Ureteral Localization of Amyloidosis

The urinary tract is one of the most frequent sites of amyloid disease (PEAR 1986). One in two patients suffering from this disease dies of renal failure (JOHNSON and ANKENMAN 1964). Ureteral involvement is rare, however, and represents 25% of urinary amyloidosis cases (fewer than 100 cases have been published), with which it is often associated (DAVIS et al. 1987; FUJIHARA and GLENNER 1981). Primary urinary amyloidosis and particularly isolated ureteral localizations are very exceptional (HAYASHI et al. 1998; THOMAS et al. 1977).

Ureteral amyloidosis is characterized by more or less diffuse amyloid infiltration of the ureter. It is usually unilateral and involves predominately the pelvic ureter; the symptoms are hematuria or lumbar pain secondary to the obstruction. The radiological aspect is one of a localized and irregular stenosis, sometimes lacunar, raising the possibility of tumoral disease (DAVIS et al. 1987). Sometimes it presents as more diffuse and irregular strictures (Fig. 10.32a–c). In some cases, these strictures are associated with linear calcification (GARDNER et al. 1971). The location outside the muscular layer of these calcifications explains the

presence of a radiolucent rim between the calcification and the opacified lumen. The presence of these radiolucent rims corresponds to mucosa and submucosa and is very indicative of the diagnosis; it allows the elimination of other ureteral parietal calcifications as the etiology (tuberculosis or bilharziosis) (LEE and DEETS 1976). The performance of CT slices at the level of the pathological zone makes it possible to detect calcifications not seen on EU. In the absence of calcifications, the diagnosis is made on the basis of a histological examination. Whether diagnostic or not, in the majority of cases these ureteral lesions require a direct therapeutic procedure, generally surgery. The possibility of obtaining a diagnosis on the basis of frozen-section histology helps to avoid a nephroureterectomy.

10.6.3
Ureteral Strictures of Analgesic Nephropathies

Ureteral stricture related to analgesics is an exceptional possibility described by MacGREGOR, who reports three cases (MacGREGOR et al. 1973). In two cases there was a bilateral tubulated stenosis of the lumbar ureter causing retroperitoneal fibrosis. One case involved a localized stenosis. Anatomopathological examination shows normal parietal fibrosis. The mechanism is unknown: The lesion is induced directly by analgesics or by an inflammatory reaction at the point of contact of a necrotized papilla impacted in the ureter (McGREGOR et al. 1979).

10.6.4
Leukoplasia and Ureteral Cholesteatomas (Keratinizing Desquamative Squamous Metaplasia)

Keratinizing desquamative squamous metaplasia (KDSM) is the term currently in use, including all postinflammatory changes that result in leukoplakia and cholesteatomas.

The ureteral mucosa can be, exceptionally, the location of an epidermoid (squamous) type of metaplasia . This squamous metaplasia is accompanied by desquamation and keratinization. The accumulation of desquamated keratin can lead to the formation of a keratin mass (cholesteatoma) or a thin keratin layer (leukoplakia). There is great confusion in the literature between the terms cholesteatoma, leukoplakia, squamous metaplasia (WILLS et al. 1981). Hertle grouped these terms under squamous desquamative and keratinizing metaplasia (HERTLE and ANDROULALAKIS

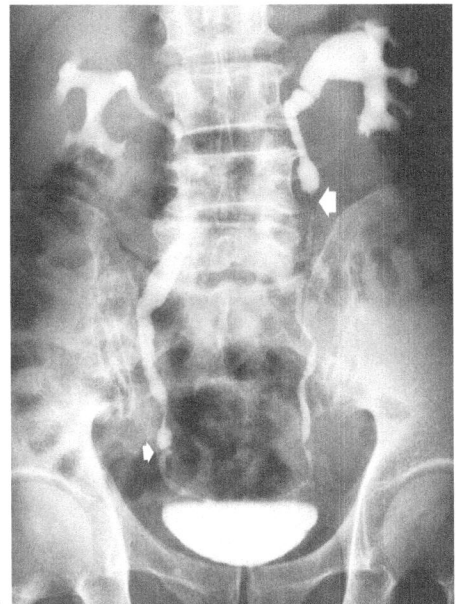

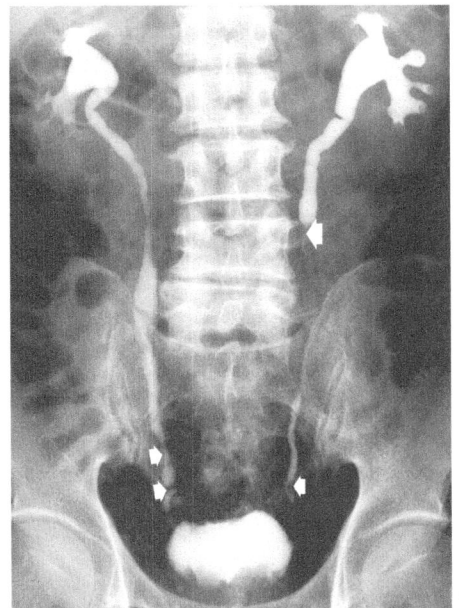

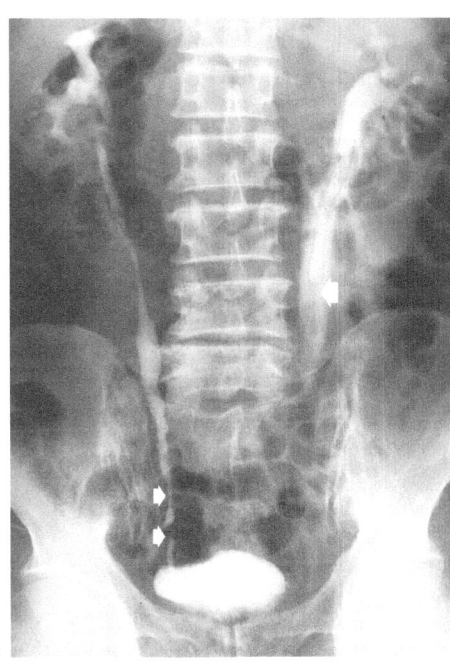

Fig. 10.32a–c. Ureteral amyloidosis. a, b EU shows multiple smooth centered stenoses of both ureters (*arrowheads*). c One month later, another EU in the same patient shows extravasation of contrast medium. Presence of periureteral CM allows evaluation of thickening of the left ureteral wall (*large arrowhead*). The right pelvic ureteral lesions are similar (*small arrowheads*)

1982). Although these were considered by some to be preneoplastic lesions (REECE and KOONTZ 1975), no malignant patterns were demonstrated and no cellular atypia was encountered. The origin of these anomalies is not clear: chronic urinary infection, lithiasis, stasis?

This disease affects mainly men over 40 years of age. Ureteral involvement is rarely isolated: it is usually concomitant with pelvicaliceal lesion. EU detects nonspecific anomalies such as multiple pyeloureteral filling defects. These filling defects are irregular and elongated, giving a striated or laminated aspect to

the ureter. Cholesteatomas are seen as solitary round lacunae of variable size, sometimes calcified, sometimes with a pseudotumoral aspect like the "goblet sign" (SHRADER and BERGREEN 1977; HAUGEN and WASSERMAN 1986). These intraluminal lacunae can be obstructive (WILLS et al. 1981; GONION and LAPERRIERE 1984). The radiological aspects are rather unspecific, and the differential diagnosis must include most causes of multiple lacunae of the ureter (WILLIAMSON et al. 1986).

Essential for the diagnosis is urinary cytology and

ureteral brushing by endoscopy, which shows the presence of desquamated urothelial cells (REECE and KOUNTZ 1975). KDSM is considered by some authors to be a premalignant lesion, and the classical treatment should be nephroureterectomy. However, in the absence of proof in this field, most authors insist on the necessity of the most conservative possible surgical treatment, with localized removal of the mass (GONION and LAPERRIERE 1984). No recurrence has been demonstrated until now in cases where the excision was total (HAUGEN and WASSERMAN 1986). Treatment of the underlying cause is essential to avoid recurrence.

10.6.5
Spontaneous Hematoma of the Ureteral Wall

Among the multiple causes of lacunar images of the ureter, one must think about spontaneous hematoma of the ureteral wall (WILLIAMSON et al. 1986). This lesion was reported by SMITH in 1974 (SMITH et al. 1974). It is a submucosal hemorrhage, the frequency of which is unknown. In fact, the presence of hematuria in a patient receiving anticoagulants is often regarded as benign in view of its frequency (40%). Investigation of these patients is generally delayed, and is then done when the radiological images have diminished. This hemorrhage normally has a pyeloureteral topography. It can be seen in patients of all ages, mostly in subjects receiving anticoagulation drugs or presenting a hemorrhage diathesis, but also in the context of urinary trauma (KAISER et al. 1975). Clinically it appears as acute lumbago, without radiation, frequently associated with macroscopic hematuria.

The diagnosis is classically made on the basis of EU: the renal pelvis and the proximal part of the ureter show multiple longitudinal, oval lacunae of varying size, presenting a broad site of implantation on the ureter wall (EISENBERG and CLARK 1976). Their contours are regular (Fig. 10.33). Two elements are important for the diagnosis: clinical context – particularly the use of anticoagulants – and the labile character of the images, which disappear in 8–15 days. In case of hematuria associated with lumbar pain, CT is increasingly being performed as the first examination. CT can be indicative of the diagnosis: There is parietal thickening of the renal pelvis and the ureter, sometimes with a spontaneous hyperdensity before injection of contrast material (Fig. 10.34a–e). There is frequently a dense infiltration of the hilar and perirenal fat (MILLER et al. 1982).

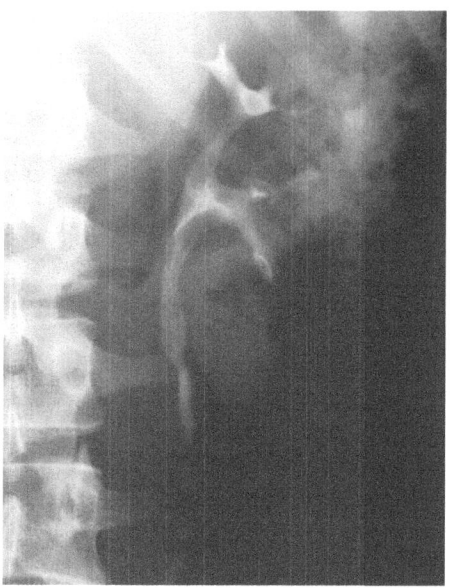

Fig. 10.33. Spontaneous hematoma of the ureter. EU shows multiple, longitudinal, oval, regular lacunae of the left pelvis and proximal ureteral wall

CT can detect another silent, associated and more frequent hemorrhagic complication (small bowel) (BELLIOL et al. 1998).

These submucosal hematomas can suggest a pyelo-ureteritis cystica (THOMPSON and McALLISTER 1975; WILLAMSON et al. 1986). In that condition, however, the lacunae are more round, regular and uniform, and nonevolutive. Nonspecific ureteritis can also be considered, but EU shows longitudinal striae with parietal haziness. In case of doubt, CT can be useful, particularly in the absence of an infectious context.

10.6.6
Ureteral Intussusception

Most exceptional cases of ureteral intussusception reported have been associated with polypoid tumors, mainly fibroepithelial polyps (FUKUSHI et al. 1983). Other authors described intussusception secondary to polypoid transitional cell carcinoma, inverted papilloma, or previous surgical intervention (COMPTON and DRUMMOND 1986). One case of retrograde intussusception was without any evident predisposing factor, except for the possibility of a vesicoureteral reflux (PARK et al. 1994). The diagnosis has to be considered in case of obstruction (mostly acute) associated with a soft tissue mass visualized at EU or RUP or on a nephrostogram.

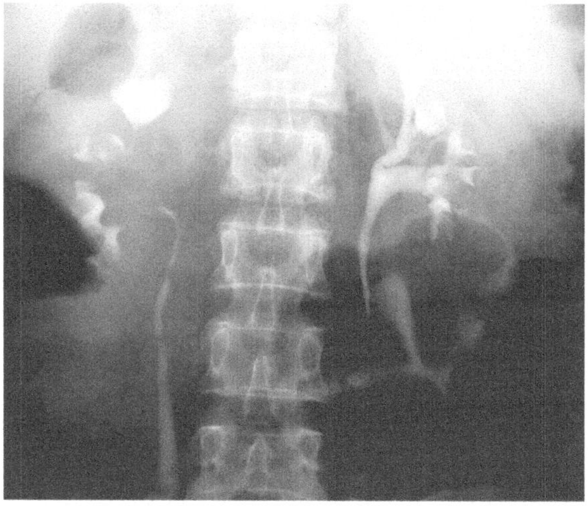

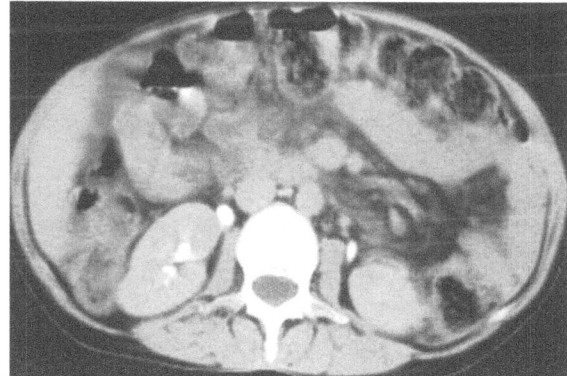

Fig. 10.34a–e. Spontaneous hematoma of the ureter. **a** EU in a patient with right lumbar pain and anticoagulant therapy. Circumferential and slightly irregular narrowing of the right pelvis and proximal ureter with multiple parietal lacunae. **b** CT without contrast medium injection: thickening of the ureteral wall with slight spontaneous hyperdensity (*arrow*). **c** CT at the same level after CM injection: The ureteral opacified lumen is surrounded by a hypodense zone inside an enhanced linear zone, probably corresponding to the ureteral adventitia. EU (**d**) and CT scan (**e**) 1 month later: total disappearance of the ureteral anomalies

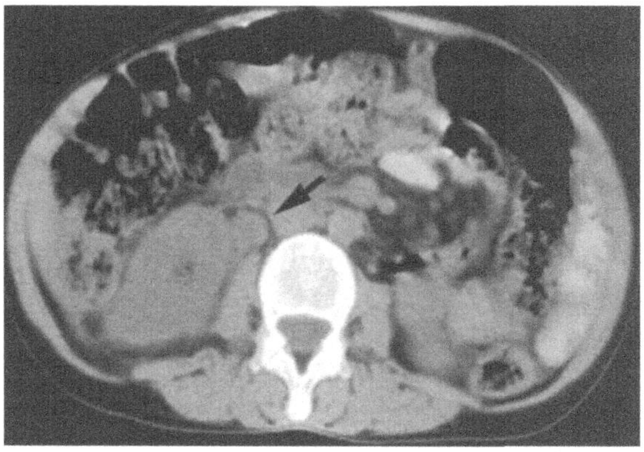

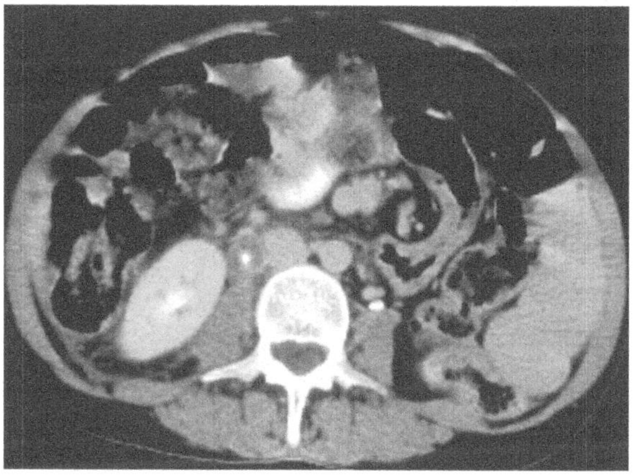

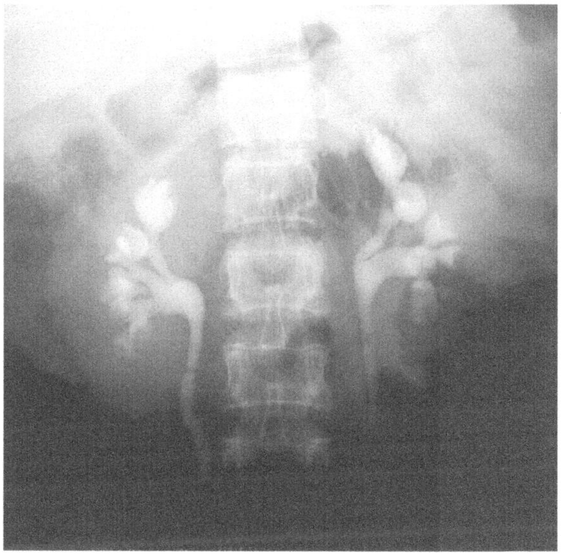

All ureteral obstruction due to a ureteral mass have to be discussed: i.e., a tumor, a radiolucent stone, a clot, a fungus ball, a sloughed papilla. The "bell-shaped" ureter has been described by MAZER as suggestive of the diagnosis (MAZER et al. 1979). Closer examination of the area at CT with thin slices and coronal reconstruction can show a cone-shaped filling defect with a small dimpled midline area (AOUN et al. 1999) (Fig. 10.35a–c).

However, definitive diagnosis is most often possible only through surgical exploration. In most cases ureteral intussusception is secondary to benign polypoid tumor, and this point has to be considered prior to surgery in order to plan conservative excision.

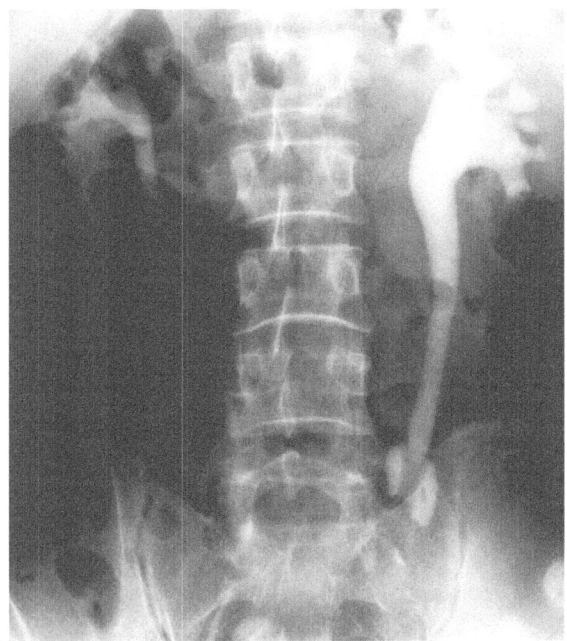

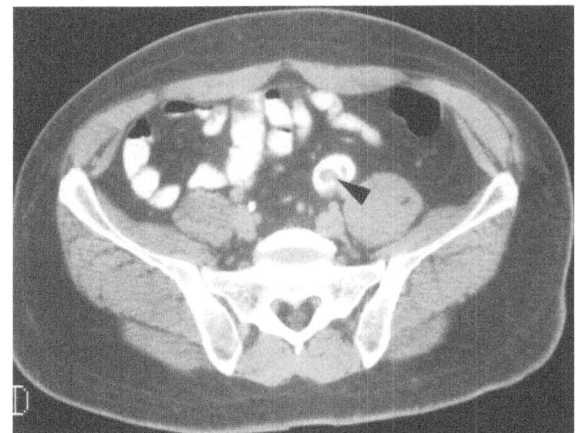

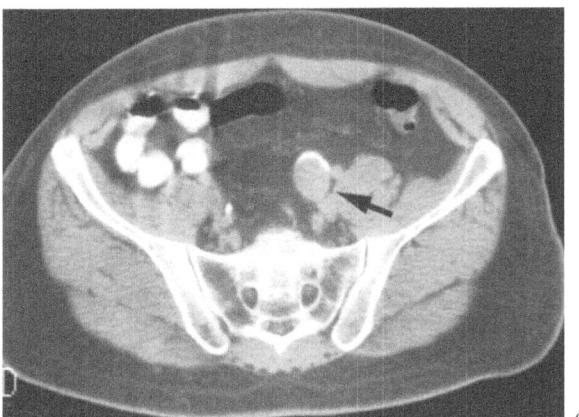

Fig. 10.35a–c. Ureteral intussusception secondary to transitional cell carcinoma (courtesy of Dr. AOUN). **a** EU for acute left renal colic shows ureteral obstruction. Above, a dilated zone presents a tubular lacuna which corresponds to the invaginated ureter. The underlying zone seems heterogeneous. **b, c** CT slices show ureteral dilatation with a central lacuna and a soft tissue mass corresponding to the invaginated ureter (*arrowhead*) and the tumor (*arrow*)

References

Adams PS (1984) Iliac artery-ureteral fistula developing after dilatation and stent placement. Radiology 152:647–648

Ahlborn TN, Birkhoff JD, Nowygrod R (1986) Common iliac artery-ureteral fistula: case report and literature review. J Vasc Surg 3:155–158

Ainsworth T, Weems WL, Merrel WH (1966) Bilateral ureteral injury due to non-penetrating external trauma. J Urol 96: 439

Amar A, Marry JP, Jougon J, et al (1989) Endometriose et sténose urétérale. A propos de 4 observations. J Chir 126:301–306

Ansong K, Khashu B, Lee WJ, et al (1985) Prophylactic use of ureteral stent in iatrogenic injuries to ureter. Urology 26: 45–49

Aoun N, Haddad-Zebouni S, Karam R, et al (1999) Invagination uretero-urétérale causée par une tumeur urothéliale maligne. J Radiol 80:317–318

Arat A, Haliloglu M, Cila A, et al (1996) Demonstration of ureterosciatic hernia with spiral CT. J Comput Assist Tomogr 20:816–817

Arciola AJ, Park T, Mallonk C, et al (1984) Multiple ureteral diverticula. J Urol 131:370

Asbeshouse BS, Asbeshouse G (1960) Endometriosis of the urinary tract: a review of the literature and a report of four cases of vesical endometriosis. J Int Coll Surg 34:63

Banner MP, Pollack HN, Ring EJ, et al (1983) Catheter dilatation of benign ureteral stricture. Radiology 147:427–431

Barasch E, Kashdam B, Rathore A (1988) Spontaneous perforation of the ureter diagnosed on ^{99m}Tc DTPA excretory urography. Urol Radiol 10:107–109

Baum ML, Baum RD, Plain L (1987) Computed tomography in the diagnosis of fistula between the ureter and iliac artery. J Comput Assist Tomogr 11:719–721

Beckley DE, Waters EA (1972) Avulsion of the pelviureteric junction – a rare consequence of nonpenetrating trauma. Br J Radiol 45:423–426

Becopoulos T, Ukourinas M, Pliotas G (1979) Spontaneous rupture of the ureter during high-dose urography. Br J Urol 51:812

Belliol E, Richez P, Barea D, et al (1998) Hematomes ureteraux compliquant un traitement anticoagulant. J Radiol 79: 49–51

Benacerraf R, Fabert G (1974) Les diverticules multiples de l'uretère. J Radiol Electrol 55:893–897

Benoit G, Boccon-Gibod L, Teyssier P, et al (1983) Traumatismes iatrogènes de l'uretère. Analyse de 47 cas. Chirurgie 109:160

Bettman MA, Murray PD, Perlmutt LM, et al (1983) Ureteroileal anastomotic leaks: percutaneous treatment. Radiology 148:95–100

Bollack C, Reinhardt W (1977) Complications urologiques de la chirurgie gynécologique. II. Les fistules urétéro-génitales. Lyon Chir 73:161–165

Borski A, Smith RA (1960) Ureteral injury in lumbar disc operations. J Neurosurg 17:925

Borkowski A, Canpliczka M (1974) Nontraumatic extravasation from the ureter. Int Urol Nephrol 5:271–275

Bright TC, Peters PC (1977a) Ureteral injuries secondary to operative procedure. Urology 9:22

Bright TC, Peters PC (1977b) Ureteral injuries due to external violence. 10 years' experience with 59 cases. J Trauma 17:616

Brueziere J, Gruner M, Firmin F, et al (1975) Rupture traumatique de l'uretère sous-pyelique après traumatisme fermé de l'enfant. J Urol Nephrol 81:582–589

Buckspan MB, Cooter NB, Goldfinger M, et al (1985) Endometriosis: an unusual cause of ureteral obstruction. Can J Surg 28:447–449

Bulkeley CJ, Carrow LA, Exjensen RD (1965) Endometriosis of the ureter. J Urol 93:139–145

Bunkin IA (1967) The ureter in obstetrics and gynecology. In: Bergman H (ed) The ureter. Hoeber Medica Division, New York, pp 527–547

Campbell CC, Mitnick JS, Bosniak MA (1982) Two cases of spontaneous ureteral rupture secondary to outlet obstruction. Urol Radiol 4:239–241

Carlton CE (1978) Injuries of the kidney and ureter. In: Harrison JH, Gittes RF, Perlmutter AD, Stamey TA, Walsh PC (eds) Campbell's urology, 4th edn. Saunders, Philadelphia

Cass AS, Odland M (1990) Uretero-arterial fistula: case report and review of literature. J Urol 143:582–583

Catalano O, Nunziata A, Cusati B, et al (1998) Retrocrural loop of the ureter: CT findings. AJR Am J Roentgenol 170:1293–1294

Cecconi RD, Lloyd L, Hawasli A, et al (1986) Bilateral transection of ureters secondary to gunshot wound to abdomen. J Trauma 26:938–940

Cochran ST, Walsman J, Barbaric ZL (1980) Radiographic and microscopic findings in multiple ureteral diverticula. Radiology 137:631–636

Compton JS, Drummond M (1986) Intussusception of the ureter by a polypoid transitional cell carcinoma. Br J Urol 58:725

Coulon A, Mandron E, Chartier-Kastler E, et al (1998) Rupture intraperitonéale spontanée de l'uretère. J Radiol 79:1401–1403

Creed LH, Post J, Hillman BJ, et al (1980) Multiple ureteral diverticula. Urol Radiol 2:29–32

Crespi R (1980) Radiodiagnostic des hernies urétérales et vésicales. Ann Radiol 23:419–424

Cullen TS (1977) Adenomyoma of the recto-vaginal septum. Bull John Hopkins Hosp 28:343

Culp OS (1947) Ureteral diverticulum: classification of the literature and report of an authentic case. J Urol 58:309–321

Curry N (1990) Hernias of the urinary tract. In: Pollack HM (ed) Clinical urography: an atlas and text book of urological imaging. Saunders, Philadelphia, pp 2570–2578

Dauplat J, Piollet H, Condat P, et al (1985) Deux cas de fistules urétéro-artérielles. J Urol 91:457–461

Davis PS, Babaria A, March DE, et al (1987) Primary amyloidosis of the ureter and renal pelvis. Urol Radiol 9:158–160

Diamond DA, Marshall FF (1982) The diagnosis and management of spontaneous rupture of the ureter. J Urol 128:808–810

Dowling RA, Corriere JN, Sandler CM (1986) Iatrogenic ureteral injury. J Urol 135:912–915

Dondelinger R, Kurdziel JL (1984) Percutaneous phenol neurolysis of the lumbar sympathetic chain with computed tomography control. Ann Radiol 27:376–379

Dufour B (1973) Les obstructions de l'uretère lombo-iliaque à l'exclusion des tumeurs urétérales. Association Française d'Urologie, Paris

Eisenberg RL, Clark RE (1976) Filling defects in the renal pelvis and ureter owing to bleeding secondary to acquired circulating anticoagulants. J Urol 116:662–663

Fagan CJ (1974) Endometriosis – clinical and roentgenographic manifestations. Radiol Clin North Am 12:109–125

Ferrie BG (1985) Ureterocolic fistula diagnosis by antegrade pyelography. Urol Radiol 7:116–118

Flynn JT, Tiptaft RC, Woodhouse CRJ, et al (1979) The early and aggressive repair of iatrogenic ureteric injuries. Br J Urol 51:454–457

Freiman DB, Ring EJ, Oleaga JA, et al (1978) Thin needle biopsy in the diagnosis of ureteral obstruction with malignancy. Cancer 42:714–716

Friedenberg RM, Ney C, Elkin M (1963) Trauma to the ureter. AJR Am J Roentgenol 90:28–36

Fritzsche P (1986) Antegrade pyelography: therapeutic applications. Radiol Clin North Am 24:573–586

Fujihara S, Glenner GG (1981) Primary localized amyloidosis of the genitourinary tract. Immunohistochemical study on eleven cases. Lab Invest 44:55–60

Fukushi Y, Orikasa S, Takeuchi M (1983) A case of ureteral intussusception associated with ureteral polyp. J Urol 129:1043–1044

Fuse H, Hara S, Ito H, et al (1985) Spontaneous rupture of the ureter of a patient with Cushing's syndrome. Eur Urol 11:346–347

Gardner KD jr, Castellino RA, Kempson R (1971) Primary amyloidosis of the renal pelvis. N Engl J Med 284:2196

Goel MC, Ramanathan R, Bannerjree G, et al (1996) Spontaneous perforation of the ureter: endourological management with renal preservation. Urol Int 57:122–125

Goldman S, Affre J, Goldman E, et al (1977) Diverticulose de l'uretère. J Radiol Electrol 58:798–800

Gonion J, Laperriere J (1984) Sténose urétérale due à une métaplasie épidermoïde de l'urothélium. J Radiol 65:207–209

Goodwin WE, Scardino PT (1980) Vesico-vaginal and uretero-vaginal fistulas: a summary of 25 years of experience. J Urol 123:370–374

Graham JB, Abad RS (1967) Ureteral obstruction due to radiation. Am J Obstet Gynecol 99:409–412

Gunther R, Marberger M, Klose K (1979) Transrenal ureteral embolization. Radiology 132:317–319

Harshman MW, Pollack H, Banner MP, et al (1982) Conservative management of ureteral obstruction secondary to suture entrapment. J Urol 127:121

Haugen SG, Wasserman NF (1986) Keratinizing desquamative squamous metaplasia of the upper urinary tract. Urol Radiol 8:211–213

Hayashi T, Kojima S, Sekine H, et al (1998) Primary localized amyloidosis of the ureter. Int J Urol 5:383–385

Heritier P, Bally G, Melka R, et al (1988) Les sténoses urétérales après colpocystopexie pour incontinence urinaire d'effort. A propos de 5 cas. J Urol 94:349–351

Hertle L, Androulalakis P (1982) Keratinizing desquamative squamous metaplasia of the upper urinary tract. J Urol 127:631–635

Higgins CC (1967) Ureteral injuries during surgery: a review of 87 cases. JAMA 199:82

Hirsch M (1985) Enhanced ascites: CT sign of ureteral fistula. J Comput Assist Tomogr 9:825–826

Holden S, Hicks CC, Walton KN (1976) Gunshot wounds of the ureter. A 15-year review of 63 consecutives cases. J Urol 116:562

Holly LE, Sumcad B (1957) Diverticular ureteral changes: a report of four cases. AJR Am J Roentgenol 78:1053–1066

Horrow MM, Tuncali K, Kirby CL (1997) Imaging of ureteroscopic complications. AJR Am J Roentgenol 168:633–637

Hospitel S, Galakhoff G, Dana A, et al (1986) Les images diverticulaires de l'uretère et du bassinet. J Radiol 67:565–572

Huffman JL (1989) Ureteroscopic injuries to the upper urinary tract. Urol Clin North Am 16:249–254

Jafri SZH, Farah J, Hollander JB (1987) Urographic and computed tomographic demonstration of uretero-arterial fistula. Urol Radiol 9:47–49

Johnson HW, Ankenman GJ (1964) Bilateral ureteral primary amyloïdosis. J Urol 92:275–277

Kaiser JA, Jacobs RP, Korobkin M (1975) Submucosal hemorrhage of the renal collecting system. AJR Am J Roentgenol 125:311–313

Kane C, Drovin P (1985) Obstructive uropathy associated with endometriosis. Am J Obstet Gynecol 151:207–211

Kaplan JH, Kudish HG (1974) Endometrial obstruction of ureter. Urology 3:327–329

Kaplan LM, Farrer JH, Lupu AN (1987) Spontaneous rupture of the ureter. Urology 29:313–316

Kelais PP (1971) Trauma to the urinary system; urinary fistulas. In: Emmet JL, Witten DM (eds) Clinical urography, 3rd edn, chap 15. Saunders, Philadelphia, p 1726

Keller FS, Barton RE, Routh WD, et al (1990) Gross hematuria in two patients with ureteral ileal conduits and double-J stents. J Vasc Interv Radiol 1:69–79

Kenney PJ, Wasserman NF (1987) Ureteral pseudodiverticulosis associated with carcinoma of renal pelvis. Urol Radiol 9:161–163

Kenney PJ, Panicek DM, Witanowski LS (1987) Computed tomography of ureteral disruption. J Comput Assist Tomogr 11:480–484

Kerr WS (1966) Endometriosis involving the urinary tract. Clin Obstet Gynecol 9:331–357

Khonsari H, Olivier JA (1971) Multiple ureteral diverticula. J Urol 58:309–321

Laberge I, Homsy YL, Dabour G (1979) Avulsion of ureter by blunt trauma. Urology 13:172–178

Lang EK (1973) Complications in the urinary tract related to treatment of cervical cancer. South Med J 66:228–236

Lang EK (1981) Diagnosis and management of ureteral fistula by percutaneous nephrostomy and anterograde stent catheter. Radiology 138:311

Lang EK (1990) Ureteral injuries. In: Pollack HM (ed) Clinical urography: an atlas and textbook of urological imaging. Saunders, Philadelphia, pp 1495–1503

Lee KT, Deeths TM (1976) Localized amyloidosis of the ureter. Radiology 120:60

Lester PD, Kyaw MM (1973) Ureteral diverticulosis. Radiology 106:77–80

Lirott SA, Ponter JS, Pierce JM (1977) Gunshot wound to the ureter: 5 years' experience. J Urol 118:551–553

Lopez AL, Pena Outeirino JM (1978) Traumatismo ureteral post-aortografia translumbar. Arch Esp Urol 31:131–138

Lucero SP, Wise HA, Kirsh G, et al (1988) Ureteric obstruction secondary to endometriosis. Report of three cases with a review of the literature. Br J Urol 61:201–204

MacGregor B, Jones N, Barraclough MA (1973) Ureteric strictures with analgesic nephropathy. Br Med J 2:271

MacGregor B, Saker BM, England EJ (1979) Ureteric stricture associated with analgesic nephropathy. Med J Aust 1:287–288

Maillet PJ, Pelle Francoz D, Leriche A, et al (1987) Fistulas of the upper urinary tract: percutaneous management. J Urol 138:1382–1385

Mattingly RF, Borkowf HI (1978) Acute operative injury to the lower urinary tract. Clin Obstet Gynecol 5:123–149

Mazer MJ, Lacys S, Kao L (1979) "Bell-shaped ureter" a radiographic sign of antegrade intussusception. Urol Rad 1:63

McGinty DM, Mendez R (1977) Traumatic ureteral injuries with delayed recognition. Urology 10:115–117

Medina D, Lavery R, Ross SE, et al (1998) Ureteral trauma: preoperative studies neither predict injury nor prevent missed injuries. J Am Coll Surg 186:641–644

Miller U, Witten DM, Shin MS (1982) Computed tomographic findings in suburothelial hemorrhage. Urol Radiol 4:11–14

Mourin-Jouret A, Squifflet JP, Cosyns JP, et al (1985) Bilateral ureteral endometriosis with end-stage renal failure. Urology 29:302–306

Nelson HN, Fried FA (1981) Iliac artery-ureteral fistula associated with Gibbon's catheter: a case report and review of the literature. J Urol 125:878–880

Newman CE, Dawson-Edwards P, Hurwatth FM (1974) Spontaneous rupture of the ureter. Br J Surg 61:458–460

Older RA (1990) Endometriosis of the genitourinary tract. In: Pollack HM (ed) Clinical urography: an atlas and textbook of urological imaging. Saunders, Philadelphia, pp 2485–2492

Orkin LA (1952) Spontaneous nontraumatic extravasation from the ureter. J Urol 67:272–283

Oyen R, Gielen J, Baert L, et al (1987) CT demonstration of a ureterosciatic hernia. Urol Radiol 9:174–176

Palmer JM, Drago JR (1981) Ureteral avulsion from nonpenetrating trauma. J Urol 125:108–111

Park J, Siegel C, Moll M, Konnk J (1994) Retrograde ureteral intussusception. J Urol 151:997–998

Parker MD, Rebsamen S, Clark RL (1989) Multiple ureteral diverticula: a possible radiographically demonstrable risk factor in development of transitional cell carcinoma. Urol Radiol 11:45–48

Pear BL (1986) Other organs and other amyloiosis. Semin Roentgenol 21:150–161

Perez-Castro Ellendt E, Martinez-Pineiro JA (1982) Ureteral and renal endoscopy. A new approach. Eur Urol 8:117

Persky L, Guerriere K (1976) Complications of Marchall-Krantz colpocystopexy. Urology 8:469–471

Persky L, Hampel N, Kedia K (1981) Percutaneous nephrostomy and ureteral injury. J Urol 125:298

Peters PC, Sagalowsky AI (1986) Genito-urinary trauma. In: Walsh PC, Gittes RF, Perlmutter AD, Stamey TA (eds) Campbell's urology, 5th edn. Saunders, Philadelphia, pp 1192–1246

Peterson NE, Schulze KA (1987) Selective diagnosis uroradiography for trauma. J Urol 137:449–451

Plous RH, Sunshine R, Goldman H, et al (1985) Ureteral endometriosis in postmenopausal women. Urology 26:408–411

Pollack HM, Willis JS (1978) Radiographic features of ureteral endometriosis. AJR Am J Roentgenol 131:627–631

Pollack HM, Popky GL, Blumberg ML (1975) Hernia of the ureter. An anatomic-roentgenographic study. Radiology 117:275–281

Presti JC, Carroll PR, McAninch JW (1989) Ureteral and renal pelvic injuries from external trauma: diagnostic and management. J Trauma 29:370–374

Purena M, Vespasiani G, Virgili G, et al (1985) Ureteral endometriosis: an endoscopic diagnosis. Urology 26:566–567

Quillin SP, Darcy MD, Picus D (1994) Angiographic evaluation and therapy of uretero-arterial fistulas. AJR Am J Roentgenol 62:873–878

Reddy AN, Evans AT (1974) Endometriosis of the ureter. J Urol 111:474

Reece RN, Koontz WW (1975) Leukoplakia of the urinary tract. A review. J Urol 114:165–171

Reiner RJ, Conway GF, Threlkeld R (1975) Uretero-arterial fistula. J Urol 113:24

Rhamy R, Stander R (1962) Pyelographic analysis of radiation therapy in carcinoma of the cervix. AJR Am J Roentgenol 87:41

Rohner TJ jr (1971) Delayed ureteral fistulas from high-velocity missiles: report of 3 cases. J Urol 63:64

Rousseau H, Gieskes L, Joffre F, et al (1996) Percutaneous treatment of peripheral aneurysms with the Cragg endopro-system. J Vasc Interv Radiol 7:35–39

Roy C, Rimmelin A, Beaujeux R (1993) Endométriose urétérale: rôle de l'imagerie médicale. J Radiol 74:165–169

Sampson JA (1940) The development of the implantation of the ovary for the origin of peritoneal endometriosis. Am J Obstet Gynecol 40:549

Sarramon JP, Serny J (1975) Lesions de l'uretère par balle. J Urol Nephrol 72:35–48

Schultz A, Kristensen JK, Bilde T, et al (1987) Ureteroscopy: results and complications. J Urol 137:865–866

Schwartz A, Caine M, Hermann G, et al (1966) Spontaneous renal extravasation during intravenous urography. AJR Am J Roentgenol 98:27

Selzman AA, Spirnak PS (1996) Iatrogenic ureteral injuries: a 20-year experience in treating 165 injuries. J Urol 155:878–881

Shingleton HM, Fowler WC, Pepper ED jr (1969) Ureteral strictures following therapy of carcinoma of the cervix. Cancer 24:77–83

Shrader DA, Bergreen PW (1977) Cholesteatoma of ureter masquerading as ureteral tumors. Urology 9:555–557

Sieben DM, Honerton L, Amin M, et al (1978) The role of ureteral stenting in the management of surgical injury of the ureter. J Urol 119:33

Smith RB (1984) Ureteral common iliac artery fistula: a complication of internal double-J ureteral stent. J Urol 132:113

Smith PJB, Williams RE (1972) Genito-urinary fistula complicating Crohn's disease. Br J Urol 44:657–661

Smith WL, Weinstein AS, Wiot JF (1974) Defects of renal collecting systems in patients receiving anticoagulants. Radiology 113:649–651

Solomons E, Levin EJ, Bauman J (1960) A pyelographic study of ureteric injuries sustained during hysterectomy for benign conditions. Surg Gynecol Obstet 3:61

Spring DB, Vandeman F, Watson RA (1983) Computed tomographic demonstration of uretero-sciatic hernia. AJR Am J Roentgenol 141:579–580

Steers WD, Corriere JN jr, Benson GS (1985) The use of indwelling ureteral stents in managing ureteral injuries due to external violence. J Trauma 25:1001

Stiehm WD, Becker JA, Weiss RB (1972) Ureteral endometriosis. Radiology 102:563–564

Talner LB (1990) Specific causes of obstruction. In: Pollack HM (ed) Clinical urography: an atlas and textbook of urological imaging. Saunders, Philadelphia, pp 1629–1751

Tencate HW (1977) Endometriosis of the urinary tract. In: Witten DM, Myers GHJR, Utz DC (eds) Emmett's clinical urography. Saunders, Philadelphia, pp 2181–2185

Teuton ME, Viner NA, Zuckerman HL (1987) Ureteroiliac vein fistula associated with a polyethylene indwelling ureteral stent. J Urol 137:975–976

Thomas SD, Sanders PW III, Pollack HM (1977) Primary amyloidosis of urinary bladder and ureter. Urology 9:586

Thompson JS, McAlister WH (1975) Subepithelial hemorrhage in the renal pelvis and ureter simulating pyeloureteritis cystica. Pediatr Radiol 3:156–157

Toolin E, Pollack HM, McLean GK, et al (1984) Uretero-arterial fistula: a case report. J Urol 132:553–554

Underwood PB Jr, Lutz MH, Smoak DL (1977) Ureteral injury following irradiation therapy for carcinoma of the cervix. Obstet Gynecol 49:663

Wasserman NF (1994) Pseudodiverticulosis: unusual appearance for metastasis to the ureter. Abdom Imaging 19:376–378

Wasserman NF, Lapointe S, Posalaky IP (1985) Ureteral pseudodiverticulosis. Radiology 155:561–566

Wasserman NF, Posalaky IP, Dykoski R (1988) The pathology of ureteral pseudodivertulosis. Invest Radiol 23:592–598

Wasserman NF, Zhang G, Posalaky IP, et al (1991) Ureteral pseudo diverticula: frequent association with uroepithelial malignancy. AJR Am J Roentgenol 137:69–72

Weinberg SR (1967) Injuries of the ureter. In: Bergman H (ed) The ureter, chap 16. Harper and Row, New York, pp 355–393

Weinberg JJ, Ansong K, Smith AD (1987) Complication of ureteroscopy in relation to experience: report of a survey and author experience. J Urol 137:384–385

Weingarten KE, D'Agostino HB, Dunn J, et al (1996) Obturator herniation of the ureter in a renal transplant recipient causing hydronephrosis: peri operative percutaneous management. J Vasc Interv Radiol 7:939–941

Weintraub JL, Pappas GM, Romano WJ, et al (2000) Percutaneous reduction of ureterosciatic hernia. AJR Am J Roentgenol 175:181–182

Wheatley JK, Ansley JD, Smith RB, et al (1981) Uretero-arterial fistula. Urology 18:498–502

Williamson B, Hartman GW, Hattery RR (1986) Multiple and diffuse ureteral filling defects. Semin Roentgenol 21:214–223

Wills JS, Pollack HM, Curtis JA (1981) Cholesteatoma of the upper urinary tract. AJR Am J Roentgenol 136:941–944

Winter CC, Williams RC (1972) Ureterocolic fistula. J Urol 108:396–398

Wrenn JJ, Assimos DG (1988) Ureteral obstruction secondary to a vena caval clip. J Urol 140:1014–1015

Zerbib M, Teyssier P, Steg A (1983) Les sténoses urétérales après traitement des cancers du col utérin: fibrose post-radiothérapique ou récidive néoplasique? J Chir (Paris) 120:503–513

Zhiri MA, Benyahia SE, Hamdouch A, et al (1987) Lesions iatrogènes de l'uretère. A propos de 13 cas. J Gynecol Obstet Biol Reprod 16:1063–1067

11 Postoperative and Posttransplantation Ureter

B. J. D'Othee, A. Gozlan, M. Soulie, F. Joffre, V. Chabbert, P. Rischman

CONTENTS

11.1
Imaging of Postoperative Ureter

Imaging of the postoperative ureter is necessary in two conditions: (a) in case of ureteral surgery (nevertheless, except from total ureterectomy in case of urothelial tumors, the indications for ureteral surgery have decreased, often replaced by interventional and endoscopic techniques) and (b) post-cystectomy ureteral derivation and reimplantation.

B. J. D'Othee, MD; A. Gozlan, MD
Service de Radiologie, Hôpital de Rangueil, 1, avenue Jean-Poulhès, 31403 Toulouse Cédex 4, France
M. Soulie, MD
Service d'Urologie, CHU Rangueil, 1, avenue Jean-Poulhès, 31403 Toulouse Cédex 4, France
F. Joffre, MD
Professor, Chef de Service, Service de Radiologie, Hôpital de Rangueil, 1, avenue Jean-Poulhès, 31403 Toulouse Cédex 4, France
V. Chabbert
Service de Radiologie, Hôpital de Rangueil, 1, avenue Jean-Poulhès, 31403 Toulouse Cédex 4, France
P. Rischman
Professor, Service d'Urologie, CHU Rangueil, 1, avenue Jean-Poulhès, 31403 Toulouse Cédex 4, France

Imaging is performed: (a) to follow the progression of the causal disease; (b) to evaluate the structural and functional integrity of the surgical reconstruction and (c) to detect postoperative complications.

Surgery for pyeloureteral junction syndrome and for VUR will not be considered in this chapter.

11.1.1
Surgical Techniques

Some principles are applicable to all techniques (Dufour 1973; Pidello et al. 1986; Hendaoui et al. 2000):

- Surgical approaches are almost always extraperitoneal and their level may vary according to the ureteral segment. Some interventions, however, can be performed by video-assisted, laparoscopic or lumboscopic surgery.
- The ureteral anatomical localization and dissection may be facilitated by preoperative retrograde double-J catheter placement. The antegrade access is usually chosen only in case the retrograde approach is difficult or impossible (Greenberg et al. 1980).
- Anastomosis should be made without tension, if possible in a healthy, well-vascularized, and not previously irradiated zone.
- Drainage techniques are focused on the operative sites and excretory tract (Pearse et al. 1985). Drainage of the operative site is the rule, especially in traumatic, hemorrhagic or infectious backgrounds. It helps to prevent urinoma and abscess formation, healing delays, and peri-ureteral fibrosis. Excretory tract drainage is usually necessary in ureteral surgery, particularly in previously dilated urinary tract, either by a surgically nephrostomy or double-J catheters, the latter being the most comfortable approach. Besides direct opacification advantages, the nephrostomy catheter also makes it possible to perform a mixed internal–external transureteral drainage, associated, however, with not insignificant infectious risks.

11.1.1.1
Ureterectomy

The ureterectomy may be segmental or total, and may be done alone or in association with a wider excision (nephroureterectomy, partial cystectomy), depending on the lesion to be treated (inflammatory or tumoral disease, benign or malignant stenosis). The surgical extent also dictates urinary tract drainage, either by derivation or by restoration of urinary tract structural continuity. The latter can be done either by uretero-ureteral anastomosis (uretero-ureterostomy) with or without kidney lowering, or by ureteral replacement using a visceral structure (mainly small bowel: uretero-ileoplasty). A uretero-ureteral anastomosis is classically beveled (ureterorgraphy) and done with ureteral stenting (double-J catheter). In distal ureteral surgery, an uretero-neocystostomy with elevation bladder technique should be performed.

11.1.1.2
Interventions that Preserve Ureteral Patency

11.1.1.2.1
Ureterotomy

A ureterotomy consists of making a localized opening through the ureteral wall. The main indication remains open lithiasis extraction, which is rarely done nowadays. It is usually done without technical difficulty unless performed in an edematous and inflammatory zone. Complications such as suture loosening and late post-operative fibrous stenosis remain possible and might be related to deficient technique, unfit anastomotic tissue, fistula formation, or insufficient post-operative drainage.

11.1.1.2.2
Ureterolysis

Ureterolysis consists of a surgical technique for ureteral release from peri-ureteral diseased tissues with preservation of its vascular pedicle (Fig. 11.1). This intervention is mainly performed for obstructive benign retroperitoneal fibrosis. If needed, it can be accompanied by either extraperitoneal or intraperitoneal (intraperitonization) external translation of the ureters distant from the fibrous plaque. The intraperitonization carries the risk of ureteral devascularization and adhesion formation when penetrating and exiting the posterior parietal peritoneum. The latter can be avoided by wrapping the ureter with epiploon after simple external extraperitoneal translation.

Post-operative ureteral opacification shows a typical ureteral deviated course, with anterior and lateral convex curves, straddling the retroperitoneal space and pelvic cavity. Urinary drainage is generally satisfactory. The risk of fistula is not negligible because of the precarious vascularization of these ureters.

11.1.1.3
Techniques of Ureteral Continuity Restoration

If anatomical and clinical conditions are favorable, they must be preferred to ureteral derivation techniques, even in patients with surgical antecedents of urinary derivation (PEARSE et al. 1985). The surgical possibilities vary with the extent and level of ureteral intervention .

11.1.1.3.1
Uretero-ureterostomy

Uretero-ureterostomy is the ideal technique. It is done by end-to-end anastomosis along an oblique section plane for ureteral lumen widening purposes (ureterorrhaphy). The essential conditions for technical success include the absence of traction on both ends, good ureteral vascularization and structural integrity (DUFOUR 1973). Upstream, an effective urinary drainage is usually necessary in order to avoid hyperpressure at the anastomotic level. Ureteral stenting is also very useful and recommended by most surgeons.

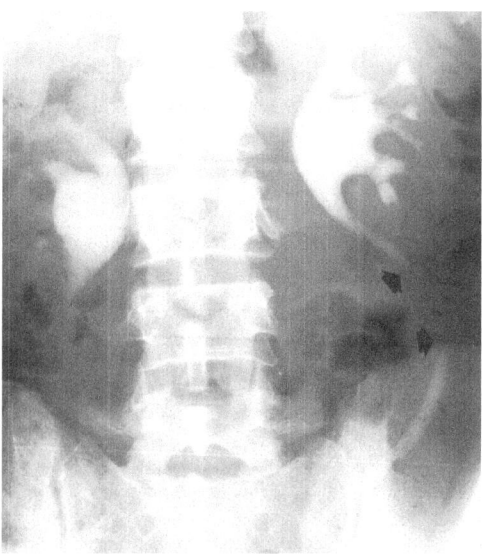

Fig. 11.1. Intraperitonization of ureter: excretory urography (EU) shows external position of the bilateral lumbar ureters (*arrows*) after ureterolysis for benign Retroperitoneal Fibrosis (RPF)

11.1.1.3.2
Mobilization

Mobilization requires a total anatomical release of the kidney and its pedicle. The kidney is then fixed by its capsule to the psoas muscle. Depending on each patient, this intervention may provide about 3–8 cm of ureteral length and may thus allow a traction-free ureteral anastomosis. In some patients, the vascular configuration and the existence of peri-nephritis (history of previous surgery or inflammatory peri-renal disease) make this impossible. Moreover, on the right side, several centimeters can be gained by vein trans-position (PEARSE et al. 1985; SARRAMON 1973).

11.1.1.3.3
Renal Autotransplantation

Renal autotransplantation is seldom used for this indication because of the risk of vascular anastomosis failure, a more serious problem compared to the other techniques of ureteral replacement (PEARSE et al. 1985).

11.1.1.3.4
Pyeloureteral or Calicoureteral Anastomoses

Pyeloureteral or calicoureteral anastomoses are used for short excision of proximal ureter. A pyeloureteral anastomosis can be technically simple or may require the creation of a tubulated pyelic flap. In fact, it is seldom feasible and failures are frequent. A calicoureteral anastomosis is carried out after partial nephrectomy using the lower calyx while raising the infracaliceal parenchyma. This technique carries the risk of secondary stenosis, a relatively frequent occurrence through the surgically created renal parenchyma crossing. This can be prevented by allowing the calyx to project the renal parenchymal section plane a few centimeters, thus allowing an extra-parenchymal anastomosis.

11.1.1.3.5
Bladder Elevation Techniques

The oldest bladder elevation technique is the Boari-Küss intervention, which makes it possible to replace up to about 8–10 cm of pelvic ureter by creating a tubulated bladder flap (Fig. 11.2). However, the iliac ureter is often technically difficult to reach. The ureter is implanted on the bladder flap termino-laterally while creating a submucosa channel for anti-reflux purposes (uretero-neocystostomy). The use of this

type of intervention has decreased as a result of the high frequency of secondary stenosis.

Another technique is the bladder psoas hitch which consists in mobilizing and raising the bladder in order to fix the homolateral vesical horn to the psoas muscle (ERLICH et al. 1978) (Fig. 11.3). This allows for an uretero-vesical anastomosis without

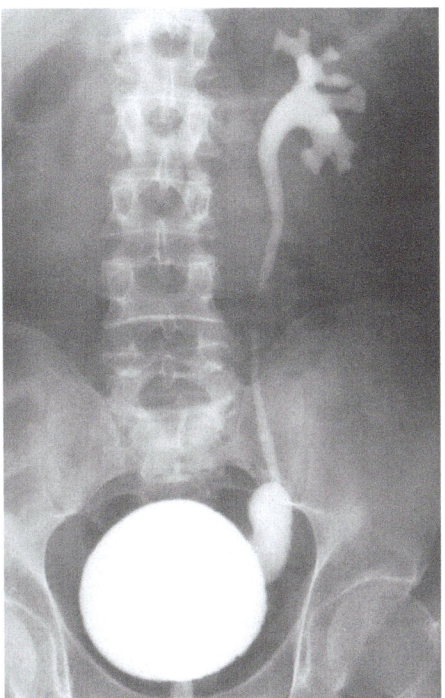

Fig. 11.2. Voiding cystouretrography (VCUG) shows a left vesico-ureteral reflux with tubular enlargement of the left pelvic ureter related to Boari-Kuss procedure

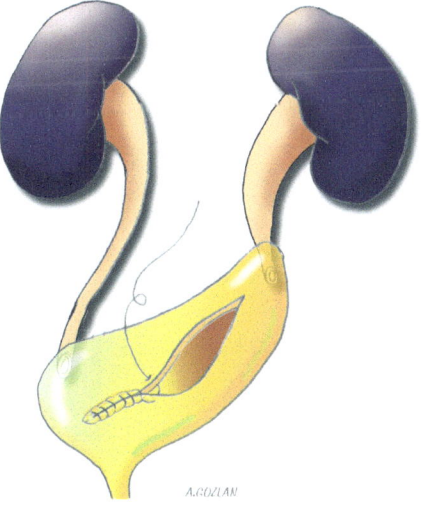

Fig. 11.3. Schematic drawing of psoas bladder hitch with fixation of the vesical horn to the psoas muscle

tension and with an anti-reflux system. It is also possible to associate the two techniques (psoatic fixation *plus* a Boari-like vesical flap) when the substance loss extends beyond the iliac vessels.

The vesical bipartition (bilateral psoas hitch with anteroposterior section of the dome) must be used in the event of bilateral ureteric lesions. In all cases, these techniques of vesical elevation require a large bladder and a good-quality and well-vascularized vesical wall.

11.1.1.3.6
The Cross-over Uretero-ureterostomy
(Transuretero-ureterostomy)

The cross-over uretero-ureterostomy consists of a transposition of the ureter immediately upstream of the obstruction from the diseased side to the other side, so as to implant it in a healthy portion of the contralateral ureter. It requires anastomosing a portion of the diseased ureter that should not be overly dilated and a sufficient ureter length to cross the midline without traction. These requirements limit this type of intervention to certain cases in spite of the appealing character of this technique. The main indication is restoring the patency of an obstructed pathological ureter in case of a rectal neoplastic lesion. Thus, this can eliminate the need for a long urologic intervention during a rectal amputation (Fig. 11.4).

11.1.1.3.7
The Methods of Replacement of the Ureter
(Ureteroplasty)

Ureteroplasties using neutral tubes are no longer in use today since the introduction of ureter intubations by double-J catheters. If attempts to intubate the ureter fail, the replacement of the ureter by an inert silicone prosthesis should be considered only in cancer patients with reduced life expectancy.

Total uretero-ileoplasty is currently the best way to replace the entire ureter (Lhez 1968) (Fig. 11.5). It is a well-codified technique and its midterm results are acceptable (Fig. 11.6). In order to obtain a caliber similar to the ureter, the width of the ileum can be reduced by longitudinal resection of the anti-mesenteric edge guided by an endoluminal tutor (Hendren 1997). Pyelo-ileal or uretero-ileal anastomoses are either termino-terminal for the renal pelvis or the dilated ureter, or termino-lateral if the ureter is healthy. The ileo-vesical anastomosis requires an anti-reflux system. However, it has been shown in animals that the intestinal peristalsis can efficiently prevent reflux (Sarramon et al. 1971). It is also possible to replace both ureters using either a U-shaped ileal graft anastomosed latero-laterally to the bladder or a cross-over intestinal segment to entirely replace both ureters. The total replacement can disturb ureteral peristalsis and there is a risk of long-term parenchymal destruction by urinary stasis.

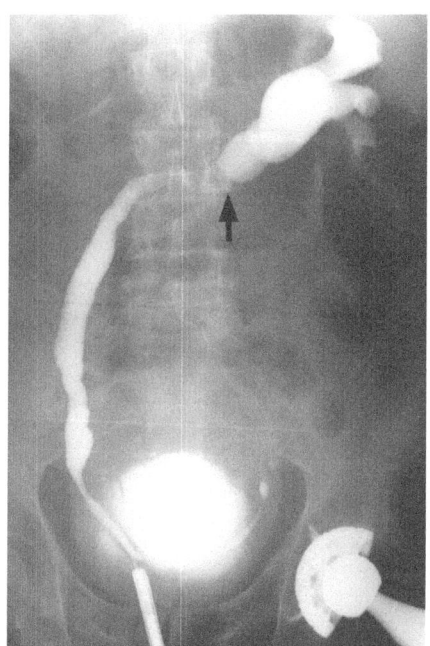 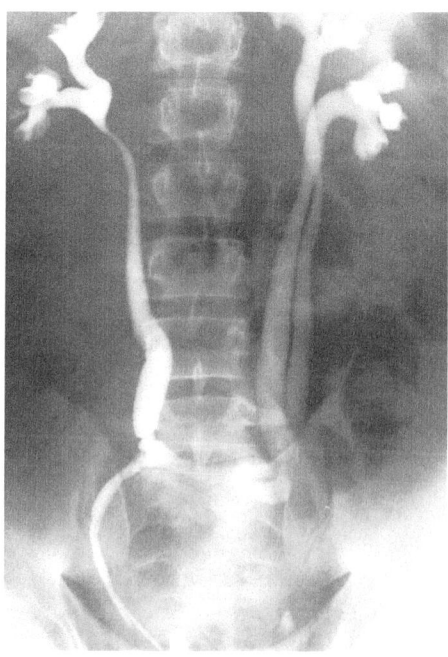

Fig. 11.4a, b. Examples of transuretero-ureter-ostomy. **a** Left to right transuretero-ureterostomy in a patient with right-side pelvic and lower-left ureter transitional cell carcinoma (TCC). Retrograde ureteropyelography (RUP) shows new localization on the left ureter before anastomosis (*arrow*). **b** Right RUP allows opacification of both upper urinary tracts by transverse uretero ureterostomy

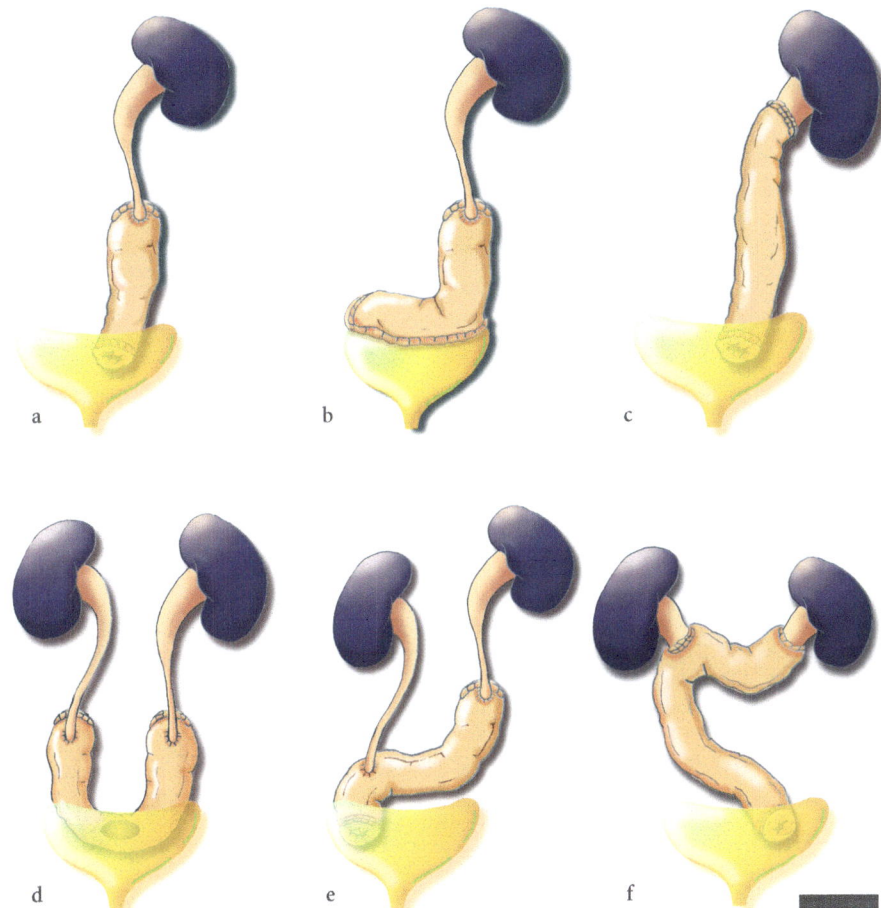

Fig. 11.5a–f. Different techniques of uretero-ileal replacement (uretero-ileoplasty). **a** Partial ileoplasty. **b** Partial ileoplasty with bladder enlargement. **c** Total ileoplasty. **d, e, f** Different procedures for bilateral uretero-ileoplasty

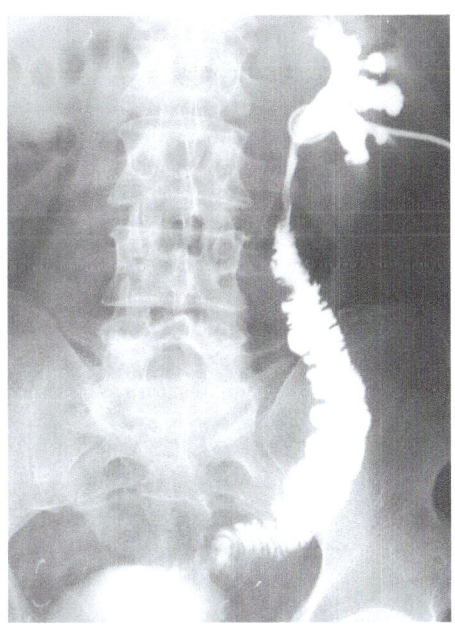

Fig. 11.6. Anterograde pyelography (AP) by percutaneous nephrostomy (PCN) allows demonstration of good patency of subtotal left ileoplasty

Partial uretero-ileoplasty is indicated when the obstruction is at the lumbar or iliac level and the pelvic ureter is healthy (LHEZ 1968; PIDELLO et al. 1986) (Fig. 11.7). Preserving the pelvic ureter prevents reflux and reducing the length of the intestinal segment decreases stasis and parietal reabsorption. In this type of indication, the ileal segment can be replaced by the appendix (uretero-appendiculoplasty). This intervention of appealing simplicity is possible only if the appendix is present. Nevertheless, the risk of stenosis is higher than with an ileal segment.

11.1.1.4
Ureteral Derivations

Some of these techniques are methods of temporary urinary derivation, the majority of which are interventional uroradiology techniques. Percutaneous nephrostomy and antegrade or retrograde ureteral intubation using double J catheters have been considered in Chap. 12. These methods have

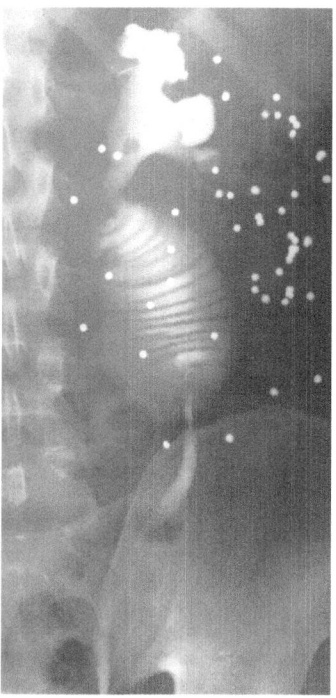

Fig. 11.7. Partial uretero-ileoplasty for gunshot traumatic lesion of left lumbar ureter. RUP shows good opacification

completely replaced temporary surgical derivations such as surgical nephrostomy and in situ ureterostomy.

Permanent ureter derivations are always currently proposed every time the bladder cannot be used (neurological bladder or for other reasons) or every time it has to be removed (tumoral pathology). These interventions share a certain number of problems (AMIS et al. 1981):

– Frequency of complications: infection (20%), fistula (3%), obstruction (10%–20%). Progressive deterioration of renal function in 10%–40% of cases, even in cases with good ureteral voiding.
– Psychological trauma and discomfort caused by the equipment of the stoma.

These numerous problems encourage the urologist to increasingly consider the restoration of continuity every time the anatomical and clinical circumstances allow it.

11.1.1.4.1
Cutaneous Ureterostomy

Cutaneous ureterostomy is the implantation of one or both ureters in the skin. The stoma is generally located in the iliac fossa. It can be intubated with a catheter, in particular when there is a risk of stenosis. In case of bilateral ureterostomy, the implantation is done on the same stoma, either with both ureters brought together side by side or in a Y formation after uretero-ureterostomy. This technique, however, is carried out much less frequently than in the past.

11.1.1.4.2
Transileal Ureterostomy (Ileal Conduit)

Transileal ureterostomy is the classic Bricker intervention which consists of isolating a pre-terminal ileal loop whose distal end is brought to the skin and whose proximal end is closed blindly by suture, and both ureters are implanted on this loop (BRICKER 1950) (Fig. 11.8). The ileal segment must be short (less than 15 cm) and must function as a contractile conduit, not as a reservoir. In general, it is seldom possible to build an anti-reflux device. However, some authors propose reconstructions, with or without ureteral tunnelization, allowing an effective reduction of reflux occurrence while decreasing the risk of post-operative stenosis. It is also possible to achieve a complex ileal invagination to decrease this reflux. The loop is left in intraperitoneal position or is placed in the retroperitoneum in order to avoid the risks of stenosis by an adhesion. The risk of anastomotic stenosis is significant (2% at 6 months, 15% at 5 years) and the entero-ureteral reflux is almost constant. Infection is frequent. As compared to the cutaneous ureterostomy, the Bricker implantation procedure makes it possible to eliminate the use of a catheter and presents the advantage of implanting the ureters in a flexible, non-irritated area.

The problems related to the continuous evacuation of the stoma have nevertheless promoted the completion of techniques using a continent reservoir (KENNEY et al. 1980). The aims of the latter techniques are to drain the stoma, to allow a discontinuous evacuation of urine by self-catheterization, and to prevent entero-ureteral reflux (SKINNER et al. 1987). Moreover, the more restrictive indications of preoperative irradiations for vesico-prostatic tumors make it possible to perform more complex reconstructions (NG and AMIS 1991).

The techniques are numerous and vary depending on the teams (AMIS et al. 1988). The reservoir must have a large capacity and the intracavitary pressure must be low in order to avoid any repercussion on the upper urinary tract (KEOGAN et al. 1997). As a general rule, these reconstructions include (a) an ileal, cecal or ileo-cecal reservoir which is not tubulated to avoid the phenomena of peristalsis and to allow enlarging; (b) an implantation of the ureters at the level of the

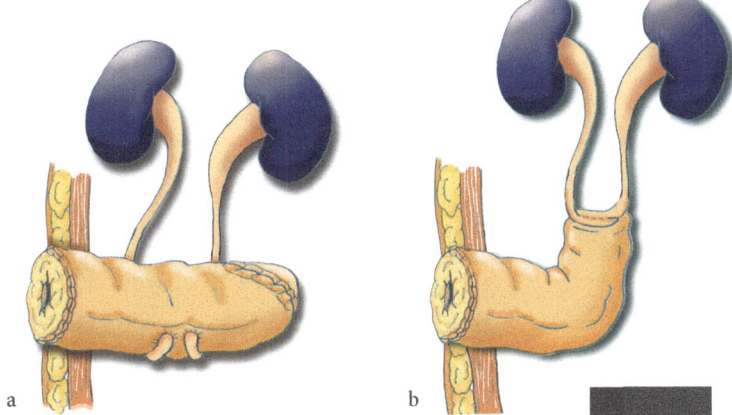

Fig. 11.8a, b. Diagrams of ileal conduit. **a** Classic Bricker derivation. **b** ileostomy with antireflux system

reservoir with an anti-reflux system (cecal implantation tunnelized at the level of the longitudinal strips of the colon (teniae); (c) a mechanism of continent stoma by ileal invagination, ileal folding or use of the ileo-cecal valve or the appendix. The continent reservoirs most frequently used are the Mainz pouch and particularly the Kock pouch, whose assembly is certainly more complex but whose results are the most significant (KOCK 1982; THUROFF et al. 1985) (Fig. 11.9). These techniques are subject to the same

early post-operative complications as other derivation techniques, and even more so as they are complex and not performed by many teams (KEOGAN et al. 1997). SKINNER reports an early complication rate of 16% of cases and the need for a reintervention in 30% of cases (SKINNER et al. 1987). These authors hope to reduce the complication rate by modifying the procedure.

The creation of a replacement neo-bladder was also proposed (CAMEY 1985) (Fig. 11.10). This technique

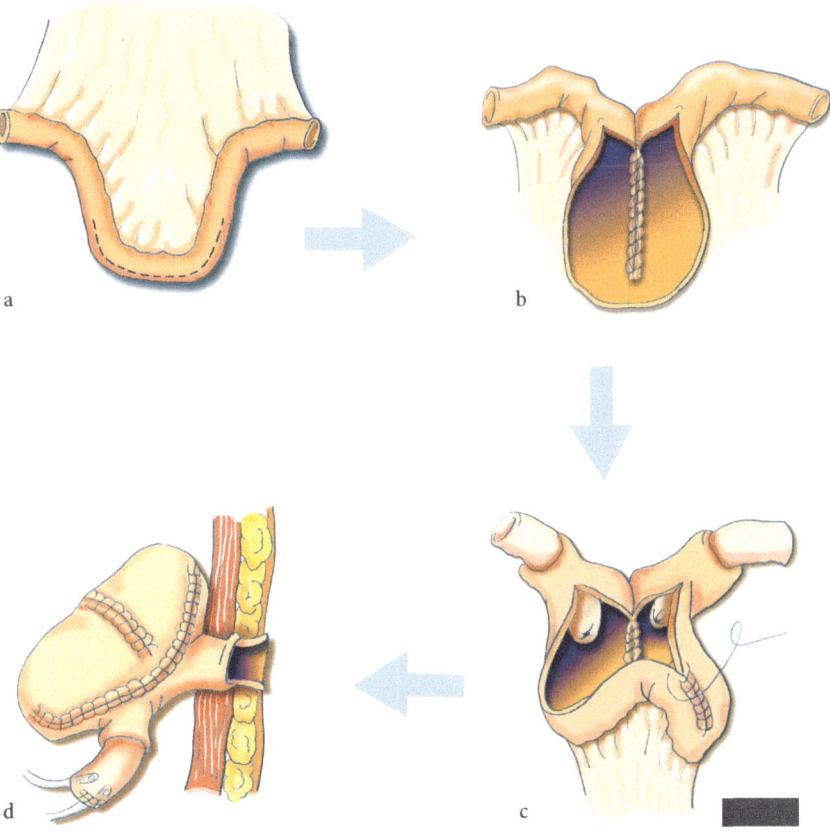

Fig. 11.9a–d. Schematic drawing of the different steps in creating a Koch pouch

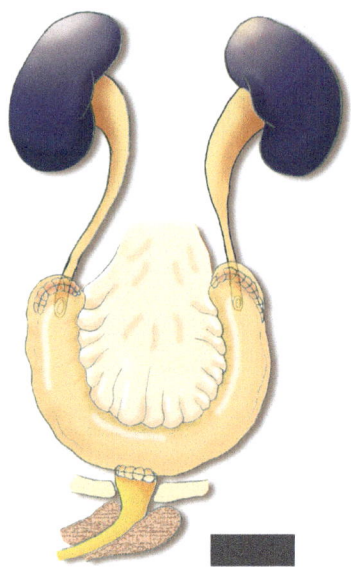

Fig. 11.10. Diagram of Camey-type enterocystoplasty

uses an ileal segment anastomosed to the posterior urethra, on which both ureters are reimplanted. This is the simplest technique of vesical replacement, but it cannot be used in women and the risk of incontinence is significant (30%–40%) (LILIEN and CAMEY 1984).

11.1.1.4.3
Ureterosigmoidostomy

This old intervention described by COFFEY (1911) has been the subject of renewed interest as a result of technical improvements and better medical supervision (PRINCENTHAL et al. 1985). It consists of anastomosing the two ureters on the sigmoid colon and performing an anti-reflux submucosal tunnelization. It is imperative that both ureters be of normal caliber (in order to decrease the risk of reflux and infection) and that the renal parenchyma be of good quality. Reflux is indeed a harmful complication as urine is always contaminated by feces. The contact of urine with the mucous membrane of the colon is responsible for electrolytic disturbances with moderate hyperchloremic acidosis and hypokalemia. Sometimes a bicarbonate infusion may be necessary. It also involves continence of the anal sphincter, but results in significant irritation. Another specific complication of this type of intervention is the secondary appearance of colic tumor whose exact mechanism is poorly known, but which is certainly related to secondary biochemical problems in contact with the urine and colic mucus. These colon cancers generally occur remotely, years after the intervention and are in general located near

the ureteral implantation area. The risk is particularly high in cases of vesical exstrophy. This requires careful colon monitoring by radiological opacification or endoscopy in these patients (ERB et al. 1990; RANDALL and PREISSIG 1974). It is preferable to avoid any enema using barium as a contrast agent. A colonoscopy and the search for hematuria must be carried out annually beginning in the third post-operative year. Even if some authors have proposed an alternative type with uretero-proctostomy to decrease some of these disadvantages, there is a trend to drop this type of derivation today (AMIS et al. 1981).

However, the high incidence of complications of alternative methods of urinary diversion, a persistent interest in simple and appliance-free techniques is reappearing . The sigma-rectum pouch (Mainz-Pouch II) is a recent example of multiple modifications proposed for ureterosigmoidostomy that seems very promising (FISCH et al. 1993). It consists in a creation of a low-pressure, high-capacity reservoir with detubularization of the sigmoid boot and side-to-side anastomosis (Fig. 11.11). Ureters are implanted via a submucosal antirefluxing tunnel and the pouch is fixed in the area of the promontory. Contraindications are pelvic radiotherapy, colonic diverticulosis or polyps.

Risks of renal complication or metabolic imbalance are largely prevented by improved surgical technique, bowel preparation, antireflux ureteral implantation, alkalinized drugs. The incidence of complications is very low. The surgical technique is simple and effective for decreasing bowel contractions. Radiological follow-up is based on renal sonography and excretory urography (EU) (Fig. 11.12). The long-term (after 5 years) risk of carcinoma in the area of uretero colic anastomosis necessitates regular pouchoscopy by a urologist (FISCH et al. 1993).

11.1.2
Radiological Techniques

Radiology is essential to appreciate the immediate post-operative result and in particular the quality of the surgical technique. It is also necessary to detect complications and evaluate the long-term results. The radiological procedure tends to become the first stage of an interventional procedure. The work-up of the surgical procedure is based on the whole set of uroradiological techniques available for the urinary tract. Certain particular technical points must, however, be underlined.

EU remains the classic basic technique and provides a good evaluation of the results in case of

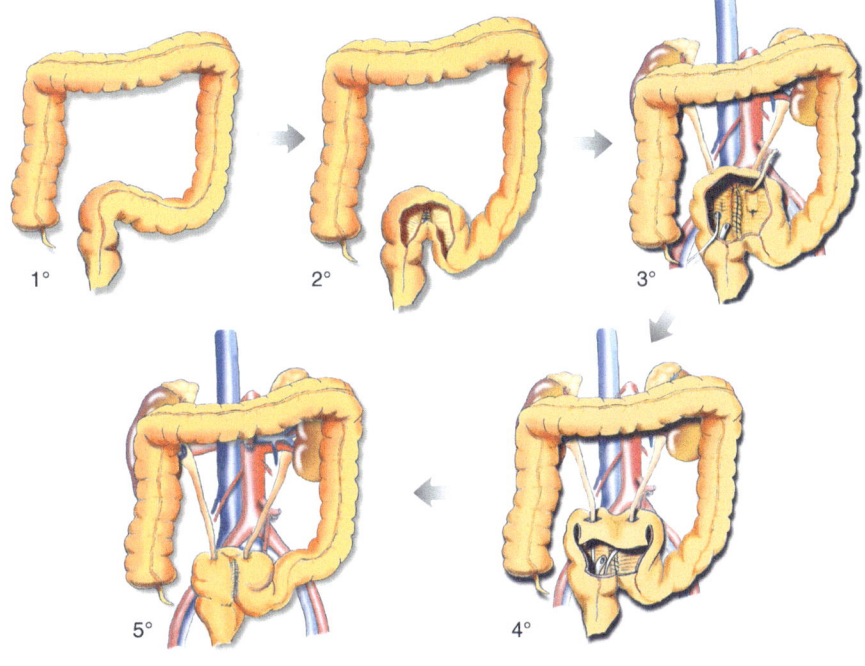

Fig. 11.11. Schematic drawing of the different steps in creating a Sigma rectum pouch

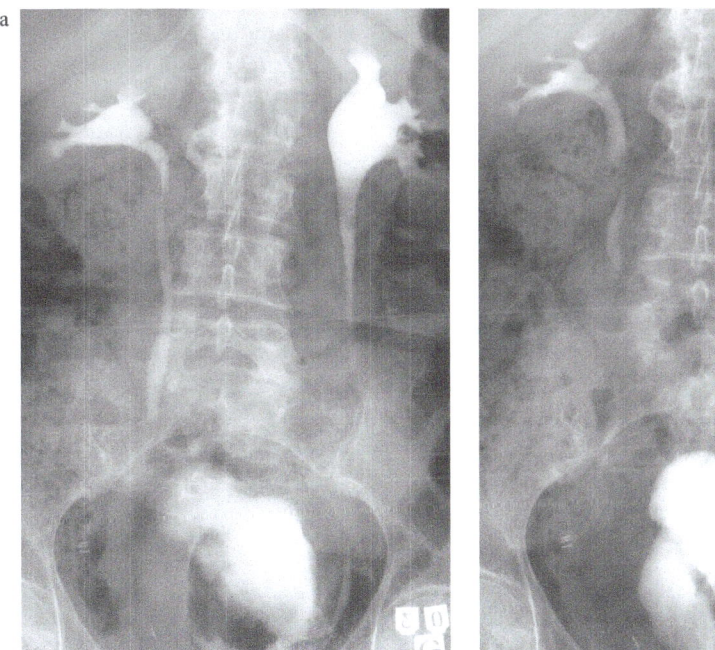

Fig. 11.12a, b. Urographic aspects (30 min after voiding) of a Sigma rectum pouch: good function of the ureterointestinal anastomoses with stasis in the pouch

uncomplicated follow-up and a screening tool for major complications (Fig. 11.13) The use of large amounts of contrast media with high iodine content is recommended, given the frequent dilution phenomena in the interposed intestinal loops. Similarly, stagnation of contrast medium may occur within intestinal pouches and should motivate the use of position changes to promote progression of the opacified urine. Prone views are particularly useful (SOLOVAY 1974).

Ultrasonography has two essential goals: first, to detect an obstruction, in particular when the EU shows an absence of opacification; and second, in certain circumstances, to detect a peri-ureteral collection (urinoma). However, the general limits of ultrasonography in the detection of an obstruction are also

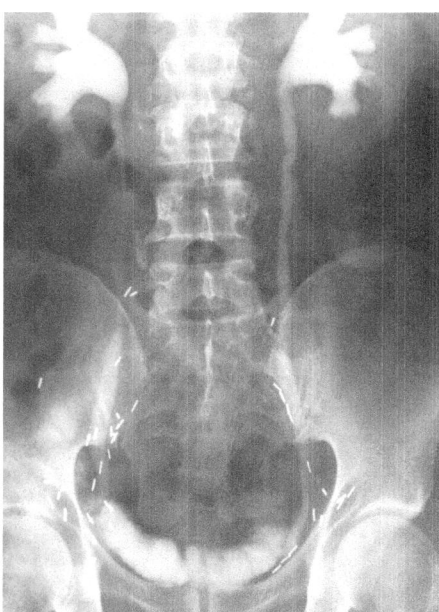

Fig. 11.13. EU in a patient presenting a Camey-type enterocystoplasty with no functional problems

present after ureteral surgery. This is even truer when the kidneys have been previously dilated or present obstructive sequelae (Cronan et al. 1986). A normal renal ultrasonography makes it possible to eliminate an obstruction in these patients. On the other hand, in transileal derivations, the number of false-positive results is near 40% (Cronan et al. 1986). This author suggests the use of opacification techniques (EU or loopography) in first intention treatment.

Direct opacification techniques should be widely used every time EU is insufficient. Retrograde techniques are seldom possible. On the other hand, antegrade pyelography has unquestionable advantages here, to affirm an obstruction as well as to perform an urodynamic examination (Whitaker's test) or a percutaneous nephrostomy (Whitaker 1973; Pfister and Newhouse 1979).

Some reservoirs may be opacified by direct catheterization. The opacification of the intestinal loop anastomosed to the skin can be easily obtained by catheterization (loopography) (Banner et al. 1984). This is performed by placement of a 14-F or 24-F Foley catheter at the level of the stoma and retrograde opacification of the loop (Montagne et al. 1978) (Fig. 11.14). This opacification is generally achieved using a slightly diluted (10%–30%) water-soluble contrast medium and low pressure (lower than 25 cm H_2O). Air opacification was proposed as a replacement solution in cases of intolerance to iodine and to promote the visualiza-

tion of poorly opaque stones. Reflux under low-pressure conditions should be considered as normal and the evacuation of the ureters should be done early. The presence of air in the urinary cavities should not be seen as abnormal. This technique is viewed as a good method to exclude an obstruction, considering that a permeable anastomosis should be opacified by reflux (Banner et al. 1984). In fact, Hudson showed that in 19% of patients an anastomosis may be permeable even if not opacified by reflux (Hudson et al. 1981). This author suggests using this technique only in cases where EU shows a progressive deterioration of the excretory tract, in a context of recurrent pyelonephritis, in case of obvious obstruction, or when the intravenous use of iodinated contrast media is contraindicated. Selective catheterization of the ureters by endoscopy of the graft can be carried out if the opacification is insufficient, provided that the ureteral openings have been located by reflux (Banner et al. 1989).

Imaging techniques of the lower urinary tract (cystography, retrograde urethrocystography) are useful to assess the status of the bladder and the anastomoses after ureteral reimplantation. These techniques are also useful when it is necessary to restore continuity after derivation. A good status of the lower urinary tract is an essential condition before its re-use (Amis et al. 1988).

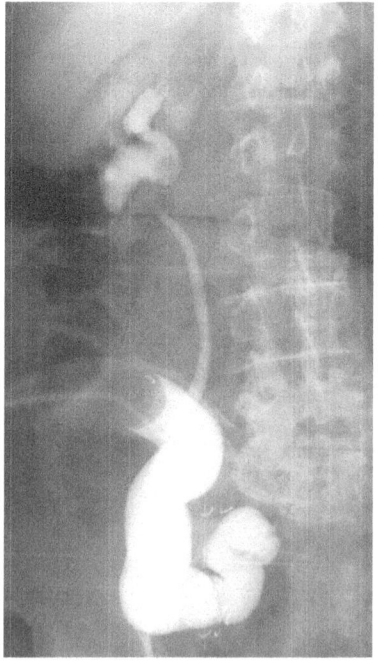

Fig. 11.14. Loopogram allows opacification of the ileal reservoir and free reflux on the upper right urinary tract. Obstruction of the left side was confirmed by AP

Radio-opaque enema can be used to look for a sigmoido-ureteral reflux and to evaluate the colonic repercussion of a Coffey's intervention. However, barium must be proscribed because of the risk of ureteral toxicity and water-soluble contrast media should be preferred (PRINCENTHAL et al. 1985).

Computed tomography (CT) plays an increasingly significant role in post-operative follow-up (ROY et al. 1993) (Fig. 11.15). In addition to its role in the monitoring of the causal pathology, it plays a major role in the early detection of complications. It requires a perfect opacification of the intestinal loops as well as a good opacification of the urinary tract, the latter being possibly completed by the placement of a drainage catheter (MIRVIS et al. 1987). Spiral CT allows rapid scanning before and after injection of contrast medium as well as 3D reconstructions (Figs. 11.16, 11.17). Additional urographic views can be acquired after CT if necessary.

Interventional radiologic procedures have an important role in the management of post-operative complication. They are detailed in Chap. 12.

11.1.3
Post-operative Follow-up

11.1.3.1
Normal Post-operative Course

Depending on the procedure performed, a simple post-operative course does not necessarily require systematic radiological follow-up. If it is necessary to carry out a radiological evaluation, it must be performed either as an emergency procedure (in case of an acute clinical presentation) or around the tenth day (theoretical date of cicatrization). The drains and drainage tubes are then clamped and withdrawn. Double-J catheters are left in place for 3–6 weeks in total.

Available techniques are antegrade pyelography by the nephrostomy tube, ultrasonography and EU (HENDAOUI et al. 2000). Antegrade pyelography is a simple procedure that provides information about the permeability of the ureter. There is, however, a septic risk and it gives no functional information. During this period, the evaluation of the excretory tract is difficult because an obstacle at the level of the operated zone often persists as a result of edema and the temporary interruption of peristalsis. Moreover, if there was a previous dilation, hypotonia of the excretory tract persists that is related to the age and size of the previous distension (MINDELL et al. 1990). Before withdrawing the nephrostomy tube, an antegrade pyelography ensures that the anastomosis is patent, even if the evacuation has not completely returned to normal However, it can detect a fistula before ablation of the drains..

An EU can be carried out on the 4th week: edema is then reabsorbed and peristalsis starts to reappear. At this time, it is possible to differentiate a residual hypotonia from a persistent obstruction. In case of hypotonia, the excretory tract is dilated but not distended and the evacuation can be completed in the standing position. The absence of secretion delay is a favorable prognostic element. In doubtful cases, however, it is necessary to wait until the 6th month to make sure that the result is favorable, particularly if the urinary tract was previously dilated. Isotopic nephrogram techniques or pyelomanometry can be useful in doubtful cases (PFISTER and NEWHOUSE 1979).

11.1.3.2
Post-operative Complications

They are particularly frequent and SCHMIDT found an 81% rate in a series of 178 patients (SCHMIDT et al. 1973). This has nevertheless clearly decreased since the generalization of ureteral intubation by double-J catheters associated or not with nephrostomy.

11.1.3.2.1
Early Complications

Early complications usually consist of pain, fever, deterioration of renal function, or a urinary leak through the drain, leading to suspicion of a problem and to perform an ultrasonography, an EU or an antegrade pyelography. The current trend is to promote direct opacification rather than EU.

Obstruction. Obstruction is generally obvious with echography and EU. It results from an overly tight anastomosis, an unrecognized obstacle downstream, or significant edema (SULLIVAN et al. 1980). It requires temporary percutaneous drainage (Fig. 11.18).

Urinary Extravasation. Although sometimes obvious on opacifications using nephrostomy tubes, urinary extravasation may appear insidiously and on late views only. It is generally caused by suture loosening or ischemic necrosis (KEOGAN et al. 1997). It can result in uretero-cutaneous, uretero-intestinal, vesical or vaginal fistulas. Prognosis depends on the size of the breach and the presence of an obstacle downstream. A urinoma can be detected by US and/or CT and interventional radiology techniques (percutane-

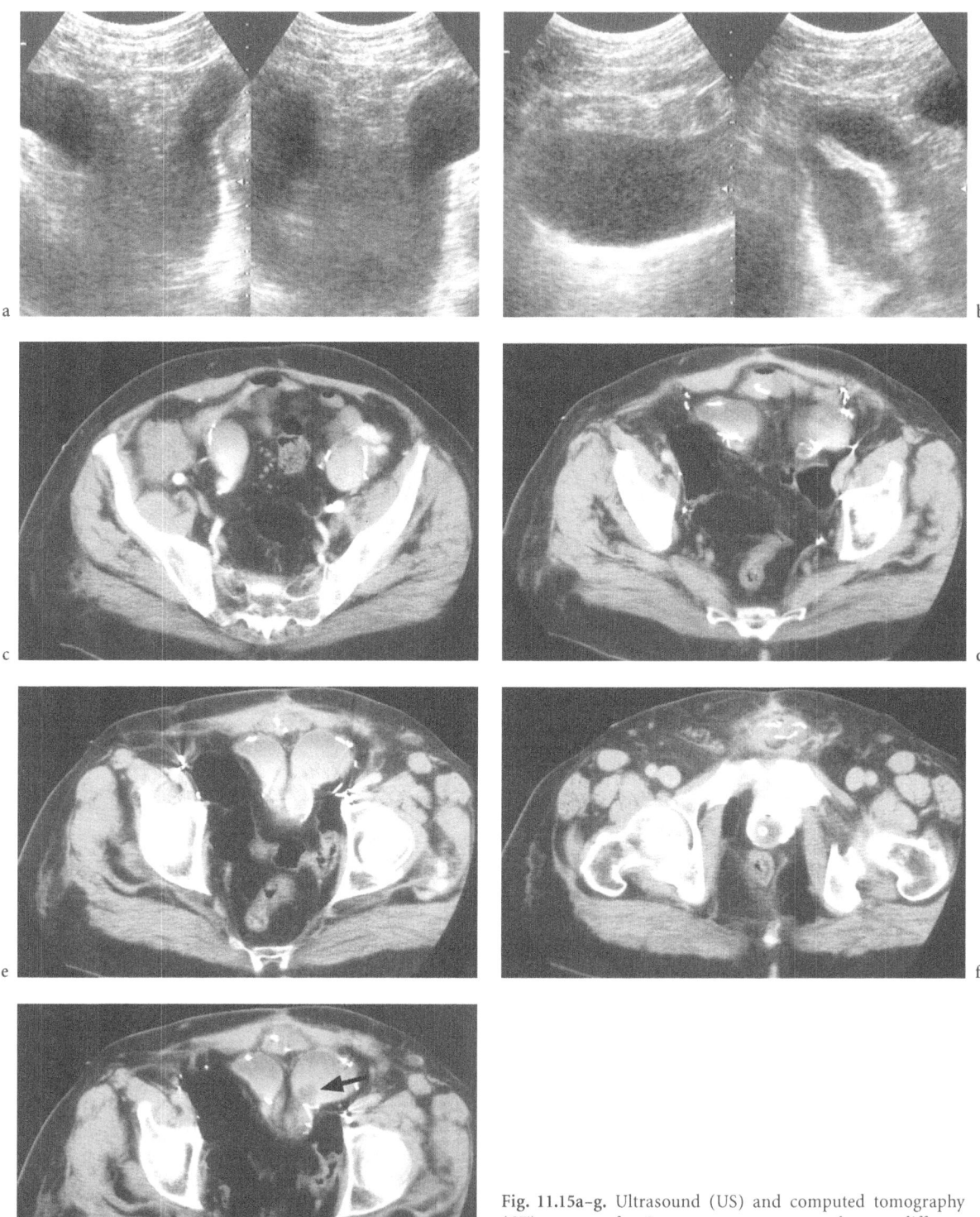

Fig. 11.15a–g. Ultrasound (US) and computed tomography (CT) aspects of a Camey-type enterocystoplasty at different levels. Presence of a filling defect in the left part of the ileal loop **g** corresponding to a recurrent transitional cell carcinoma (TCC) (*arrow*)

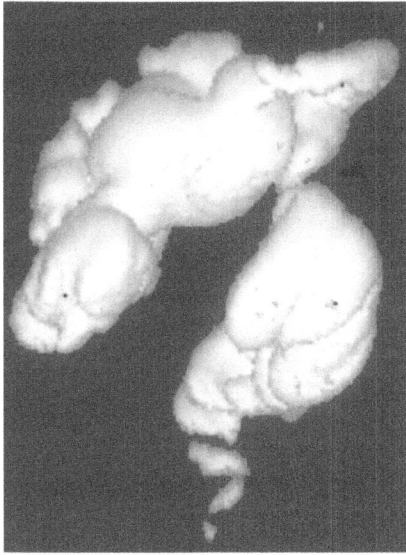

Fig. 11.16. Shaded surface display (SSD) reconstruction after CT of a patient with a Bricker-type intervention on a transplanted kidney. Dilatation of upper urinary tract secondary to an anastomotic stenosis (*white arrowhead*)

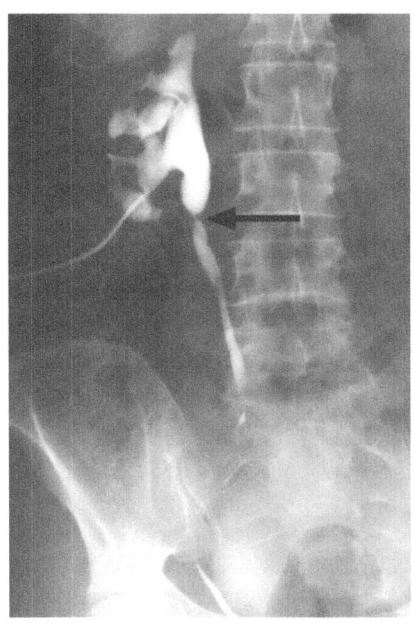

Fig. 11.18. AP via a nephrostomy catheter: right lumbar ureter stenosis after ureterotomy for stone extraction (*white arrow*)

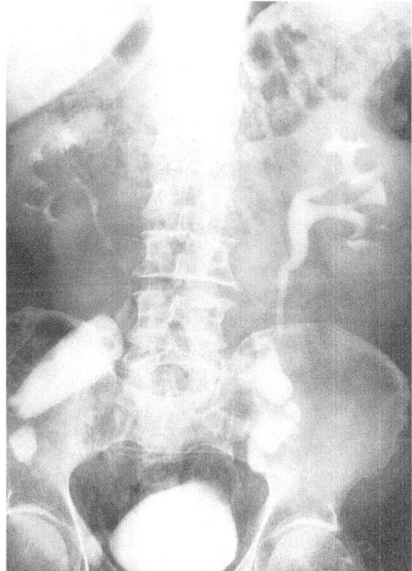

a

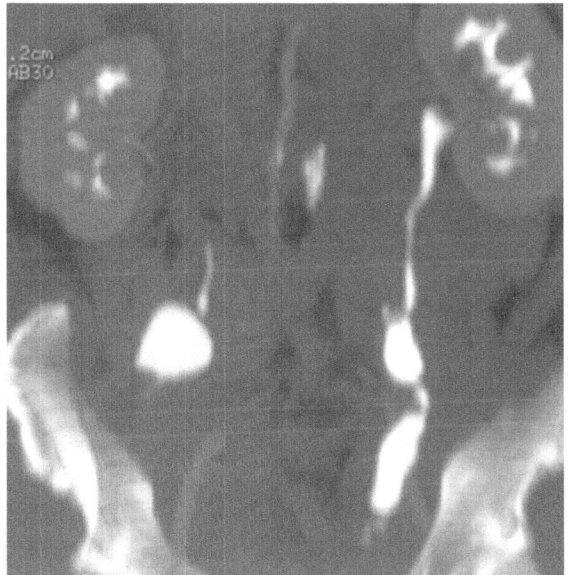

b

Fig. 11.17a, b. Partial bilateral uretero-ileoplasty with good drainage of urine. a Urographic view. b Maximum intensity projection (MIP) reconstruction after CT

ous nephrostomy, double-J tubes) are increasingly advantageous. A simple percutaneous nephrostomy is sometimes sufficient if the fistula is small. In other cases, ureteral intubation by a double-J tube has two advantages: it favors urothelial proliferation around the ureteral gap and prevents excessive scar stenosis. In some large fistulas, an upstream ureteral occlusion by a small balloon catheter is useful in association with an upstream urinary drainage (see Chap. 12).

Post-operative Suppurations. Post-operative suppurations are much less frequent since the generalization of the antibiotic prophylaxis and the use of double-J intubation. Their diagnosis and treatment may benefit from new imaging techniques (ultrasound and CT) and from interventional radiological techniques (percutaneous drainage). These early complications are usually treated by non-invasive techniques and seldom require repeat surgical intervention.

11.1.3.2.2
Late Complications

The same complications as described in the preceding sections may occur with delay (SULLIVAN et al. 1980).

Obstructions are frequent (approximately 20% of cases). They occur particularly in uretero-intestinal anastomoses (Fig. 11.19). The most frequent cause of obstruction is the occurrence of a stenotic scar at the terminal portion of the ureter, upstream of the anastomosis and related to a fibrosis secondary to postoperative and post-radiotherapy ischemia (Figs. 11.20, 11.21). It occurs early, often in the first 6 post-operative months. Less frequent causes include peri-ureteral fibrosis or an intrinsic or extrinsic obstruction related to the natural progression of the causal neoplasm.

Lastly, stenoses of the stoma and stenoses of the ileal loop by inflammatory reaction of unspecified cause (infection or chronic irritation due to the presence of alkaline urine) have exceptionally been described (MITCHELL 1977). Some cases of volvulus of the intestinal loop resulting in bilateral ureteral obstruction have also been described (FLANAGAN et al. 1995). All of these obstructions may be responsible for complications (infection, lithiasis, deterioration of renal function). Their surgical treatment is often difficult because of the local anatomical modifications due to the previous intervention or possibly to radiotherapy. It is well-known that stenoses detected early (before the 6th month) can respond favorably to dilation by a small balloon catheter, whereas failures are much more frequent beyond this time period (BANNER et al. 1983; LANG 1986). However, the treatment of a post-operative cicatricial stenosis by dilation must always be followed by placement of a double-J catheter in order to maintain the dilated zone open (SHAPIRO et al. 1988) (Fig. 11.22). The double-J catheter must be kept in place for several months (MARTIN et al. 1982).

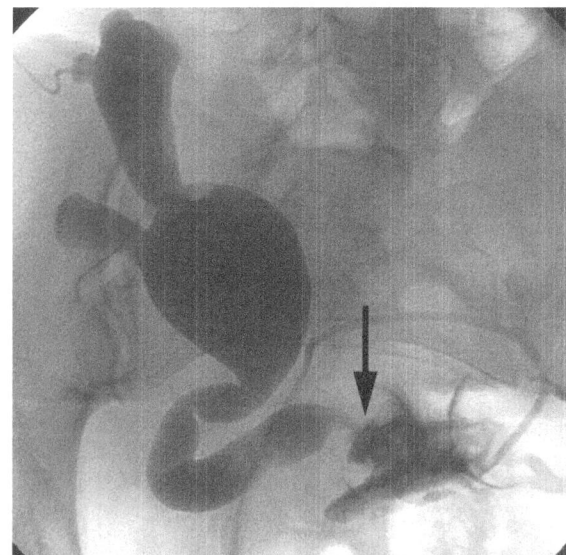

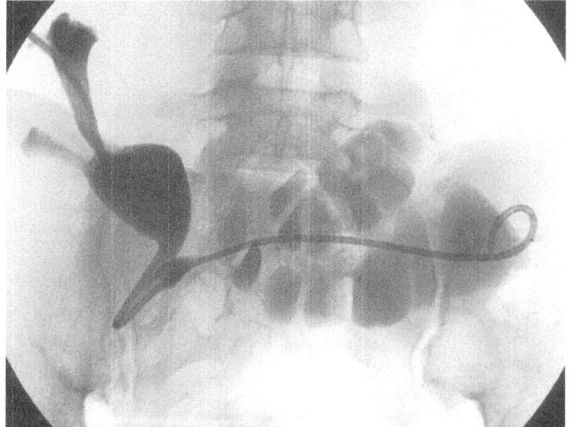

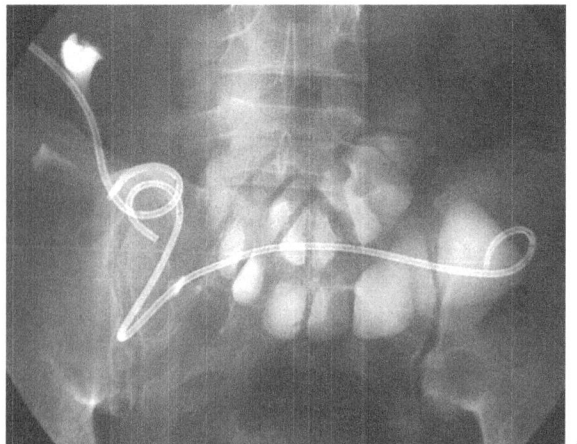

Fig. 11.19a–c. a AP on a transplant recipient with obstruction of the ureteroileal anastomosis after Bricker procedure (*arrow*). **b, c** Nephrostogram after temporary treatment by placing a double-J catheter: better opacification of the ileal loop

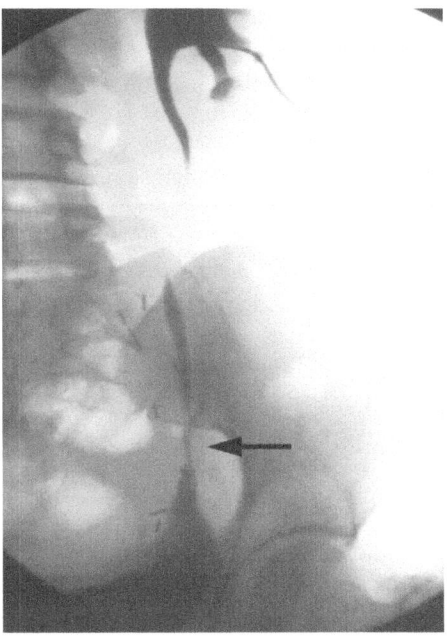

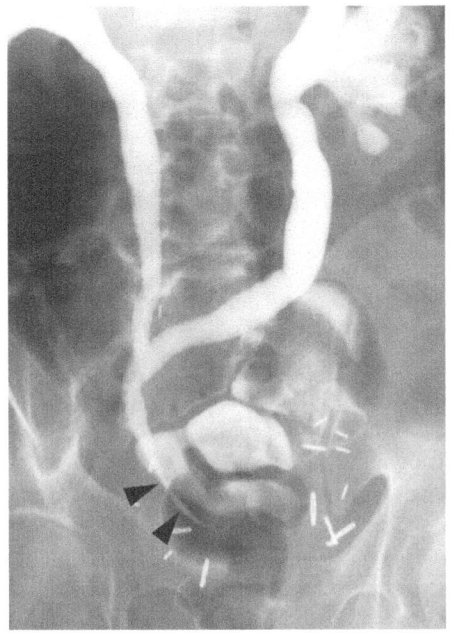

Fig. 11.20. Nephrostogram in a patient with a psoas hitch and post-radiotherapy narrowing of the distal ureter (*arrow*)

Fig. 11.21. Trans uretero-ureterostomy and right uretero sigmoidostomy (Coffey-type): post-radiotherapy stenosis of the right lower ureter (*arrowheads*)

This therapeutic strategy is nevertheless frequently disappointing and it is often necessary to propose either a ureterotomy by endourologic approach or a surgical reimplantation (SHAPIRO et al. 1988).

Fistulas are less frequent. They generally consist of early fistulas that have been unrecognized and whose late clinical consequence is a urinoma. Only the occur-

rence of a liquid retroperitoneal mass, compressing or not the excretory tract, often in an infectious context will make diagnosis possible. The diagnosis is performed by ultrasonography and CT, both of which offer the advantage of guiding a diagnostic and therapeutic puncture.

– Vesico-ureteral or entero-ureteral reflux must be

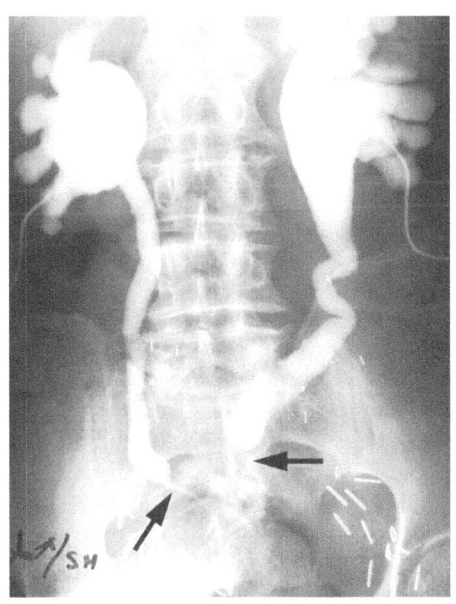

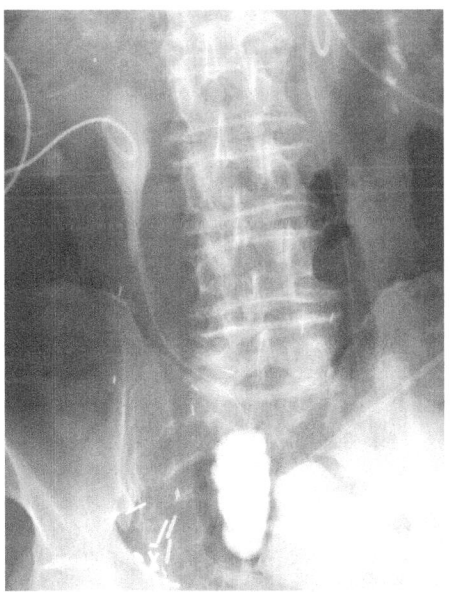

Fig. 11.22a, b. a Bilateral nephrostograms show obstruction of the uretero-intestinal anastomosis of a Koch pouch (*arrows*).
b Relief of obstruction by placement of bilateral double-J catheters

searched for every time an ureteral reimplantation is performed in the bladder or in extra-vesical position. It is constant in certain interventions but must be monitored. Although often well tolerated by the kidney in some interventions (such as a Bricker or a replacement bladder), it is sometimes poorly tolerated in other cases (such as the Coffey intervention) with a risk of acute pyelonephritis related to repeated ascending infections.

- Lithiatic complications. Their frequency is not insignificant (10%). Lithiasis may originate from multiple causes: unrecognized preexisting lithiasis, obstruction, infection, or migration of surgical staples. They can also be seen in cases of ureteral surgery using intestinal segments whose anastomoses have been performed with automatic suturing devices. These stones can migrate along the urinary tract (WEBSTER et al. 1987).
- Infectious complications (pyelonephritis, pyonephrosis, etc.) are the consequence of an obstruction or a vesico-ureteral reflux.

Complications of the operated ureter involve a certain number of requirements for a solution adapted to the arising problems:
- The radiologist must know the various types of possible interventions, their risks and how to monitor them.
- The diagnosis is often based on traditional opacification methods, but percutaneous access to the upper excretory tract for opacification and drainage plays an increasingly significant role.

The difficulty of surgical reinterventions implies a perfect radio-urological collaboration in order to determine the best initial approach and the best therapeutic choice.

11.2
Ureter of the Transplanted Kidney

The ureter is the target of most urological complications of renal transplants. These complications may originate in the operative procedure itself, in immunologic manifestations that surround the intervention, and in the pathology of the transplanted kidney itself. As compared to post-operative ureteral complications of the native ureter, these complications raise specific problems (SCHIFF 1978). They concern a solitary kidney, they raise difficult diagnostic problems, in particular with transplant

rejection, and the transplanted patients are fragile, immunodepressed, sensitive to infection and prone to poor healing. Their occurrence rate varies from 5% to 15% according to published series (JASKOWSKI et al. 1987; BENNETT et al. 1986; MUNDY et al. 1981). This frequency seems stable, although some authors have noted a significant decrease concomitant to the emergence of dose reductions in corticotherapy and to the advent of cyclosporin therapy. The incidence rate does not appear to increase in patients undergoing repeated transplantations and it decreases in well-trained transplantation teams. Other authors claim this frequency does not vary whereas the gravity and morbidity of complications decreases (LOUGHLIN et al. 1984). The overall seriousness of these complications is undisputed. Statistics show that surgical treatment of these complications is responsible for transplant loss in approximately 30% of cases and patient death may occur in 20% of cases (SCHIFF 1978). Palestrant notes that 12% of transplant kidney failures are related to urological complications (PALESTRANT and DEWOLF 1982). Nevertheless, the emergence of new imaging methods and interventional uroradiological techniques has resulted in a dramatic reduction of morbidity and mortality.

11.2.1
Guidelines

Early diagnosis of ureteral complications of the kidney transplant is clearly of the utmost importance. This diagnosis is based on radiological techniques, the choice of which will be decided as a function of clinical presentation, type of surgical reconstruction and the results of other biological and radiological examinations.

11.2.1.1
Surgical Technique

In most cases restoration of the urinary continuity is achieved by uretero-vesical anastomosis (ureteroneocystostomy). Submucosal tunneling following the Leadbetter-Politano technique has been abandoned for an extravesical anti-reflux course (SARRAMON et al. 1985). This has the advantage of reducing surgical opening of the bladder and therefore decreases the amount of time required for drainage. This technical choice resulted in a significant reduction in urologic complications. The uretero-ureteral termino-terminal anastomosis on a double-J catheter may be considered if the vesical wall is damaged and/or if the ureter is short and poorly vascularized. It is contraindicated in cases of pre-existing reflux in the recipient. The pelvi-ureteral anastomosis is used exclusively in cases with pre-existing pelvic dilation in the donor. The renal fossa must be systematically drained, especially in plethoric patients. Some authors propose temporary placement of a double-J catheter, which seems to reduce morbidity (HERON et al. 1995). Careful dissection is very important during sampling with respect to vascularization and peri-ureteral fat as well as are the shortest ischemic time possible and careful hemostasis (RISCHMAN 1983).

11.2.1.2
Radiological Follow-up

The need for early diagnosis requires a rigorous but adapted protocol for each case. Ultrasonography plays a major role in the early detection of complications (LOUGHLIN et al. 1984; GRENIER et al. 1994). Superficial location of the transplanted kidney is favorable for a precise and complete examination. Ultrasonography evaluates the renal parenchyma and its vasculature well, detects dilatation of the urinary tract, and detects peri-renal and peri-ureteral collections (GERBENS et al. 1980). The basic strategy consists of a weekly ultrasonographic follow-up during the 1st month, associated with an EU performed 1 month after transplantation. Later, yearly ultrasonography is usually sufficient. This scheme may vary depending on clinical events that follow the transplantation: urinary leak through the drain, fever, sometimes with signs of urinary infection, a palpable mass in the transplant fossa, oliguria, and an increase in the plasma creatinine level. Pain in the transplant area is rarely found as a result of denervation.

Indications of EU are decreasing. Unless contraindicated by overly severe renal failure, EU provides precise information on ureteral patency (Fig. 11.23), the existence of a dilation of the urinary tract as well as the potential of a peri-renal collection.

DTPA (95^{mtc} diethylene triamine pentacetic acid) isotopic scans have been used by several teams to detect ureteral obstruction and to differentiate it from rejection (FRODIN and WICKLLIND 1981). However, their reliability appears less than that of ultrasonography (SMITH et al. 1988a): they only allow a diagnostic suspicion and carry a significant false-negative rate, especially in cases of renal insufficiency. Computed tomography is useful when there is a suspicion of a peri-renal collection (whether or not it is associated with a urinary fistula) or a space-occupying lesion that compresses the ureter (NOVICK et al. 1981). New three-

dimensional reconstruction techniques allow coronal imaging of the urinary tract in different projections, particularly helpful in cases of dilation.

Suspicion of ureteral disease on the basis of abnormalities found on clinical, ultrasonographic and/or urographic findings requires antegrade or retrograde direct opacification techniques. The first preferred approach should be the antegrade pyelography (STREEM et al. 1988; SMITH et al. 1988; SCHIFF et al. 1979) by urinary tract puncture guided by fluoroscopy and/or ultrasonography. It makes it possible to confirm the ureteral obstruction with certainty and carries a low risk (GLASS et al. 1982; BARBARIC and THOMPSON 1978). The percentage and gravity of hemorrhagic complications is minimal (LIEBERMAN et al. 1982). As reported by other authors, it also allows pressure measurements (Whitaker test) in cases where there is doubt about a potential obstruction (ZOLLIKOFER et al. 1985; WHITAKER 1979). The percutaneous approach to pelvicaliceal cavities makes interventional uroradiologic procedures easier than the retrograde approach does, should the need for such interventions arise (PFISTER and NEWHOUSE 1979). The aims of these procedures include decompression of the excretory tract, urine derivation (percutaneous nephrostomy), transitory bypass of an ureteral obstruction or breach (ureteral intubation by a double-J catheter), treatment of a ureteral stenosis (dilation followed by a ureteral intubation), and retrieval of ureteral calculi (percutaneous nephrolithotomy). It also can evaluate renal function and recovery possibilities of the transplanted kidney.

Retrograde catheterization of the ureter has several drawbacks in the kidney transplant patient: technical

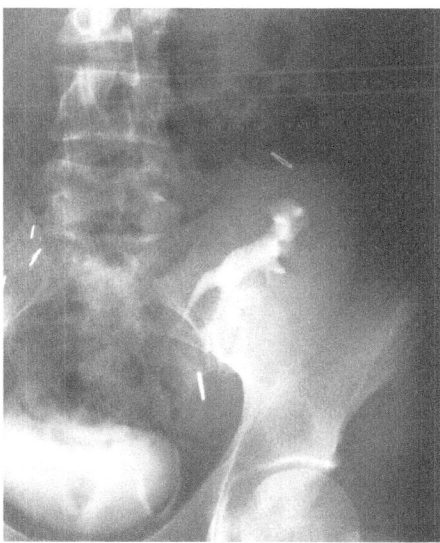

Fig. 11.23. Normal EU of a left transplanted kidney

failures are frequent as the creation of a ureteroneocystostomy often results in a highly and antero-laterally located neomeatus, which is more difficult to visualize and to catheterize (SCHMELLER et al. 1985). The use of hydrophilic guidewires nevertheless allows retrograde catheterization by an experienced endoscopist. Even if this catheterization is successful, assessment of the stenosis remains difficult: the opacification of the suprastenotic ureter is difficult in cases of tight stenoses and taking multiple incidence X-ray pictures becomes delicate. Furthermore, the risk of infection is not insignificant in these immunodepressed patients.

11.2.2
Ureteral Fistulas

Ureteral fistulas may be found in 2%–10% of cases according to different series, mainly in cases of uretero-ureteral anastomoses (JASKOWKI et al. 1987; MUNDY et al. 1981). They are responsible for a significant morbidity and mortality (SCHIFF et al. 1976). Depending on the mechanism and time of occurrence, early and delayed fistulas must be distinguished:

Early fistulas occur before the 6th post-transplantation day. They are seldom due to a ureteral injury and more frequently related to an ischemic necrosis of the ureter secondary to a defective dissection or an abnormality of the ureteral vascularization.

Delayed fistulas happen between the 10th and 15th post-operative day. The role of ureteral ischemia may be invoked, but immunologic phenomena – gathered under the term "ureteral rejection" – are also possibly involved (WOODS et al. 1973). This ureteral rejection reaches the terminal portion of the donor ureter and may sometimes be the only manifestation of a rejection, i.e. without any renal extent. It evolves towards regression, stenosis or necrosis.

Whatever the occurrence timing, clinical presentation is identical. The patient has fever and may present a mass in the transplant fossa with diffuse tenderness of the corresponding lower quadrant. Urinary diuresis is reduced and plasma creatinine level increases. Urinary leak through the drain is frequently observed. Imaging has a triple objective: (a) to detect, locate and assess the importance of the fistula, (b) to look for a possible para-renal collection, and (c) to intervene radiologically, should the need arise.

EU, even in cases where renal function is preserved, is often insufficient to show the CM leak (SPIGOS et al. 1977). In some cases the kidney and/or the ureter may be pushed away and compressed by a peri-renal mass syndrome. The opacification by contrast medium depends on whether the fistulous tract is closed.

Antegrade pyelography is the method of reference. It allows opacification of the urinary tract when renal function is impaired and invariably shows the extravasation of contrast medium (STREEM et al. 1988; SMITH et al. 1988b). The breach size and the status of the overlying ureter must be assessed (Fig. 11.24). This is mandatory for therapeutic decision-making. Antegrade pyelography represents the first step of urinary drainage and potential further ureteral intubation. In difficult cases, it can solve diagnostic problems that may arise regarding potential rejection or tubulopathy (BECKER and KUTCHER 1978).

a 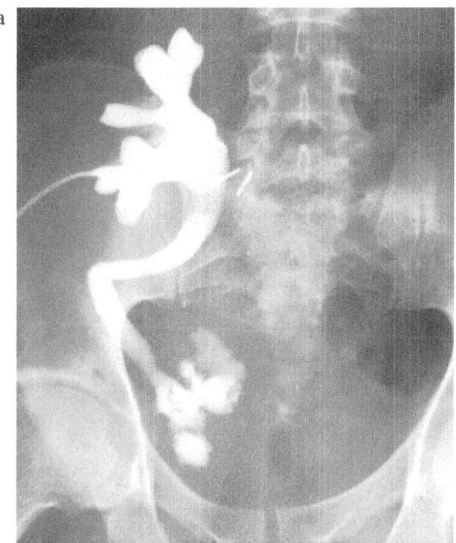 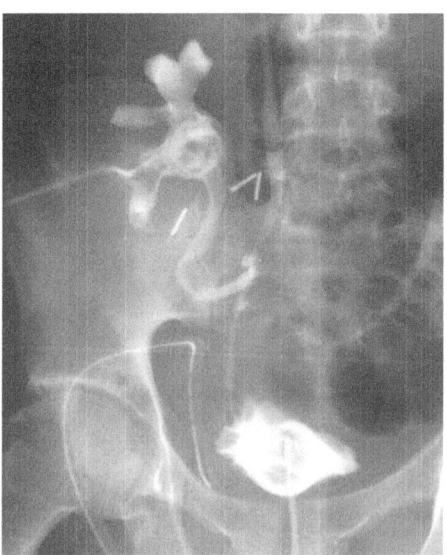 b

Fig. 11.24a, b. Post-rejection ureteral fistula. a AP via the nephrostomy catheter shows pyelocaliceal and ureteral dilatation with extravasation of contrast medium (CM) before the anastomotic site. Absence of bladder opacification. b AP control after surgical derivation by uretero-ureteral anastomosis on the native right ureter. Normal opacification of the bladder

US and CT may be useful in the hypothesis of a significant collected urinoma with or without communication with the ureter (Gerbens et al. 1980). The collection can be exactly located (most frequently subperitoneal) and percutaneous drainage possibilities can be determined (Glanz et al. 1985). CT can also reveal the urinary leak (Spigos et al. 1977). 3D reconstruction after helical CT acquisition permits an accurate depiction of the location of the leak and evaluation of the site, relationships and morphology of the urinoma (Fig. 11.25). Treatment varies according to the teams. Some authors prefer surgical repair (Guerin et al. 1990). However, the current trend is to propose uroradiological interventional techniques in first intention as a definitive treatment or as a preliminary treatment before surgery (see also Chap. 12). Uroradiological interventional techniques have several objectives: (a) to dry up the fistula, (c) to preserve renal function (c) to drain the urinoma, (d) to prevent against infection, and (e) to restore ureteral continuity (Rischman 1983).

Percutaneous nephrostomy is the first therapeutic step and is sometimes sufficient if the fistula is small. Ureteral catheterization with a floppy and/or hydrophilic guidewire should be gently attempted and a ureteral intubation by an internal–external drainage catheter or by a double-J tube should be performed if possible (Streem et al. 1988). However, in case of a proximal fistula without opacification of the underlying ureter, the breach loss is probably significant and ureteral intubation is then likely to fail. In such a case, only surgery remains possible. It is the case in extensive necrosis that imposes pyeloureteral anastomosis by using the recipient's native ureter (Fig. 11.24).

It is important to carefully supervise the long-term ureteral patency after treatment of a fistula, as the occurrence of a further stenosis always remains possible. Delay in the diagnosis reduces the chances of success for further dilation. Percutaneous drainage of an urinoma must be considered in case it appears well collected (Glanz et al. 1985).

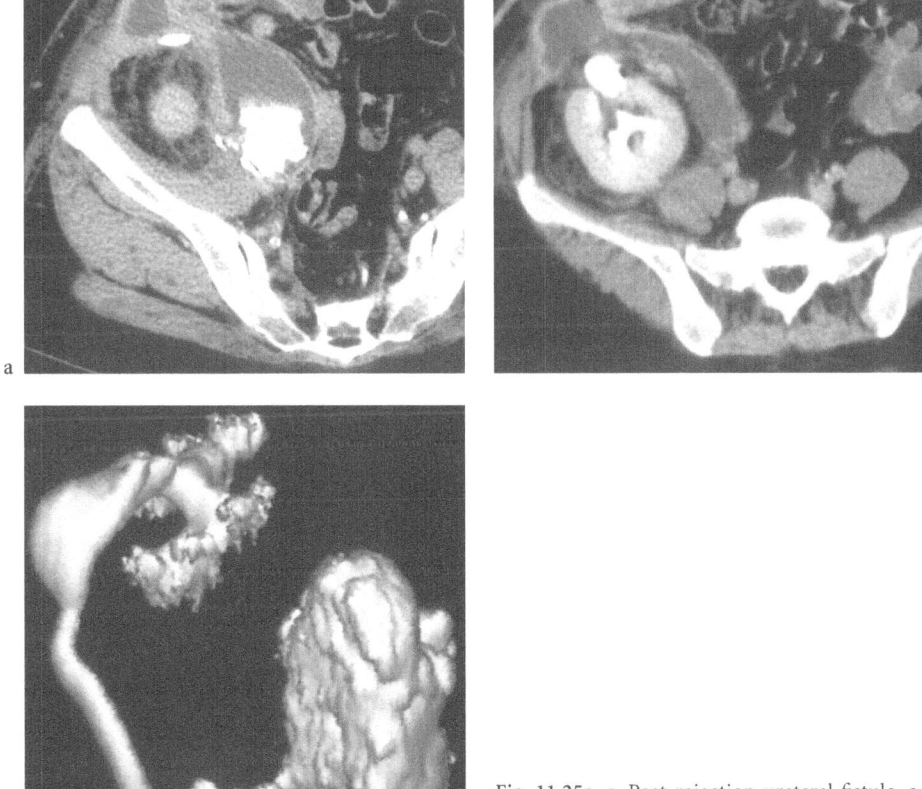

Fig. 11.25a–c. Post-rejection ureteral fistula. **a, b** Axial CT slices showing perirenal urinoma with extravasation of CM in the bottom of the collection. **c** SSD reconstruction showing the fistula (arrow), the opacification of the urinoma and the absence of CM in the lower ureter

11.2.3
Ureteral Stenoses

They represent the most frequent ureteral complication of the transplanted kidney. They occur in 2%–
8% of cases according to published series (CANTON et
al. 1987; JASKOWSKI et al. 1987). Screening of ureteral
stenosis largely depends on ultrasonography, which
easily detects dilatation of the upper urinary tract
(Fig. 11.26) Their mechanism and pathophysiology
are discussed as follows.

Stenoses by Ureteral Fibrosis. Stenoses by ureteral fibrosis appear to be the most frequent etiology (MUNDY et

al. 1981). They affect the juxta-anastomotic portion of
the distal ureter and mostly occur between the 1st and
3rd months after transplantation (Fig. 11.27). A more
delayed occurrence is possible but remains exceptional, although one case of stenosis was reported
5 years after transplantation (ZINCKE et al. 1977).
More rarely, the ureter is almost completely involved
and presents a long and tubular stenosis, which can
also extend up to the renal pelvis (LAMASTERS et al.
1980). The diagnostic discussion mainly focuses on the
respective roles of rejection and ischemia. According
to some authors (PALMER and CHATTERJEE 1978;
SCHWEIZER et al. 1977), the role of ureteric ischemia,
by destruction of the vascularization, seems to be

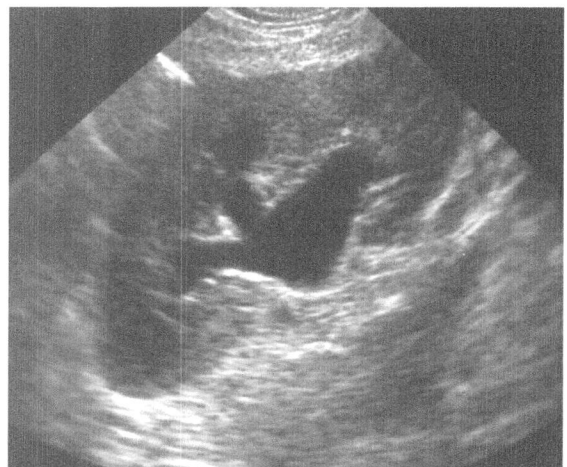
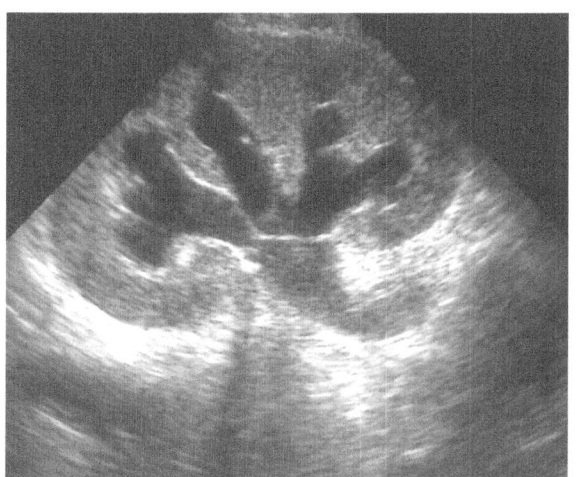

Fig. 11.26a, b. Some ultrasonographic aspects of uretero-hydronephrosis in transplanted kidneys

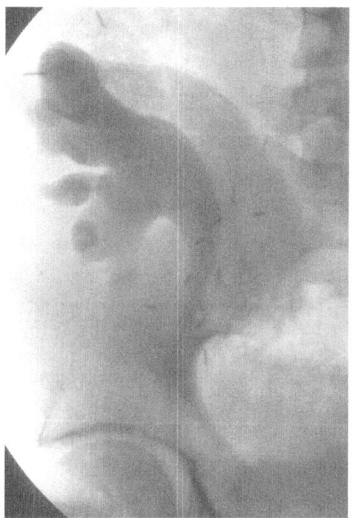
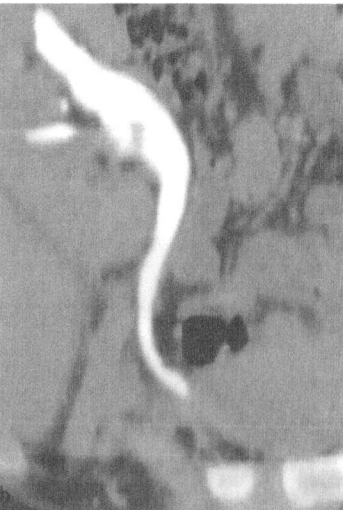
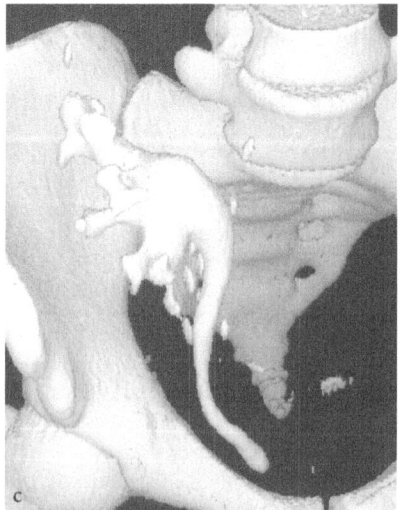

Fig. 11.27a–c. Post-operative stenosis of the uretero-vesical anastomosis. Comparison between EU and CT. **a** Ureterohydrone-
phosis on EU. **b, c** CT coronal reconstruction showing ureterohydronephrosis with absence of CM in the bladder and ureterovesical stenosis (**b,** multiplanar reformation, MPR; **c,** SSD)

of major importance. Ischemia of ureter is secondary to undue tension on the ureteroneocystostomy or post-dissection devascularization of the donor ureter. Ischemia leads to ureteral necrosis or stricture formation (GHASEMIAN et al. 1996). Unrecognized anatomical abnormalities of the transplanted kidney could play a predisposing factor in the pathogenesis of vascular lesions (bifidity, UPJ, unrecognized inferior polar artery) (JASKOWSKI et al. 1987). Similarly, a difficult dissection, an already ischemic ureter and a difficult vesical approach may all be predisposing factors for ureteric ischemia. For others, rejection would have a major role, as suggested by some functional and morphological ureteric deteriorations observed by HRICAK in experimental rejections (HRICAK et al. 1986). This damage, and in particular the urodynamic disorders, could be responsible for a moderate obstruction of functional origin (BELITZKI et al. 1972). This atony can be observed using fluoroscopic analysis and the Whitaker test (ZOLLIKOFER et al. 1985).

However, the exact role of rejection in the occurrence of a fibrous ureteral stenosis has never been proven. The accompanying ischemic phenomena could play a predisposing role (TEXTER et al. 1974).

Stenoses by Peri-ureteral Fibrosis. The occurrence of stenoses by peri-ureteral fibrosis is more delayed, most frequently during the first year (QUINIBI et al. 1982). They consist of extrinsic stenoses secondary to a peri-ureteral sclerosis of variable significance: simple band or sclerotic bulky mass responsible for an extended stenosis. The origin of the sclerosis is difficult to determine: post-operative urohematoma or immunologic process?

Stenoses by Extrinsic Compression. Stenoses by extrinsic compression are sometimes related to post-operative collections (lymphocele, urinoma), more rarely to compression by pre-existing anatomical structures: spermatic cord, polar artery (MUNDY et al. 1981) (Figs. 11.28, 11.29).

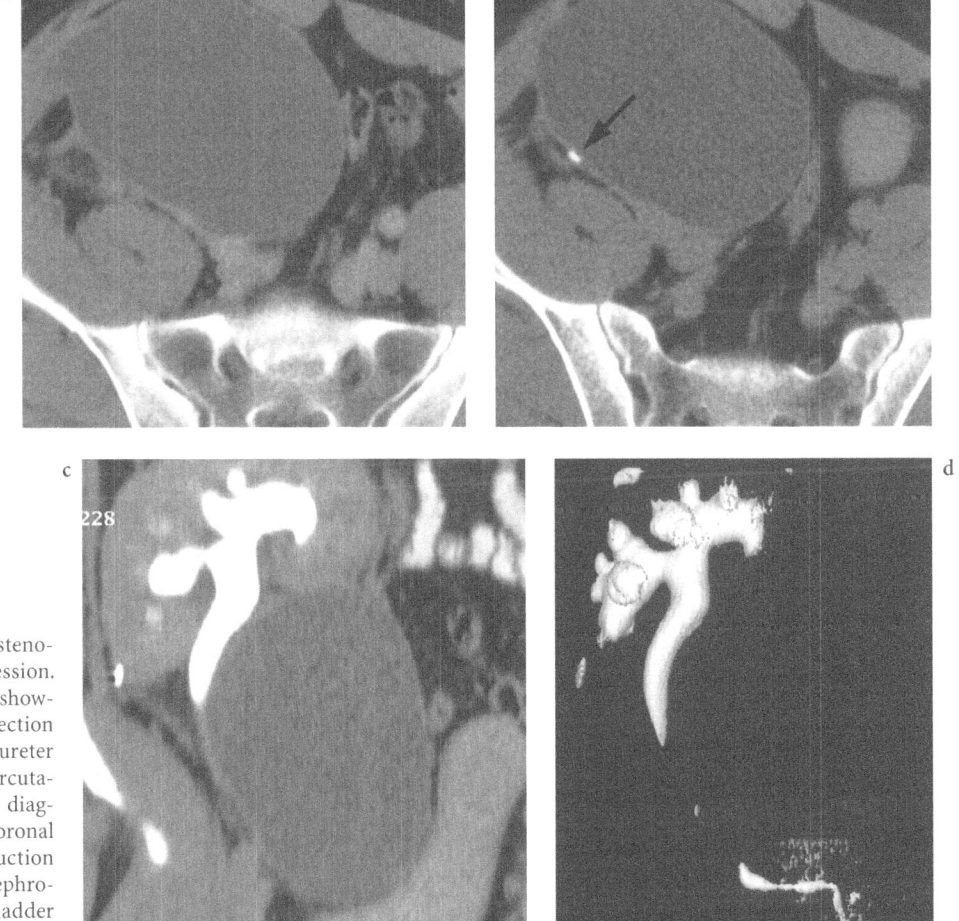

Fig. 11.28a–d. Ureteral stenosis by external compression. a, b Axial CT slices showing a hypodense collection with compression of ureter (**arrow**); subsequent percutaneous puncture allows diagnosis of urinoma. c Coronal multiplanar reconstruction shows uretero-hydronephrosis with ureteral and bladder compression by the urinoma. d SSD reconstruction

Fig. 11.29a–e. Ureteral stenosis by external compression. a, b Longitudinal and transversal ultrasonographic views demonstrating ureterohydronephrosis of the transplanted kidney. c This echographic view shows the external compression of the ureter (+) by an anechoic mass corresponding to the collection (*) (lymphocele confirmed by puncture). d, e MPR view showing ureterohydronephrosis and external compression of the ureter by the lymphocele (*)

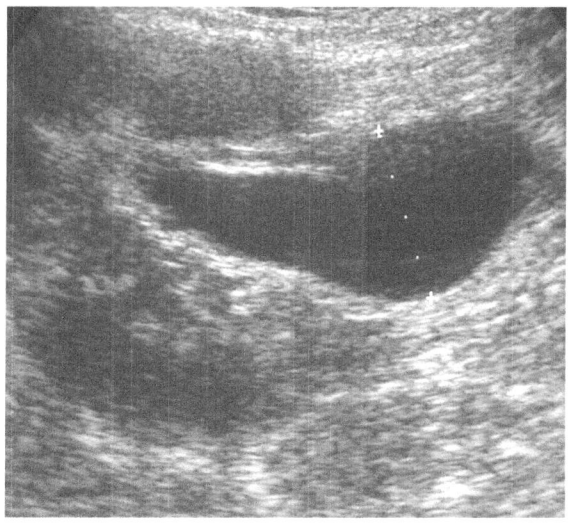

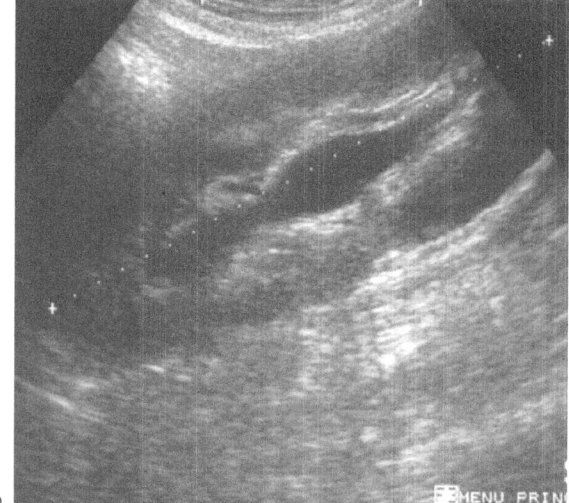

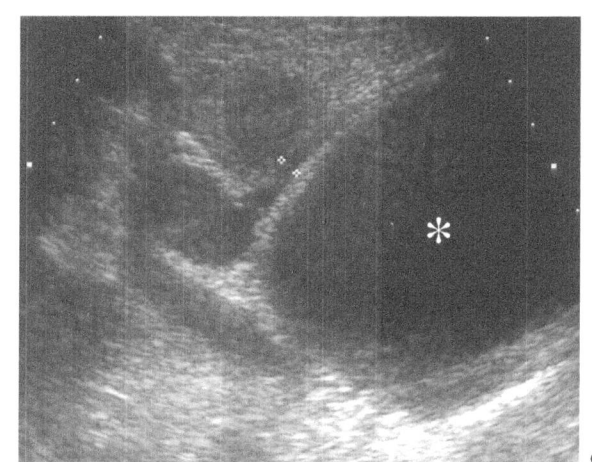

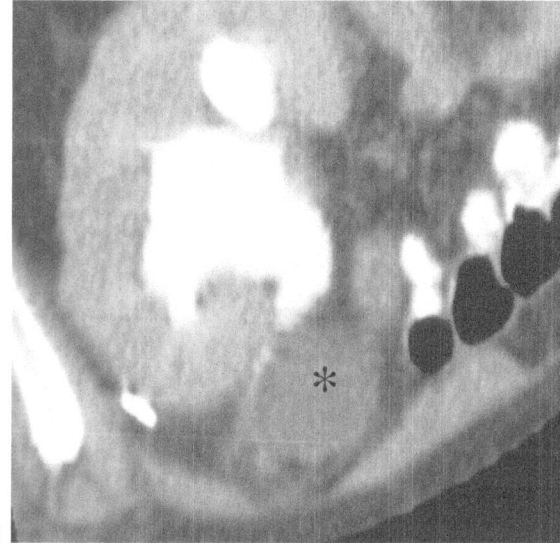

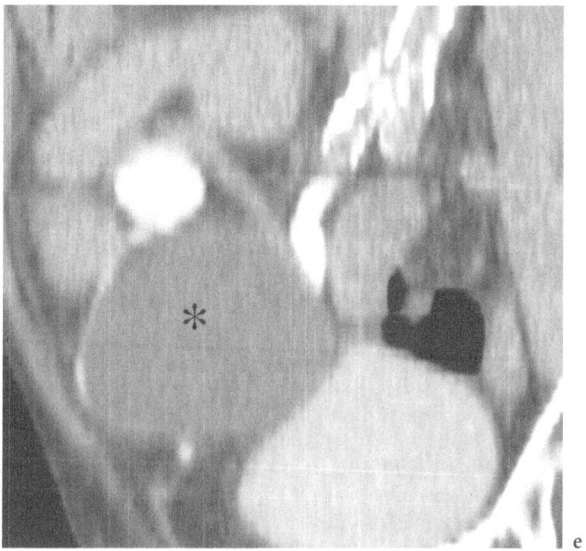

Stenoses Related to a Defective Surgical Reconstruction. Folding, kinking or torsion of the ureter stenoses at the ureterovesical junction can result from defective reconstruction of the anti-reflux system (SCHIFF 1978). They lead to acute or chronic obstruction depending on the degree of torsion (Figs. 11.30, 11.31). Most frequently they appear as a short and mild stenosis of the middle third without folding, but which can lead to an intraluminal obstruction (blood clot).

Pre-existing Stenoses. Pre-existing stenoses consist of UPJ syndromes that were not recognized during sampling and transplantation procedures. Intra-

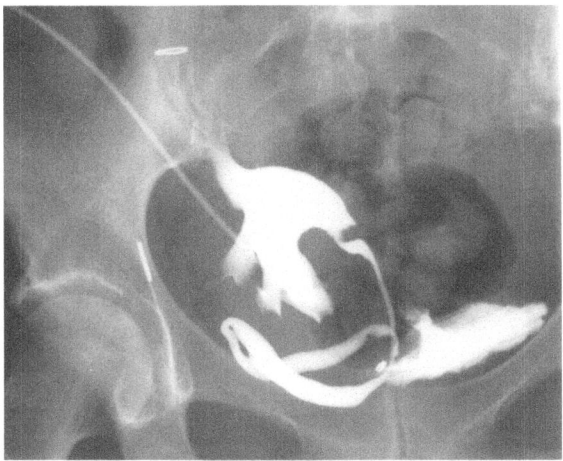

Fig. 11.30. Antegrade pyelography performed to determine the cause of hydronephrosis: opacification shows multiple sinuosities of the ureter with kinking due to excessive ureteral length

operative discovery requires either a pelvi-ureteral anastomosis or a cure of the junctional zone while taking care not to deteriorate the ureteric vascularization.

Clinical presentation is variable. Sometimes it is an acute presentation with fever and acute renal failure, in particular in early stenoses. In most cases, the progressive emergence of renal insufficiency with reduced diuresis and increased plasma creatinine levels will motivate the search for an obstruction (ZINCKE et al. 1977). The differential diagnosis with chronic rejection may be difficult, since some rejections may be accompanied by hypotonia of the excretory tract (ZOLLIKOFER et al. 1985). Obstruction and rejection may also be associated (GLASS et al. 1982). These problems involve the systematic completion of an antegrade pyelography every time a dilation is suspected at ultrasonography (ZINCKE et al. 1977; QUIGG et al. 1986). Indeed, the diagnosis is based mainly on the association between ultrasonography and antegrade pyelography. EU is often not sufficient as soon as renal function is impaired. Isotopic nephrogram is used by some authors, but the false-negative proportion is high, about 80% (SMITH et al. 1988a). This can be explained by the impairment in renal function.

Ultrasonography must be systematically performed as soon as an obstruction is suspected, as it confirms the existence of the latter in approximately 85% of cases (GERBENS et al. 1980). However, other authors have recognized that the presence of a dilation of the pelvicaliceal cavities without coexist-

a

b

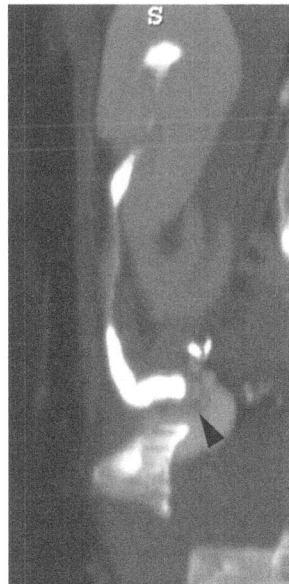
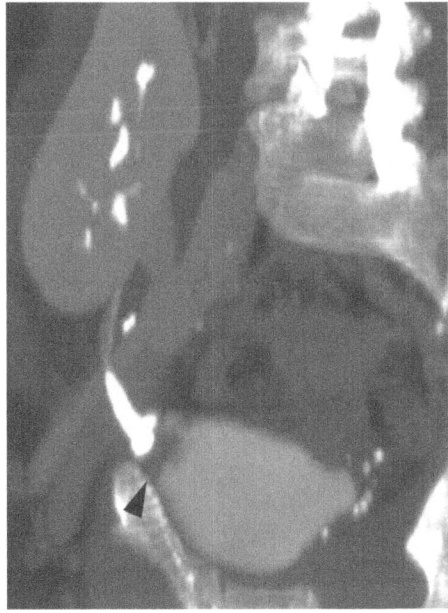

Fig. 11.31a, b. Post-operative anastomotic stenosis related to Teflon injection for vesico-ureteral reflux treatment. MPR CT slices show the presence of moderate ureteral dilatation with uretero-vesical stenosis and filling defect image of the anastomotic region (*arrowheads*)

ing obstruction could be noted in half of the cases (BALCHUNAS et al. 1982; STRATTON et al. 1989). The existence of an isolated dilation of the renal pelvis is particularly frequent and can be explained by hypotonic phenomena on the excretory tract related to a rejection or by a pre-existing anomaly in the morphology of the urinary tract (HECKEMAN et al. 1979). TEXTER claims that multiple episodes of rejection could result in a non-stenosing fibrosis of the ureter that decreases the peristalsis (TEXTER et al. 1974). These pelvic dilations should, however, be carefully followed up as one-third evolve to a true obstruction. On the other hand, a dilation can be hidden in case of renal edema. All these reasons explain why antegrade pyelography must be used every time the diagnosis remains doubtful (LIEBERMAN et al. 1982). With its effectiveness and its low risk rate (thanks to the use of a fine needle less than 1 mm in diameter), this technique is the examination of choice in this kind of situation. Its reliability is 100% (Fig. 11.32). It makes it possible to study intrarenal perfusion pressures using the Whitaker test in cases where the diagnosis of obstruction remains ambiguous, although this test has low reproducibility. According to ZOLLIKOFER, it also assesses peristalsis throughout the ureter in fluoroscopy (ZOLLIKOFER et al. 1985). The morphological information provided by direct ureter opacification remains limited for the purpose of etiological diag-

nosis and the mechanism of the obstruction can be difficult to confirm. The presentation mode, the time since transplantation, the length of the stenosis, and the topographical location are the only elements of orientation.

CT, eventually guided by antegrade pyelography, can show signs of extrinsic compression (spermatic cord, peri-ureteral collection) or peri-ureteral fibrosis and provides a 3D visualization of the obstructed urinary tract after reconstruction (LETOURNEAU et al. 1987). Recently, MR urography has been proposed to assess ureteral obstruction of transplanted kidneys (SCHUBERT et al. 2000) (Fig. 11.33). The information is similar with CT, but the use of enhancement with gadolinium can provide functional information (DORSAM et al. 1997).

Etiological orientation is important for the future therapeutic decision. The treatment relies on the kind of lesion, the time of onset, the consequences

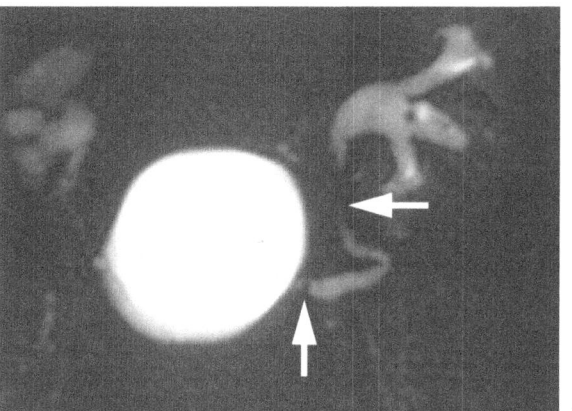

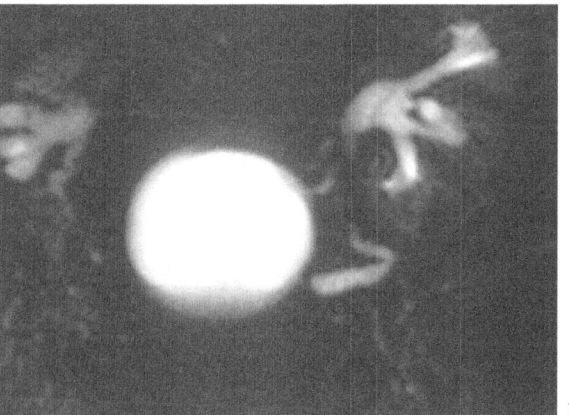

Fig. 11.33a, b. UroMR with single-shot fast spin echo or turbo spin echo (SSTSE) sequence: presence of moderate ureterohydronephrosis of the left transplanted kidney. Double stenoses are demonstrated at the mid portion and immediately upstream the uretero-vesical anastomosis (*white arrows*). Visualization of a right nonfunctional previously transplanted kidney

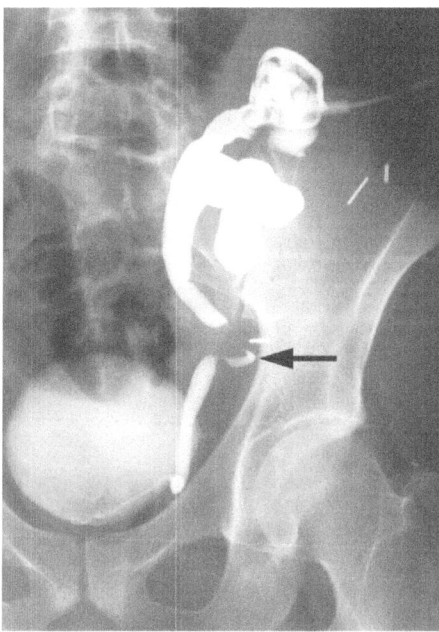

Fig. 11.32. Ureteral stenosis by periureteral fibrosis: AP (antegrade pyelography) shows ureterohydronephrosis due to tight stenosis of the mid part of the ureter with angulation and external deviation (*arrow*)

on the upstream urinary tract and renal function, and the existence of an associated urinary infection or rejection. The emergence of interventional radiology has completely modified the therapeutic strategy in ureteral obstructions. Surgical treatment is accompanied by a significant morbidity with loss of the kidney in 10% of cases, and by a significant operative mortality. Surgery is difficult indeed in these fragile patients and often results in ureterolysis and considering an ureteral replacement by ileoplasty or appendicoplasty (SARRAMON et al. 1985). It is systematic in some cases (kinking, extrinsic compression), as well as in failures of ureteral intubation.

Percutaneous nephrostomy is currently a fundamental therapeutic procedure that settles the urinary cavities, reduces edema, controls infection, and assesses renal function, whatever the next planned therapeutic step (HUNTER et al. 1983). It is performed by the antero-lateral approach of the transplanted kidney with echographic guidance. CO_2 insufflation of the excretory tract is very useful to locate and approach the excretory tract through the anterior calices (SMITH et al. 1988a). This percutaneous approach is the first step of endoluminal treatment of ureteric stenoses. Use of vascular catheterization techniques enables transstenotic placement of a tube more easily than through a retrograde approach. This intubation may be performed by placement of either a double-J tube or an internal–external drainage catheter (LIEBERMAN et al. 1981). The latter option is warranted in case of transitory drainage as an adjuvant treatment for an extrinsic ureteral compression (pararenal collection, vascular compression). Currently, in most cases, when ureteral intubation is possible, a ureteral dilation must be attempted (VOEGELI et al. 1988). This dilatation is done using balloon catheters that are available for transluminal angioplasty and allow high pressure inflations (above 15 atm). Balloons are 6–8 mm in diameter. Dilation is prolonged (3–5 min) and repeated. A double-J catheter is invariably left in place for a time period ranging between 1 and 3 months. Results vary according to teams and treated lesions. Generally, the technique provides a 45% success rate with a follow-up longer than 1 year (STREEM et al. 1988). All failures occur during the 1st year. No relation seems to appear between failure occurrence and age of the obstruction, contrary to benign stenoses of native ureters. VOEGELI describes normal patency at 1 year in 11 of 14 cases (79%), with two consecutive dilations in three cases (VOEGELI et al. 1988). This success rate might be explained by early detection and treatment,

but this author indicates that four of his patients were successfully treated despite symptoms aging from 6–13 years. This therapeutic protocol may be applied every time it is possible, even if success is not constantly observed. Afterwards, these patients must be regularly followed up by blood sample tests and ultrasonography.

11.2.4
Ureteral Lithiasis and Other Ureteral Diseases

Urinary lithiasis of the transplanted kidney is rare (AFFRE et al. 1978). It occurs in less than 1% of cases, but its frequency is increasing with the greater life expectancy of renal transplants (VAN GANSBEKE et al. 1985; HERON et al. 1995). Transplanted kidney lithiasis is most frequently caliceal lithiasis and usually asymptomatic (LERUT et al. 1979). True ureteral lithiasis is much less frequent. It results from the migration of an upper urinary tract lithiasis. The pathology of transplanted kidney stones is widely discussed (ROSENBERG et al. 1975; BRIEN et al. 1980). There is often a lithogenic metabolic factor: hypercalciuria secondary to hyperparathyroidism due to prolonged corticotherapy, hyperuraturia induced by the use of cyclosporin, and renal tubular acidosis (STRUCK et al. 1986). These factors may be worsened by disturbances in pelviureteral motoricity of the transplanted kidney. Lithiasis can be secondary to a chronic obstruction, possibly associated with a chronic urinary infection related to the obstruction. The predisposing role of anastomoses using nonresorbable thread has also been reported.

The diagnosis of ureteral lithiasis should be evoked in case of acute renal function impairment or, more rarely, progressive renal failure with a decrease in urinary output. Renal colic is seldom noted. Ultrasonography may detect a lithiasis obstruction. Plain abdominal X-ray may show radio-opaque lithiasis. The diagnosis is scarcely based on EU but rather on antegrade pyelography, which most often is followed by percutaneous nephrostomy (Fig. 11.34). As for native kidneys, unenhanced CT allows detection on tiny ureteral stones (Fig. 11.35). In cases where access to the calculus may be achieved, a percutaneous nephrolithotomy may be attempted. If possible, the retrograde approach can complete treatment by ureteroscopy or push back the calculus toward the renal pelvis, thereby allowing access for further extracorporeal lithotripsy. This may, however, become difficult as a result of the interposition of the iliac crests.

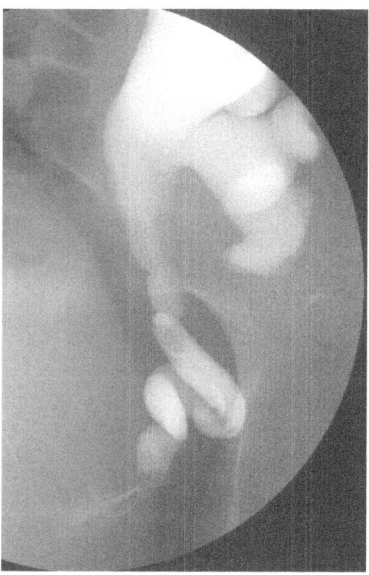

In some rare occasions the ureter presents endoluminal obstruction due to clots or mycelial fragments related to a urinary candidosis. Finally, the longer lifetime of the graft means one can consider the possible occurrence of a pathological condition proper to the ureter such as a tumor. The possibility of a pre-existing excreto-urinary tumor on the donor kidney should also be kept in mind.

Defective reconstruction of the anti-reflux system can occur and voiding cysto-ureterocystography is very useful to demonstrate vesico-ureteral reflux, particularly in cases of infectious parenchymatous disease of the transplanted kidney (Fig. 11.36).

Fig. 11.34. Uratic lithiasis of the uretero-vesical junction. AP shows ureterohydronephrosis and a lacunar image of the terminal part of the ureter

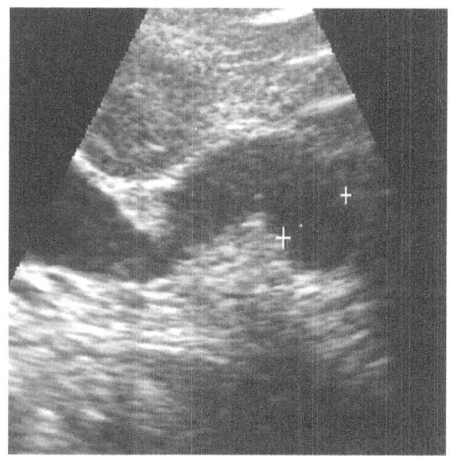
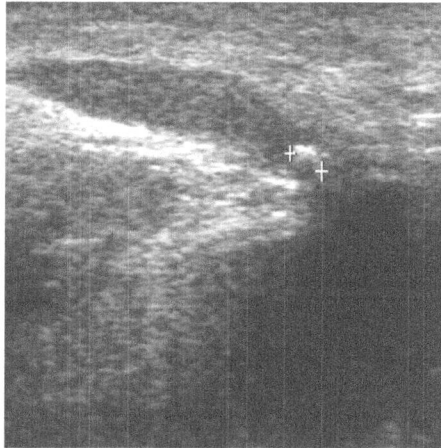

Fig. 11.35a–d. Uratic lithiasis of the uretero-vesical junction. **a** Dilatation of the ureter on ultrasonography. **b** Hyperechoic image of the terminal part of the ureter without evident acoustic shadowing. **c, d** Unenhanced CT axial slices showing the hyperdense intra-ureteral images (*arrows*) within the dilated ureter

a,b

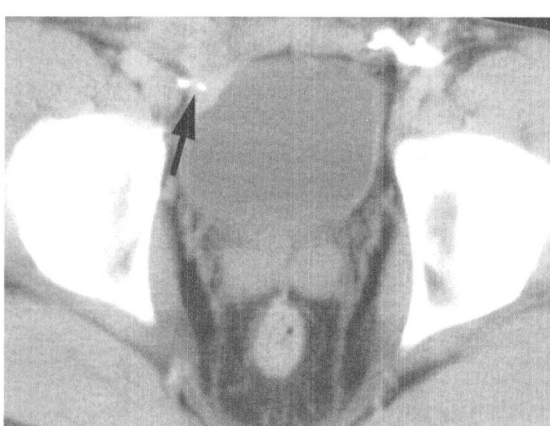
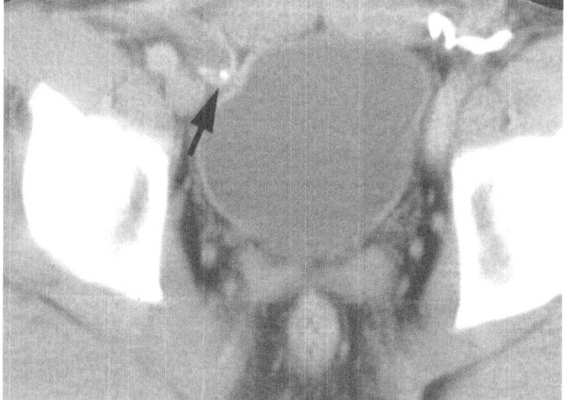

c   d

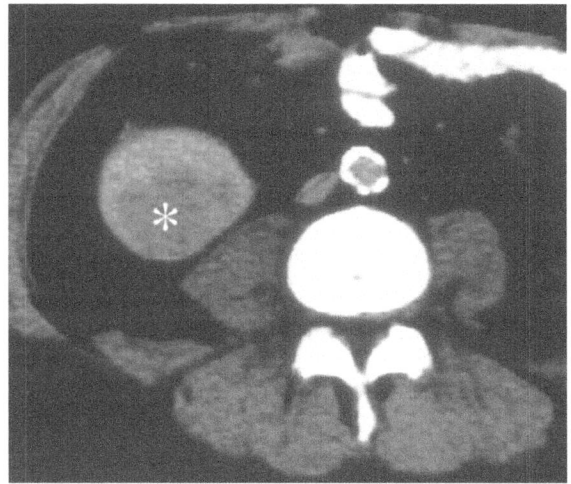
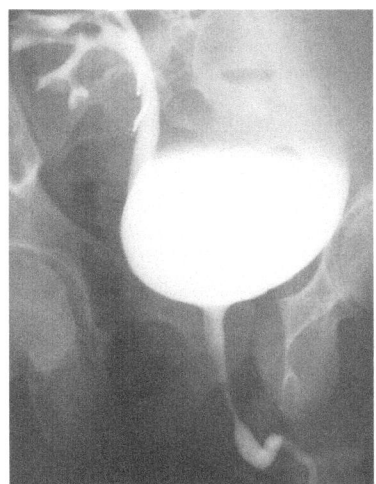

Fig. 11.36a, b. a axial CT slice on a male transplant recipient with symptoms of acute pyelonephritis. Presence of hypodense parenchymatous area of the upper pole of the kidney corresponding to focal pyelonephritis (*). b VCUG shows severe vesico-ureteral reflux

a,b

References

Affre J, Moreau JF, Kreis H et al (1978) Lithiase urinaire après transplantation rénale. Nouv Presse Med 7:3223

Amis ES, Pfister RC, Hendren WH (1981) Radiology of urinary undiversion. Urol Radiol 5:161–169

Amis ES Jr, Newhouse JH, Olsson CA (1988) Continent urinary diversions: review of surgical procedures and radiologic imaging. Radiology 168:395–401

Balchunas WR, Hill MC, Isikoff MB et al (1982) The clinical significance of dilatation of the collecting system in the transplanted kidney. J Clin Ultrasound 10:221–225

Banner MP, Pollack HM, Ring EJ et al (1983) Catheter dilatation of benign ureteral strictures. Radiology 147:427–433

Banner MP, Pollack HM, Bonavita JA et al (1984) The radiology of urinary diversions. Radiographics 4:885–913

Banner MP, Amendola MA, Pollack HM (1989) Anastomosed ureters: fluoroscopically guided transconduit retrograde catheterization. Radiology 170:45–49

Barbaric ZL, Thompson KR (1978) Percutaneous nephropyelostomy in the management of obstructed renal transplants. Radiology 126:639–642

Becker JA, Kutcher R (1978) Urologic complication of renal transplantation. Semin Roentgenol 13:341–351

Belitsky P, Klauber GT, Toth J et al (1972) Ureteral dynamics in human renal transplantation. A cineradiographic study. JAMA 220:1087–1089

Bennett LN, Voegeli DR, Crummy AB et al (1986) Urologic complications following renal transplantation: role of interventional radiologic procedures. Radiology 160:531–536

Brien G, Scholz D, Oesterwitz H et al (1980) Urolithiasis after kidney transplantation: clinical and mineralogical aspects. Urol Res 8:211–218

Bricker EM (1950) Bladder substitution after pelvic evisceration. Surg Clin North Am 30:1511–1521

Camey M (1985) Bladder replacement by ileal cystoplasty following radical cystectomy. World J Urol 3:161–166

Canton F, Gelet A, Bouchou F et al (1987) Les stenoses ureterales après transplantation rénale. J Urol 93:117–121

Coffey RC (1911) Physiologic implantation of the severed ureter or common bile duct in the intestine. JAMA 56:397

Cronan JJ, Amis ES, Scola FM et al (1986) Renal obstruction in patients with ileal loops: US evaluation. Radiology 158:647–648

Dorsam J, Knopp MV, Carl S et al (1997) Ureteral complications after kidney transplantation: evaluation with functional magnetic resonance urography. Transplant Prov 29:132–135

Dufour B (1973) Les obstructions de l'uretère lombo-iliaque. Association Française d'Urologie, Paris

Erb RE, Kaufman AJ, Kolhm O et al (1990) Adenocarcinoma in a sigmoid conduit: case report. Urol Radiol 12:115–117

Erlich RM, Melman A, Shinner DG (1978) The use of vesico psoas hitch in urologic surgery. J Urol 119:322–325

Fisch M, Wammack R, Steinbach F et al. (1993) Sigma-rectum pouch (Mainz Pouch II) Urol Cl North Amer 20:561–569

Flanagan FL, Fenlon HM, Breatnach E (1995) Ileal loop volvulus: a rare but reversible cause of bilateral ureteric obstruction. Clin Radiol 50:177–179

Frodin L, Wicklund H (1981) Computed tomography, ultrasonography and gamma camera scintigraphy after renal transplantation. Scand J Urol Nephrol 15:299–309

Gerbens D, Teyssou H, Manteau G et al (1980) Echotomographie et complications chirurgicales du rein transplanté. J Radiol 61:405–410

Ghasemian SM, Guleria AS, Khawand NY et al (1996) Diagnosis and management of urologic complications of renal transplantation. Clin Transplant 10:218–223

Glanz S, Rotter MR, Gordon DH et al (1985) Interventional radiologic procedures in the management of the renal transplant patient. Urol Radiol 7:97–105

Glass NR, Fisher DT, Lieberman R et al (1982) Management of ureteral obstruction after transplantation by percutaneous antegrade pyelography and pyelo-ureterostomy. Urology 20:15–19

Greenberg SH, Ring EJ, Oleaga JP et al (1980) Antegrade ureteral catheterization prior to complicated ureteral surgery. Urol Radiol 2:99–101

Grenier N, Douws C, Brichaux JC et al (1994) Imagerie du transplant rénal: technique radiologique. J Radiol 75: 19–24

Guerin C, Heritier P, Levigne F (1990) Les fistules urinaires après transplantation rénale. J Urol 96:75–80

Heckemann R, Hartman HG, Eickeniberg HW (1979) Combined ultrasound radiographic detection of ureteral obstruction in renal transplants. Urol Radiol 1:233–235

Hendaoui L, Hamida K, Souissia-M et al (2000) Radiologie de l'appareil urinaire opéré. Encycl Med Chir 34.380 A-10 21p

Hendren WH (1997) Historical perspectives of the use of bowel in urology. Urol Clin North Am 24:703–711

Heron SP, O'Brien DP, Whelchel JD et al (1995) Ureteral obstruction due to calculi in the early post-operative period in renal cadaveric transplantation: a case report and discussion of ureteral obstruction in the renal transplant patient. J Urol 153:1211–1213

Hricak H, Mark AS, Alpers CE et al (1986) Sonographic evaluation of the rejecting ureter. Urol Radiol 8:25–31

Hudson HC, Kramer SA, Anderson EE (1981) Identification of ureteroileal obstruction by retrograde loopography. Urology 17:147–148

Hunter DN, Castaneda-Zuniga WR, Coleman CC et al (1983) Percutaneous techniques in the management of urological complication in renal transplant patients. Radiology 148:407

Jaskowski A, Jones RM, Murie JA et al (1987) Urological complications in 600 consecutive renal transplants. Br J Surg 74:922–925

Kenney PJ, Hamrick KM, Samuels LJ et al (1980) Radiologic evaluation of continent urinary reservoirs. Radiographics 10:455–466

Keogan MT, Carr L, McDermott VG et al (1997) Continent urinary diversion procedures: radiographic appearance and potential complications. AJR 169:173–178

Kock NG (1982) Urinary diversion via a continent ileal reservoir: clinical results in 12 patients. J Urol 128:469

LaMasters D, Katzberg RW, Confer DJ et al (1980) Ureteropelvic fibrosis in renal transplants: radiographic manifestations. AJR 135:79–82

Lang EK (1986) Transluminal dilatation of uretero-pelvic junction strictures, ureteral strictures, and strictures at ureteroneocystostomy sites. Radiol Clin North Am 24: 601–613

Lerut J, Lerut T, Gruwez JA et al (1979) Case profile: donor graft lithiasis. Unusual complication of renal transplantation. Urology 14:627–628

Letourneau JG, Day DL, Feinberg SB (1987) Ultrasound and computed tomographic evaluation of renal transplantation. Radiol Clin North Am 25:267–279

Lhez A (1968) Les remplacements de l'uretère. Association Française d'Urologie, Paris

Lieberman RP, Crummy AB, Glass NR et al (1981) Fine needle antegrade pyelography in the renal transplants. J Urol 126: 155–158

Lieberman SF, Glass NR, Crummy RB et al (1982) Nonoperative percutaneous management of urinary fistulas and strictures in renal transplantation. Surg Gynecol Obstet 155:667

Lilien OM, Camey M (1984) 27 years experience with replacement of human bladder (Camey procedure). J Urol 132:886–891

Loughlin KR, Tilney NL, Richie JP (1984) Urologic complications in 718 renal transplant patients. Surgery 95:297–302

Martin EC, Fankuchen EI, Casarella WJ (1982) Percutaneous dilatation of ureteroenteric strictures or occlusions in ileal conduits. Urol Radiol 4:19–21

Mindell HJ, Quiogue T, Lebowitz RL (1990) Post-operative uroradiological appearances. In: Pollack HM (ed) Clinical urography. An atlas and text book of uro-radiological imaging, vol 3. Saunders, Philadelphia, pp 2510–2538

Mirvis SE, Whitley NO, Javadpour N et al (1987) Computed tomography of Kock and modified Kock continent ileal reservoir. Urology 29:361–367

Mitchell MF (1977) Ileal loop stenosis: a late complication of urinary diversion. J Urol 118:957–961

Montagne JP, Kressel HY, Moss AA et al (1978) Radiologic evaluation of the continent (Kock) ileostomy. Radiology 127:325–329

Mundy AR, Podesta ML, Bewick M et al (1981) The urological complications of 1000 renal transplants. Br J Urol 53:397–402

Ng C, Amis ES (1991) Radiology of continent urinary diversion. Radiol Clin North Am 29:557–569

Novick AC, Irish C, Steinmuller D et al (1981) The role of CT in renal transplantation patients. J Urol 125:15–18

Palestrant AM, de Wolf WC (1982) The pseudo-stricture of transplant ureteral torsion. Radiology 145:49–50

Palmer JM, Chatterjee SN (1978) Urologic complications in renal transplantation. Surg Clin North Am 58:305–319

Pearse HD, Barry JM, Fuchs EF (1985) Intra-operative consultation for the ureter. Urol Clin North Am 12:423–437

Pfister RC, Newhouse JH (1979) Interventional percutaneous pyeloureteral techniques I. Antegrade pyelography and ureteral perfusion. Radiol Clin North Am 17:351–363

Pidello R, Coulange C, Huguet JF (1986) Radiologie de l'appareil urinaire post-opéré chez l'adulte. Feuill Radiol 26:449–469

Princenthal RA, Lowman R, Zeman RK et al (1985) Ureterosigmoidostomy: the development of tumors, diagnosis and pitfalls. AJR 141:77–81

Quigg RJ, Idelson BA, Greengield A et al (1986) Transplant ureteral obstruction masquerading as recurrent rejection episodes. Management by percutaneous antegrade balloon dilatation. Am J Kidney Dis 8:67–70

Quinibi WY, Chavez A, Guerriero WG et al (1982) Renal transplant ureteric obstruction by peri-ureteric fibrosis. Am J Nephrol 2:91

Randall S, Preissig M (1974) The increased incidence of carcinoma of the colon following ureterosigmoidostomy. AJR 4:806–810

Rischman P (1983) Complications chirurgicales de la transplantation rénale. Doctoral thésis, University of Toulouse

Rosenberg JC, Arnstein Aring IS, Pierse JM Jr et al (1975) Calculi complicating a renal transplant. Am J Surg 129: 326–330

Roy C, Denys B, Campos M et al (1993) Tomodensitometrie de l'appareil urinaire opéré. Feuill Radiol 33:458–470

Sarramon JP (1973) Chirurgie de la voie excrétrice et abaissement rénal. J Urol Nephrol. 79:264–268

Sarramon JP, Conte J, Bouissou H (1971) Uretéro-iléoplastie: incidences urologiques et néphrologiques. Etude expérimentale chez 13 chiens. J Urol Nephrol 78:579–593

Sarramon JP, Lazorthes F, Lhez JM (1985) Restauration de la continuité urinaire et transplantation rénale. Ann Urol 19: 269–271

Schweizer RT, Bartus AS, Kahn CS (1977) Fibrosis of a renal transplant ureter. J Urol 117:125–126

Schiff M Jr (1978) Ureter in renal transplantation. Urology 12:256–260

Schiff M Jr, McGuire EJ, Weiss RM et al (1976) Management of urinary fistulas after renal transplantation. J Urol 115:251

Schiff M Jr, Rosenfield AT, McGuire FJ (1979) The use of percutaneous antegrade renal perfusion in kidney transplant recipients. J Urol 122:246–248

Schmeller NT, Schuller J, Hofstetter A et al (1985) Fine needle antegrade pyelography of transplanted kidney. Urol Radiol 7:19–22

Schmidt JD, Hawtrey CE, Flocks RH et al (1973) Complications, results and problems of ileal conduit diversion. J Urol 109:210–216

Schubert RA, Gockeritz s, Mentzel HJ et al (2000) Imaging in ureteral complications of renal transplantation: value of static fluid MR urography. Eur Radiol 10:1152–1157

Shapiro MJ, Banner MP, Amendola MA et al (1988) Balloon catheter dilation of ureteroenteric strictures: long-term results. Radiology 168:385–387

Skinner DG, Lieskowsky G, Boyd SM (1987) Continuing experience with continent ileal reservoir (Kock pouch) as an alternative to cutaneous urinary diversion: an update after 250 cases. J Urol 137:1140–1145

Smith TP, Hunter DW, Letourneau JG et al (1988a) Urinary obstruction in renal transplants: diagnosis by antegrade pyelography and results of percutaneous treatment. AJR 151:507–510

Smith TP, Hunter DW, Letourneau JG et al (1988b) Urine leaks after renal transplantation: value of percutaneous pyelography and drainage for diagnosis and treatment. AJR 151:511–513

Solovay J (1974) Advantages of the prone position for the excreting urogram in ileal conduit urinary diversion. J Urol 4:530–537

Spigos DG, Tan W, Pavel DG et al (1977) Diagnosis of urine extravasation after renal transplantation. AJR 129:409–413

Stratton JA, McMillan A, Morley P (1989) Ultrasound in suspected obstruction complicating renal transplantation. Br J Radiol 62:803–806

Streem SB, Novick AC, Steinmuller DR et al (1988) Percutaneous treatment of urologic complications following renal transplantation. World J Urol 6:95–100

Stuck KJ, Jafri SZH, Adler DD et al (1986) Ultrasound evaluation of uncommon renal transplant complication. Urol Radiol 8:6–12

Sullivan JW, Grabstald H, Whitmore WJ Jr (1980) Complications of uretero-ileal conduit with radical cystectomy: review of 336 cases. J Urol 124:797–801

Texter JH Jr, Bobinsky G, Broecker B (1974) Ureteral rejection in isolated allograft ureter. Urology 4:37

Thuroff JW, Alken P, Riedmiller H et al (1985) The Mainz Pouch (mixed augmentation ileum and caecum) for bladder augmentation and continent diversion. World J Urol 3:179–184

Van Gansbeke D, Zalcman M, Matos C et al (1985) Lithiasic complications of renal transplantation. The donor graft lithiasis concept. Urol Radiol 7:157–160

Voegeli DR, Crummy AB, McDermott JC et al (1988) Percutaneous dilation of ureteral strictures in renal transplant patients. Radiology 169:185–188

Webster GD, Henry HH, Tomlin EM (1987) Calculus formation and ureteral obstruction after ileal conduit constriction using autosuture and strapping devices. Urology 30:571–573

Whitaker RH (1973) Method of assessing obstruction in dilated ureter. Br J Urol 45:15–22

Whitaker RH (1979) The Whitaker test. Urol Clin North Am 6:529–539

Woods JE, Deweerd JH, Leary FF (1973) The allograft ureter. J Urol 109:958

Zincke H, Woods JE, Hattery RR et al (1975) Experience with lymphocele after renal transplantation. Surgery 77:444–450

Zincke H, Woods JE, Hattery RR et al (1977) Late ureteral obstruction mimicking rejection after renal transplantation. Urology 9:504–508

Zollikofer CL, Bruhlmann WF, Baumgartner D (1985) Antegrade pyelography, percutaneous nephrostomy and ureteral perfusion Whitaker test for the renal transplant recipient. ROFO Fortschr Geb Rontgenstr Nuklearmed 142:193–200

12 Interventional Radiology of the Ureter

H. Rousseau, M. I. Millan, L. Bouchard, M. Soulie, F. Joffre, T. Smayra

More than 40 years have passed since Goodwin reported on "percutaneous trocar (needle) nephrostomy in hydronephrosis" (Goodwin et al. 1955). The introduction and acceptance of this procedure as a safe and effective alternative to surgical nephrostomy served as the impetus for the development and expansion of an ever-increasing number of techniques that are encompassed by the term "interventional uroradiology". Percutaneous nephrostomy (PCN) has become an indispensable part of the diagnosis and management of a wide variety of urologic problems. This simple technique can be performed under local anesthesia and should be part of every radiologist's training. Percutaneous renal access makes it possible to perform many endourologic procedures: urinary diversion in supravesical obstruction or fistula management, adjunct therapy for complex infections, treatment of calculus disease in primary therapy or combined with extracorporeal shock-wave lithotripsy (ESWL), and diagnostic or therapeutic nephroscopy and ureteroscopy. Among these, ureteral interventions are the most frequent.

H. Rousseau, MD; M. I. Millan, MD; L. Bouchard, MD; F. Joffre, MD; T. Smayra, MD
Service de Radiologie, Hôpital de Rangueil, 1, avenue Jean-Poulhès, 31403 Toulouse Cédex 4, France
M. Soulie, MD
Service d'Urologie, CHU Rangueil, 1, avenue Jean-Poulhès, 31403 Toulouse Cédex 4, France

12.1
Principles of Percutaneous Renal Access

The main prerequisite to interventional uroradiologic procedures is the creation of an appropriate PCN tract. The reasons for and the potential complications of the intervention should be discussed with the patient. Familiarity with basic renal anatomy is necessary to select a safe route for renal entry. Posterior relationships with the 12th rib, pleural reflection line, colon, spleen, liver, and lobar vascular distribution are important points to take into account (Joffre et al. 1995).

The percutaneous access must follow certain important rules to avoid problems and/or complications (Dyer et al. 1997): (a) The posterior calices of the middle part are the best site for a safe and efficient approach to ureter. (b) The puncture site should be generally below the 12th rib at the lateral border of the paraspinal muscle. (c) A transparenchymal posterolateral approach is mandatory near Brodel's avascular line.

For accessing the intrarenal collecting system and guiding the puncture, all imaging modalities have been used (Joffre et al. 1990). Both ultrasonography and fluoroscopy have their advantages. The best situation is to have both modalities available. In a very dilated collecting system, ultrasound may be used alone. In the less dilated system, while ultrasound is good for directing the needle into the calyx, fluoroscopy is helpful to confirm the final needle position. Fluoroscopy may be used alone following intravenous contrast opacification. However, when the kidney is obstructed or poorly functioning, opacification of the collecting system may be delayed or insufficient. Direct opacification by fine-needle antegrade pyelography or by retrograde catheterization is useful in certain circumstances, particularly for antegrade endoureteral intervention in the nondilated upper collecting system. It may help to distend the collecting system to facilitate guidewire entry into the renal pelvis.

CT scanning may be useful for placing the definitive puncture needle in patients with renal ectopia or pathologic renal displacement (Barbaric et al. 1997;

Bohlman et al. 1998; Lemaitre et al. 2000). MR guidance has been studied experimentally and could have the advantage of accurately guiding the puncture even in the nondilated urinary tract (Nolte-Ernsting et al. 1999).

Local anesthesia, intravenous sedation, and analgesia are generally used. General anesthesia is rarely necessary, except for complex endourologic interventions. Care should be taken to prevent overdistension of the obstructed collecting system, especially if infection is present (Pollard and Nicholson 1994). Urine should be aspirated and a lesser volume of contrast medium used for opacification to prevent extravasation of infected urine with potential bacteremia. The plasma creatinine level and urinalysis are needed to determine the most appropriate diagnostic and therapeutic strategy. A severe disposition to bleeding or abnormal clotting parameters are relative contraindications, but they are usually correctable with vitamin K or fresh-frozen plasma and platelet infusion.

12.2
Ureteral Interventions

12.2.1
Ureteral Strictures

When planning therapy for a ureteral stricture, the first question to answer is whether the stricture is due to benign or malignant disease. Interventional diagnostic techniques such as endoluminal brushing or percutaneous guided biopsy at the site of the stricture have been proposed to determine the exact nature of the stricture.

Ureteral strictures caused by extrinsic compression, ureteral encasement, or direct invasion from a malignancy are generally approached by retrograde techniques, using an internal 2-J catheter to relieve obstruction. Retrograde ureteral catheterization without cystoscopic assistance has been described but remains reserved for centers without urologic facilities or for patients with uretero-ileal anastomosis (Babel and Winterkorn 1993; Banner et al. 1989; Wetton and Gedroyc 1995; Zaleski et al. 1998). If retrograde 2-J placement is not successful or presumed difficult, antegrade ureteral catheterization can be done (Fig. 12.1a, b). In patients with multiple sites of obstruction, or in cases of obstruction associated with very dilated and tortuous ureters, a primary antegrade approach may be useful (Kenny et al. 1995). In case of pyonephrosis the choice of an antegrade approach is still being debated.

Malignant strictures generally require permanent internal drainage. Permanent external nephrostomy drainage is usually done if internal drainage is unsuccessful (Banner et al. 1991). Most patients prefer internal drainage over a PCN catheter for obvious practical, psychological, and cosmetic reasons (Evans et al. 1988). However, patients with severe bladder disease are better managed with permanent PCN.

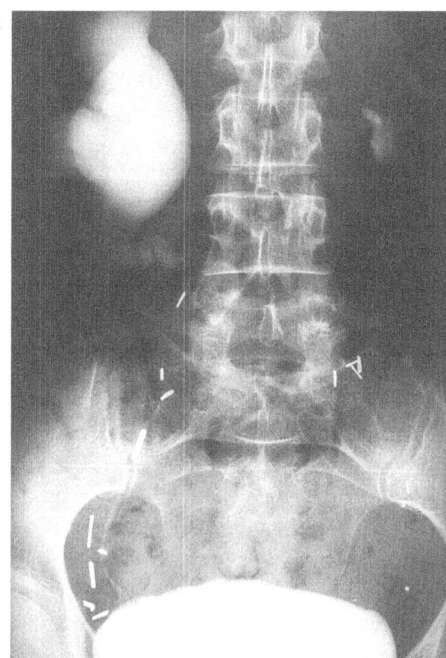
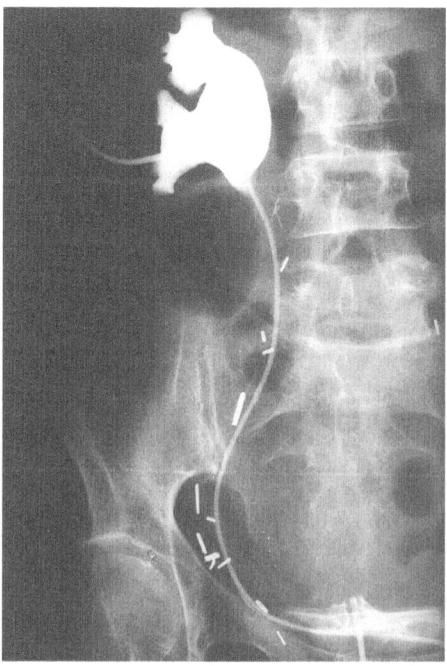

Fig. 12.1. a EU shows a chronic obstruction of the upper urinary tract secondary to postoperative recurrence of a retroperitoneal malignant histiosarcoma. **b** Antegrade pyelography via the nephrostomy catheter, after ureteral intubation with a 2-J pyelovesical catheter. Antegrade approach was used after failure of retrograde catheterization

Most strictures (80%) can be crossed by using standard curved angiographic catheters, such as multipurpose or cobra catheters, and a hydrophilic-coated guidewire (DYER et al. 1997). In patients with markedly dilated and tortuous ureters, external urinary drainage for several days, possibly in combination with corticosteroids (prior to a new attempt at ureteral negotiation), often improves ureteral architecture and the chance for ureteral catheterization. If a distal ureteral malignant stricture is difficult to cross, a paraureteral tract can be made by perforating the bladder wall with a stiff guidewire or a transseptal stylet (LANG 1987) or by electrocauterization of the tract, creating a ureteroneocystostomy (CORNUD et al. 1991).

Once the catheter and guidewire have been successfully advanced into the bladder, the guidewire is removed and contrast medium is injected to confirm the intravesical position. A stiff guidewire is then advanced through the angiographic catheter, which is removed after the distance between pelvis and bladder has been measured. If the stricture is very tight, is it often helpful to pre-dilate before internal drainage catheter placement. In addition, inserting a thin-walled sheath through the cutaneous tract into the renal pelvis or proximal ureter often facilitates 2-J placement (MITTY et al. 1986). Also available are long peel-away sheaths that can be used for stiffening purposes, when placed throughout the urinary tract from the PCN tract to the distal ureter. In very tight obstructions a "through-and-through" technique is performed, with endoscopic retrieval of the guidewire from the bladder and through the urethra, allowing retrograde placement of the 2-J with control of the guide at the flank and the urethral sites (HOLMES et al. 1993) (Fig. 12.2a–f.). The drainage catheter is then passed over the guidewire and the distal loop is allowed to form in the bladder. The proximal position of the stent is then assessed fluoroscopically. The guidewire is withdrawn as the pusher deploys the proximal loop in the renal pelvis. In case of inadequate catheter positioning the interventionist can pull back the 2-J with a removable suture attached to the proximal extremity of the catheter. An external catheter is routinely left in the intrarenal collecting system for 24–48 h following internal drainage. A nephrostogram is performed to confirm adequate positioning of the proximal and distal loop of the 2 J. After 12–24 h of external drainage to allow clearance of blood and debris, the nephrostomy tube can be clamped to assess antegrade flow via the newly placed drainage catheter. Before the nephrostomy tube is removed, a contrast nephrostogram should be obtained to verify catheter permeability. Nephrostomy tube removal should be done under fluoroscopic guidance to prevent inadvertent dislodgment of the 2 J. Routine 2 J exchange can be done by cystoscopy.

For patients with malignant strictures, ureteral catheter drainage is the appropriate technique, but a preceding multidisciplinary discussion is desirable to assess the benefit of drainage with regard to the presumed survival of the patient (GASPARINI et al. 1991; KENNY et al. 1995). Ureteral catheter drainage is not the optimal therapy for benign strictures, many of which are suitable for balloon catheter dilatation and/or endourologic incision. Balloon dilatation of the stricture followed by uretero-intestinal drainage may provide long-term success, defined as the absence of recurrence after 6 months (LANG and GLORIOSO 1988). Three main factors have an important influence on patency: duration and length of the stenosis, vascular supply status of the ureter: A short (less than 3 cm), recent (less than 3 months old), distal, postoperative stenosis without significant devascularization is the best indication for ureteral dilatation. Old, cicatricial, post-radiation strictures are more refractory to this treatment approach. While encouraging results were reported, with a primary success rate superior to 70% after a 1-year follow-up, the majority of authors postulate that the recurrence rate is better than 50% (SHAPIRO et al. 1988; RAVERY et al. 1998). Despite these variable results, it is worthwhile to propose this therapeutic approach for all benign strictures, combined with ureteral stenting, which represents the main alternative therapeutic choice in case of failure and is preferable to additional surgery (Figs. 12.3a–e; 12.4a–c)

Once the stricture has been crossed by the guidewire, the balloon dilatation catheter is advanced across the stricture and then inflated under fluoroscopic control (BECKMAN et al. 1989). Inflation usually lasts 1 min, and several sessions may be necessary (KWAK et al. 1995). Balloon dilatation is performed with high-pressure balloons 6–8 mm in diameter at more than 15 atm (JOHNSON et al. 1991). After dilatation, an 8-F internal drainage catheter is kept in place for 6 weeks to maintain luminal patency while the ureteral musculature heals (POCOCK et al. 1986). If the post-dilatation pyelographic control is acceptable, ureteral intubation can sometimes be avoided (Fig. 12.5). When further manipulations are necessary, an internal-external drainage catheter is used. These internal-external drains are useful for patients who require long-term stenting or for whom difficult cystoscopic maintenance is anticipated.

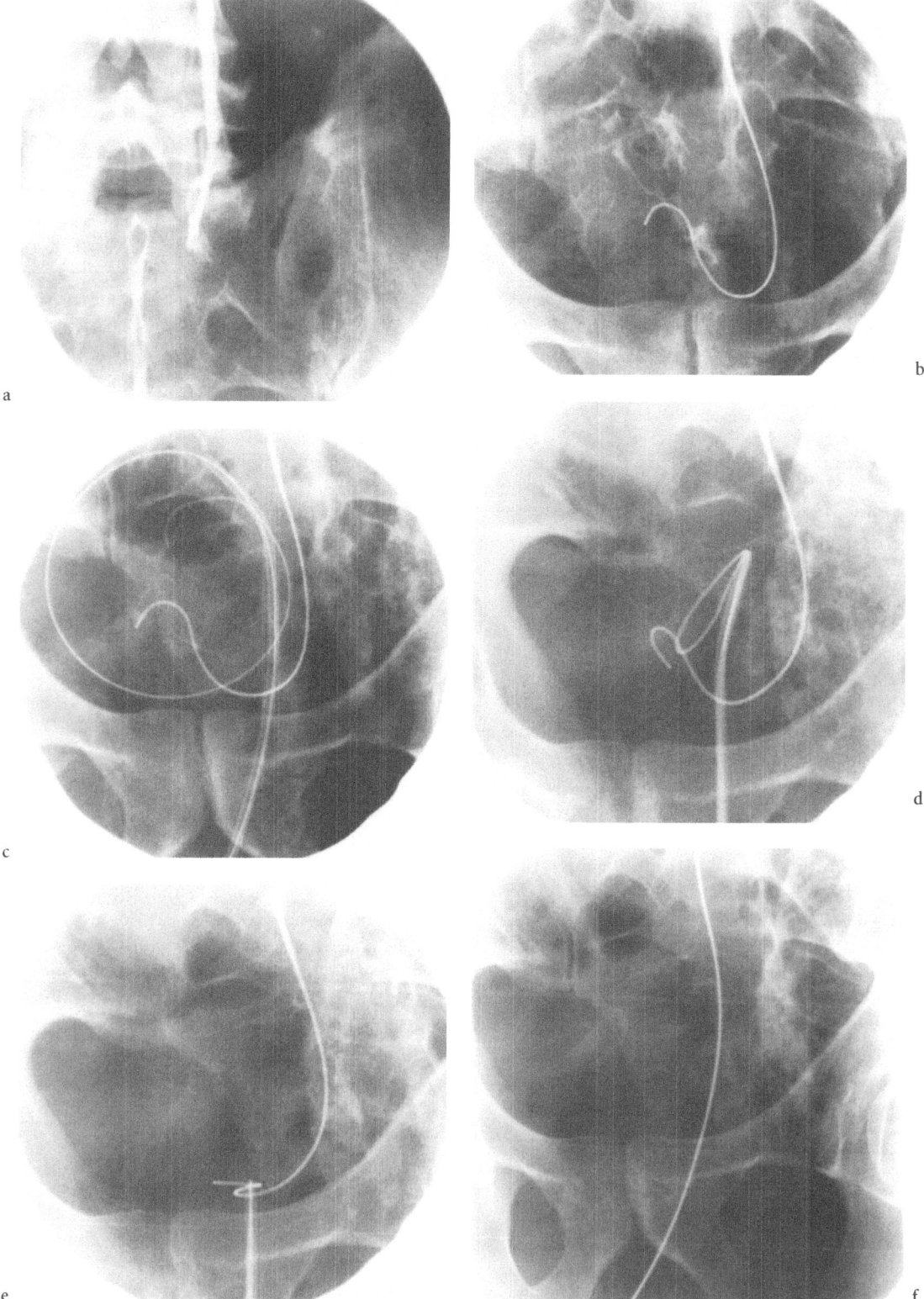

Fig. 12.2. a "Through and through" technique without endoscopy for a distal and total neoplastic ureteral stenosis in a female patient. **b** This stenosis was negotiated with only a hydrophilic guidewire, which was placed into the bladder. **c** Transurethral placement of a catheter into the bladder. **d** Introduction of a snare guidewire in the bladder. **e** The snare grasps the ureteral guidewire. **f** Transurethral extraction of the ureteral guidewire, which will allow the retrograde introduction of a 2-J catheter

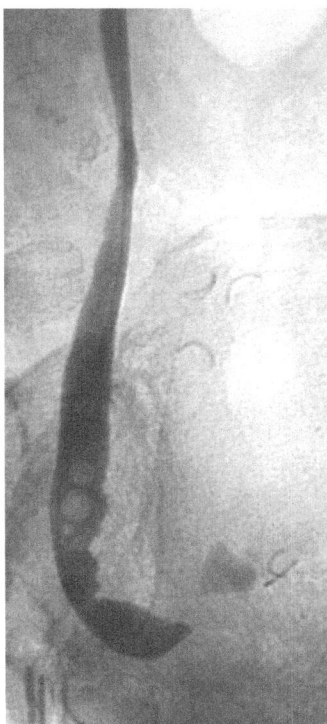

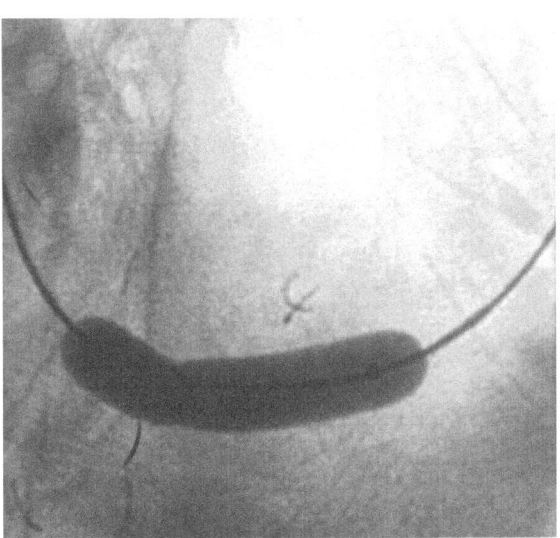

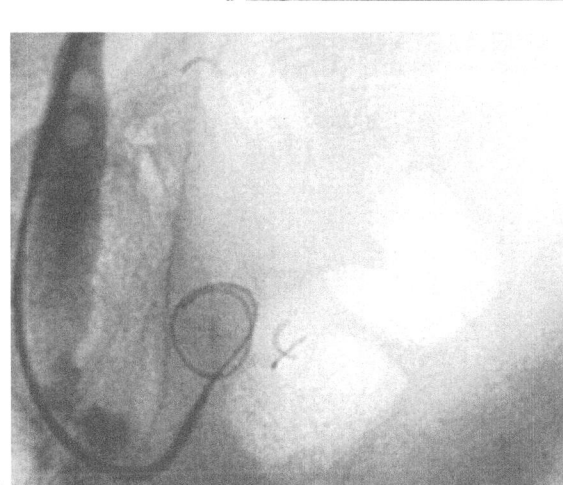

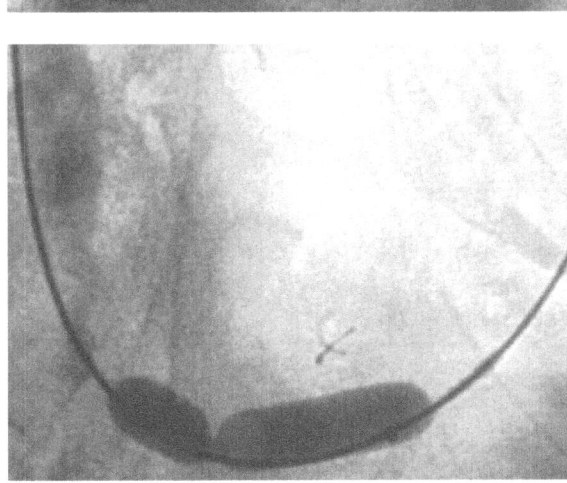

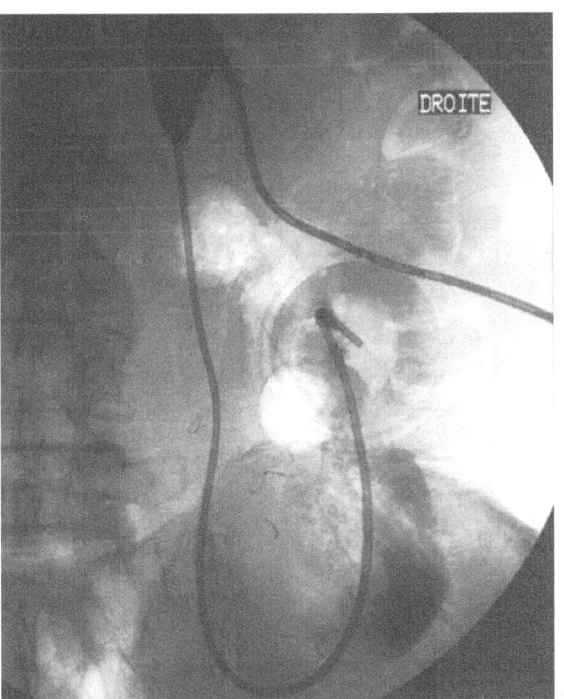

Fig. 12.3a–e. Dilatation of a right stenotic uretero-enteric anastomosis. **a** Antegrade pyelography (prone position) showing absence of opacification of the anastomosis. **b** Catheterization with a cobra catheter and a hydrophilic guidewire. **c** Balloon dilatation (6 atm) of the stenotic area: presence of a wasp-waisted print related to a tight stenosis. **d** Disappearance of the print after high pressure inflation. **e** Control after 2-J catheter placement (prone proposition)

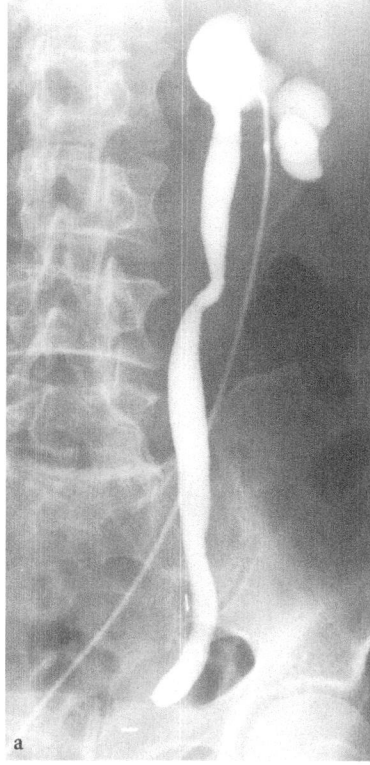
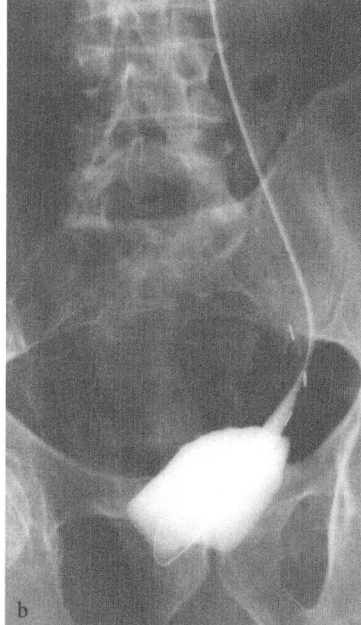
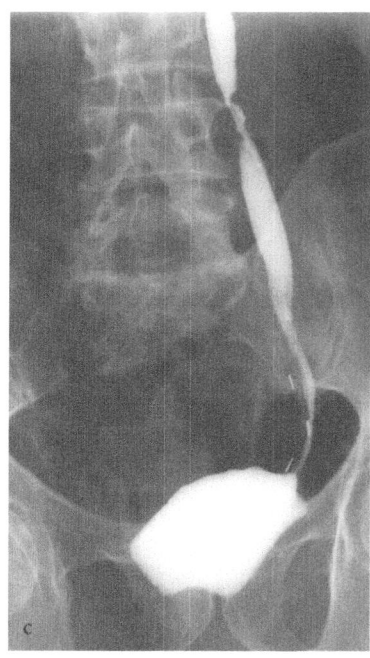

Fig. 12.4a–c. Dilatation of a right benign postoperative stenosis after surgery and radiotherapy for carcinoma of the cervix. **a** Antegrade pyelography (prone position) showing total occlusion of the distal part of the ureter. **b** High-pressure dilatation (15 atm) of the stenotic area. **c** Control after 2-J catheterization: poor patency of the distal ureter

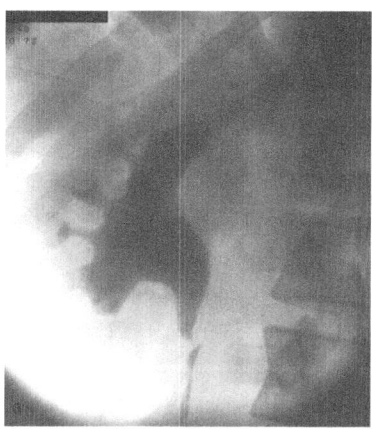
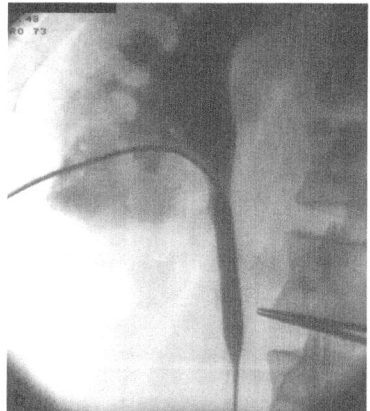
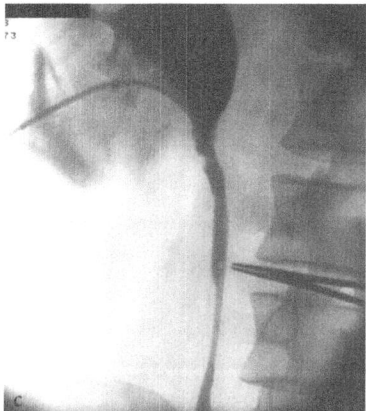

Fig. 12.5a–c. Ureteral stenosis secondary to ureterotomy for lithiasis. **a** Urographic demonstration of a centered and localized stenosis of the proximal lumbar ureter. **b** Balloon dilatation of the stenotic area. **c** Pyelographic control shows excellent patency, making it unnecessary to perform 2-J placement

Balloon dilatation with 2-J placement appears to be the appropriate initial therapy for most benign ureteral strictures and does not preclude later surgical intervention. After successful treatment, careful monitoring is mandatory because a clinically silent recurrence is possible.

The use of a ureteral internal drainage catheter can be associated with complications. Microscopic hematuria, pyuria, lower abdominal pain, dysuria, urinary frequency, nocturia, and flank pain on voiding are frequent. Catheter migration and secondary ureteral fibrosis can occur (CULKIN et al. 1992). Catheter encrustation is unavoidable with all types of 2-J catheters but can be minimized with a high output of noninfected acid urine (SALTZMAN 1988). 2-J catheters should be replaced at least every 6 months, and more frequently in patients who form stones (SOMERS 1996). Bladder disease (fistula, hemorrhagic or radiation cystitis, large tumoral involvement) or pelvic masses with bladder compression are generally contraindications to internal ureteral drainage.

The effectiveness of the internal drainage catheter is not completely understood but is probably linked to drainage around the catheter. This is one of the reasons why internal ureteral drainage catheters may not drain kidneys as well as PCN. In case of persistent hydronephrosis, 2-J obstruction should be suspected. No universally accepted method exists for determining 2-J patency (DYER et al. 1997). It was recently demonstrated that the identification of encrustation of ureteral stents is possible with detection of twinkling artifact using color-flow Doppler ultrasonography (TRILLAUD et al. 2001). Cystoscopic 2-J exchange is often required when the issue cannot be resolved. Fluoroscopically guided 2-J exchange is possible mainly in women (BREEN and COWAN 1995) (Figs. 12.6a–d; 12.7a–e). For better patient comfort and to avoid multiple exchange of ureteral catheters, a radiosurgical technique was described which consists of a subcutaneously placed catheter between the pelvis and the bladder (COCKBURN et al. 1997).

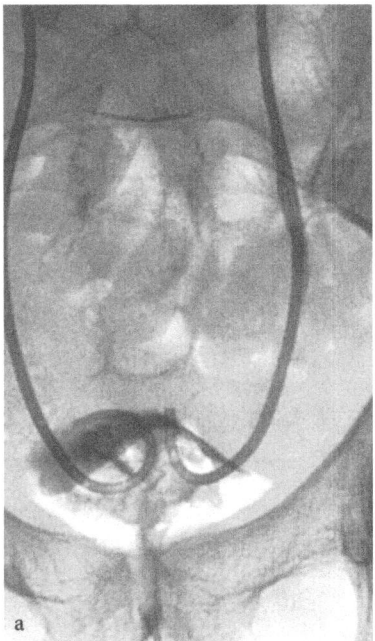
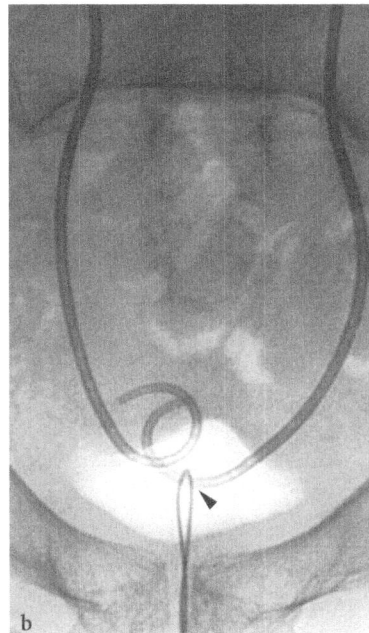
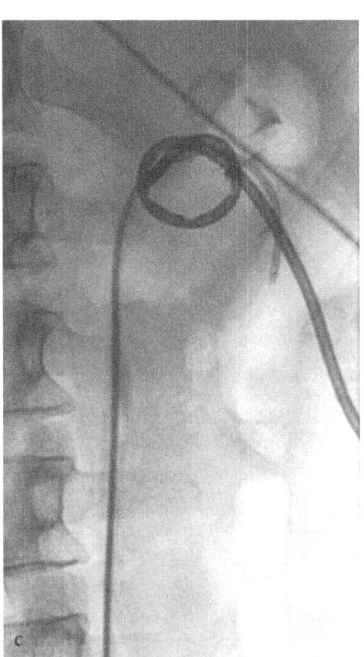
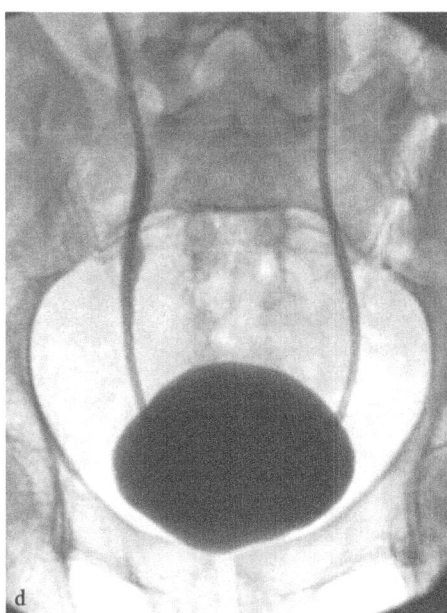

Fig. 12.6a–d. Transurethral retrograde replacement of an occluded 2-J catheter in a woman. a Occlusion of the 2-J catheter. b Transurethral extraction of the 2-J catheter with a snare guidewire (*arrowhead*). c Retrograde placement of a guidewire into the left pelvis to place a new 2-J catheter. d Control after changing the left 2-J catheter

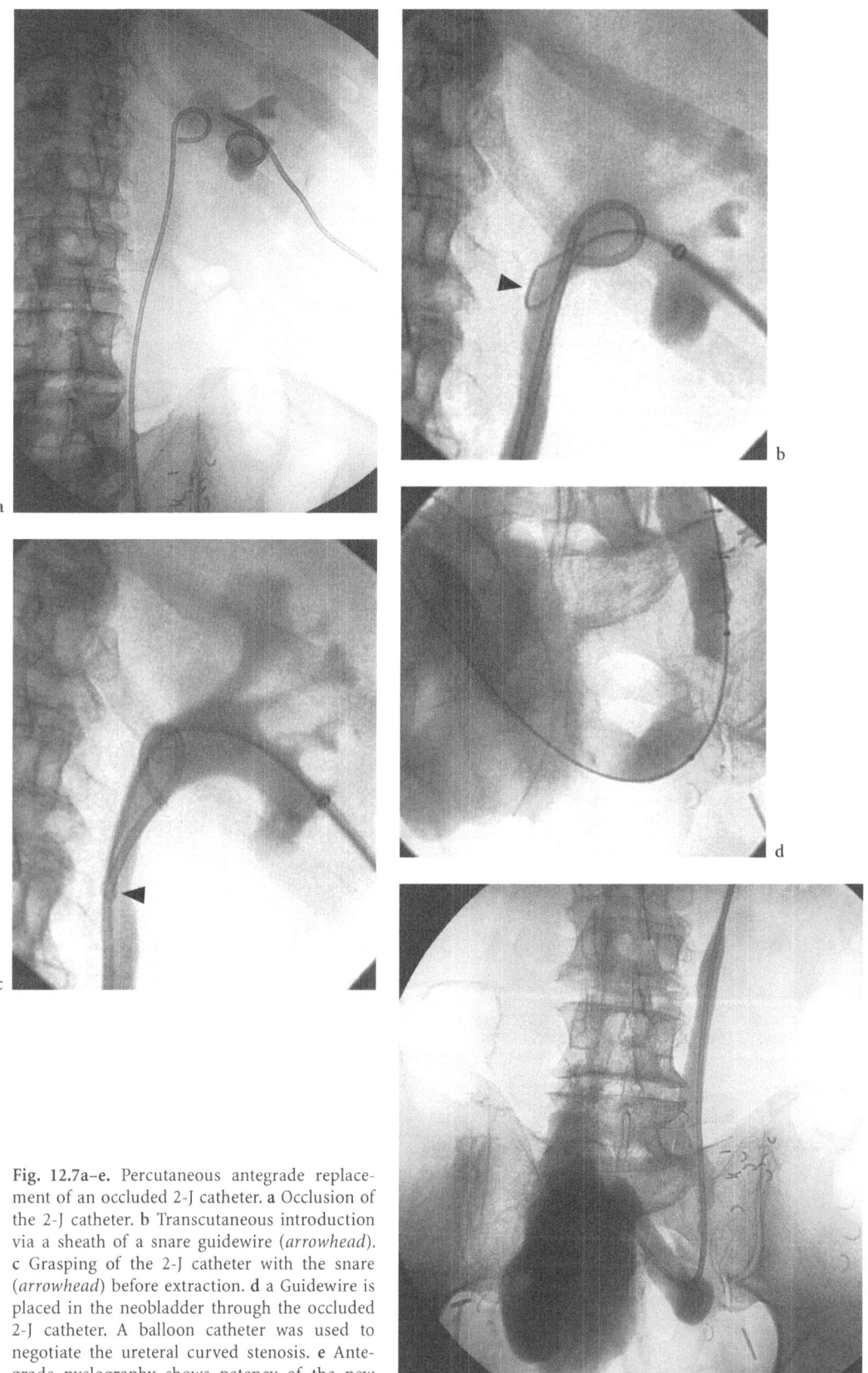

Fig. 12.7a–e. Percutaneous antegrade replacement of an occluded 2-J catheter. **a** Occlusion of the 2-J catheter. **b** Transcutaneous introduction via a sheath of a snare guidewire (*arrowhead*). **c** Grasping of the 2-J catheter with the snare (*arrowhead*) before extraction. **d** A guidewire is placed in the neobladder through the occluded 2-J catheter. A balloon catheter was used to negotiate the ureteral curved stenosis. **e** Antegrade pyelography shows patency of the new 2-J catheter

The high potential for failure or recurrence after balloon dilatation has led to the proposal of other technical modalities, such as electroincision or placement of a metallic stent.

Electroincision was first proposed by CORNUD (CORNUD et al. 1992). Recently, this author reported a series of 37 patients with strictures of uroenteric anastomoses percutaneously treated with a cutting balloon catheter that had a long-term actuarial patency of 77% at 1 year and 62% at 3 years. This percutaneous technique is much simpler than retrograde endoscopic guidance (CORNUD et al. 2000). The procedure is safe if CT has confirmed the absence of potentially risky neighboring vital structures such as aorto-iliac vessels (KABALIN 1997).

The use of metallic stents in ureteral stenosis has been described by several authors (REINBERG et al. 1994; VAN SONNENBERG et al. 1994). These self-expanding metallic stents usually have a diameter of 7 mm and a length adapted to the length of the stenosis. Post-implantation experimental studies showed acute hyperplasia inside the stent (HEKIMOGLU et al. 1996). The main reason probably is the radial pressure against the wall, which causes irritation and inhibition of peristalsis (MURPHY 1999). Moreover, encrustation of the stent and tumor overgrowth through the wire meshes may affect its use and long-term patency. The mid-term patency is similar (64% at 6 months) or inferior to that of 2-J catheters (31% at 1 year) (LUGMAYR and PAUER 1996; POLLAK et al. 1995) (Fig. 12.8a–e). These poor results explain why almost all authors never use metallic stents for benign stenosis. In case of malignant stenosis, the results seem better, particularly if temporary 2-J catheters are used. Metallic stents can then play a palliative role in the treatment of some of these patients (MURPHY 1999; FLUECKIGER et al. 1993)

12.2.2
Urinary Fistulae

Urinary fistulae of ureteral origin in patients with advanced (and often incurable) abdominal, retroperitoneal, or pelvic malignancies are among the most difficult therapeutic problems for the interventional radiologist. They occur most often in patients with recurrent uterine or colorectal malignancies, most of whom have previously undergone many surgical procedures and/or radiation therapy for local cancer recurrence. Surgical treatment of fistulae is often difficult and leads to a 20% nephrectomy rate. Failure of retrograde intubation occurs in approximately

40%–60% of cases (DRUY et al. 1983). Percutaneous treatment has several advantages (MAILLET et al. 1987):
- Possibilities of antegrade opacification, which allows fistula follow-up,
- Less risk of infection,
- Catheter-induced endothelialization and remodeling of the defect.

Small leaks are often successfully managed by simple external urinary drainage (DYER et al. 1997). When large ureteral leaks occur without obstruction, stent placement across the site of leakage is beneficial in many ways (Fig. 12.9a, b). Antegrade placement is more easy and accurate compared with the retrograde approach, but in difficult cases combined antegrade and retrograde techniques with the internal "rendezvous" technique, using a loop snare, can be considered (DE BAERE et al. 1995).

The presence of the catheter accelerates bridging of the ureteral defect by transitional epithelium growth. It reduces outflow through the defect and provides a strut to prevent stricture during the healing process (MAILLET et al. 1987). Urinary leaks can be associated with a urinoma: Percutaneous drainage of it may be helpful to reduce distortion of the segments proximal and distal to the site of leakage and can therefore facilitate catheterization. An internal-external or preferably 2 J catheter is favored for these patients (CHANG et al. 1987). External drainage is removed only when closure of the fistula is confirmed by contrast studies. Using Lang's criteria (closure of the fistula, absence of ureteral stenosis, persistence of a functioning kidney), a successful intervention can be expected in approximately 70% of cases (LANG 1984). However, the cause and age of the fistula influence the rate of success: A higher rate of failure is observed in patients with a history of gynecologic surgery for cancer than in patients with fistulae secondary to uretero-intestinal anastomosis. Persisting fistulae were noted in 43% of a series of 72 cancer patients. Residual ureteral stenosis occurred in 19%. These results can be explained largely by the history of previous surgery and/or radiotherapy (DE BAERE et al. 1995). In case of nonevolutive disease, patients with persisting fistulae can be referred to surgery for ureteral diversion.

Special care should be taken in patients with ureteroenteric anastomosis leaks. Draining tubes must be of sufficient length to bring the distal draining portion into the pyeloureterostomy bag, with no holes in the stent along the ureteroenteric leak or within the bowel conduit, because mucus forming

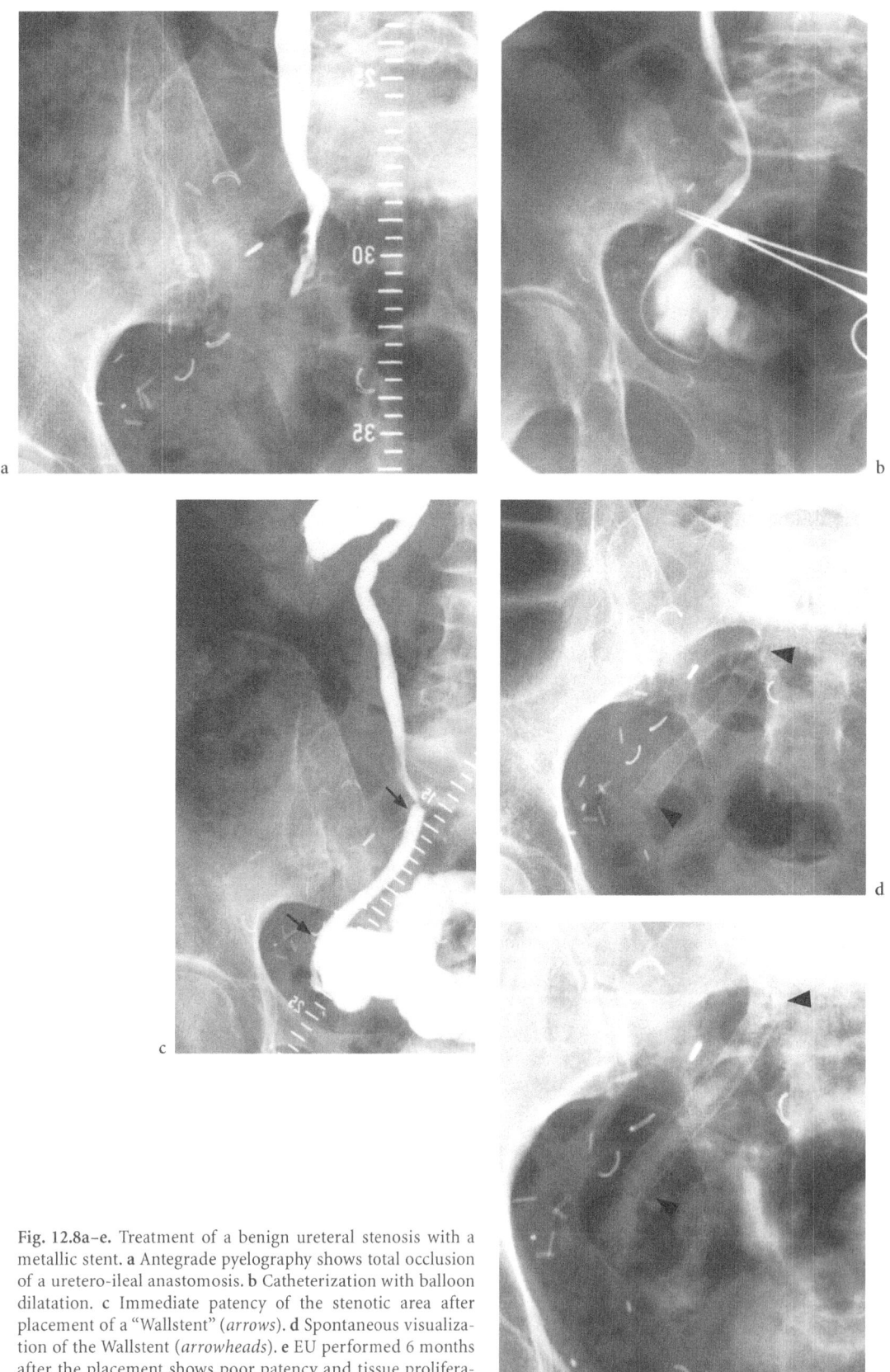

Fig. 12.8a–e. Treatment of a benign ureteral stenosis with a metallic stent. **a** Antegrade pyelography shows total occlusion of a uretero-ileal anastomosis. **b** Catheterization with balloon dilatation. **c** Immediate patency of the stenotic area after placement of a "Wallstent" (*arrows*). **d** Spontaneous visualization of the Wallstent (*arrowheads*). **e** EU performed 6 months after the placement shows poor patency and tissue proliferation inside the stent (*arrowheads*)

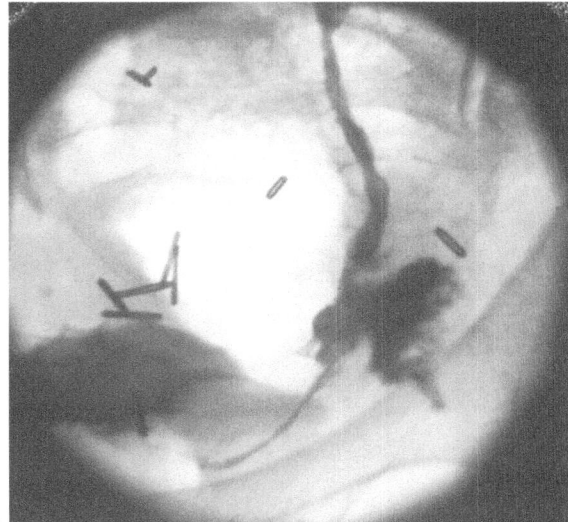

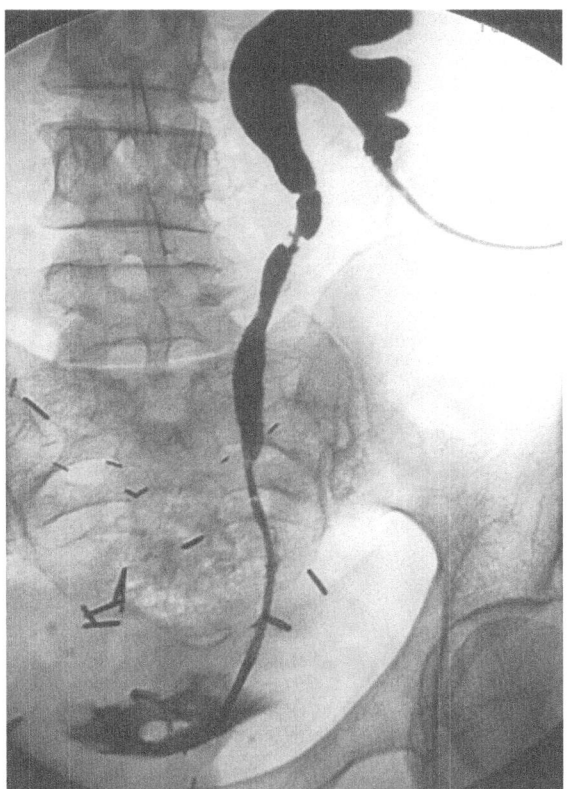

Fig. 12.9. a Antegrade pyelography shows a postoperative ureteral fistula. b Disappearance of the leakage after placement of a 2-J pyelo-vesical catheter

within the conduit can obstruct the holes, and this may lead to acute urinary tract obstruction and sepsis. Percutaneous endourologic management of urinary fistula requires patience. Complete closure of the fistula may require several months.

Temporary or permanent ureteral occlusion may be necessary for some patients in whom fistulae develop. Temporary occlusions with special catheter techniques, including occlusion with a nondetachable balloon catheter, may be appropriate for patients in whom rapid healing is anticipated, or in cases of large leak or after failure of a 2 J (PAPANICOLAOU et al. 1985) (Fig. 12.10a, b). In patients with high-output fistulae, for which conservative management has been ineffective, or in patients too ill for more radical interventions, permanent occlusion of the ureter may be more appropriate. Methods of permanent occlusion with detachable balloons, tissue adhesives, electrocautery and "nest" of coils, and Gelfoam, as well as percutaneous ureteral clipping have been described (BING et al. 1992; CASTANEDA et al. 1989; CRAGG et al. 1989) (Figs. 12.11a–c; 12.12a, b). All these techniques imply permanent external urinary drainage after ureteral occlusion, except in cases of poorly functioning or nonfunctioning kidneys.

Renal arterial embolization is yet another technique for managing intractable ureteral fistulae by obliterating renal function (SCHILD et al. 1994). Bilateral temporary ureteral occlusion with a similar technique can be useful in case of large bladder fistula.

12.2.3
Percutaneous Procedures for Lithiasis

ESWL has established itself as the preferred method of treatment for most symptomatic renal and proximal ureteral calculi (CHAUSSY et al. 1984); it can effectively treat 70%–80% of such cases. When combined with adjunctive endourologic and percutaneous procedures, ESWL can be used to treat over 90% of patients with lithiasis. Distal ureteral calculi are best managed by retrograde ureteroscopy, with ESWL emerging as a viable alternative in selected cases and lithotripter installations, primarily with second-generation lithotripters that offer improved fluoroscopic imaging and more versatile patient positioning.

Paradoxically, calculus disease represents the one area in which there is a decrease rather than an increase in the use of interventional uroradiology. Since the introduction of ESWL and ureteroscopy, there is no longer any need for primary percutaneous nephrolithotomy (PCNL) for most renal and ureteral

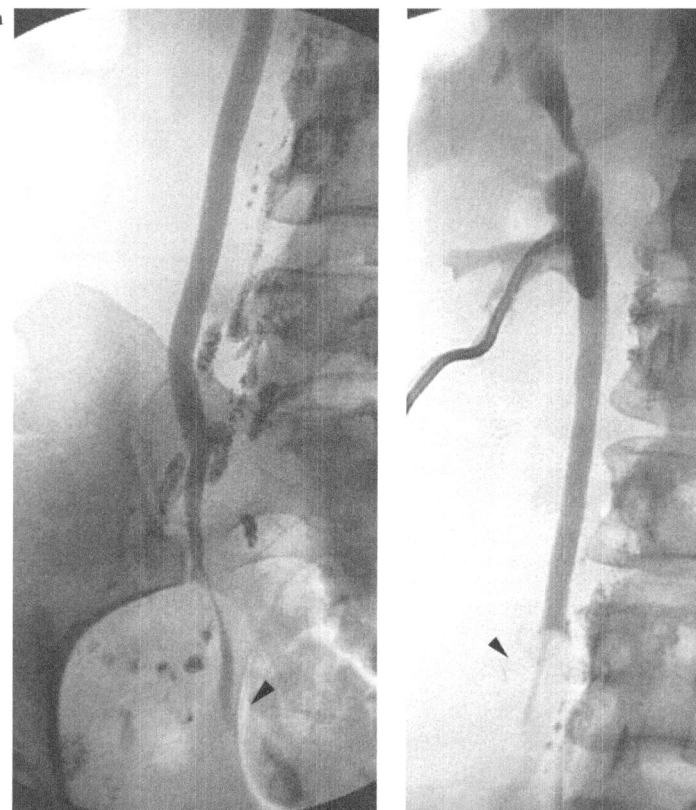

Fig. 12.10. a Antegrade pyelography shows a left uretero-vaginal fistula after radical hysterectomy for carcinoma (*arrowhead*). b Temporary occlusion with ureteral balloon (*arrowhead*) catheter associated with external drainage

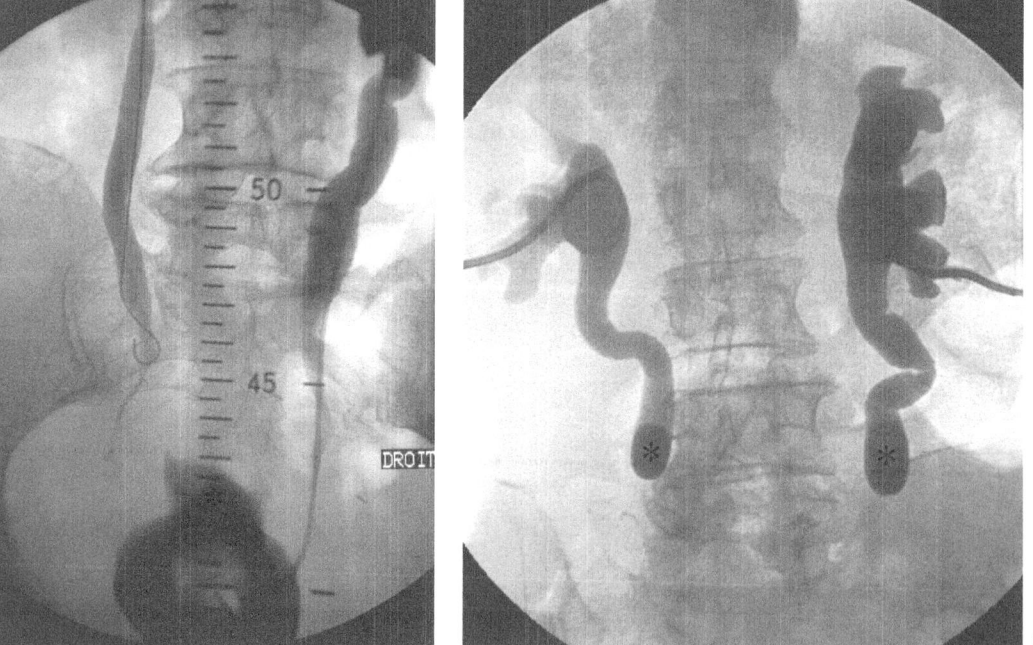

Fig. 12.11a, b. Definitive bilateral ureteral occlusion for a vesico-rectal fistula. a Bilateral antegrade pyelography shows bilateral obstruction with stenosis of both pelvic ureters secondary to cancer recurrence. Left ureter was impossible to catheterize. A 2-J catheter was placed on the right side. The cystogram shows simultaneous opacification of the rectum (*asterisk*). b The patient's condition requires a bilateral ureteral occlusion with detachable balloons (*asterisks*) and permanent bilateral nephrostomy

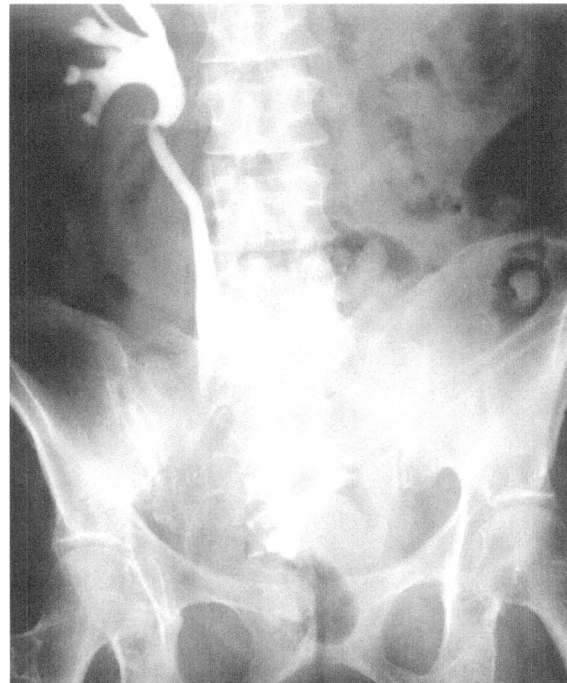
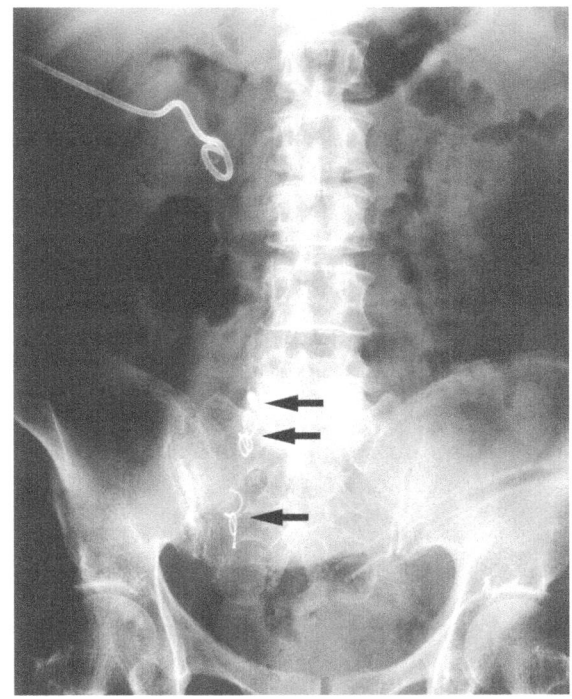

a

b

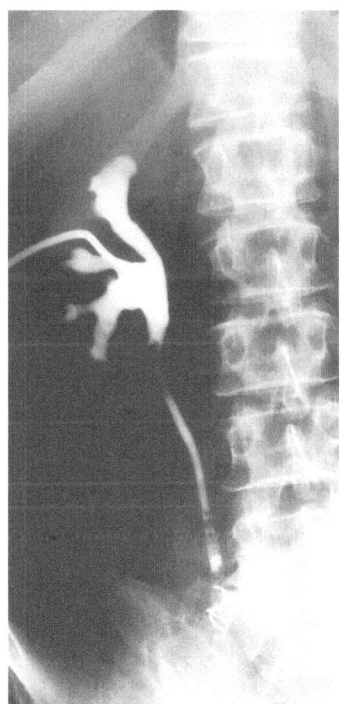

c

Fig. 12.12. a Postoperative uretero-cutaneous fistula shown on antegrade pyelography of the right kidney. The left kidney is absent. b Occlusion of the right ureter with coils and detechable balloon (*arrows*). c Pyelographic control via the permanent percutaneous nephrostomy. (Courtesy of Dr. HUGUET)

calculi which, for the first half of the 1980s, constituted a significant component of the interventional radiologist's work (VAN CANGH and DARDENNE 1990) (Figs. 12.13, 12.14).

Percutaneous techniques for accessing and/or decompressing the kidney, as well as for extracting

or disintegrating some calculi, are still needed, both as primary therapy for patients with selected stones, abnormal urinary tract morphology, or unusual clinical circumstances, and as secondary therapy when ESWL or ureteroscopy are ineffective (SMITH and CASTANEDA-ZUNIGA 1990).

Percutaneous techniques are important as an initial or additional procedure in the following circumstances (VAN CANGH and DARDENNE 1990); however these circumstances are exceptional in case of ureteral lithiasis:

- Large stone volume (single stone larger than 2 cm in diameter or multiple renal calculi with an aggregate diameter of 2.5 cm). However, as more urologists have adopted routine pre-ESWL ureteral drainage for large stones, the need for adjunctive PCNL has correspondingly diminished, except for very large calculi.
- Stones associated with compromised urinary drainage (Fig. 12.15a, b). In these cases, percutaneous stone therapy may be combined with endourologic treatment for the underlying obstructive process, such as endopyelotomy for ureteropelvic junction (UPJ) stenosis and balloon dilatation for infundibular or ureteral stricture. In these cases,

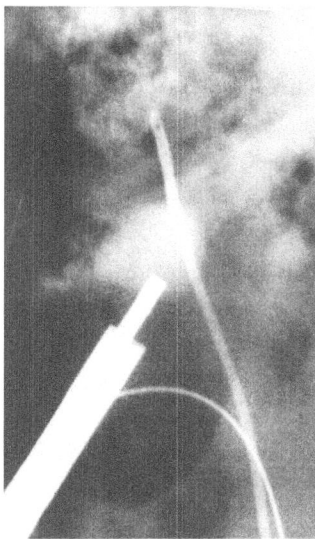

Fig. 12.13. Percutane-
ous nephrolithotomy
of a pelvic stone
refractory to ESWL

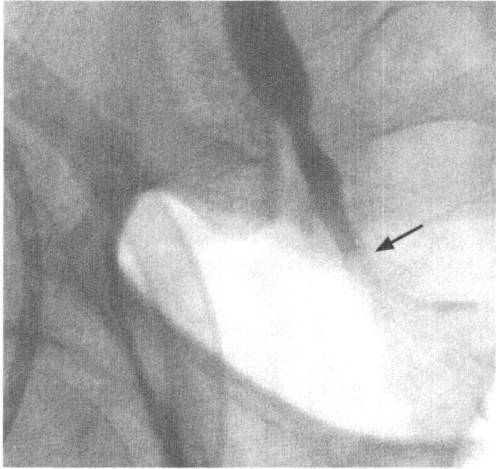

a

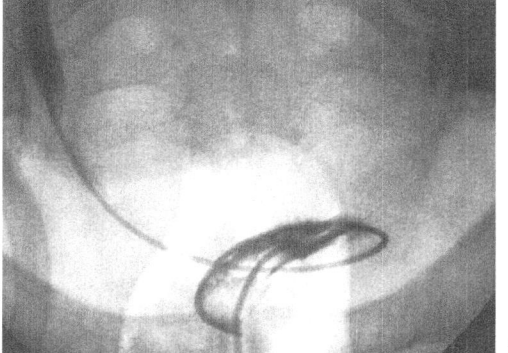

b

Fig. 12.15a, b. Percutaneous antegrade catheterization for
acute renal failure secondary to a right ureteral stone on a
single kidney and after failure of retrograde catheterization.
a Cupula-shaped occlusion of the pelvic ureter on antegrade
pyelography (*arrow*). b 2-J catheter in place in the bladder

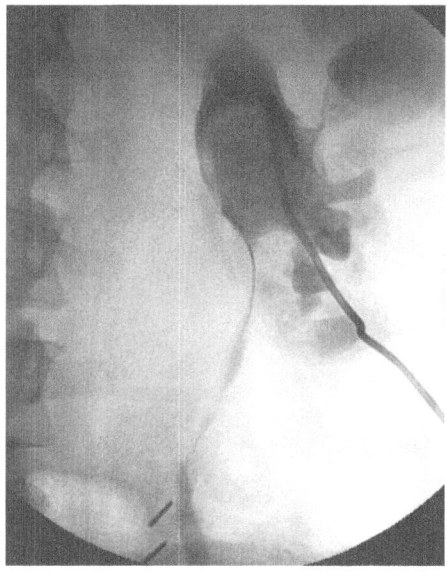

Fig. 12.14. Percutaneous nephrostomy as a first step of PCNL
for a staghorn calculus of the right kidney

post-ESWL ureteral migration can occur.

– When treated with ESWL, cystine calculi char-
acteristically fragment into large pieces rather
than small fragments. Percutaneous ultrasonic
lithotripsy and/or topical irrigation with various
solutions via PCN catheters to dissolve residual
cystine fragments are then indicated. Topical che-
molysis may also exceptionally be employed with
residual uric acid or struvite fragments (Dretler
et al. 1979) (Fig. 12.16a, b).

– Stone-bearing patients whose body habitus renders

them physically unsuitable for treatment by ESWL.
Patients with anomalous, ectopic, or transplanted
kidneys can, on the other hand, be readily managed
by ESWL in most cases, but an occasional indication for PCN with or without PCNL will arise. Renal
calculi diagnosed during pregnancy can usually be
managed expectantly (with or without ureteral
drainage), but if treatment cannot be deferred,
PCNL or ureteroscopy are preferred instead of
ESWL for obvious reasons.

– When renal decompression is needed and endoscopic attempts have not been successful. This
can occur either prior to lithotripsy or following
it, e.g., in patients who develop an obstructing or
otherwise symptomatic ureteral "Steinstrasse" following ESWL of upper tract calculi.

– Stones that do not adequately fragment with
ESWL or ureteroscopy

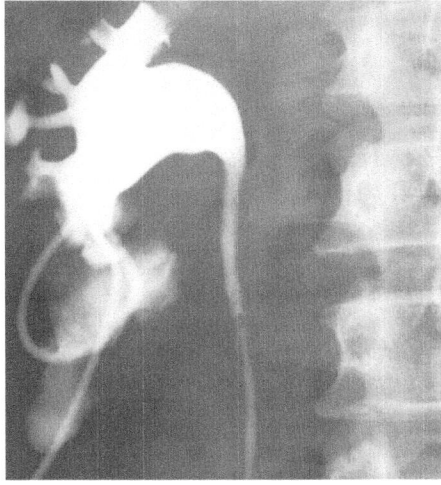
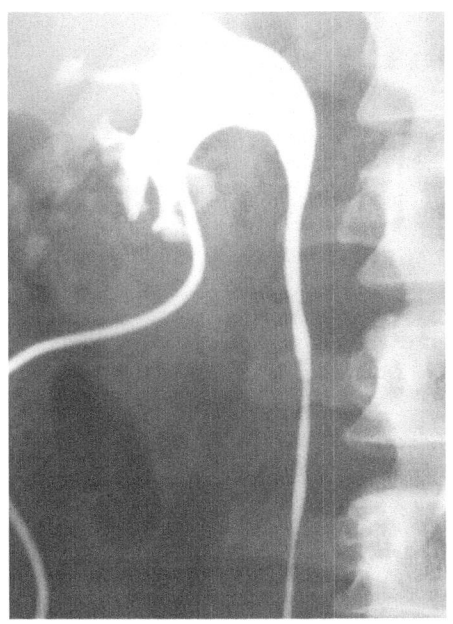

Fig. 12.16. a Right nephrostomy for acute renal colic with fever. Opacification shows a small lacunar, rounded uratic stone in the lumbar ureter. b Control after alkaline irrigation via the nephrostomy catheter shows disappearance of the stone

12.2.4
Other Procedures

Various endoureteral manipulations can be performed by the percutaneous antegrade route, such as the removal of foreign bodies or the replacement of occluded 2-J catheters (Fig. 12.17a–e). Loop snare, baskets, grasping forceps, and balloon catheters can be used, via an antegrade or a retrograde approach (YEDLICKA et al. 1991).

12.3
Role of Interventional Radiology of the Ureter in Renal Transplantation

Renal transplantation is an effective and widely applied treatment for end-stage renal disease. Advances in the management of graft rejection have led to improved graft and patient survival rates. Thus, although surgical complications remain rare (2%–13%), the relative importance of these patients as a group of subjects with potentially reversible morbidity and mortality has increased significantly (LOJANAPIWAT et al. 1994).

The most frequent urologic complications are ureteral stenosis or obstructions and leaks (BECKER and RUTCHER 1978). Delay in the treatment of these complications may result in allograft loss or loss of life. Therefore, they must be diagnosed early and rapidly differentiated from rejection: Delays in accurate

diagnosis and inappropriate antirejection therapy may result in loss of the transplanted kidney as well as in increased patient morbidity (IRVING and KASHI 1992).

The cause of ureteral stenosis or necrosis remains open to speculation, although vascular insufficiency seems very likely. The blood supply to the terminal ureter in renal allografts is clearly vulnerable to surgical trauma, as it is derived entirely from the main renal artery, but vasculitis due to preservation injury, rejection, or even cyclosporine toxicity have all been suggested as alternative pathogenic mechanisms (FONTAINE et al. 1997).

Ureteral complications of the transplanted kidney have traditionally been treated with surgical techniques. However, surgical repair is associated with considerable morbidity and mortality. Due to postoperative periureteral fibrosis, surgical dissection is difficult, leading to a high rate of leakage, recurrence of obstruction, and kidney loss (LOJANAPIWAT et al. 1994). With the development of percutaneous techniques, such as antegrade ureteral stent placement, interventional radiology offers a viable alternative treatment to surgery, with lower complication rates.

12.3.1
Obstructions

The key to early diagnosis of ureteral obstruction is serial ultrasound scanning. The use of ultrasonography to detect collecting system dilation has long been established, but the significance of this finding

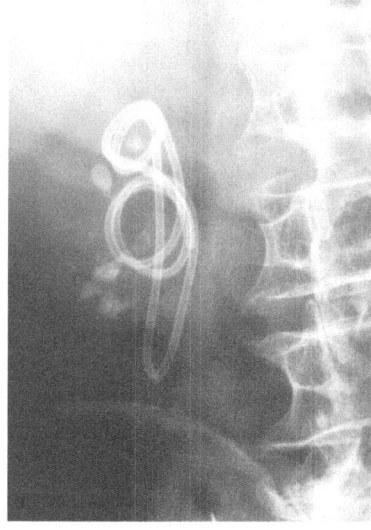
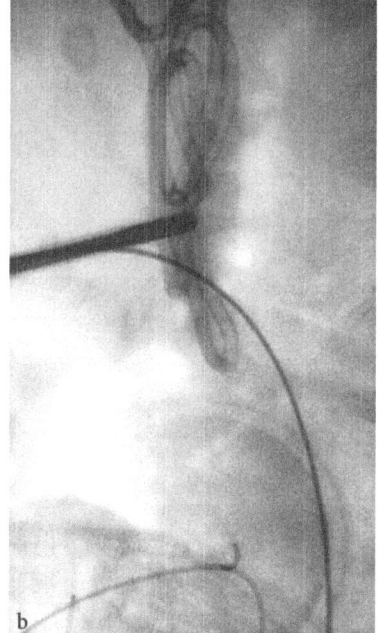
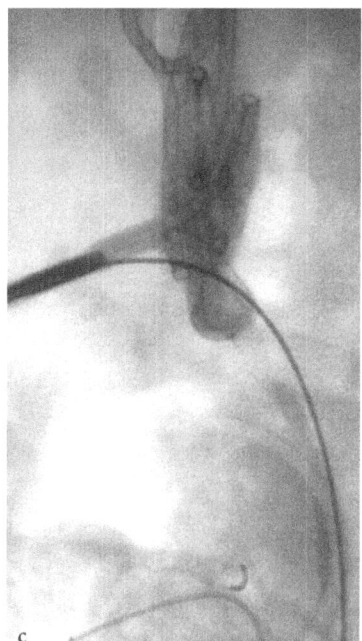
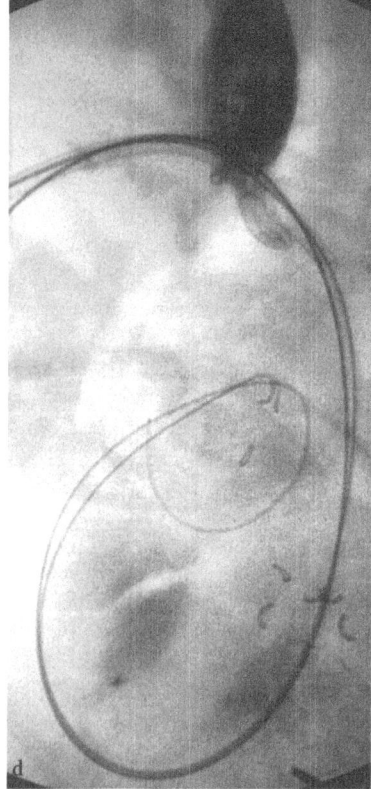
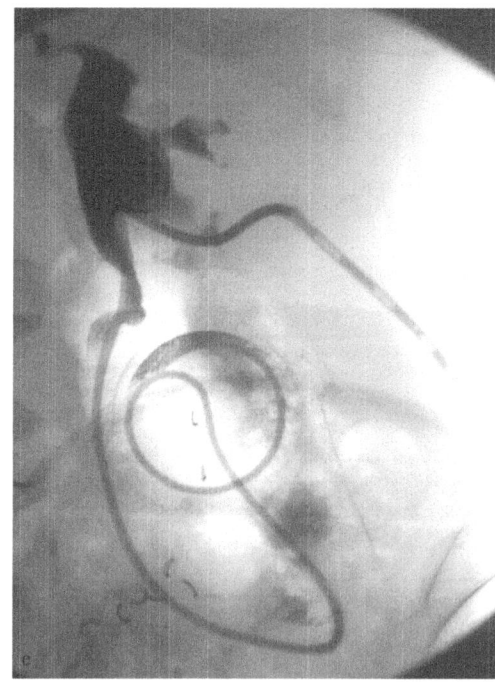

Fig. 12.17a–e. Percutaneous extraction of a dislodged 2-J catheter and replacement. **a** Upper spontaneous migration of a 2-J catheter in the right renal pelvis. **b** Percutaneous catheterization of the right ureter with a guidewire. Introduction, via the same route, of a forceps for grasping the catheter. **c-d** Extraction of the catheter via the percutaneous route. **e** Control after replacement of a new 2-J catheter through the uretero-ileal anastomosis

in the early postoperative period has been subject to some uncertainty. In the absence of pelvicaliceal dilation and in the presence of good or improving renal function, the chances of obstruction are very low. Furthermore, even in the presence of poor or deteriorating renal function, a normal ultrasound scan provides a sensitivity of 93% and specificity of 99% in the diagnosis of ureteral obstruction (IRVING and KASHI 1992).

Collecting system dilation may occur even in the absence of obstruction. While the causes of such a clinical situation are not known, etiologic possibilities include preexisting dilation in the donor system or dilation due to a resolving rejection process. Most grafts with mechanical ureteral obstruction can be rescued by appropriate management.

Obstruction is suspected clinically when there is tenderness over the kidney, elevation of serum creatinine, and/or decreasing urine output. An ultrasound scan must be performed and, if dilation of the collecting system has developed or increased in severity compared with the baseline or previous scan, antero-grade pyelography should be performed (BECKER and RUTCHER 1978).

An antegrade pyelogram provides anatomic infor-mation and also permits an assessment of the rate of flow of contrast down the ureter into the bladder. It also allows percutaneous treatment at the same time if advisable. The presence or absence of partial or complete ureteral obstruction is usually obvious, but the addition of pressure-flow studies (Whitaker test) provides a more objective assessment of impedance to urine flow (SMITH et al. 1988).

When obstruction is suspected on the basis of the antegrade pyelogram, a percutaneous nephros-tomy should be performed to relieve excessive pain, restore renal function, and gain time during which the options for the most appropriate form of therapy can be discussed by the surgeon and radiologist (SMITH et al. 1988).

Further management of these patients depends upon the exact cause of the obstruction. Early postoperative obstruction may be due to edema at the uretero-neocystostomy site and may resolve spontaneously after a few days of external drainage.

Other causes are surgically related: ureteral clotting, external compression by hematoma. In these patients, repeated nephrostograms to confirm urinary tract patency are followed by a period of "catheter clamp-ing" prior to definitive catheter withdrawal. If the obstruction at the uretero-neocystostomy site per-sists, insertion of a 2-J stent, with or without bal-loon dilatation of the stricture, is the treatment of choice (LIEBERMAN et al. 1982; BHAGAT et al. 1998; KIM et al. 1993) (Fig. 12.18a–c.). The uretero-vesical anastomosis is the most frequent site of obstruction; ischemic problems and surgical manipulations occur most often at this site. Balloon dilatation using high-pressure angioplasty balloons, 4–6 mm in diameter, is performed when there has been any difficulty in pass-ing an 8-F catheter through the stricture. This should always be followed by 2-J internal drainage (VOEGELI et al. 1988). Stents are left in place for at least 3 months and up to 6 months, during which close monitoring of both serum creatinine levels and ultrasound appear-ance are mandatory to detect whether the ureteric stricture recurs. Late obstructions are secondary to localized or diffuse fibrosis resulting from ischemia or rejection. The possibility of resolving obstruction with stenting is less likely in this situation and the rate of failure and recurrence is very high, leading to a noninterventional solution (ORONS and ZAJKO 1995).

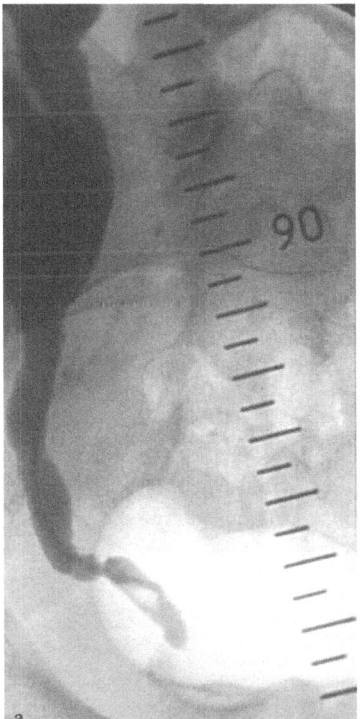
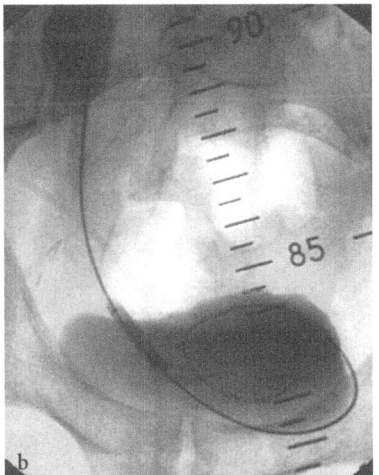
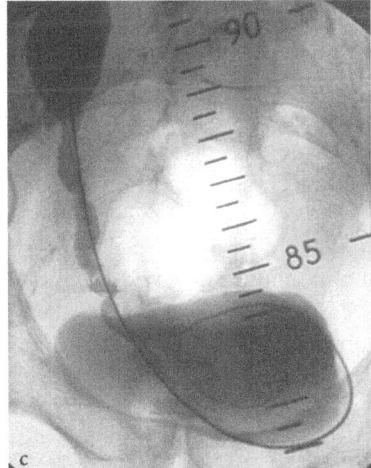

Fig. 12.18. a Antegrade pyelography on a transplanted kidney: presence of a distal ureteral stenosis on the ureteroneocystostomy site with absence of passage. b Balloon dilatation of the stenotic area. c Control after dilatation

Other causes of ureteral obstruction that can be managed percutaneously include obstruction due to a stone, for which percutaneous ureterolithotomy can be performed, postsurgical obstruction at a pyeloureterostomy, and ureteral compression by a fluid collection, with success rates for percutaneous therapy alone of more than 70% (GEDROYC et al. 1989).

However, not all causes of obstruction are amenable to interventional radiology; long ischemia-related ureteral strictures, obstructions due to tumors, such as immunosuppression-induced lymphoma, and recurrent ureteroneocystostomy strictures are likely to necessitate a surgical approach (HUNTER et al. 1983).

12.3.2
Urinary Leakage

Leaks are usually the result of ureteral necrosis due to rejection or vascular insufficiency. Clinical suspicion of urinary leakage is based on low urine output, a rise in serum creatinine, detection of a perirenal fluid collection, or a leak from the wound. Leaks usually occur in the first 2–3 weeks after kidney transplantation and almost invariably within 5–6 weeks post-transplantation. Prompt leakage diagnosis and treatment are necessary, because delays result in increased morbidity and mortality. Urinary extravasation can lead to infection and sepsis, especially in such immunocompromised patients. The mortality due to an untreated leak can be as high as 50% (BECKER and RUTCHER 1978). A voiding cystogram may demonstrate a leak from the site of neocystostomy, which can be treated by continuing drainage via the urethral catheter, with surgical repair if the leak fails to resolve. If a leak at the ureteroneocystostomy site is demonstrated, or if no leak is detected at cystography, an anterograde pyelogram is performed (FONTAINE et al. 1997). If a leak is confirmed, the percutaneous approach relies on diversion of the urinary flow away from the leak by means of a PCN catheter (BHAGHAT et al. 1998). A subsequent nephrostogram will show whether there is total ureterovesical discontinuity, in which case surgical repair is mandatory, or whether some persisting communication exists. In the latter case, an attempt can be made to pass a guidewire into the bladder so that antegrade 2-J insertion can be performed. The rate of complication is very low, largely less than that of surgery. The transplant survival is 100% after 2-J placement and 87% after surgery, which has a failure rate as high as 30% (BHAGHAT et al. 1998).

References

Babel SG, Winterkorn KG (1993) Retrograde catheterization of the ureter without cystoscopic assistance: preliminary experience. Radiology 187:547–549

Banner M, Amendola MA, Pollack HM (1989) Anastomosed ureters: fluoroscopically guided transconduit retrograde catheterization. Radiology 170:45–49

Banner M, Ramchandani P, Pollack H (1991) Interventional procedures in the upper urinary tract. Cardiovasc Intervent Radiol 14:267–284

Barbaric Z, Hall T, Cochran S, et al (1997) Percutaneous nephrostomy: placement under CT and fluoroscopy guidance. AJR Am J Roentgenol 169:151–155

Becker JA, Rutcher R (1978) Urologic complications of renal transplantation. Semin Roentgenol 13:341–351

Beckman CF, Roth RA, Bihrce W (1989) Dilatation of benign ureteral strictures. Radiology 172:437–441

Bhagat V, Gordon R, Osorio R, et al (1998) Ureteral obstructions and renal leaks after renal transplantation: outcome of percutaneous antegrade ureteral stent placement in 44 patients. Radiology 209:159–167

Bing KT, Hicks ME, Picus D, et al (1992) Percutaneous ureteral occlusion with use of Gianturco coils and gelatin sponge, part II. Clinical experience. J Vasc Intervent Radiol 3:319–321

Bohlman M, Khazan R, Regan F (1998) Rapid nephrostomy tube placement using a CT-guided non-fluoroscopic, single-stick technique. J Intervent Radiol 13:101–105

Breen D, Cowan N (1995) Fluoroscopically guided retrieval of ureteric stents. Clin Radiol 50:860–863

Castaneda F, Moradian GP, Epstein DH, et al (1989) A new technique for complete temporary occlusion of the ureter. AJR Am J Roentgenol 155:81–82

Chang R, Marshall FF, Mitchell S (1987) Percutaneous management of benign ureteral strictures and fistulas. J Urol 137:1126–1131

Chaussy C, Schmiedt E, Jocham D, et al (1984) Extracorporeal schock-wave lithotripsy for treatment of urolithiasis. Urology 23:59–66

Cockburn JF, Borthwick-Clarke A, Hanaghan J (1997) Radiologic insertion of subcutaneous nephrovesical stent for inoperable ureteral obstruction. AJR Am J Roentgenol 169:1588–1590

Cornud FE, Casanova JMP, Bonnel DH, et al (1991) Impassable ureteral strictures: management with percutaneous uretero-neocystostomy. Radiology 180:451–454

Cornud F, Mendelsberg M, Chretien Y, et al (1992) Fluoroscopically guided percutaneous transrenal electroincision of uretero-intestinal anastomotic strictures. J Urol 147:578–581

Cornud F, Chretien Y, Helenon O, et al (2000) Percutaneous incision of stenotic uroenteric anastomoses with a cutting balloon catheter: long-term results. Radiology 214:358–362

Cragg AH, Castaneda F, Amplatz K, et al (1989) Percutaneous ureteral clipping. Technique and results. Semin Intervent Radiol 6:176–181

Culkin DJ, Zitman R, Bundrick WS, et al (1992) Anatomic, functional and pathologic changes from internal ureteral stent placement. Urology 40:385–390

De Baere T, Roche A, La Grange C (1995) Combined percutaneous antegrade and cystoscopic retrograde approach in the treatment of distal ureteral fistula. Cardiovasc Intervent Radiol 18:349

Dretler SP, Pfister RC, Newhouse JH (1979) Renal stone dissolution via percutaneous nephrostomy. N Engl J Med 300: 341–343

Druy EM, Gharib M, Finder CA (1983) Percutaneous nephro-ureteral drainage and stenting for post-surgical ureteral leaks. AJR Am J Roentgenol 141:389–394

Dyer B, Assimos D, Regan J (1997) Update on interventional uroradiology. Urol Clin North Am 24:623–651

Evans P, Nisbert H, Saxton H (1988) Antegrade ureteric stents in malignant disease. J Intervent Radiol 3:9–13

Flueckiger F, Lammer J, Klein GE, et al (1993) Malignant ureteral obstruction: preliminary results of treatment with metallic self-expandable stents. Radiology 186:169–173

Fontaine AB, Nijjar A, Rangaraz R (1997) Update on the use of percutaneous nephrostomy/balloon dilatation for the treatment of renal transplant leak/obstruction. J Vasc Intervent Radiol 8:649–653

Gasparini M, Caroll P, Stoller M (1991) Palliative percutaneous and endoscopic urinary diversion for malignant ureteral obstruction. Urology 38:408–412

Gedroyc WMW, MacIver D, Joyce MRL, et al (1989) Percutaneous stone and stent removal from renal transplantation. Clin Radiol 40:174–177

Goodwin WE, Casey WE, Woolf W (1995) Percutaneous trocar (needle) nephrostomy in hydronephrosis. JAMA 157:891–894

Hekimoglu B, Men S, Punar A, et al (1996) Urothelial hyperplasia complicating use of ureteral stent in malignant ureteral obstruction. Eur Radiol 6:675–681

Holmes SAU, Christmas TJ, Rickards D (1993) Ureteric stents. In: Rickards D, Jones S, Thomson KR, Rifkin MD (eds) Pratical interventionnal uroradiology. Arnold, London, pp 55–65

Hunter DW, Castaneda-Zuniga WR, Coleman CC, et al (1983) Percutaneous techniques in the management of urological complications in renal transplant patient. Radiology 148: 407–412

Irving H, Kashi H (1992) Complications of renal transplantation and the role of interventional radiology. J Clin Ultrasound 20:545–552

Joffre F, Plante P, Tregant PH (1990) Techniques d'opacification radiologique directe des voies excrétrices supérieures. Editions Techniques Encycl Méd Chir Paris, France. Radiodiagnostic V, 34015 B10, 12, 1–6

Joffre F, Tregant PH, Rousseau H (1995) Radiologie interventionnelle urinaire des voies excrétrices supérieures. Editions Techniques Encycl Méd Chir Paris, France. Radiodiagn Urol Gynécol 34–350 A 10, 1–14

Johnson CD, Oke FJ, Dunnick NR, et al (1991) Percutaneous balloon dilatation of ureteral stricture. AJR Am J Roentgenol 148: 181–184.

Kabalin JN (1997) Acucise incision of uretero-enteric strictures after urinary diversion. J Endourol 11:37–40

Kenny B, Lynch N, Hurley G (1995) Antegrade stenting of malignant ureteral strictures. Eur Radiol 5:623–625

Kim J, Banner M, Ramchandani P (1993) Balloon dilatation of ureteral strictures after renal transplantation. Radiology 186:717–722

Kwak S, Leef J, Rosenblum J (1995) Percutaneous balloon catheter dilatation of benign ureteral strictures. Effect of multiple dilatation procedures on long-term patency. AJR Am J Roentgenol 165:97–100

Lang EK (1984) Antegrade ureteral stenting for dehiscence, strictures and fistulae. AJR Am J Roentgenol 143:795–801

Lang EK (1987) Percutaneous management of ureteral stricture. Semin Intervent Radiol 4:79–89

Lang KK, Glorioso LW (1988) Antegrade transluminal dilatation of benign ureteral stricture. Long-term results. AJR Am J Roentgenol 150:131–134

Lemaitre L, Mestdagh P, Marecaux-Delomez J, et al (2000) Percutaneous nephrostomy: placement, index laser guidance and renal-time CT fluoroscopy. Eur Radiol 10:892–895

Lieberman SF, Keller FS, Barry JM, et al (1982) Percutaneous antegrade transluminal ureteroplasty for renal allograft ureteral stenosis. J Urol 128:122–124

Lojanapiwat B, Mital D, Fallon L, et al (1994) Management of ureteral stenosis after renal transplantation. J Am Coll Surg 179:21–24

Lugmayr HF, Pauer W (1996) Wallstents for the treatment of extrinsic malignant ureteral obstruction. Mid-term result. Radiology 198:105–108

Maillet PJ, Pelle-Francoz D, Leriche A, et al (1987) Fistulas of the upper urinary tract: percutaneous management. J Urol 138:1382–1385

Mitty HA, Train JS, San SJ (1986) Placement of ureteral stents by antegrade and retrograde technique. Radiol Clin North Am 24:587–600

Murphy GJ (1999) What is the place for self-expanding metal stents in the ureter? J Intervent Radiol 14:189–192

Nolte-Ernsting CL, Bucker A, Neverburg JM, et al (1999) MR imaging-guided percutaneous nephrostomy and use of MR-compatible catheters in the nondilated porcine urinary tract. J Vasc Intervent Radiol 10:1305–1314

Orons PD, Zajko AB (1995) Angiography and interventional aspects of renal transplantation. Radiol Clin North Am 33: 461–477

Papanicolaou N, Pfister RC, Yoder IC (1985) Percutaneous occlusion of ureteral leaks and fistulas using nondetachable balloon. Urol Radiol 7:28–31

Pocock R, Stower M, Ferro M, et al (1986) Double J stent. A review of 100 patients. Br J Urol 58:629–633

Pollak JS, Rosenblatt MM, Egglin TK, et al (1995) Treatment of ureteral obstruction with the Wallstent endoprosthesis: preliminary results. J Vasc Intervent Radiol 6:417–425

Pollard A, Nicholson D (1994) Percutaneous nephrostomy – how to do it. J Intervent Radiol 9:129–141

Ravery V, de Lataille P, Hoffmann P, et al (1998) Balloon catheter dilatation in the treatment of ureteral and uretero-enteric stricture. J Endourol 12:335–340

Reinberg Y, Ferral H, Gonzalez R, et al (1994) Intraureteral metallic self-expanding endoprosthesis (Wallstent) in the treatment of difficult ureteral strictures. J Urol 151: 1619–1622

Saltzman B (1988) Ureteral stents. Urol Clin North Am 15: 481–491

Schild HH, Gunther R, Thelen M (1994) Trans-renal ureteral occlusion: results and prognosis. J Vasc Intervent Radiol 5:321–325

Shapiro MJ, Banner MP, Amendola MA, et al (1988) Balloon catheter dilatation of uretero-enteric strictures: long-term results. Radiology 168:385–387

Smith TP, Hunter DW, Letourneau JG, et al (1988) Urinary obstruction in renal transplants: diagnosis by antegrade pyelography and results of percutaneous treatment. AJR Am J Roentgenol 151:507–510

Smith TP, Castaneda-Zuniga W (1990) Percutaneous management of stones in the urinary tract. In: Dondelinger RF,

Rossi P, Kurdziel JC, Wallace S (eds) Interventional radiology. Thieme, Stuttgart, pp 262–280

Somers WJ (1996) Management of forgotten or retained indwelling ureteral stents. Urology 47:431–435

Trillaud H, Pariente JL, Rabie A, et al (2001) Detection of encrusted indwelling ureteral stents using a twinkling artefact revealed on color Doppler sonography. AJR Am J Roentgenol 176:1446–1448

Van Cangh PJ, Dardenne A (1990) Endoscopic management of stones in the urinary tract. In: Dondelinger RF, Rossi P, Kurdziel JC, Wallace S (eds) Interventional radiology. Thieme, Stuttgart, pp 255–260

Van Sonnenberg F, D'Agostino HB, O'Laoide R, et al (1994) Malignant ureteral obstruction: treatment with metal stents – technique, results and observations with percutaneous intraluminal US. Radiology 191:765–768

Voegeli DR, Crummy AB, McDermott JC, et al (1988) Percutaneous dilatation of ureteral stricture in renal transplant patient. Radiology 169:185–188

Wetton C, Gedroyc W (1995) Retrograde radiological retrieval and placement of double-J ureteric stents. Clin Radiol 50: 562–565

Yedlicka JW Jr, Aizpuru R, Hunter DW (1991) Retrograde replacement of internal double J ureteral stents. AJR Am J Roentgenol 156:1007–1009

Zaleski G, Funaki B, Newmark G (1998) Placement of retrograde nephroureteral stent through ileal conduits. AJR Am J Roentgenol 170:1275–1278

13 Strategy for Ureteral Imaging

J. P. Sarramon, F. Joffre, B. Janne d'Othee, L. Bouchard, Ph. Otal, P. Plante

CONTENTS

Because of its topography and the length of its course, the involvement of the ureter in pathologic conditions is variable, including both diseases of the ureter itself and extension of pathologic processes from surrounding structures. This wide variety contrasts with the paucity and lack of specificity of clinical signs. Some signs point immediately towards the urinary tract; in other cases, the clinical presentation of an extraurinary disease leads the clinician to search for the origin of a symptom at the level of the urinary tract, or a deleterious upstream consequence. In still other cases urinary disease is discovered fortuitously.

J. P. Sarramon, MD
Service d'Urologie, CHU PURPAN, place Baylac, 31059 Toulouse Cédex, France
F. Joffre, MD, B. Janne d'Othee, MD; L. Bouchard, MD; Ph. Otal, MD
Service de Radiologie, Hôpital de Rangueil, 1, avenue Jean-Poulhès, 31403 Toulouse Cédex 4, France
P. Plante, MD
Service d'Urologie, CHU Rangueil, 1, avenue Jean-Poulhès, 31403 Toulouse Cédex 4, France

Except in some particular circumstances, the lack of specificity of most clinical signs makes it necessary to carry out a first-line screening radiological examination that allows a fast and effective evaluation of the whole urinary tract.

For a long time, EU has played a guiding role in revealing urinary pathology (POLLACK and BANNER 1985). However, its disadvantages, its risks, and the limited information it provides in case of renal insufficiency often result in ultrasonography being chosen as the first-line imaging modality, in particular when the search is for an obstruction (which is the main mode of expression of ureteral diseases). Any diagnostic algorithm for ureteral disease must take into account the technical progress and the multiple possibilities offered by new reconstruction imaging techniques (CHOYKE 1992; BIGOT 1995; MOREAU 1995; AMIS 1999).

In all clinical situations, it is necessary to keep in mind an essential element that will direct the strategy: the renal functional status. Be it evaluated by biological sampling or suspected on the basis of first-line imaging data, the level of parenchymal deterioration seen on an echography or on unenhanced CT enables one to roughly estimate the quality of the opacification likely to be obtained.

13.1
Clinical Presentation

13.1.1
Urinary Manifestations

Ureteral disease can be revealed by isolated or associated urinary signs that do not always point towards the ureter but will result in a complete examination of the whole urinary tract. Macroscopic hematuria, either associated with other symptoms or especially if isolated, is a common symptom that should initially raise suspicion of a tumoral disease. The discovery of microscopic hematuria rather evokes a nephrological disease, especially when it is associated with proteinuria, but it can also be met in some conditions affecting the urinary tract. Urinary infection – whether it is only biological or clinically expressed as a severe acute pyelonephritis – can also be the consequence of a ureteral disease, in particular obstructive, or can be accompanied by radiological anomalies of the ureter. Acute painful symptomatology – such as in classical renal colic – is one of the most frequent signs and points initially towards ureteral disease. Chronic lumbar pain is frequent but less specific. The existence of renal insufficiency must suggest a ureteral obstruction, either bilateral or unilateral on a single functional kidney. It may be either oligoanuric acute renal failure or chronic renal insufficiency with preserved diuresis. The use of iodinated CM depends on the presence and the level of renal insufficiency. Anomalies of the urinary sediment or proteinuria may be found. Any sign that points to the lower urinary tract should lead us to make sure that the ureter is not affected by a lower urinary tract pathology. The occurrence of a trauma in the urinary tract, the performance of surgical operations on the ureter, or a transplantation make it particularly important to check the integrity of the ureter.

13.1.2
Extraurinary Signs

The presence of systemic clinical signs such as an isolated fever or an impaired general status should suggest a urinary etiology. Some retroperitoneal and/or pelvic diseases also prompt a search for ureteral involvement. This may be found in the case of retroperitoneal tumors, aneurysms of the abdominal aorta, and benign or malignant RPF (digestive, gynecological, urological). The preoperative assessment of pelvic tumors must include a search for possible ureteral involvement. Today this is done with echography. Similarly, the monitoring of these patients after treatment must include an evaluation of the upper urinary tract.

13.1.3
The Incidental Discovery of a Disease

The multiplication of indications for modern imaging techniques of the abdominal cavity results more and more often in the fortuitous discovery of a pathologic condition of ureteral origin.

13.1.4
The Current Clinical Practice

In current practice, the majority of symptoms or conditions generally lead to an ultrasonographic examination of the urinary tract which has the merit of being able to detect a distension of the urinary tract, in particular when there is renal insufficiency. Ultrasonography may also help to assess the extent of possible parenchymal atrophy and thus to determine a therapeutic strategy. The reliability of ultrasonography is questionable only in the case of acute obstructive syndrome. Thus, it is rare today to begin the search for a ureteral pathology with EU, except in cases where patients present with a macroscopic hematuria. In some situations, this examination may be carried out as a complement to ultrasonography or CT.

In practice, one may face two possibilities: Either there is an obstructive syndrome or there is not. In case of obstruction, the classical strategy consists of exploring the urinary tract either by EU, possibly supplemented by a direct antegrade and/or retrograde opacification of the urinary tract. Direct opacification is often essential for two reasons. It makes it possible to better visualize the ureter at the level of the obstacle, and it is often the first step in external ureteric drainage by nephrostomy or internal drainage by intubation of the ureter with a 2J catheter. When the opacification is insufficient to determine the cause of the obstruction, a CT examination of the stenotic zone provides the most valuable information by pointing towards an extraureteral or ureteral origin of the obstruction (MEGIBOW et al. 1982).

Today, a more modern attitude may be proposed, particularly in some difficult situations. The principle is to explore by helical CT, or possibly by MRI, the whole ureteral course (ROY et al. 1998). The choice between the two techniques is still under evaluation and each modality has its own advantages and drawbacks. The presence of a contraindication to the use of iodinated contrast media (allergy, renal insufficiency) or to the use of X-rays rather favors the use of MRI, but it should be kept in mind that 3D reconstructions after helical CT acquisition can be achieved without injection of contrast medium. A complete scan of the whole abdomen before injection enables spontaneous visualization of detectable anomalies. After injection of contrast medium, volumetric acquisition makes it possible to visualize the totality of the ureter and its environment and to provide a urographic picture (LEMAITRE et al. 2000). This last option can be performed by taking plain films after CT, by post-CT urographic multiplanar reconstructions, or by adapted MRI sequences.

The typical example of this new approach is the new diagnostic strategy for renal colic. This strategy does not remove the need for completing direct antegrade or retrograde opacification of the urinary tract, should the need arise, particularly before ureteral intubation.

If there is no obstruction, it is of the utmost importance to opacify the urinary tract in the presence of symptoms that evoke a ureteral pathology. In these cases, EU remains always powerful. Direct opacification is also useful but can mask small-sized lesions as a result of the hyperpressure they may produce. It can be the first step of a brushing or an endoscopic sampling. CT may be less useful here for the diagnosis but sometimes provides etiologic arguments, in particular to distinguish between an intraluminal or parietal disease of the ureter itself (in particular lithiasis or tumor) and a periureteric pathologic condition.

13.2
The Main Radiological Presentations and Their Diagnostic Strategy

The radiological signs that prompt suspicion of a ureteral disease are extremely varied. They can be grouped in two main categories: direct signs that reflect the existence of a ureteral pathology, and indirect signs corresponding to the upstream impact of the ureteral lesion on the urinary tract. Both categories may be associated, but in fact, the indirect signs of obstruction are more frequent and should be considered first, as their discovery provides the impulse to seek and detect a ureteral lesion.

13.2.1
Signs of Obstruction

We have described the symptomatology for either acute, chronic, or intermittent obstructions (TALNER 1990). Similarly, we have discussed the existence or not of an obstruction in case of ureteric dilation. The multiplicity and ambiguity of the terms used illustrate the difficulty of this problem and the frequent confusion regarding the terminology. In practice, the diagnosis is easier with EU than with echography, thanks to the functional information provided. In any case, as soon as there is a doubt, it is essential to determine whether an obstruction exists, its level, and its origin. Direct opacification has its place here. But CT study of the obstructive site can provide much information useful for the whole diagnosis. The existence

of dilation affecting all of one or both ureters must suggest an obstruction of vesico-prostatic origin.

13.2.2
Specific Radiological Signs of Ureteral Disorders

The diagnostic value of radiological signs is highly variable as a result of their unequal specificity (PFISTER and NEWHOUSE 1978). Some signs point immediately towards a precise etiology. Others may correspond to multiple causes.

13.2.2.1
Abnormal Opacities of the Ureter

The confirmation of their ureteral origin is not always easy (MARGOLIN and COHEN 1982; SINGH and MALEK 1982). No matter whether they are discovered on plain roentgenograms (KUB) or by CT, some features of abnormal opacities may favor ureteral lithiasis, such as their topography, morphology, and associated signs (thickening of the ureteric wall). However, one should be aware of the topographic anomalies of the ureter in order to avoid missing a ureteral origin (FRIEDENBERG et al. 1966). Similarly, pelvic phleboliths in helical CT were considered above. Once the ureteral topography has been confirmed, either after classic urographic opacification or on CT, it should be remembered that an abnormal opacity is not always lithiasic and that some tumors can be calcified.

13.2.2.2
Topographic Abnormalities of the Ureter

Topographic abnormalities are frequent anomalies that evoke either a constitutional malposition (Table 13.1) or, more frequently, an extrinsic compression phenomenon (CUNAT and GOLDMAN 1986). Before diagnosing ureteric compression, one should take care to remember the wide mobility of the ureters and the numerous topographic variations that may be observed depending on the subject, the side, and the patient's position (ADAM et al. 1985; ESHO and CASS 1973; SALDINO and PALUBINSKAS 1972). The subject's muscular status can favor a more medial position of the ureters as a result of the hypertrophy of psoas muscles (BREE et al 1976; LEVINE et al. 1969). EU shows well both the topographic anomalies of the ureter and the associated signs. It is possible to miss an anterior or posterior compression which may be responsible for a false widening of the ureter and might be detectable on the profile view only, but this type of deviation is seldom isolated.

Table 13.1. Causes of abnormal ureteral position

	Medial deviation	Lateral deviation
Upper third	Lower pole renal mass	Malrotation of kidney
	Retroperitoneal mass:	Horseshoe kidney
	tumor, abscess, urinoma, hematoma	Postoperative
		Lymphadenopathies (testis – right side)
		Dilated nonopacified upper duplicated ureter
		Distended duodenal loop (right side)
		Pancreatic pseudocyst (left side)
		Medial retroperitoneal mass
Middle third	Retroperitoneal fibrosis	Lymphadenopathies
	Retrocaval ureter (right side)	Aortic aneurysm
	Psoas muscle hypertrophy	Medial retroperitoneal mass
	Retroperitoneal mass:	Psoas hypertrophy or mass
	tumor, abscess, urinoma, hematoma	
	Psoas mass:	
	tumor, abscess, hematoma	
Lower third	Iliac artery aneurysm or tortuosities	Pelvic tumor (central):
		uterus, rectum, ovary
	Abdominal-perineal surgery (rectum)	Fecal impaction
	Bladder diverticulum	Sciatic hernia
	Iliac lymphadenopathy	Bladder diverticulum
	Pelvic lipomatosis	Ureteral suspension
	Pelvic fibrosis	Pelvic surgery
	Pelvic collection:	Distended bladder
	hematoma, abscess, urinoma, lymphocele	
	Pelvic tumor (lateral):	
	ovary, uterine fibromyoma	
	Infiltrating neoplasm	
	Uterine prolapse	
	Prostatic hypertrophy	

The compressive character of a ureteric deviation must be considered if the following criteria are present simultaneously: localized arciform deviation with large curvature radius, compression of the ureter in the different space planes, upstream suppression distension of the urinary tract. CT examination provides valuable information by showing the cause of the compressive phenomenon (JOFFRE and PORTALEZ 1984). Direct opacification may be misleading in the case of moderate compressive phenomena, as the hyperpressure secondary to the injection may mask indirect signs. The causes of these topographic anomalies are highly variable but are mostly represented by compressive tumoral pathology (CUNAT and GOLDMAN 1986).

13.2.2.3
Filling Defects

Filling defects appear as a lucency of the ureteric lumen when opacification techniques are performed. They can be isolated or can result in a ureteric narrowing which will cause upstream dilation. They can be missed in particular if the technique is inappropriate, such as

insufficient opacification; on the other hand, too dense opacification may also result in them being missed (FEIN and McCLENNAN 1986). Any number of factors can be the cause of filling defects in the ureter:

- Radiolucent calculi
- Blood clots
- Sloughed papillae
- Inflammatory and infectious diseases
    - Ureteritis and ureteritis cystica
    - Fungus ball
    - Tuberculosis of the ureter
    - Malakoplakia
    - Leukoplasia and cholesteatomas
- Tumors
    - Fibroepithelial polyps
    - Transitional cell and squamous cell carcinomas
    - Ureteral metastases
    - Connective tumors of the ureter (hemangioma)
- Foreign bodies
- Air bubbles
- Vascular impressions
- Parietal hematoma
- Amyloidosis

The analysis of the ureter should make it possible to specify the single or multiple character, the size, the regularity of the edges, the relationship with the wall, the topography, the uni- or bilateral nature, and the mobility (WILLIAMSON et al. 1986). One of the most significant points is to specify the intraluminal, parietal, or extrinsic origin, which often allows etiologic orientation.

Intraluminal filling defects classically have sharp edges and are completely surrounded by contrast medium in all incidences (and/or on CT slices). The contact angle with the wall is obtuse. Lucencies of parietal origin present a wide base connecting them to the wall and are not completely encircled by contrast medium. The dimensions of the implantation base to the wall are variable and the value of the contact angle with the wall varies according to these dimensions. It may be acute in case of a pedicle of small diameter, but it does not have to exceed 90° in theory. Lacunar images secondary to an extrinsic compression are usually characterized by fuzzy edges, in particular when the lucency is seen *en face*. The implantation base is broad when the lucency is seen on a profile view. The contact angle with the wall is most often obtuse and closer to 180° than to 90°. The opacification techniques appear better than the urographic reconstruction techniques for the visualization of small lacunar images. However, the latter can provide information on the origin of the image, and the association of the various imaging techniques is often necessary to specify the different characteristics of lacunar images. Nonetheless there are cases where only endoscopy or examination of the anatomic specimen after surgery will yield the etiology of the lucency.

13.2.2.4
Ureteral Narrowing

Ureteral narrowing is the most frequent anomaly, almost always responsible for upstream obstructive phenomena and often associated with topographic abnormalities of the ureter, with periureteric or ureteric parietal changes, or even with lacunar images.

The radiological appearance at the time of EU or direct opacification is highly variable, depending on the etiology. Analysis of the narrowing is always essential to progress in the diagnosis. One should specify the exact topography, the unilateral or bilateral, centered or eccentric, regular or irregular character. The length of the narrowing and the junctions with adjacent normal ureteric portions should be described, as well as the associated abnormalities, in particular the topographic modifications or parietal anomalies. The type of upstream obstruction and the degree of functional impact on the renal parenchyma are also valuable for etiologic orientation.

Narrowing often presents without particular characteristics, and this absence of specificity prompts analysis of the narrowed zone by CT. CT often facilitates attribution of the narrowing to a ureteric or periureteric pathologic condition.

13.2.2.5
Parietal Thickening on Cross-sectional Imaging

Thickening is seldom visible by ultrasonography, except at the level of the pelvic ureter (where it may be seen by endocavitary ultrasound in particular). It has various causes:
- Ureteral tumors
  - Transitional cell carcinoma
  - Periureteral and ureteral metastasis
  - Ureteral lymphoma
- Inflammatory diseases
  - Nonspecific ureteritis
  - Radiation therapy
  - Periureteral fibrosis
  - Long-standing ureteral stents
  - Iatrogenic and noniatrogenic trauma
  - Specific ureteritis (tuberculosis, schistosomiasis)
  - Vasculitis, amyloidosis
- Stone-induced ureteral edema
- Chronic obstruction

Thickening is most often detected by CT and was also described in MRI (MEGIBOW et al. 1982; ROY et al. 1998). The symptoms analysis must focus on specifying the extension in height and width, topography, enhancement after contrast injection, visualization or not of the opacified lumen, and extension to the periureteric fat. All these anomalies are not specific and can correspond to quite different pathologies. Comparison with the images of ureter opacification is very useful. The context of occurrence and the evolution under medical treatment can also be arguments for diagnosis. In case of persisting diagnostic doubt, endoscopy or – more frequently – surgical exploration will allow the diagnosis.

13.2.3
Periureteric Diseases

Ureteric modifications seen by opacification techniques are often suggestive, but the cross-sectional imaging techniques are decisive for the diagnosis when they point towards the nature of the retroperitoneal and/or pelvic disease. In such pathologic conditions, two kinds of problems may arise:

1. Preservation of the renal function in case of severe obstruction: Radiourologic drainage techniques allow decompression of the obstructed kidneys by ureteric intubation while waiting for the diagnosis and a possible definitive treatment of the cause of the obstruction.

2. Diagnosis of nature of the periureteral lesion: Whenever imaging cannot yield the possible diagnosis, either a guided biopsy or a surgical operation must be considered. Biopsy is proposed in case of previous neoplastic history, multifocal or expansive disease, contraindication to surgery, or retroperitoneal fibrosis (BARBARIC and MCINTOSH 1981). Surgery is proposed in the remaining situations.

13.3
The Future of EU

"EU is not dead but changing." Nowadays, the usefulness and future of EU raise many controversies (BECKER et al. 2001; AMIS 2001; DALLA PALMA 2001). "Urographic" visualization of the ureter can be achieved by standard EU, by urographic films made after CT, by urographic "scout films" made during abdominal CT, and by urographic-like images made with multiplanar reconstructions after CT or MRI.

Still, the highlighting of very precise details on the urinary tract level and in particular on the ureteral level [for assessment of hematuria or to search for a transitional cell tumor (TCC), for post-treatment follow-up or for searching of rare ureteral disease] can be achieved only with high-quality urographic

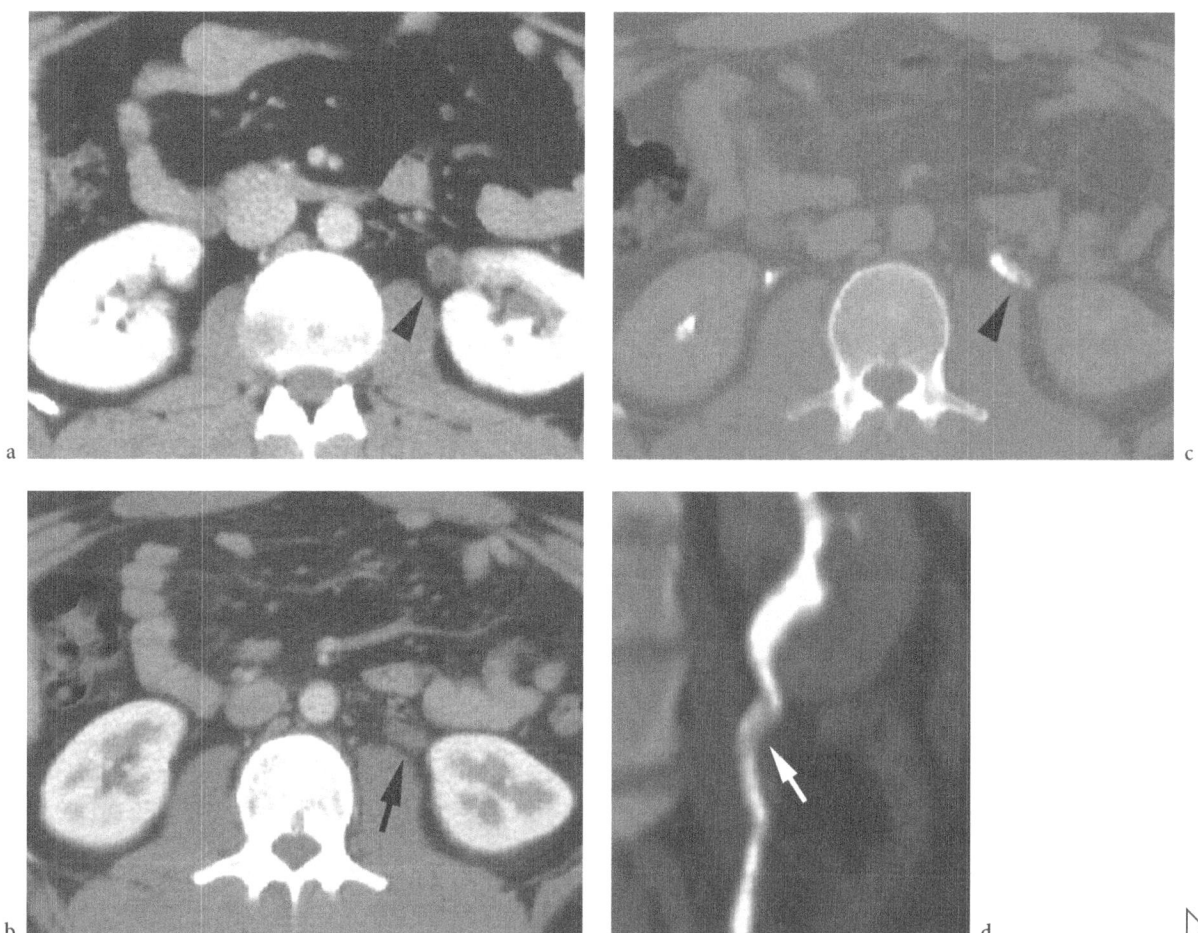

Fig. 13.1a–h. Comparison between EU and single-row helical CT with reconstructions. A 19-year-old patient with previous left renal colic. **a, b** Early post CM axial CT slices show a diffuse thickening of the ureteral wall (*arrowhead*) and the presence of a soft tissue mass in the ureteral area (*arrow*). **c** Late post-CM axial CT slice shows a filling defect in the same area (*arrowhead*). **d–f** Several views after MPR and MIP CT reconstructions allow depiction of few details of the filling defect (*arrows*). **g, h** Post-CT urographic views show an intraluminal and irregular filling defect. The oblique view reveals...

imaging (Fig. 13.1). The question is: Will technological or reconstruction advances and in particular digital "scout images" with a multidetector row CT allow equal or better ureteral imaging compared with standard EU? This comparison is necessary and it will have to consider imaging performances in terms of not only pathology detection but also cost-effectiveness ratio, the accessibility of the new alternative techniques, and their respective risk, in particular the patient's exposure to radiation.

If this evaluation confirms that the advantages of the urographic images carried out at the same time as the helical CT are indisputable, one can propose two types of ureteral urographic imaging. The current indications for urographic imaging of the ureter are:

1. Gross evaluation of the urinary tract with CT or MRI reconstruction
   - Obstructive uropathy
   - Congenital anomalies of the urinary tract
   - Mapping of the urinary tract prior to percutaneous, endourological, or surgical procedures
   - Follow-up after ureteral surgical procedures
2. Precise evaluation of the urinary tract (EU or post-CT urographic scout films)
   - Suspicion of urothelial tumor, especially in the follow-up of bladder TCC
   - Hematuria of unknown origin
   - Suspicion of tuberculosis, ureteritis and other parietal ureteral disorders
   - Follow-up after ureteral surgical procedures

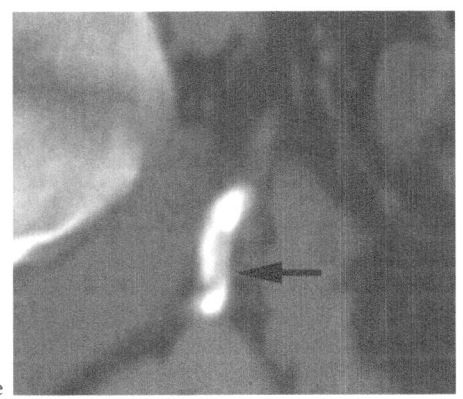

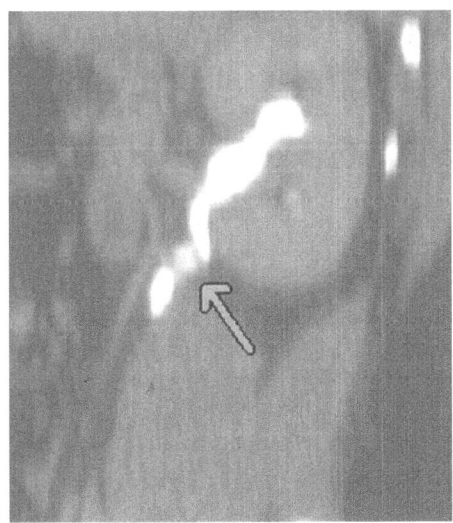

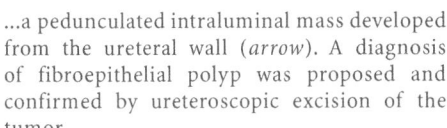

...a pedunculated intraluminal mass developed from the ureteral wall (*arrow*). A diagnosis of fibroepithelial polyp was proposed and confirmed by ureteroscopic excision of the tumor

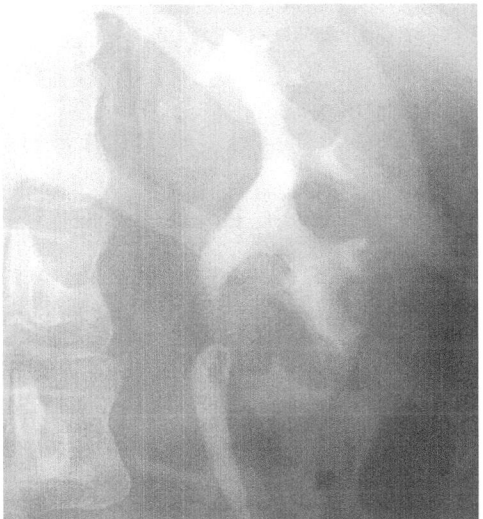

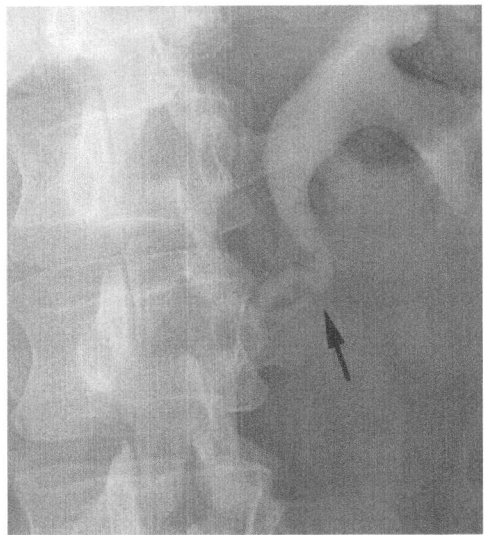

References

Adam EJ, Desai SC, Layton G (1985) Racial variations in normal ureteric course. Clin Radiol 36:373–375

Amis ES jr (1999) Epitaph for the urogram. Radiology 213:639–640

Amis ES jr (2001) Replay to "urography survives". Radiology 218:299–300

Barbazic ZI., McIntosh PK (1981) Periureteral thin-needle aspiration biopsy. Urol Radiol 2:181–185

Becker JA, Pollack HM, McClennan BL (2001) Urography survives (letter). Radiology 218–299

Bigot JM (1995) Que reste-t-il de l'urographie en 1995? J Radiol 76:987–988

Bree RL, Green B, Keiller DL, et al (1976) Medial deviation of the ureter secondary to psoas muscle hypertrophy. Radiology 118:691–695

Choyke PL (1992) The urogram: are rumors of its death premature? Radiology 184:33–36

Cunat JS, Goldman SM (1986) Extrinsic displacement of the ureter. Semin Roentgenol 21:188–200

Dalla Palma L (2001) What is left of i.v. urography? Eur Radiol 11:931–939

Esho JO, Cass AS (1973) Medial deviation of ureters following abdomino-perineal resection carcinoma of large bowel. Urology 2:658–659

Fein AB, McClennan BL (1986) Solitary filling defects of the ureter. Semin Roentgenol 21:214–223

Friedenberg RM, Ney C, Lopez F (1966) Clinical significance of deviations of the pelvic ureter. J Urol 96:146–151

Joffre F, Portalez D (1984) Apport de la scanographie dans l'exploration des voies urinaires supérieures. Radiologie J CEPUR 4:21–24

Lemaitre L, Ala Edine C, Dubrulle F (2000) Retroperitoneum and ureters. In: Ferrier F, Grossholz M, Becker CD (eds) Spiral CT of the abdomen. Springer-Verlag, Berlin Heidelberg New York, pp 277–317

Levine RB, Forrester D, Halpern M (1969) Ureteral deviation due to iliopsoas hypertrophy. AJR Am J Roentgenol 107:756–759

Margolin EG, Cohen LH (1982) Genitourinary calcifications: an overview. Semin Roentgenol 17:95-102

Megibow AJ, Mitnick JS, Bosniak MM (1982) The contribution of computed tomography to the evaluation of obstructed ureter. Urol Radiol 4:95–104

Moreau JF (1995) Défense et illustration de l'urographie. J Radiol 76:989

Pfister RC, Newhouse JH (1978) Radiology of ureter. Urology 1:15–39

Pollack HM, Banner MP (1985) Current status of excretory urography. A premature epitath? Urol Clin North Am 12:585–601

Roy C, Saussine C, Guth S (1998) MR Urography in the evaluation of urinary in the evaluation of urinary tract obstruction. Abdom Imaging 23:27–34

Saldino RM, Palubinskas AJ (1972) Medial placement of the ureter: a normal variant which may simulate retroperitonel fibrosis. J Urol 107:582–585

Singh EO, Malek RS (1982) Calculus disease in the upper urinary tract. Semin Roentgenol 27:113–132

Talner LB (1990) Obstruction uropathy. In: Pollack HM (ed) Clinical urography: an atlas and text book of uroradiological imaging, vol 2. Saunders, Philadephia, pp 1535–1629

Williamson B, Hartman GW, Hattery RR (1986) Multiple and diffuse ureteral filling defects. Semin Roentgenol 21:214–223

Subject Index

List of Abbreviations

AIA	Aorto iliac aneurysm
AP	Antegrade pyelography
CM	Contrast media
CSF	Cerebro-spinal fluid
CT	Computed tomography
DMSA	99^{mtc} dimercapto succinic acid
DTPA	99^{mtc} diethylene triamine pentaacetic acid
EPI	Echoplanar imaging
ESR	Erythrocytes sedimentation rate
ESWL	Extracorporeal shock wave lithotripsy
EU	Extretory urography
FOV	Field of view
FSE	Fast spin echo
Gd	Gadolinium
GRE	Gradient recalled echo
HASTE	Half-Fourier acquisition single-shot turbo spin echo
HCT	Helical computed tomography
HIV	Human immunodeficiency virus
HOCM	High osmolality contrast media
HU	Hounsfield unit
IV	Intravenous
IVC	Inferior vena cava
KDSM	Keratinizing desquamative squamous metaplasia
KUB	Kidney, ureters, bladder
LOCM	Low osmolality contrast media
MAG 3	99^{mtc} mercapto triacetylglycine
MHZ	Megahertz
MIP	Minimal intensity projection
MPR	Multiplanar reconstruction
MPVR	Multiplanar volume rendering
MRI	Magnetic resonance imaging
MURSC association	Mullerian duct, unilateral renal agenesis, and anomalies of the cervico-thoracic somites
NSAID	Non steroid antiinflammatory drug
PCN	Percutaneous nephrostomy
PCNL	Percutaneous nephrolithotomy
PIF	Perianeurysmal inflammatory fibrosis
PPV	Predictive positive value
RARE	Rapid acquisition with relaxation enhancement
RCC	Renal cell carcinoma
RI	Resistive index
ROE	Renal output efficiency
ROI	Region of interest
RP	Retrograde pyelography
RPF	Retroperitoneal fibrosis
RUP	Retrograde ureteropyelography
SSD	Surface shaded display
SSFSE	Single shot fast spin echo
SSTSE	Single shot turbo spin echo
STIR	Short Tl inversion recovery
TCC	Transitional cell carcinoma
TE	Time of echo
UPJ	Uretero-pyelic junction
US	Ultrasonography
UTI	Urinary tract infection
UVJ	Uretero-vesical junction
VACTERL association	Vetebral anomalies, and atresia, congenital heart disease, tracheo-oesophageal fistula or oesophageal atresia, reno-urinary anomalies and limb defects
VCUG	Voiding cysto-urethrography
VRT	Volume rendering technique
VUR	Vesico-ureteral reflux

List of Contributors

MEDHI BENNACEUR, MD
Service de Radiologie
CHU Rangueil
1, avenue Jean-Poulhès
31403 Toulouse Cédex 4
France

LOUIS BOUCHARD, MD
6239 Dumas
Montreal, Québec
H4E 2Z8
Canada

VALÉRIE CHABBERT, MD
Service de Radiologie
CHU Rangueil
1, avenue Jean-Poulhès
31403 Toulouse Cédex 4
France

KATIA CHAUMOIRE, MD
Service de Radiologie
Hôpital Nord
Chemin des Bourrelys
13915 Marseille Cédex 20
France

RAMI CHEMALI, MD
Service de Radiologie
Hôpital Saint Georges
Achrafieh
Beirut
Lebanon

PATRICIA CHEMLA, MD
Service de Radiologie
CHU Rangucil
1, avenue Jean-Poulhès
31403 Toulouse Cédex 4
France

MICHEL CLAUDON, MD
Professor, Service de Radiologie
CHU Nancy Brabois
rue du Morvan
54511 Vandoeuvre Les Nancy
France

PHILIPPE DEVRED, MD
Professor, Service de Radiologie
Hôpital Enfant de la Timone
264 rue Saint Pierre
13385 Marseillie Cédex 05
France

GHISLAINE ESCOURROU, MD
Service d'Anatomo-pathologie
CHU Rangueil
1, avenue Jean-Poulhès
31403 Toulouse Cédex 4
France

ALEXANDRE GOZLAN, MD
Service de Radiologie
CHU Rangueil
1, avenue Jean-Poulhès
31403 Toulouse Cédex 4
France

NICOLAS GRENIER, MD
Professor, Service de Radiologie
G. Hosp. Pellegrin Tripode
place Amélie Raba Léon
33076 Bordeaux Cédex
France

MURIEL IRSUTTI, MD
Service de Radiologie
CHU Rangueil
1, avenue Jean-Poulhès
31403 Toulouse Cédex 4
France

BERTRAND JANNE D'OTHEE, MD
Medical Center
Department of Radiology CC308
One Deaconess Road (West Campus)
Boston, MA 02215-5400
USA

FRANCIS JOFFRE, MD
Professor, Chef de Service
Service de Radiologie
Hôpital de Rangueil
1, avenue Jean-Poulhès
31403 Toulouse Cédex 4
France

FRANÇOIS LEFEVRE, MD
Service de Radiologie
CHU Nancy Brabois
rue du Morvan
54511 Vandoeuvre Les Nancy
France

BERNARD MALAVAUD, MD
Service d'Urologie
CHU Rangueil
1, avenue Jean-Poulhès
31403 Toulouse Cédex
France

CATHERINE MAZEROLLES, MD
Service d'Anatomo-pathologie
CHU PURPAN
place Baylac
31059 Toulouse Cédex
France

MARIA INES MILLAN, MD
Calle A Resid Tamarindo
Apt 92 La Alameda
Caracas 1080
Venezuela

SIDI MOUSSOUNI, MD
Service de Radiologie
CHU Rangueil
1, avenue Jean-Poulhès
31403 Toulouse Cédex
France

PHILIPPE OTAL, MD
Service de Radiologie
CHU Rangueil
1, avenue Jean-Poulhès
31403 Toulouse Cédex
France

JEAN LOUIS PARIENTE, MD
Service de Radiologie
G. Hosp. Pellegrin Tripode
place Amélie Raba Léon
33076 Bordeaux Cédex
France

MICHEL PANUEL, MD
Professor, Service d'Imagerie Médicale
Hôpital Nord
Chemin des Bourrelys
13915 Marseille Cédex 20
France

PIERRE PLANTE, MD
Professor, Service d'Urologie
CHU Rangueil
1, avenue Jean-Poulhès
31403 Toulouse Cédex 4
France

PASCAL RISCHMAN, MD
Professor, Service d'Urologie
CHU Rangueil
1, avenue Jean-Poulhès
31403 Toulouse Cédex 4
France

HERVÉ ROUSSEAU, MD
Professor, Service de Radiologie
CHU Rangueil
1, avenue Jean-Poulhès
31403 Toulouse Cédex 4
France

JEAN-PIERRE SARRAMON, MD
Professor, Service d'Urologie
CHU Rangueil
1, avenue Jean-Poulhès
31403 Toulouse Cédex 4
France

PHILIPPE SEGUIN, MD
Service d'Urologie
CHU Rangueil
1, avenue Jean-Poulhès
31403 Toulouse Cédex 4
France

TAREK SMAYRA, MD
Hotel Dieu de France Beth Israel Deaconess
Service de Radiologie
Rue Alfred Naccache
Beyrouth
Lebanon

MICHEL SOULIE, MD
Service d'Urologie
CHU Rangueil
1, avenue Jean-Poulhès
31403 Toulouse Cédex 4
France

HERVÉ TRILLAUD, MD
Service de Radiologie
Hôpital Saint André
1 rue Jean Burguet
33000 Bordeaux
France

GÉRARD VICTOR, MD
Service de Médecine Nucléaire
CHU Rangueil
1, avenue Jean-Poulhès
31403 Toulouse Cédex 4
France

MEDICAL RADIOLOGY   Diagnostic Imaging and Radiation Oncology

Titles in the series already published

DIAGNOSTIC IMAGING

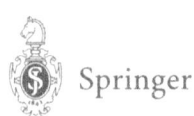

Springer

MEDICAL RADIOLOGY Diagnostic Imaging and Radiation Oncology

Titles in the series already published

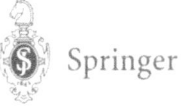

Springer

The manufacturer's authorised representative in the EU is Springer
Nature Customer Service Centre GmbH, Europaplatz 3, 69115 Heidelberg,
Germany. If you have any concerns regarding our products, please
contact ProductSafety@springernature.com

Printed and bound by CPI Group (UK) Ltd, Croydon, CR0 4YY

29/04/2026

02099553-0004